I0888554

Environmental Factors in Carcinogenesis:

Exposome-Driven Insights Into Cancer Risk and Prevention

Ramya Raghavan
Sri Sathya Sai University for Human Excellence, India

IGI Global
Scientific Publishing
Publishing Tomorrow's Research Today

Vice President of Editorial	Melissa Wagner
Director of Acquisitions	Mikaela Felty
Director of Book Development	Jocelynn Hessler
Production Manager	Mike Brehm
Cover Design	Jose Rosado

Published in the United States of America by
IGI Global Scientific Publishing
701 East Chocolate Avenue
Hershey, PA, 17033, USA
Tel: 717-533-8845
Fax: 717-533-7115
Website: https://www.igi-global.com E-mail: cust@igi-global.com

Copyright © 2026 by IGI Global Scientific Publishing. All rights reserved. No part of this publication may be reproduced, stored or distributed in any form or by any means, electronic or mechanical, including photocopying, without written permission from the publisher.

Product or company names used in this set are for identification purposes only. Inclusion of the names of the products or companies does not indicate a claim of ownership by IGI Global Scientific Publishing of the trademark or registered trademark.

Library of Congress Cataloging-in-Publication Data

LCCN: 2025941856 (CIP Data Pending)
ISBN13: 979-8-3373-5796-6
Isbn13Softcover: 979-8-3373-5797-3
EISBN13: 979-8-3373-5798-0
British Cataloguing in Publication Data
A Cataloguing in Publication record for this book is available from the British Library.

All work contributed to this book is new, previously-unpublished material.
The views expressed in this book are those of the authors, but not necessarily of the publisher.
This book contains information sourced from authentic and highly regarded references, with reasonable efforts made to ensure the reliability of the data and information presented. The authors, editors, and publisher believe the information in this book to be accurate and true as of the date of publication. Every effort has been made to trace and credit the copyright holders of all materials included. However, the authors, editors, and publisher cannot assume responsibility for the validity of all materials or the consequences of their use. Should any copyright material be found unacknowledged, please inform the publisher so that corrections may be made in future reprints.

Table of Contents

Detailed Table of Contents

Cervical cancer remains a significant public health concern, particularly in low- and middle-income countries. While human papillomavirus (HPV) infection is a well-established primary cause, emerging research highlights the role of environmental exposures, lifestyle factors, and socioeconomic conditions in modulating carcinogenesis. This chapter explores the concept of cancer exposomics in the context of cervical cancer, emphasizing the cumulative impact of chemical pollutants, dietary habits, occupational hazards, and lifestyle factors on disease progression. The interplay between HPV infection, environmental toxins (such as endocrine disruptors and heavy metals), and immune system modulation is discussed. Additionally, the chapter highlights the significance of early screening, vaccination, and personalized interventions in mitigating the risk. By integrating exposomic research with molecular epidemiology, this study provides insights into novel preventive and therapeutic strategies for cervical cancer management.

Endocrine disruptors, which are environmental chemicals, interfere with hormone regulation and increase health risks. This chapter examines the DNA-damaging effects of EDs, which lead to mutations, genomic instability, and the development of cancer. Key molecular mechanisms include oxidative damage, epigenetic alterations, and receptor-mediated abnormalities that result from EDs exposure and associated health issues. It also discusses the risks of endocrine disruptors for pregnant women and children, as well as other vulnerable population groups. The discussion encompasses public health implications as well as regulatory standards for risk evaluation and methods to minimize exposure. Future directions include advancing biomarker development, refining risk assessment models, and designing safer chemical alternatives to reduce exposure.

Prostate cancer (PCa), especially androgen-resistant PCa (ARPC), poses a major global health burden shaped by both genetics and environmental exposures. This chapter examines how toxicants like endocrine disruptors, POPs, and xenobiotics contribute to PCa progression through exposomics, toxicogenomics, and multi-omics approaches. It highlights mechanisms such as AR signaling disruption, mitochondrial dysfunction, metabolic shifts, and epigenetic changes driving therapy resistance. Using cell models and spatial transcriptomics, it explores how exposures promote metastasis. The chapter also discusses tools like eDNA, epigenetic biomarkers, and predictive models for early detection and prevention, underscoring the importance of integrating environmental risk into precision oncology.

Breast cancer remains one of the most prevalent malignancies worldwide, with chemotherapy serving as a cornerstone of treatment despite its substantial toxicity risks. Carboxylesterase 1 (CES1), a critical drug-metabolizing enzyme, plays a central role in the activation and clearance of various chemotherapeutic agents, including capecitabine. Genetic polymorphisms in CES1, together with environmental exposures such as pollutants, diet, and lifestyle factors, contribute to the interindividual variability in chemotherapy metabolism and toxicity profiles. This chapter examines the complex gene–environment interplay influencing treatment outcomes in breast cancer and highlights emerging strategies for integrating genetic and environmental assessments. A deeper understanding of these interactions paves the way for precision

Preface

Understanding your health has never been more crucial in a world of information. But what if the key to a longer, healthier life isn't just in your genes? Environmental Factors in Carcinogenesis offers a detailed overview of current exposomic research, emphasizing its potential to transform disease prevention, personalize medicine, and guide public health strategies. The authors aspire to contribute to a future where environmentally-driven diseases are mitigated and human health is safeguarded against the challenges of our ever-evolving environment. We begin by synthesizing the critical role of environmental exposures across a lifetime in shaping cancer risk. The multi-omics data and systems biology approaches unravel the gene-environment effects that reinforce oncogenesis. From the basic principles to potential applications, present book displays how genetic predispositions interact with environmental exposures. Our comprehensive volume is an essential resource for many readers, including undergraduate and graduate students pursuing careers in environmental health sciences, toxicology, epidemiology, and precision medicine. The chapters are also designed to benefit experienced researchers, clinicians, public health professionals, and policymakers. Its pedagogical approach ensures accessibility for adolescents and young adults grappling with health decisions. The contents with robust scientific depth fulfill the unmet need of aspiring parents seeking to optimize preconception health and fetal development. The scientific information backed by research is for all ages interested in disease susceptibility and cancer prevention.

The study of gene-environment interactions in cancer development recognizes that genetic predispositions seldom function independently. Certain demographic groups, such as developing fetuses, infants, children, and those with significant occupational or environmental exposures, display increased susceptibility. Environmental and lifestyle factors in carcinogenesis examined are the influence of chemical pollutants, dietary habits, and occupational hazards. While germline mutations in high-penetrance genes contribute to a minority of familial cancers, the vast majority of sporadic cancers are attributable to a complex interplay between an individual's genetic variations and social determinants of health. Parental and fetal exposures play a significant role in shaping genetic variation during embryonic development. The developmental origins of health and disease illustrate how early life exposures, both prenatal and postnatal, shape an individual's long-term health outcomes. Exposure to harmful substances by paternal and maternal germ cells and during pregnancy can elevate the risk of cancer. The case studies aren't just about understanding the problem; it's about empowering you with knowledge. The exposome and complex interactions between genes and the environment drive innovative research and provide valuable insights for evidence-based clinical practices.

Environmental factors in carcinogenesis influence toxicity and drug response, laying a foundation for understanding health disparities. Xenobiotic metabolism explains how the body processes foreign compounds. A crucial aspect of environmental toxicology, includes techniques like metabolomics and transcriptomic analyses, focusing on cytochrome enzymes. High-throughput sequencing techniques identify genetic variations in drug metabolism enzymes and transporters. Spatial omics and microfluidics elucidate the molecular and cellular effects of carcinogenic agents. The biotechnology tools offer cutting-edge in vitro models, computational toxicology, and advanced bioinformatics in simulating and dissecting complex environment-driven carcinogenesis. Additionally, the molecular mechanisms of gene-environment interactions advance environmental health and cancer research for a more equitable future for all.

Gene-environment interactions (GxE) in carcinogenesis are an essential topic that explores how an individual's genetic makeup influences their response to environmental exposures. By identifying how specific genetic polymorphisms modify the biological response to environmental carcinogens, we can delineate precise cellular pathways that lead to malignant transformation. Next-generation sequencing continues to be a cornerstone technology in cancer genomics. They unequivocally create opportunities to investigate tumor initiation and progression mechanisms, effectively linking epidemiological observations with mechanistic data. Adopting a digital age approach, they are set to integrate diverse datasets to clarify causal relationships and identify promising biomarkers for cancer treatment. The computational algorithms decisively enable the classification of cancers into subtypes and significantly enhance survival predictions. As research in cancer biology continues to evolve, we expect further advancements in high throughput technologies, data integration methods, and AI-driven analysis tools. The book chapters will articulate the next generation of challenges and opportunities in the field. An urgent need is enhanced computational tools and artificial intelligence/machine learning algorithms to manage and interpret the colossal datasets generated by exposomic studies. Future directions include the development of novel, high-throughput exposure assessment technologies from traditional environmental monitoring and digital exposome tools.

Upcoming discussions will extend to refining biomarkers of exposure and effect, which are crucial for precise risk stratification and early disease detection.

INTRODUCTION TO EXPOSOME: EXPOSOME IN GAMETOGENESIS, TERATOGENESIS AND CANCER

In Chapter 1, we embark on a journey that lays the groundwork for understanding the essential role of environmental exposures from the earliest stages of life. By identifying crucial exposure windows and vulnerable genetic profiles, public health campaigns can be effectively designed to mitigate environmental burdens. Everyday exposures contribute to health outcomes like cancer, and understanding social determinants empowers our communities. You'll find insights and actionable knowledge that apply directly to long-term well-being. Early-life environmental exposures can permanently reprogram gene expression and epigenetic states, increasing the penetrance of tumor-suppressor gene defects and cancer susceptibility later in life. The role of the exposome in gametogenesis and teratogenesis highlights the impact of internal and external exposures on reproductive health and predisposition to cancer. The topic sets the stage by introducing the exposome concept and its critical relevance during the most vulnerable developmental stages. The discussion encompasses public health implications to minimize exposure to cancer risks.

SECTION 2: DISEASE-SPECIFIC APPLICATIONS OF EXPOSOME INTO CANCER RISK PREDICTION

Disease specific applications explore the environmental factors contributing to cervical, breast, and prostate cancers through the lens of toxicogenomics. Identifying and validating reliable biomarkers that indicate exposure and cancer risk is paramount. Advanced techniques such as spatial transcriptomics, mass spectrometry, and imaging-based proteomics allow for in-depth molecular profiling. Multiomics advancements allow protein expression analyses, interactions, post-translational modifications, and metabolic profiling. A significant focus is placed on dynamic models that simulate interactions within cancer cells to advance personalized therapy. Additionally, research on health disparities reveals how socioeconomic status and environmental exposures play a critical role in the differing incidence and outcomes of cancer across various populations.

Cervical Cancer Exposomics and the Impact of Environmental and Lifestyle Factors on Carcinogenesis:

Cervical cancer can be the cumulative impact of chemical pollutants, dietary habits, occupational hazards, and lifestyle factors. Presenting a specific example illustrates how exposomics is applied to understand the environmental and lifestyle drivers of cervical cancer. The discussion highlights the critical interactions between virus infections, environmental toxins, endocrine disruptors, and heavy metals and their impact on the regulation of the immune system. Additionally, the chapter underscores the value of early screening, vaccination, and tailored interventions as effective strategies for reducing cervical cancer risks. The epidemiological patterns of disease are considered, emphasizing their interplay with infectious agents, such as Human Papillomavirus (HPV) infection, in the context of carcinogenesis. Strategies for prevention are also addressed.

Endocrine Disruptors and DNA Damage: Mechanisms, Risks, And Public Health Implications

The exposome includes all occupational and non-occupational exposures that impact health. Endocrine disruptors and environmental chemicals interfere with hormone regulation and increase health risks. DNA-damaging effects, can lead to mutations, genomic instability, and cancer development. The interaction between endocrine-disrupting chemicals (EDCs) and DNA integrity exposes the associated health risks and the resultant public health implications.

Chapter 3 elaborates on endocrine disruptors that can induce epigenetic modifications, such as DNA methylation and histone changes, to alter gene expression in tumors and surrounding cells. EDCs disrupt DNA repair, cell cycle control, and immune responses, contributing to cancer risk. The link between EDCs, DNA damage, and cancer, reproductive disorders, metabolic dysfunction contributes to the global disease burden. Due to their association with human cancer, specific attention is given to exposome-related metabolites, including endocrine disruptors and DNA adducts formed by polycyclic aromatic hydrocarbons. The review emphasizes the risks that endocrine disruptors pose to pregnant women, children, and other vulnerable population groups. Chapter 3 describes breast cancer exposomics and risk factors with epidemiology and prevention methods.

Deciphering the Role of Environmental Exposures in Androgen-Resistant Prostate Cancer: Insights from Exposomics, Toxicogenomics, and Integrative Multi-Omics Approaches

Chapter 4 showcases exposomic and multi-omics insights into androgen-resistant prostate cancer. The primary goal here is to clarify the contribution of environmental exposures to androgen-resistant prostate cancer. Another disease-specific example demonstrates the use of toxicogenomics contributions to prostate cancer. The authors emphasize paternal environmental exposure's timing and cumulative effects in cancer incidence of offsprings. Researchers have linked persistent organic pollutants and heavy metals to altered epigenetic modifications that may raise cancer susceptibility.

The chapter leverages exposomics, toxicogenomics, and multi-omics approaches to provide insights into androgen-resistant prostate cancer (PCa). The discussion highlights underlying mechanisms such as androgen receptor (AR) signaling disruption, mitochondrial dysfunction, metabolic shifts, and epigenetic changes that drive therapy resistance in PCa. What specific exposures disrupt critical pathways like AR signaling, leading to cellular dysfunction and therapy resistance in prostate cancer? Disparities in cancer incidence can often be traced back to specific demographic groups, which may be influenced by unique genetic allele frequencies or varying environmental exposures. Understand the role of environmental factors, such as endocrine disruptors, persistent organic pollutants, and xenobiotics, in advancing prostate cancer (PCa) progression and contributing to the unequal rates of cancer incidence. By examining environmental influences, we can work towards strategies that address disparities and cancer prevention and treatment efforts.

The Interplay Between CES1 Gene Polymorphisms and Environmental Exposures in Chemotherapy Toxicity in Breast Cancer: CES1 Variants and Environment in Chemo Toxicity

Chapter 5 details explicitly the role of Carboxylesterase 1 (CES1) gene polymorphisms and their interplay with environmental exposures in influencing chemotherapy toxicity in breast cancer. Gene-environment interactions, pharmacogenomics, and next-generation sequencing represent the future of chemotherapy for breast cancer. This case study is the interaction between CES1 gene polymorphisms and chemotherapy toxicity in breast cancer patients. Research underscores gene-environment interaction can significantly affect therapeutic outcomes. Moreover, findings contribute to the advancement of medical services by promoting personalized medicine, early detection, and more effective cancer treatments.

The discussion also highlights the foundational role of next-generation sequencing, including whole exome sequencing and whole genome sequencing, as cornerstone technologies in cancer genomics. The chapter goes in-depth about CES1 gene polymorphisms and the context of chemotherapy toxicity in breast cancer. The significant impact of genetic variations on drug metabolism is their role in adverse reactions like hand-foot syndrome. By connecting genetic predispositions and environmental factors to drug response and toxicity, the chapter establishes a solid foundation. Exposomics understanding is crucial for advancing personalized medicine approaches and also addressing health disparities effectively.

SECTION 3: EXPOSOME-DRIVEN INSIGHTS INTO HEALTH DISPARITIES AND CANCER PREVENTION

Research on health disparities underscores the significant role that socioeconomic status and environmental exposures play in influencing the incidence and outcomes of cancer. A nuanced understanding of gene-environment interactions is essential for informing public health initiatives aimed at developing more effective disease prevention strategies.

By integrating exposomics knowledge, stakeholders can tailor interventions that specifically address the unique needs of communities, reducing health inequities.

Toxicogenomics and Pharmacogenomics Research in Health Disparities

Toxicogenomics and Pharmacogenomics research in Chapter 6 delves into how environmental exposures and genetic variations contribute to health disparities. A primary emphasis is placed on health disparities and social determinants of health, acknowledging the differential impact of environmental exposures on vulnerable demographic groups. Targeted therapies for at-risk populations and vulnerable genetic profiles. It also calls for precision medicine during critical exposure windows. The health disparities highlight socioeconomic status and environmental factors predisposed variations in cancer incidence and outcomes. Developmental toxicogenomics and pharmacogenomics examine how parental and fetal exposures influence genetic variation during embryological development. It then transitions to the basic principles, potential applications, and associated issues. Toxicogenomics and pharmacogenomics establish strong connections between genetic predispositions and environmental exposures, significantly influencing both toxicity and drug responses. It aligns with core public health principles by promoting prevention, addressing health inequalities, and improving population health. Furthermore, discussions of ethical, social, and policy implications and applications is provided. There are practical insights into utilizing exposome data for personalized health interventions and environmental risk assessments, in toxicology and drug response contexts. Exposomic maps can aid the systems biology approach by addressing the cumulative impacts of exposures on population health. The review also examines future directions, including the prospect of exposome-based interventions for public health applications.

Exposome Insights to Action: A Unified Call for Cancer Prevention and a Vision for Precision Prevention

The final chapter summarizes the applications of exposomics research for public health interventions. A comprehensive understanding of GxE interactions empowers public health initiatives to develop more effective disease prevention strategies. The authors highlight how the exposome can inform global public health policy and provide recommendations for international organizations. Thus, cancer exposomics promotes a collaborative approach integrating diverse fields to advance epidemiology and promote a healthier future.

The final chapter summarizes the key insights and emphasizes the need for action in cancer prevention. It focuses on community-based interventions that assess the cumulative environmental impacts on health and enhance our understanding of disease causes. The chapter also highlights the importance of identifying reliable biomarkers for early detection and targeted prevention. Additionally, it addresses the ethical, legal, and societal implications of using exposomic data, including data privacy, health disparities, and equitable access to personalized prevention. Exposomics necessitates transparent communication, robust policy frameworks. Collaborative efforts among researchers, policymakers, healthcare providers, and communities ensure the exposomics lead to cancer prevention. Ultimately, exposomics research serves as a call to action for a transformative shift in cancer prevention. It envisions a future in which exposome-informed precision prevention is not just a theoretical concept but a reality. In future, individuals know their unique gene-environment effects, for healthy lifestyle modifications. Additionally targeted chemoprevention, and robust environmental regulations safeguard vulnerable populations.

We are a pioneer in publishing a book on exposomes that aims to display the multi-omics approach and interdisciplinary collaborations. The book explores innovative research and case studies emphasizing a holistic understanding of environmental impacts on human health.

- Advanced Methodological Coverage: The text explores advanced methodologies and technologies for exposome study, including mass spectrometry, metabolomics, and data analytics.
- Ethical and Policy Examination: The content includes a discussion of ethical, social, and policy implications of exposome research and applications.
- Translational Utility: Practical insights are provided for leveraging exposome data in personalized health interventions and environmental risk assessment.
- Actionable Research Applications: The publication discusses practical applications of exposomics research for disease prevention and environmental health.

This book explores the practical applications of exposomics research. It aims to examine multi-omics about environmental factors in carcinogenesis and cancer prevention. Combining omics data provides insight into informed decisions to mitigate environmental factors influence cancer development and precision treatment outcomes. Our work will serve as a vital resource for researchers, clinicians, and public health professionals, bridging the gap between scientific research and cancer prevention.

With Best Wishes for a Health and Happy Life

Ramya Raghavan
Sri Sathya Sai University for Human Excellence, India

Section 1
Exposomics and Environmental Factors in Carcinogenesis

Chapter 1
Introduction to Exposome in Gametogenesis Teratogenesis and Cancer

Christopher Oloruntoba Akintayo
https://orcid.org/0009-0008-3446-466X
Achievers University, Nigeria

Samuel O. Onyekweli
https://orcid.org/0000-0002-4715-7932
Lagos University Teaching Hospital, Idi-Araba, Nigeria

Gloria Osayamen Omoruyi
Obafemi Awolowo University Teaching Hospital Complex, Nigeria

Tobi O. Olaleye
Achievers University, Nigeria

Oluwakemi M. Olowomeye
Achievers University, Nigeria

Victor O. Osundele
Osun State Ministry of Health, Nigeria

Paul A. Oyewole
Obafemi Awolowo University Teaching Hospital Complex, Nigeria

ABSTRACT

Risk factors provides a chance to comprehend the cancer formation, and its molecular classification. The exposome represents a thorough evaluation of all environmental factors that affect a person throughout their life, including biological, research has demonstrated the connection between adverse developmental outcomes, including growth restriction, preterm birth, and morphological and functional abnormalities, and environmental chemical exposures for both the mother and the father prior to, during, and following conception. According to recent studies, human pregnancy and

DOI: 10.4018/979-8-3373-5796-6.ch001

Copyright © 2026, IGI Global Scientific Publishing. Copying or distributing in print or electronic forms without written permission of IGI Global Scientific Publishing is prohibited.

development can be significantly impacted by environmental exposures to chemical, biological, and physical variables that both the mother and the father experience. Exposures associated with poor developmental outcomes include metals, volatile and persistent organics, chemicals in food, occupational exposures, agricultural chemicals, and pollution of the air and water. Premature birth, mortality, growth restriction, and structural and functional abnormalities are developmental endpoints linked to these exposures.

INTRODUCTION

The dynamic interplay between environmental factors and biological systems represents a frontier in understanding the etiology of developmental and proliferative disorders across the human lifespan. Gametogenesis, teratogenesis, and carcinogenesis are processes governing reproductive cell development, embryonic formation, and neoplastic transformation, respectively. They exhibit remarkable sensitivity to exogenous influences at critical developmental windows. Despite extensive progress in genomic medicine, contemporary epidemiological evidence reveals that modifiable environmental and occupational exposures contribute to approximately 60% of global mortality, with nine million deaths annually attributed to pollution alone (Landrigan *et al.,* 2018). This striking environmental burden substantially exceeds the explanatory power of genetic variation, particularly for common multifactorial conditions (Ioannidis *et al.,* 2009). The exposome concept, introduced by Wild in 2005, provides a comprehensive framework to systematically characterize the "environmental complement to the genome", encompassing the totality of non-genetic exposures throughout the life course, from chemical pollutants and dietary constituents to psychosocial stressors and physical factors (Wild, 2012). This paradigm transcends traditional reductionist approaches by capturing both external exposures and their corresponding internal biological perturbations. As Rappaport and Smith (2010) articulated, these exposures are not limited to exogenous chemicals entering the body but include compounds produced through inflammation, oxidative stress, lipid peroxidation, and microbiome interactions, all of which can disrupt critical molecular pathways governing cellular differentiation, embryonic development, and tissue homeostasis (Rappaport & Smith, 2010). The succeeding chapters aim to examine how the exposome paradigm, coupled with technological advances in high resolution mass spectrometry (HRMS) and network medicine (Barabási & Oltvai, 2004), illuminates the chemical-biological interface in three interconnected domains where environmental influences may be particularly consequential: the formation and maturation of gametes, the development of embryonic and fetal tissues, and the dysregulated cellular proliferation characteristic of neoplastic disease.

Gametogenesis, Teratogenesis, and Cancer: Definitions and Environmental Susceptibility

Gametogenesis encompasses the complex cellular processes through which specialized haploid cells, spermatozoa and oocytes are produced through meiotic division and cytodifferentiation. This process exhibits sexual dimorphism in timing and vulnerability windows: oocyte development begins prenatally and remains suspended in meiotic prophase for decades, while spermatogenesis occurs continuously throughout adult reproductive life (Edson *et al.,* 2009). The extended duration of female gametogenesis creates prolonged windows for environmental insults to accumulate, potentially compromising genomic integrity and epigenetic programming.

Teratogenesis refers to the disruption of normal embryonic or fetal development resulting in structural or functional abnormalities. The developing embryo undergoes precisely orchestrated morphogenetic events during organogenesis, creating defined windows of susceptibility when environmental exposures can derail developmental trajectories. The thalidomide tragedy of the 1950s-60s dramatically illustrated this principle, as exposure during specific gestational days (days 20 to 36 post-conception) resulted in characteristic limb malformations, while exposure outside this window produced different or no effects (Vargesson, 2013). Cancer represents a collection of diseases characterized by uncontrolled cellular proliferation, invasion, and metastasis, arising from progressive accumulation of genetic and epigenetic alterations that disrupt normal regulatory mechanisms. While traditionally viewed through a genetic lens following Knudson's "two-hit hypothesis" (Knudson, 1971), contemporary evidence increasingly recognizes carcinogenesis as a complex process where environmental exposures interact with genetic susceptibility throughout an individual's entire developmental trajectory (Miller and Joes, 2014).

THE EXPOSOME CONCEPT: FROM DEFINITION TO APPLICATION

The concept of the exposome emerged as a response to the imbalance between genomic and environmental research methodologies. As it has been noted, "the ease of genotyping following the introduction of the PCR in the late 1980s and 1990s saw a major shift in effort and resources, away from development of accurate exposure biomarkers towards the conduct of gene-disease association studies." This methodological disparity created what Wild metaphorically described as resembling "the male fiddler crab (Uca pugnax), a species characterized by one huge well-developed claw, waved proudly to attract a mate, but contrasting almost comically with its second, apparently underdeveloped one". Wild initially defined the exposome as encompassing "life-course environmental exposures (including lifestyle factors), from the prenatal period onwards" (Wild, 2012). This definition has since been refined by Miller and Jones (2014) to include "the cumulative measure of environmental influences and associated biological responses throughout the lifespan, including exposures from the environment, diet, behavior, and endogenous processes." This expanded definition importantly incorporates three key elements: cumulative biological responses to external challenges, behavioral factors beyond lifestyle choices, and endogenous processes including the complex biochemistry of internal metabolic reactions (Miller & Jones, 2014).

The exposome framework provides a comprehensive approach to studying environmental influences across three complementary domains:

(1) the general external exposome, encompassing broader social, economic, and psychological influences;
(2) the specific external exposome, including specific environmental agents, pollutants, diet, lifestyle factors, and infections; and
(3) the internal exposome, comprising internal biological responses including inflammation, oxidative stress, metabolism, and the microbiome (Rappaport, 2011; Wild, 2012).

As Miller and Jones (2014) argued, "The revised definition makes this demonstrably clear, and indicated that exposome research can begin to provide the tangible and quantifiable entities that medicine and public health desperately need." They further noted that "elucidating the exposome, i.e., developing an integrated science of nurture, will help fulfill the promises of the Human Genome Project." This sentiment echoes Francis Collins' statement upon publication of the first draft human genome: "What more powerful form of study of mankind could there be than to read our own instruction book?" To which Miller and Jones (2014) respond: "The answer, of course, is to read the subsequent chapters that explain the interactions between our genes and our environment that determine health and disease." Overall, the exposome encompasses the totality of internal and external environmental exposures; chemical, physical, biological, behavioral, and psychosocial experienced dynamically across the lifespan. It integrates temporal dimensions (e.g., developmental windows, cumulative dose effects) and spatial contexts, operating bidirectionally with the genome and epigenome to shape molecular adaptations or damage. Measurable through multi-omics profiling, geospatial modeling, and longitudinal biomonitoring, it quantifies both exposure sources (e.g., pollutants, diet) and biological imprints (e.g., DNA adducts, epigenetic changes). This systems level framework transcends siloed risk factors, unifying gene environment interplay to decode mechanisms in gametogenesis, teratogenesis, and carcinogenesis. By bridging molecular signatures with population level data, it offers a reproducible, actionable lens for precision prevention and health equity.

Technological Advances Enabling Exposome Research

The characterization of the exposome presents formidable technical challenges, as it represents "a highly variable and dynamic entity that evolves throughout the lifetime of the individual". However, as Wild notes, "the methodologic challenge may not be more daunting than the one faced two decades ago of investigating an estimated 10 million single nucleotide polymorphisms in the human genome" (Wild, 2012). Recent technological advances in high-throughput screening and 'omics' methodologies now enable more comprehensive assessment of environmental exposures. Wild (2012) suggests that "the new 'omics' technologies of transcriptomics, proteomics, and metabolomics can help unlock the problem of environmental exposure assessment." These approaches offer the potential to identify "specific signatures or fingerprints of environmental exposures across a broad spectrum of mechanisms of action, both genotoxic and nongenotoxic" (Wild, 2012). Early examples supporting this approach include the identification of gene expression patterns in peripheral blood cells that differentiate smokers from non smokers, and metabonomic profiling that detected changes in plasma metabolites following transition from a non-soy to soy-containing diet. These preliminary studies demonstrate that 'omics' technologies can potentially detect signatures of environmental exposures in accessible biological samples. The integration of exposome data with genome wide association studies (GWAS) enables more comprehensive investigation of gene-environment interactions. While GWAS have revealed genetic associations that improve understanding of disease, "these still account for only a fraction of disease risk" (Miller & Jones, 2014). By incorporating exposome data, environment wide association studies (EWAS) could become "much more powerful and complement GWAS and deep sequencing studies" (Miller & Jones, 2014).

RELEVANCE TO GAMETOGENESIS, TERATOGENESIS, AND CANCER

The exposome concept holds particular relevance for understanding gametogenesis, teratogenesis, and carcinogenesis due to several shared characteristics of these processes. First, all three exhibit heightened sensitivity during specific developmental windows when cellular differentiation, morphogenesis, or tissue homeostasis can be permanently altered by environmental influences. Second, these effects often manifest after considerable latency periods, complicating traditional epidemiological approaches to causation. Third, each process involves complex interactions between exposures and genetic susceptibility factors that cannot be fully elucidated without comprehensive assessment of both components. For gametogenesis, exposome research offers opportunities to identify previously unrecognized environmental contributors to declining fertility rates observed in many highly industrialized nations. For teratogenesis, exposome-based approaches may enable more comprehensive assessment of the thousands of industrial chemicals to which pregnant women are exposed but which have undergone limited safety testing (Woodruff *et al.,* 2011). For carcinogenesis, the exposome framework provides tools to address what Hiatt and Brody (2018) describe as the "exposome-genome continuum" in cancer etiology, where environmental exposures and genetic susceptibility interact throughout a lifetime to determine cancer risk (Hiatt & Brody, 2018). As Wild (2012) notes, "Developing reliable measurement tools for such a complete exposure history is extremely challenging." However, "as with the genome, even a partial, targeted understanding of exposure can provide substantial advances." The application of exposome research to these three interconnected domains offers promising directions for advancing our understanding of how environmental influences shape human development and disease risk.

DEFINING THE EXPOSOME

Historical Context and Evolution of the Concept

The notion that environmental factors shape human health traces back to antiquity. In "On Airs, Waters, and Places" (circa 400 BCE), Hippocrates meticulously cataloged how climate, geography, and water quality influenced disease patterns. He observed that cities exposed to hot winds and marshy waters suffered higher rates of digestive disorders and epilepsy, while mountainous regions with cold winds bred robust but arthritic populations (Hippocrates, 400 BCE). This ancient text laid the groundwork for environmental epidemiology by positing that health disparities arose not from divine wrath but from tangible, measurable elements of one's surroundings. Hippocrates' insistence that physicians "consider the seasons, winds, and waters" underscores an early recognition of the interconnectedness between external environments and biological outcomes, a precursor to the modern exposome. The 19th and 20th centuries saw pivotal advances bridging environmental observation with scientific rigor. John Snow's 1854 investigation of London's cholera outbreak linked contaminated water to disease transmission, revolutionizing public health by demonstrating that specific environmental exposures could be mapped and mitigated (Snow,1855). By the late 20th century, the "Barker Hypothesis" emerged, positing that fetal undernutrition and low birth weight predisposed individuals to cardiovascular disease in adulthood. This theory shifted focus to "critical windows of susceptibility", illustrating how early life environmental insults could manifest decades later. These milestones crystallized the idea that health was a lifelong dialogue between biological systems and external conditions, a concept demanding a framework to capture cumulative exposures. In 2005, molecular epidemiologist Christopher Paul Wild formalized this framework by coining the term "exposome", defining it as "the totality of human environmental (non-genetic) exposures from conception onwards, complementing the genome". Wild's definition emerged from frustration with the genomic era's imbalance; while the Human Genome Project had sequenced DNA by 2003, tools to quantify environmental influences remained rudimentary. He argued that just as genomics revealed genetic risk variants, the exposome could decode how pollutants, diet, and social stressors interacted with biology across time. A decade later, Miller and Jones (2014) expanded this definition to include endogenous processes such as metabolism, oxidative stress, and gut microbiome activity, emphasizing that the exposome encompassed not just external exposures but also their "biological imprints", such as epigenetic modifications and protein adducts. Today, the exposome is quantified through technologies unimaginable to early pioneers. High-resolution mass spectrometry (HRMS) detects thousands of chemicals in biological samples, from pesticides to microbial metabolites, while wearable sensors track real time air pollution and UV exposure (Vermeulen *et al.,* 2020). Network science maps interactions between exogenous chemicals and cellular pathways, revealing how endocrine disruptors alter metabolic networks or how particulate matter synergizes with genetic susceptibility in cancer (Vermeulen *et al.,* 2020). These tools fulfill Wild's vision, transforming the exposome from a theoretical construct into a measurable entity. By integrating multi-omics data, geospatial modeling, and longitudinal biomonitoring, modern exposomics bridges Hippocrates' observational wisdom with 21st-century systems biology, offering a lens to dissect environmental contributions to gametogenic defects, teratogenesis, and carcinogenesis.

Components of the Exposome:

Internal Exposome

The internal exposome encompasses endogenous biochemical processes that occur within an organism, including metabolism, inflammation, oxidative stress, and microbiome interactions. These processes are not static but exist in dynamic equilibrium, continuously shaped by genetic predispositions, developmental stages, and critically external environmental exposures (Jirtle & Skinner, 2007; Halliwell,

2007). Unlike the external exposome, which focuses on exogenous factors, the internal exposome represents the body's biochemical "response landscape," reflecting the integration of both intrinsic physiological mechanisms and adaptive reactions to external stimuli.

Key Endogenous Processes and Their Environmental Interplay

Metabolism lies at the core of the internal exposome, orchestrating energy production, detoxification, and signaling. However, metabolic pathways are highly susceptible to environmental perturbations. For example, maternal dietary intake of methyl donors (e.g., folate, choline) during pregnancy alters DNA methylation patterns in offspring, as demonstrated in the seminal Agouti mouse model (Jirtle & Skinner, 2007). This association highlights how external nutritional inputs can reprogram endogenous epigenetic regulation, blurring the distinction between internal and external influences. Oxidative stress, traditionally viewed as an intrinsic imbalance between reactive oxygen species (ROS) production and antioxidant defenses, is increasingly recognized as a mediator of environmental toxicity. While mitochondrial respiration generates ROS as a byproduct (Halliwell, 2007), exogenous factors such as air pollution or heavy metals exacerbate oxidative damage, leading to DNA adducts and lipid peroxidation. The duality of oxidative stress are both a physiological process and a pathological trigger underscores its role as a bridge between endogenous biology and environmental insult. Inflammation, another pillar of the internal exposome, exemplifies this convergence. Chronic low-grade inflammation, often rooted in immune dysregulation, can be amplified by external agents like pathogens or particulate matter. For instance, persistent exposure to polycyclic aromatic hydrocarbons (PAHs) activates the aryl hydrocarbon receptor, provoking pro-inflammatory cytokine release and epigenetic silencing of tumor suppressor genes (Jirtle & Skinner, 2007). Such interactions illustrate how environmental toxins co-opt endogenous signaling pathways to drive disease. Th0e microbiome, though technically a community of exogenous organisms, functions as a quasi-endogenous system. Gut microbiota modulates host metabolism by producing short-chain fatty acids (SCFAs) that influence immune responses and epigenetic modifications (Sender *et al.*, 2016). Dietary shifts, antibiotics, or environmental toxins can disrupt microbial diversity, altering SCFA profiles and triggering systemic inflammation, a phenomenon linking external exposures to internal metabolic rewiring. Is oxidative stress truly an endogenous process when its magnitude hinges on airborne pollutants? Can inflammation be deemed "internal" if initiated by a lifetime of inhaled toxins? These questions underscore a central debate in exposomics: where to delineate intrinsic biology from environmentally induced alterations. The Agouti mouse study epitomizes this ambiguity, that the maternal diet (external) reshapes fetal epigenetics (internal), yet the resulting phenotype is a product of both (Jirtle

& Skinner, 2007). Similarly, mitochondrial ROS production, though endogenous, becomes pathological under the burden of exogenous heavy metals (Halliwell, 2007). This interplay challenges reductionist categorizations, suggesting that the internal exposome is less a fixed entity than a fluid interface between genes and environment.

External Exposome

The external exposome encompasses all exogenous factors encountered throughout life, ranging from environmental pollutants to socioeconomic conditions. Unlike the internal exposome, which focuses on endogenous processes, the external exposome represents the totality of exposures originating outside the body, yet capable of reshaping biological systems through direct toxicity, epigenetic modulation, or systemic inflammation. These exposures are further categorized into specific (e.g., chemicals, radiation) and general (e.g., diet, lifestyle) domains, each contributing uniquely to disease etiology.

Specific External Exposures

Pollution remains one of the most pervasive environmental threats. Airborne particulate matter (PM2.5), heavy metals, and industrial chemicals like polycyclic aromatic hydrocarbons (PAHs) are linked to respiratory diseases, cardiovascular dysfunction, and epigenetic alterations. For instance, PM2.5 exposure induces global DNA hypomethylation, particularly in genes regulating inflammation (e.g., IL-6), as shown in urban populations (Jirtle & Skinner, 2007; Landrigan *et al.,* 2018). Water and soil contamination by arsenic or lead further exacerbate these effects, with prenatal exposure to lead correlating with lifelong cognitive deficits, a stark example of temporal vulnerability. Radiation, both ionizing (e.g., radon, medical imaging) and non-ionizing (e.g., UV light), illustrates the dose-dependent duality of external exposures. While low-dose ionizing radiation is a known carcinogen, damaging DNA via double-strand breaks and oxidative stress (Halliwell, 2007), UV radiation's role in vitamin D synthesis underscores its context-dependent impact. The Chernobyl cohort studies revealed that prenatal radiation exposure disproportionately increased thyroid cancer risk compared to adult exposure, highlighting critical windows of susceptibility. Pathogens such as Helicobacter pylori and human papillomavirus (HPV) exemplify biologically active external exposures. H. pylori induce gastric cancer through chronic inflammation and epigenetic silencing of tumor suppressors like CDKN2A, while HPV integrates into host DNA, disrupting genomic stability (IARC, 2012). Notably, pathogenicity often intertwines with the internal exposome; for example, gut microbiome dysbiosis amplifies H. pylori-induced damage, illustrating host-environment-microbe crosstalk (Sender *et al.,* 2016).

General External Exposures

Diet serves as a double-edged sword, acting as both a source of nutrients and xenobiotics. The Mediterranean diet, rich in antioxidants and fiber, reduces oxidative stress and modulates microbiome derived metabolites like butyrate, which enhances DNA repair (Hu *et al.,* 2003). Conversely, processed diets high in advanced glycation end products (AGEs) promote inflammation and metabolic syndrome. The Agouti mouse model demonstrated that maternal high-fat diets predispose offspring to obesity via altered DNA methylation at metastable epialleles, a legacy of prenatal nutritional programming (Jirtle & Skinner, 2007). Socioeconomic Status (SES) transcends traditional exposure categories, acting as a systemic modifier of risk. Lower SES correlates with higher pollution exposure, limited healthcare access, and nutrient poor diets, a phenomenon termed "toxic social environments" (Krieger, 2007). For example, low income neighborhoods in urban centers often face elevated PM2.5 levels, compounding respiratory and cardiovascular risks. A debate persists: Should SES be classified as a core exposome component or merely a contextual modifier? Its pervasive influence across multiple exposure pathways argues for the former (Krieger, 2007). Lifestyle factors, including smoking, alcohol consumption, and physical inactivity, contribute to 40% of cancer deaths globally. Synergistic effects are evident; smoking combined with asbestos exposure multiplies lung cancer risk by 50 folds. However, lifestyle choices are rarely independent of SES. For instance, smoking prevalence is higher in low income populations, reflecting socioeconomic constraints on health behavior, a nuance often overlooked in individualized risk models (Krieger, 2007).

TEMPORAL DYNAMICS: PRENATAL VS. ADULT EXPOSURES

The timing of exposure critically determines health outcomes. Prenatal exposure to air pollution alters fetal glucocorticoid receptor methylation, predisposing offspring to metabolic disorders (Jirtle & Skinner, 2007). In contrast, adult exposure to benzene primarily impacts hematopoietic cells, increasing leukemia risk (Landrigan *et al.,* 2018). These temporal hierarchies underscore the need for life-course exposomics, integrating sensitive developmental periods into risk assessment.

Methodological Challenges and Innovations

Mapping the exposome, whether internal or external demands navigating a labyrinth of dynamic interactions, temporal variability, and biological complexity. Traditional tools like metabolomics and biomarker assays (e.g., urinary PAH metabolites or 8-OHdG for oxidative stress) have identified critical exposure-disease linkages but falter in capturing real-time fluctuations or disentangling endogenous processes from exogenous insults (Halliwell, 2007). For instance, distinguishing microbiome-derived short-chain fatty acids from dietary metabolites requires advanced isotopic labeling, while geographic information systems (GIS) often fail to account for microenvironments, a person's commute through polluted streets versus their home air filtration (Sender *et al.,* 2016). Latent effects pose another hurdle: prenatal lead exposure may manifest as cognitive decline decades later, eluding conventional biomarker timelines. Emerging technologies, however, are revolutionizing exposomics. Wearable sensors now track both external exposures (real-time PM2.5, UV radiation) and internal responses (cortisol in sweat, glucose fluctuations), bridging the divide between environmental inputs and biological outcomes. Multi-omics integration, such as pharmaco-metabonomics, which predicts drug toxicity using pre-dose metabolic profiles which deciphers interactions between gut microbiota, host metabolism, and pollutants (Jirtle & Skinner, 2007). Machine learning models further untangle socioeconomic gradients; for example, clustering algorithms reveal how low SES amplifies dietary and pollution risks, transforming SES from a confounder to a quantifiable exposome component (Krieger, 2007). Together, these innovations herald a paradigm shift from static snapshots to dynamic, life-course exposomics are essential for personalized prevention and equitable health solutions.

METHODOLOGIES FOR EXPOSOME ASSESSMENT

The systematic characterization of environmental influences on human health represents one of the most formidable challenges in modern biomedical research. Unlike genomics, where a relatively static set of approximately 25,000 genes can be sequenced with standardized technology, the exposome encompasses a vast, dynamic array of external and internal factors throughout the lifespan. This section explores the methodological landscape of exposome assessment, highlighting both the significant challenges and innovative solutions that have emerged in recent years. Understanding these methodologies is particularly crucial when investigating how environmental exposures may influence gametogenesis, contribute to teratogenic effects, or promote carcinogenesis processes that often involve complex exposure-response relationships across critical developmental windows.

Challenges in Measuring the Exposome
Complexity of Environmental Exposures

The exposome concept was initially proposed to complement genomics research by providing a framework for comprehensive assessment of non-genetic factors in disease etiology. As Safarlou and colleagues note, exposomics aims "to enable the analysis of the complete complexity of exposures and their corresponding biological responses as an alternative to taking a piecemeal approach". Sarfalou also notes that "because we cannot continuously measure and analyze everything 'nongenetic' in the universe, a discovery-driven approach to the whole environment should limit what is measured based on at least a) the capacity of measurement technology, and b) the requirements of data analytics". This observation highlights the fundamental challenge of prioritizing which exposures to measure when comprehensive monitoring remains technologically unfeasible. This endeavour immediately confronts the extraordinary diversity of environmental agents from industrial chemicals and air pollutants to dietary components and psychosocial stressors that may influence human biology through multiple mechanistic pathways. The numerical scale of this challenge is daunting. Of the approximately 140,000 registered industrial chemicals, fewer than 5,000 have been well-characterized regarding their health effects. Moreover, these compounds do not exist in isolation but combine in complex mixtures that may produce synergistic, antagonistic, or additive biological effects. For instance, in studies of reproductive toxicology, mixtures of endocrine-disrupting chemicals at individually innocuous doses have demonstrated significant impacts on gonadal development when administered together. This phenomenon, known as the "something from nothing" effect, underscores the limitations of traditional single-chemical toxicological approaches. Low-dose effects present another layer of complexity. Traditional toxicological paradigms often fail to capture non-monotonic dose-response relationships, particularly relevant for endocrine disruptors like bisphenol A that may affect gametogenesis at concentrations below regulatory thresholds. These low-dose effects may induce subtle epigenetic alterations in gametes that manifest as transgenerational phenotypes, highlighting the need for sensitive biomarkers that can decode multifactorial interactions at the molecular level. Further complicating this landscape is the phenomenon of biological transformation. Environmental chemicals undergo metabolic processing within the body, potentially generating metabolites with greater toxicity than their parent compounds. The classic example is benzo[a]pyrene in cigarette smoke, which requires metabolic activation to form DNA-reactive epoxides capable of initiating carcinogenesis. Similarly, the pesticide DDT metabolizes to DDE, which possesses greater persistence and endocrine-disrupting potential, with documented effects on reproductive development. These transformation processes create a moving target for exposure assessment, demanding methods capable of capturing both parent compounds and their biologically relevant metabolites. The dynamic, life-course nature of environmental exposures presents another layer of complexity. Critical windows of susceptibility during gametogenesis, fetal development, puberty, or other transitional periods may dramatically amplify the biological significance of even low-dose exposures. This temporal dimension necessitates longitudinal approaches to exposure assessment, particularly when investigating developmental origins of health and disease. For example, maternal exposure to endocrine disruptors during specific gestational windows may permanently alter the reproductive capacity of offspring through epigenetic reprogramming of developing gametes, a process undetectable to cross-sectional assessment methods.

Data Integration Challenges

Modern exposome research generates unprecedented volumes of heterogeneous data from targeted biomonitoring of specific chemicals to untargeted metabolomic profiles, from questionnaire-based lifestyle assessments to high resolution environmental monitoring. Integrating these diverse data streams presents formidable methodological challenges that require innovative computational approaches. Systems biology has emerged as a crucial framework for conceptualizing and analyzing these multi-dimensional datasets. Rather than examining individual exposure-outcome relationships in isolation, systems approach attempts to model complex networks of interactions among exposures, biological responses, and health endpoints. For example, in investigating how environmental exposures influence spermatogenesis, researchers might integrate data on chemical exposures, seminal fluid metabolomics, testicular transcriptomics, and clinical parameters of sperm quality. However, these integrative analyses demand sophisticated statistical methods capable of handling high-dimensional, often sparse, and frequently correlated data structures. The harmonization of disparate measurement scales and data types represents a persistent challenge in exposome research. Molecular data (metabolomics, transcriptomics, epigenomics) typically derive from standardized laboratory protocols with defined units and quality control procedures. In contrast, environmental measurements may come from diverse sources, with varying levels of precision, detection limits, and spatiotemporal resolution. For instance, air pollution data might combine fixed-site monitoring stations, satellite remote sensing, and personal exposure sensors, each with distinct characteristics and limitations. Reconciling these differences requires careful consideration of measurement error structures and development of appropriate data transformation methods. Statistical approaches for exposome data analysis must address the multiple testing problem inherent in examining thousands of potential exposure-outcome associations. Traditional methods control false discovery rates but may lack power to detect modest but biologically significant effects. Recent methodological innovations include sparse regression techniques, Bayesian model averaging, and machine learning approaches that can identify patterns in high-dimensional exposome data. For example, exposome-wide association studies (ExWAS) have been employed to screen hundreds of exposures simultaneously against health outcomes, identifying novel associations for targeted investigation. Network-based analytical methods offer particular promise for exposome research by explicitly modeling the complex interrelationships among exposures and biological responses. Chemical similarity networks can identify structural analogues with potentially shared toxicological mechanisms, while biochemical pathway networks can reveal how environmental perturbations propagate through biological systems. A noteworthy application is the adverse outcome pathway (AOP) framework, which maps mechanistic links from molecular initiating events (e.g., receptor binding) through key events to adverse outcomes (e.g., impaired gametogenesis). These structured approaches help translate exposome data into biologically meaningful insights with relevance to human health.

Temporal and Spatial Variability

Environmental exposures vary dramatically across time and space, creating substantial complexity for exposome assessment. This variability occurs across multiple scales, from diurnal fluctuations in air pollution levels to seasonal changes in dietary patterns to life-course transitions in exposure profiles. Capturing this temporal dimension requires thoughtful study design and sampling strategies tailored to the biological processes under investigation. The HELIX project (Human Early Life Exposome) exemplifies this approach, following mother-child pairs across Europe from pregnancy through childhood with repeated biological sampling and environmental monitoring. This longitudinal design enables researchers to identify critical windows during development when exposures may have particularly profound and lasting effects. For instance, HELIX investigators documented distinct patterns of exposure to endocrine-disrupting chemicals across pregnancy trimesters, with implications for fetal development. Such timing-specific effects would remain invisible to cross-sectional study designs or aggregate exposure metrics. Implementing longitudinal exposure assessment presents numerous practical challenges. Biospecimen collection must balance participant burden against the need for temporal resolution, often leading to strategic sampling during hypothesized critical windows. Analytical methods must account for time-varying confounders and complex correlation structures in repeated measures data. Furthermore, measurement technologies may evolve over extended study periods, necessitating careful cross-calibration to maintain comparability. These methodological considerations are particularly significant for studies of reproductive and developmental effects, where exposures during discrete biological windows may exert disproportionate influence. Spatial variability in environmental exposures introduces another dimension of complexity. Individuals traverse multiple microenvironments daily homes, workplaces, transportation corridors, recreational spaces—each with distinct exposure profiles. Geographic information systems (GIS) have become essential tools for characterizing this spatial dimension, integrating diverse geospatial data sources to model exposure distributions. For example, studies of prenatal teratogen exposure might combine residential history, land use regression models of air pollution, water quality monitoring networks, and occupational history to construct comprehensive spatial exposure assessments. Time-activity patterns further modulate individual exposure profiles by determining the duration and intensity of contact with environmental agents across different settings. Traditional time-activity questionnaires provide valuable but imprecise information about these patterns. Emerging technologies, including smartphone-based GPS tracking and proximity sensors, offer more objective and detailed characterization of human mobility and microenvironmental exposures. These digital approaches can document exposure-relevant behaviors with high temporal resolution while minimizing recall bias. For example, Shih *et al.* (2019) deployed smartphone-based activity tracking in a cohort of reproductive age women, revealing previously unrecognized patterns of exposure to traffic-related air pollution during daily commutes (Shih, *et al.,* 2019). Similarly, Zare Sakhvidi *et al.* (2021) combined personal sensor data with GPS coordinates to create time-weighted exposure estimates for reproductive toxicants that accounted for both spatial concentration gradients and individual movement patterns. Integration of these mobility data with environmental monitoring networks enables development of dynamic exposure models that reflect the complex interplay between human behavior and spatiotemporally variable environmental conditions, a crucial consideration when investigating exposures that may affect vulnerable biological processes such as gametogenesis or embryonic development (Sakhvidi *et al.,* 2022).

Tools and Technology for Exposome Assessment

High-Throughput Analytical Techniques

The technological revolution in analytical chemistry has dramatically expanded our capacity to detect and quantify environmental exposures. Mass spectrometry-based approaches, particularly liquid chromatography-mass spectrometry (LC-MS) and gas chromatography-mass spectrometry (GC-MS), have emerged as cornerstone technologies in exposome research due to their sensitivity, specificity, and multiplexing capabilities. These platforms enable simultaneous measurement of hundreds to thousands of chemicals in biological samples, supporting both targeted analysis of known compounds and untargeted discovery of novel exposures. High-resolution mass spectrometry (HRMS) has been particularly transformative, allowing precise measurement of chemical signatures at environmentally relevant concentrations. For example, Andra *et al.* (2015) demonstrated the application of HRMS to detect over 700 xenobiotic compounds in maternal-fetal biological matrices, providing unprecedented insights into prenatal chemical exposures that may influence gametogenesis and embryonic development (Andra *et al.,* 2015). Similarly, Wang *et al.* (2018) employed HRMS-based metabolomics to identify specific chemical signatures associated with impaired spermatogenesis, revealing potential biomarkers of reproductive toxicity (Wang *et al.,* 2018).

Sensor Technologies and Personal Exposure Monitoring

Traditional environmental monitoring often relies on fixed-site sampling stations that may not accurately reflect individual exposure profiles. Recent advances in wearable sensor technology have enabled more personalized exposure assessment, allowing researchers to track environmental exposures with high temporal and spatial resolution (Nieuwenhuijsen *et al.,* 2015). These devices range from simple passive samplers that accumulate chemical exposures over time to sophisticated real-time monitors with wireless data transmission capabilities. The MyExposome personal exposure monitor exemplifies this approach, utilizing silicone wristbands embedded with adsorbent materials to capture a broad spectrum of organic compounds in an individual's personal environment (O'Connell *et al.,* 2014). In reproductive toxicology research, such devices have been deployed to characterize preconception exposures to endocrine-disrupting chemicals, providing more accurate exposure estimates than environmental modeling alone. Researchers have utilized wearable samplers to document correlations between personal exposure to phthalates and altered reproductive hormone profiles in both men and women planning pregnancy.

Biomonitoring Advances

Biological monitoring provides direct evidence of chemical exposures through measurement of environmental agents or their metabolites in tissues or biofluids. Recent innovations in biomonitoring include expanded panels of exposure biomarkers, improved analytical sensitivity, and novel matrices that enable retrospective exposure assessment. Non-invasive biomonitoring approaches have gained particular traction in developmental and reproductive research, where traditional sampling methods may be ethically or practically challenging. Analysis of shed deciduous teeth can reveal prenatal and early childhood exposure to metals and other persistent chemicals through growth layer-specific sampling (Arora & Austin, 2013). This technique has documented associations between early-life heavy metal exposures and subsequent reproductive abnormalities, suggesting potential transgenerational effects mediated through gamete damage. Similarly, hair analysis provides a temporal record of exposure to mercury and other persistent compounds, with particular relevance for assessing maternal exposures during gametogenesis and pregnancy (Appenzeller *et al.,* 2020). Molecular biomarkers of exposure effect represent another frontier, linking chemical exposures to early biological perturbations that may precede clinical manifestations. Adductomics, the comprehensive analysis of chemical modifications to DNA and proteins can reveal exposure-induced molecular damage with potential implications for gamete integrity and carcinogenesis (Balbo *et al.,* 2014). Studies have identified specific patterns of DNA adducts in sperm associated with occupational exposure to mutagenic chemicals, providing potential mechanistic links between environmental exposures and paternally-mediated developmental effects.

Omics Technologies in Exposome Research

The integration of exposome assessment with multi-omics technologies has created unprecedented opportunities to elucidate how environmental factors influence biological systems at multiple organizational levels. These approaches generate comprehensive molecular profiles that can serve as intermediate biomarkers between external exposures and health outcomes. Transcriptomics and epigenomics have proven particularly valuable in reproductive and developmental exposome research by revealing how environmental chemicals may reprogram gene expression in gametes or developing tissues. For instance, Soubry *et al.* (2017) employed genome-wide DNA methylation profiling to demonstrate that paternal preconception exposure to organophosphate pesticides induces specific epigenetic alterations in sperm that persist in fetal tissues following fertilization (Soubry *et al.,* 2017). Similarly, Hou *et al.* (2019) used RNA sequencing to identify transcriptional signatures in primordial germ cells exposed to endocrine-disrupting chemicals, providing insights into potential mechanisms of transgenerational inheritance (Hou *et al.,* 2021). Proteomics and metabolomics extend these investigations to functional endpoints, characterizing how exposures perturb protein expression and metabolic pathways relevant to reproduction and development. Metabolomics has proven especially valuable as an integrative readout of exposome influences, reflecting both external chemical exposures and endogenous metabolic responses. In the context of carcinogenesis, metabolomic profiling has identified specific molecular signatures associated with chemical carcinogen exposure, potentially enabling earlier detection of cancer-promoting environmental factors.

Exposure Assessment Methodologies

Questionnaire-Based Assessment

Despite technological advances, questionnaires and interviews remain essential tools for exposome research, providing contextual information about lifestyle factors, occupational exposures, and other determinants of environmental exposure that may not be captured by biomonitoring or sensor technologies. Structured questionnaires enable systematic documentation of exposure histories across diverse domains, including diet, consumer product use, and residential history. In reproductive health research, specialized questionnaires have been developed to capture exposures during critical windows such as preconception and pregnancy. For example, the LIFE Study (Longitudinal Investigation of Fertility and the Environment) implemented detailed exposure assessment questionnaires that documented associations between occupational solvent exposure and reduced fecundity in both men and women (Louis *et al.*, 2016). Similarly, questionnaire-based assessment in the Agricultural Health Study revealed links between specific pesticide exposures and aberrant fetal development, highlighting the value of occupation-specific exposure assessments. The accuracy of self reported exposure information varies considerably across exposure domains, with more salient or discrete exposures (e.g., smoking) generally reported more reliably than ambient or ubiquitous exposures (e.g., passive air pollution). Validation studies comparing questionnaire responses to objective exposure measurements have documented both under- and over-reporting of environmental exposures, underscoring the importance of multi-method assessment approaches (Vrijheid *et al.*, 2014). Despite these limitations, questionnaires provide crucial contextual information that complements biomonitoring data and may help identify sources of exposure for intervention.

Environmental Modeling and Remote Sensing

Sophisticated modeling approaches have significantly enhanced researchers' ability to characterize environmental exposures across populations and geographies. Land use regression models combine measurement data with geographic predictors to estimate spatial exposure patterns for air pollutants and other environmental contaminants. These models have documented associations between maternal air pollution exposure and adverse birth outcomes, suggesting potential teratogenic effects mediated through placental dysfunction or direct fetal toxicity (Zhang *et al.*, 2016, 2017). Remote sensing data from satellites provides another dimension of environmental exposure assessment, offering broad spatial coverage and temporal resolution for certain exposures. For instance, satellite-derived measures of particulate matter have been incorporated into studies of prenatal exposure effects, enabling researchers to retrospectively estimate air pollution exposures during specific developmental windows. Similarly, remote sensing of vegetation indices and land surface temperature has informed assessments of heat exposure during pregnancy, revealing potential links to birth defects and altered fetal development. Atmospheric transport and dispersion models enable reconstruction of historical exposure patterns, particularly valuable for investigating reproductive or developmental effects of industrial emissions, chemical spills, or other discrete environmental events. Scinetists also employed such models to characterize prenatal exposure to perfluoroalkyl substances from industrial facilities, subsequently linking these exposures to altered reproductive development in offspring. These modeling approaches provide particular value when combined with biomarker data in integrated exposure assessment frameworks.

Integrated Exposure Assessment Frameworks

The complexity of the exposome demands integrated assessment approaches that combine multiple data streams to develop more comprehensive exposure profiles. The exposome-wide association study (ExWAS) paradigm exemplifies this approach, systematically evaluating relationships between comprehensive exposure measures and health outcomes of interest (Patel *et al.,* 2010). This methodological framework has revealed novel associations between environmental chemicals and reproductive parameters, including semen quality, ovarian function, and pregnancy outcomes. The concept of the "personal exposome" emphasizes integration across external exposure measurements, internal biomarkers, and biological response indicators to characterize individual exposure profiles with unprecedented detail. For example, the HELIX project combined external exposure assessment from environmental monitoring, internal exposure measurement through biospecimen analysis, and molecular response profiling to characterize how the early-life exposome influences child development (Vrijheid *et al.,* 2014). This integrated approach has identified specific chemical exposures during prenatal development that may predispose individuals to reproductive abnormalities and increased cancer susceptibility later in life. Computational approaches for integrating diverse exposome data continue to evolve rapidly. Machine learning methods have proven particularly valuable for identifying patterns in high-dimensional exposome datasets and prioritizing exposures for mechanistic investigation. In recent times reserchers employed machine learning algorithms to identify combinations of prenatal chemical exposures associated with altered reproductive development, revealing interaction effects not detectable through traditional statistical approaches. These computational advances, coupled with expanding technological capabilities, promise to further enhance our understanding of how environmental exposures influence gametogenesis, teratogenesis, and carcinogenesis across the life course. The advancement of integrated exposure assessment faces several methodological challenges that have sparked both debate and innovation in the field. A central concern is the lack of standardized protocols for harmonizing sensor data across studies, which limits data comparability and meta-analysis opportunities. Li *et al.* (2021) highlighted how this methodological heterogeneity has impeded the development of comprehensive exposure databases and reference ranges crucial for reproductive toxicology research. In response, significant innovations have emerged, notably the development of MetFrag software for spectral matching in high-resolution mass spectrometry (HRMS), which has enabled more consistent identification of environmental chemicals across laboratories (Ruttkies *et al.,* 2016). Similarly challenging is the integration of multi-omics data, particularly the overlap between endogenous metabolites and environmental chemicals that complicates the distinction between exposure and biological response signatures. Vermeulen *et al.* (2020) demonstrated this challenge in a study of maternal exposures during pregnancy, where chemical signatures in maternal serum were difficult to distinguish from pregnancy-related metabolic changes. Network science approaches have provided promising solutions, with Barabási *et al.* (2011) pioneering methods to map chemical-protein interactions that reveal how environmental agents may perturb biological pathways relevant to gametogenesis and embryonic development (Barabási *et al.,* 2011). These methodological advances are gradually enabling more sophisticated exposome characterization, though the field continues to grapple with balancing technical innovation against the need for standardization and reproducibility.

EXPOSOME AND GAMETOGENESIS

The sophisticated cellular and molecular processes that govern the formation of gametes; spermatogenesis in males and oogenesis in females, represent a critical juncture in reproductive biology where environmental influences can significantly impact developmental outcomes. While the genetic blueprint provides the foundational architecture for gametogenesis, the exposome encompassing the totality of environmental exposures throughout the lifespan modulates these genetic instructions in ways that can profoundly affect gamete quality and, consequently, reproductive health (Wild, 2012). This aspect aims to examine the complex interplay between environmental exposures and gametogenesis, with particular emphasis on mechanisms of action, biomarkers of effect, and implications for human fertility and transgenerational health. Recent advancements in analytical technologies, including high-throughput screening methods, metabolomics, and epigenomic profiling, have enhanced our ability to characterize the exposome and its effects on reproductive function. These methodological innovations have facilitated more comprehensive assessments of exposure-response relationships and revealed previously unrecognized mechanisms through which environmental factors can disrupt gametogenesis.

Impact on Sperm Development

Environmental Factors Affecting Spermatogenesis

Spermatogenesis represents a continuous process of cell proliferation and differentiation that is exquisitely sensitive to environmental perturbations. Among the most well documented environmental factors affecting sperm development are agricultural chemicals, which have shown consistent associations with altered semen parameters across numerous studies. It was demonstrated that men from agrarian regions (mid-Missouri) exhibited significantly reduced sperm concentration and motility compared to men from urban centers, with specific pesticides emerging as potential culprits. Metabolites of herbicides including alachlor and atrazine, and the insecticide diazinon, were significantly elevated in men with poor semen quality, with striking odds ratios of 30.0, 11.3, and 16.7, respectively. These findings align with historical occupational exposure studies documenting profound effects of certain agricultural chemicals on male fertility, including the nematocide dibromochloropropane, which affected over 26,000 plantation workers worldwide, leaving 64% with reduced sperm concentrations and 28% involuntarily childless. More recent research has expanded our understanding of the range of pesticides that may affect male reproductive function. Organophosphate pesticides, commonly used in both agricultural and residential settings, have been associated with reduced sperm concentration, motility, and normal morphology in numerous studies (Mehrpour *et al.*, 2014). A meta-analysis study identified consistent negative associations between organophosphate exposure and multiple semen parameters across diverse study populations. Heavy metals constitute another critical class of reproductive toxicants, with lead, cadmium, and mercury demonstrating particular potency in disrupting spermatogenesis. These metals can compromise the blood-testis barrier, induce oxidative stress in testicular tissue, and directly impair Sertoli and Leydig cell function (Wirth & Mijal, 2010). Occupational exposures in battery manufacturing, welding, and metal recycling industries have been associated with dose-dependent decreases in sperm concentration, motility, and normal morphology, even at blood levels below established occupational safety thresholds (Telišman *et al.*, 2007). Recent studies have highlighted the importance of cadmium as a reproductive toxicant, demonstrated that even low-level environmental cadmium exposure was associated with impaired sperm function, likely through interference with calcium channels critical for capacitation and acrosome reaction. Similarly, it was found out that, there were significant inverse correlations between seminal cadmium concentrations and sperm count, motility, and morphology in men attending fertility clinics. Endocrine-disrupting chemicals (EDCs) represent perhaps the most mechanistically complex class of reproductive toxicants, given their ability to interfere with hormonal signaling pathways essential for testicular development and function. Bisphenol A (BPA), phthalates, polychlorinated biphenyls (PCBs), and certain pesticides can mimic, block, or otherwise interfere with androgen and estrogen signaling, disrupting the delicate hormonal balance required for spermatogenesis (Gore *et al.,* 2015). These compounds are ubiquitous in modern environments are found in plastics, personal care products, food packaging, and building materials, making exposure virtually universal in industrialized societies. The reproductive effects of phthalates have received particular attention due to their widespread use and endocrine-disrupting properties. There were significant inverse associations between urinary phthalate metabolite concentrations and sperm concentration, motility, and morphology in men attending fertility clinics. These associations were strongest for mono-(2-ethylhexyl) phthalate (MEHP), the primary metabolite of di-(2-ethylhexyl) phthalate (DEHP), suggesting particular reproductive toxicity of this common plasticizer. Emerging research has identified per- and polyfluoroalkyl substances (PFAS) as potential reproductive toxicants. These persistent synthetic chemicals, used in non-stick cookware, stain-resistant fabrics, and food packaging, have been detected in human seminal plasma and associated with reduced sperm concentration and motility (Di Nisio *et al.,* 2019). A Danish cohort study found that men with higher serum PFAS concentrations had significantly higher proportions of morphologically abnormal sperm (Joensen *et al.,* 2009). Lifestyle factors, including smoking, alcohol consumption, psychological stress, and nutritional status, also substantially influence spermatogenesis. Cigarette smoke contains numerous reproductive toxicants, including cadmium, lead, benzene, and polycyclic aromatic hydrocarbons, which collectively impair all aspects of sperm function (Dia *et al.,* 2015). Alcohol's reproductive effects appear dose-dependent, with moderate to heavy consumption associated with decreased testosterone production, abnormal spermatogenesis, and reduced sperm quality (Muthusami & Chinnaswamy, 2005). Emerging evidence suggests that psychological stress may impair spermatogenesis via hypothalamic-pituitary-gonadal axis dysregulation, oxidative stress mechanisms, and inflammatory pathways (Nargund, 2015). The importance of nutrition in male reproductive health has gained increasing recognition. Both under- and overnutrition can negatively impact spermatogenesis, with obesity emerging as a significant risk factor for impaired sperm production and function (Sermondade *et al.,* 2013). A meta-analysis of 21 studies found that obese men had significantly higher rates of oligozoospermia and azoospermia compared to normal-weight men, with odds ratios of 1.42 and 1.81, respectively (Sermondade *et al.,* 2013). These effects appear mediated through multiple mechanisms, including altered reproductive hormone profiles, increased testicular temperature, and systemic inflammation. Physical factors, including elevated testicular temperature (from occupational heat exposure, tight clothing, or laptop computer use), ionizing radiation, non-ionizing electromagnetic fields, and air pollution, represent an often-overlooked category of reproductive exposures. The testicular environment requires temperatures approximately 2-4°C below core body temperature for optimal spermatogenesis, and even moderate temperature elevations can significantly reduce sperm production and quality (Durairajanayagam *et al.,* 2015). Occupational heat exposure has been associated with reduced sperm count and altered morphology in numerous studies. A meta-analysis found consistent negative associations between occupational heat exposure and semen parameters across diverse populations. Similarly, habitual use of saunas, hot tubs, and even prolonged seated positions (as in professional driving) has been associated with reduced sperm production and quality (Durairajanayagam *et al.,* 2015).

Effects on Sperm Quality

Environmental exposures manifest their effects on sperm through alterations in conventional semen parameters (concentration, motility, morphology) and more subtle functional and molecular characteristics. Sperm concentration (count) appears particularly vulnerable to environmental insults, with longitudinal studies suggesting significant global declines in sperm counts over the past five decades, potentially attributable to increasing environmental chemical exposures (Levine *et al.,* 2017). However, men from agricultural regions had significantly lower sperm concentrations compared to urban counterparts, with strong associations between specific pesticide metabolites and reduced counts. A comprehensive meta-analysis by Levine and colleagues (2017) found a 52.4% decline in sperm concentration among men from North America, Europe, Australia, and New Zealand between 1973 and 2011, with the rate of decline accelerating in recent decades (Levine *et al.,* 2017). While the causes of this decline remain debated, increasing environmental chemical exposures represent a plausible contributing factor. Sperm motility is essential for navigating the female reproductive tract and penetrating the oocyte, which could be similarly susceptible to environmental disruption. The mitochondria-rich midpiece that powers sperm motility is vulnerable to oxidative damage from numerous environmental toxicants. Pesticides including diazinon and chlorpyrifos can inhibit acetylcholinesterase activity in sperm cells, disrupting energy metabolism and calcium signaling necessary for coordinated flagellar movement. Heavy metals, particularly cadmium and lead, disrupt mitochondrial function and deplete cellular antioxidant capacity, resulting in ATP depletion and impaired motility (Wirth & Mijal, 2010). A recent study by Smarr and colleagues (2018) found significant associations between air pollution exposure and reduced sperm motility in a cohort of fertile men. Specifically, increased exposure to particulate matter less than 2.5 micrometers in diameter (PM2.5) was associated with decreased progressive motility, potentially due to oxidative stress mechanisms. Sperm morphology represents another critical parameter affected by environmental exposures. Normal morphology requires precise genetic and epigenetic regulation during spermiogenesis, the final stage of spermatogenesis involving extensive nuclear condensation and cytoplasmic remodeling. Endocrine disruptors can interfere with this process by disrupting androgen signaling, resulting in increased proportions of abnormally shaped sperm cells with defects in the head, midpiece, or tail regions. Phthalate exposure has been particularly associated with abnormal sperm morphology. Study also found that men with higher urinary concentrations of monoethyl phthalate (MEP) had significantly higher proportions of sperm with abnormal morphology. Similarly, occupational exposure to solvents and pesticides has been associated with increased rates of morphologically abnormal sperm. DNA integrity, while not assessed in routine semen analysis, represents perhaps the most significant functional parameter affected by environmental exposures. Sperm DNA fragmentation has been associated with numerous toxicants, including pesticides, heavy metals, air pollutants, and lifestyle factors such as smoking and alcohol consumption (Aitken *et al.,* 2015). The mechanisms underlying environmentally-induced DNA damage include oxidative stress, defective apoptosis, and impaired DNA repair. Unlike somatic cells, sperm have limited DNA repair capacity, making them particularly vulnerable to genotoxic insults. Importantly, sperm DNA damage may not affect conventional semen parameters but can significantly impact fertilization, embryo development, and offspring health. Recent research has highlighted the importance of sperm DNA integrity in reproductive outcomes. A meta-analysis study found that high levels of sperm DNA fragmentation were associated with significantly reduced pregnancy rates in both natural conception and assisted reproductive technology cycles. Similarly, study also found that sperm DNA fragmentation levels were significantly higher in infertile men compared to fertile controls, regardless of conventional semen parameters. Emerging evidence suggests that environmental exposures may also affect sperm factors beyond conventional parameters and DNA integrity. For example, specific proteins involved in sperm-oocyte interaction, such as IZUMO1 and JUNO, may be affected by environmental toxicants, potentially compromising fertilization capacity without altering standard semen parameters (Aitken, 2020).

Epigenetic Alterations in Sperm

Beyond direct effects on semen parameters and DNA integrity, environmental exposures can induce epigenetic modifications in sperm that may affect embryo development and offspring health. DNA methylation patterns, which regulate gene expression without altering the underlying DNA sequence, appear particularly susceptible to environmental influences during spermatogenesis. Heavy metals (particularly lead and cadmium), pesticides, endocrine disruptors, air pollutants, and lifestyle factors including diet, smoking, and alcohol consumption have all been associated with altered sperm DNA methylation profiles (Donkin & Barrès, 2018). It was reported that men with low sperm counts exhibited aberrant DNA methylation patterns at imprinted genes, suggesting potential epigenetic mechanisms underlying some forms of male infertility. Similarly, it was found that occupational exposure to organophosphate pesticides was associated with altered DNA methylation at specific genomic loci in sperm. Paternal nutritional status appears capable of inducing significant epigenetic alterations in sperm. Animal studies have demonstrated that both undernutrition and overnutrition can modify sperm DNA methylation patterns, with potential implications for offspring metabolic health (Donkin & Barrès, 2018). In humans, it was found that obese men had significantly different sperm DNA methylation patterns compared to normal-weight men, particularly at genes involved in growth and development. Histone modifications represent another critical epigenetic mechanism affected by environmental exposures. While most histones are replaced by protamines during spermiogenesis, approximately 5-15% of the sperm genome remains histone-bound, particularly at developmentally important loci (Lambrot *et al.,* 2019). This retained histone fraction appears selectively vulnerable to environmental influences, with exposure to endocrine disruptors such as BPA and phthalates associated with altered histone acetylation and methylation patterns at key developmental genes (Stouder & Paoloni-Giacobino, 2010). Studies by Urdinguio and colleagues (2015) have demonstrated that retained histones in human sperm are enriched at developmental promoters and genes involved in embryonic development, suggesting a functional role in early embryogenesis. Environmental exposures that alter histone modifications at these loci may therefore affect offspring development through epigenetic mechanisms. Non-coding RNAs, including microRNAs, long non-coding RNAs, and piwi-interacting RNAs, constitute an emerging class of epigenetic regulators increasingly recognized as targets of environmental toxicants. These RNA species can be transferred to the oocyte during fertilization and influence early embryonic gene expression (Krawetz *et al.,* 2011). Environmental exposures that alter sperm non-coding RNA profiles may therefore affect offspring development through epigenetic mechanisms that bypass direct DNA sequence alterations. A study by Ostermeier and Krawetz (2005) demonstrated that sperm deliver specific RNAs to the oocyte during fertilization, potentially influencing early embryonic development. More recent research has shown that paternal exposure to environmental toxicants can alter sperm microRNA profiles, with potential implications for offspring phenotypes (Marczylo *et al.,* 2012). The transgenerational implications of environmentally-induced epigenetic alterations in sperm are profound. Unlike genetic mutations, epigenetic modifications are potentially reversible but can nonetheless be transmitted across generations if they affect the germline. Animal studies have demonstrated that exposure to endocrine disruptors, pesticides, and other environmental chemicals can induce epigenetic changes in sperm that manifest as disease phenotypes in unexposed subsequent generations, raising significant concerns about the long-term health impacts of current environmental exposures (Nilsson & Skinner, 2015). The landmark studies by Anway and colleagues (2005) demonstrated that exposure to the fungicide vinclozolin during critical periods of fetal development induced epigenetic alterations in the male germline that persisted for at least four generations in the absence of additional exposure. These epigenetic changes manifested as increased rates of various disease phenotypes, including testicular abnormalities, prostate disease, and kidney disease, in unexposed descendants of exposed individuals. Human studies have begun to provide evidence of environmentally-induced transgenerational epigenetic effects. Thus, it was found that paternal smoking during the slow growth period before puberty was associated with increased body mass index in sons but not daughters, suggesting potential sex-specific transgenerational effects mediated through epigenetic mechanisms in the male germline. The determination of "safe" exposure thresholds for endocrine disruptors represents one of the most contentious areas in reproductive toxicology, with significant implications for regulatory policy and public health. Traditional toxicological paradigms assume monotonic dose-response relationships with identifiable thresholds below which no adverse effects occur. However, endocrine disruptors frequently display non-monotonic dose-response curves, wherein low doses may exert effects distinct from or even opposite to those observed at higher doses (Vandenberg *et al.,* 2012). This phenomenon challenges conventional risk assessment approaches and has fueled debate regarding appropriate regulatory frameworks. A comprehensive review by Vandenberg and colleagues (2012), identified numerous examples of non-monotonic dose responses for endocrine disruptors, with hormetic effects (beneficial at low doses, harmful at high doses) and U-shaped or inverted U-shaped dose-response curves observed for various reproductive endpoints (Vandenberg *et al.,* 2012). These patterns reflect the complex nature of endocrine signaling, wherein low doses of exogenous compounds may mimic or antagonize endogenous hormones through receptor-mediated mechanisms, while higher doses may elicit cytotoxic effects through different pathways. Methodological challenges further complicate threshold determination for endocrine disruptors. Reproductive outcomes often manifest after substantial latency periods, making causal attribution difficult in epidemiological studies. Additionally, the timing of exposure may be as important as the dose, with specific developmental windows exhibiting heightened vulnerability. For instance, fetal and peripubertal exposures often exert more profound effects on reproductive development than equivalent adult exposures (Diamanti-Kandarakis *et al.,* 2009). Traditional toxicity testing protocols may fail to capture these developmental sensitivities or low-dose effects, potentially underestimating risks. The scientific community remains divided on how to address these challenges. Some researchers advocate for the "endocrine disruptor low-dose hypothesis," which posits that exogenous chemicals can interfere with endogenous hormone signaling at environmentally relevant concentrations far below established regulatory thresholds (Vandenberg *et al.,* 2012). Others contend that while non-monotonic dose responses occur in controlled laboratory settings, their relevance to real-world human exposures remains uncertain (Rhomberg & Goodman, 2012). This scientific uncertainty has contributed to disparate regulatory approaches internationally, with the European Union adopting a more precautionary stance compared to the United States.

The complexity of real-world exposures further complicates threshold determination. Humans are simultaneously exposed to numerous potential endocrine disruptors that may act additively, synergistically, or antagonistically. Current regulatory frameworks predominantly assess chemicals individually, potentially underestimating cumulative effects. The recent "mixture hypothesis" suggests that combinations of endocrine disruptors, each at individually ineffective concentrations, may collectively induce adverse reproductive outcomes (Kortenkamp *et al.,* 2012). It was demonstrated that mixtures of antiandrogens at doses below individual no-observed-adverse-effect levels (NOAELs) could induce significant reproductive abnormalities when administered collectively. Similarly, it was found that mixtures of endocrine disruptors at low doses could induce developmental abnormalities not observed with individual compounds at equivalent doses, supporting the concept of additive or synergistic effects.

Impact on Oocyte Development

Environmental Factors Affecting Oogenesis

Oogenesis differs fundamentally from spermatogenesis in its temporal dynamics; while spermatogenesis continues throughout adult life, oogenesis initiates during fetal development with a finite pool of primordial follicles established prenatally. This distinct developmental timeline creates unique vulnerabilities, as environmental exposures during critical prenatal and early postnatal periods can irreversibly affect female reproductive potential. Moreover, oocytes remain arrested in prophase I of meiosis for decades before maturation, providing an extended window for environmental insults to accumulate. The environmental factors affecting oogenesis largely parallel those impacting spermatogenesis, though often with distinct mechanisms and consequences. Agricultural chemicals, including pesticides, herbicides, and fungicides, have demonstrated adverse effects on ovarian folliculogenesis and oocyte quality in both animal models and epidemiological studies. Organochlorine pesticides, organophosphates, and certain herbicides can disrupt ovarian steroidogenesis, alter follicular development, and compromise oocyte maturation, potentially contributing to reduced fecundity and increased time to pregnancy observed in agricultural communities. A prospective cohort study found that women exposed to pesticides through agricultural work had significantly longer time to pregnancy and increased risk of infertility compared to unexposed women. However, it was found that women who used herbicides and fungicides had significantly increased odds of infertility compared to non-users, with odds ratios of 3.8 and 3.3, respectively. Heavy metals exhibit particular ovotoxicity, with lead, cadmium, mercury, and arsenic implicated in premature ovarian insufficiency, altered cyclicity, and reduced oocyte quality. These metals can accumulate in ovarian follicular fluid, where they induce oxidative stress, disrupt mitochondrial function, and impair the complex bidirectional communication between oocytes and surrounding granulosa cells essential for normal folliculogenesis (Bloom *et al.,* 2012). Study revealed that women with higher blood lead levels had significantly lower antral follicle counts, suggesting potential effects on ovarian reserve. Similarly, increased blood cadmium levels were associated with longer menstrual cycles and reduced odds of ovulation, potentially reflecting disrupted folliculogenesis. Endocrine disruptors may exert particularly profound effects on oogenesis given the central role of hormonal signaling in female reproductive function. BPA, phthalates, dioxins, and perfluorinated compounds can interfere with estrogen, progesterone, and androgen signaling pathways critical for follicular recruitment, development, and ovulation. These compounds may also disrupt hypothalamic-pituitary-ovarian axis function, resulting in altered gonadotropin secretion and ovulatory dysfunction. BPA exposure has been associated with reduced ovarian response to stimulation in women undergoing in vitro fertilization. Research found that women with higher urinary BPA concentrations had significantly fewer oocytes retrieved and lower peak estradiol levels during ovarian stimulation. Increased urinary BPA levels were associated with lower antral follicle counts in women undergoing fertility evaluation. Phthalate exposure has been linked to various adverse reproductive outcomes in women. Studies found that women with higher urinary phthalate metabolite concentrations had increased odds of implantation failure during in vitro fertilization. Similarly, Louis and colleagues (2013) found that increased urinary phthalate metabolite levels were associated with longer time to pregnancy in a prospective cohort of women attempting conception. Maternal factors, including diet, psychological stress, and age, represent a category of exposures particularly relevant to oogenesis. Maternal undernutrition or micronutrient deficiencies can compromise primordial follicle formation and oocyte quality, potentially programming lifelong reproductive dysfunction in female offspring. Similarly, maternal psychological stress appears capable of altering fetal ovarian development through glucocorticoid signaling pathways, with transgenerational implications. Advanced maternal age constitutes a significant risk factor for oocyte chromosomal abnormalities, potentially exacerbating the effects of environmental exposures through compromised cellular repair mechanisms and accumulated oxidative damage. Animal studies have demonstrated that maternal undernutrition during pregnancy can reduce primordial follicle numbers in female offspring, potentially compromising future reproductive potential. Similarly, maternal micronutrient deficiencies, particularly folate and vitamin B12, have been associated with altered DNA methylation patterns in oocytes, suggesting potential epigenetic mechanisms underlying nutritional effects on oogenesis (Steegers-Theunissen *et al.,* 2013). Psychological stress may affect oogenesis through multiple mechanisms, including hypothalamic-pituitary-adrenal axis activation, oxidative stress, and inflammatory pathways. Lynch and colleagues (2014) found that women reporting high levels of perceived stress had significantly lower antral follicle counts compared to women reporting low stress levels. It was also observed that women with higher psychological stress scores had significantly fewer oocytes retrieved during in vitro fertilization and lower pregnancy rates.

Effects on Oocyte Quality

Oocyte quality, encompassing nuclear and cytoplasmic maturation, chromosomal integrity, and metabolic competence, represents a critical determinant of fertility and embryonic developmental potential. Environmental exposures can compromise multiple aspects of oocyte quality, with consequences ranging from reduced fertilization rates to early pregnancy loss and developmental abnormalities (Machtinger & Orvieto, 2014). Meiotic maturation, the process by which oocytes resume meiosis and progress to metaphase II arrest prior to fertilization, appears particularly vulnerable to environmental disruption. Endocrine disruptors, heavy metals, and certain pesticides can interfere with the carefully orchestrated signaling cascades that regulate meiotic resumption, spindle formation, and chromosome segregation. BPA, for example, has been shown to induce meiotic aberrations including altered spindle morphology, chromosomal misalignment, and aneuploidy—potentially contributing to the increased incidence of chromosomal abnormalities observed in human oocytes compared to sperm (Hunt *et al.,* 2003). A study by Hunt and colleagues (2003) found that exposure to environmentally relevant BPA concentrations during meiotic maturation induced significant increases in chromosomal abnormalities in mouse oocytes. It was revealed that BPA exposure during in vitro maturation of mouse oocytes disrupted spindle formation and chromosome alignment, potentially explaining the increased aneuploidy rates observed in BPA-exposed oocytes. Cytoplasmic maturation, involving organelle reorganization, mRNA accumulation, and post-transcriptional modifications, is similarly susceptible to environmental perturbations. Mitochondria, which provide the energetic support for oocyte maturation, fertilization, and early embryonic development, represent primary targets for numerous environmental toxicants. Heavy metals, air pollutants, and certain pesticides can compromise mitochondrial membrane potential, induce reactive oxygen species production, and disrupt ATP synthesis, potentially explaining associations between these exposures and reduced fertilization rates in assisted reproductive technology outcomes. A study by Machtinger and colleagues (2018) found that women with higher urinary phthalate metabolite concentrations had oocytes with reduced mitochondrial membrane potential and increased reactive oxygen species production. Study demonstrated that cadmium exposure during oocyte maturation disrupted mitochondrial distribution and function, potentially compromising energy production necessary for fertilization and early embryonic development. Chromosomal integrity remains perhaps the most significant aspect of oocyte quality affected by environmental exposures. Aneuploidy rates in human oocytes exceed 20% even under optimal conditions and increase dramatically with advanced maternal age. Environmental toxicants appear capable of exacerbating this inherent vulnerability, with endocrine disruptors, heavy metals, and oxidative stressors linked to increased rates of chromosomal abnormalities. These effects likely reflect disruption of spindle assembly checkpoint mechanisms, cohesin complex function, and DNA repair pathways essential for maintaining chromosomal integrity during the protracted meiotic arrest characterizing human oocytes. Hence, BPA exposure during meiotic maturation disrupted the meiotic spindle assembly checkpoint, potentially explaining the increased aneuploidy rates observed in exposed oocytes. Similarly, in vitro exposure of human oocytes to BPA induced significant increases in spindle abnormalities and chromosomal misalignment. Recent research has highlighted the importance of epigenetic integrity in oocyte quality. However, environmental exposures during oocyte growth and maturation could alter DNA methylation patterns at imprinted genes, potentially affecting embryonic development and offspring health. Thus, endocrine disruptors could induce aberrant histone modifications in oocytes, potentially compromising epigenetic regulation of early embryonic development.

Epigenetic Alterations in Oocytes

Epigenetic programming in oocytes exhibits distinct patterns and dynamics compared to sperm, with potentially profound implications for environmentally-induced alterations. Unlike sperm, which undergo extensive epigenetic reprogramming during spermatogenesis, oocytes establish much of their epigenetic landscape during the growth phase preceding ovulation. This extended developmental window provides multiple opportunities for environmental exposures to disrupt normal epigenetic programming. DNA methylation patterns in oocytes appear particularly vulnerable to environmental influences, with nutritional factors, endocrine disruptors, and heavy metals all capable of altering methylation at specific genomic loci. These effects appear most pronounced at imprinted genes, those expressed in a parent-of-origin-specific manner—potentially explaining associations between maternal environmental exposures and imprinting disorders in offspring. Notably, maternal periconceptional folate status can significantly influence DNA methylation patterns in oocytes, highlighting the importance of nutritional factors in epigenetic programming (Steegers-Theunissen *et al.,* 2013). It was also found out that women with higher urinary BPA concentrations exhibited altered DNA methylation patterns at imprinted genes in their oocytes. Similarly, Piyasena and colleagues (2016) demonstrated that maternal dietary folate deficiency during oocyte growth induced aberrant DNA methylation at imprinted genes in mouse oocytes, potentially explaining associations between maternal nutrition and offspring developmental outcomes. Histone modifications in oocytes represent another critical epigenetic mechanism susceptible to environmental disruption. Unlike sperm, oocytes retain their histones throughout development, creating an extended window for environmentally-induced alterations in histone acetylation, methylation, and other post-translational modifications. BPA, for example, has been shown to alter histone methylation patterns in mouse oocytes, with consequent effects on gene expression and developmental competence. These alterations may affect not only oocyte quality but also early embryonic development, as maternal histones persist until embryonic genome activation. A study by Chao and colleagues (2012) found that exposure to environmentally relevant BPA concentrations during oocyte growth altered histone methylation patterns at developmentally important genes in mouse oocytes. Similarly, Machtinger and Orvieta (2014) demonstrated that exposure to endocrine disruptors during oocyte maturation induced aberrant histone acetylation patterns, potentially compromising epigenetic regulation of early embryonic development. Non-coding RNAs in oocytes, including microRNAs and long non-coding RNAs, constitute an emerging area of investigation regarding environmental influences on epigenetic regulation. These RNA species play critical roles in post-transcriptional gene regulation during oocyte maturation and early embryonic development. Environmental toxicants including

BPA, phthalates, and certain pesticides have been shown to alter non-coding RNA expression profiles in oocytes, potentially disrupting the complex regulatory networks governing maternal-to-embryonic transition. A study by Machtinger and Orvieta (2014) found that women with higher urinary phthalate metabolite concentrations exhibited altered microRNA expression profiles in their oocytes, potentially explaining associations between phthalate exposure and reduced fertilization rates. It was established that BPA exposure during oocyte growth altered expression of specific microRNAs involved in cell cycle regulation and apoptosis, potentially compromising oocyte quality and developmental competence. Transgenerational inheritance through maternal germline exposure represents a particularly significant aspect of oocyte epigenetics. The oocyte cytoplasm contains not only nuclear material but also mitochondria and other organelles that are transmitted exclusively through the maternal lineage. Environmental exposures that affect mitochondrial DNA, RNA species, proteins, and metabolites in oocytes may therefore exert transgenerational effects independent of nuclear genetic or epigenetic alterations, creating a "maternal exposome legacy" that can influence offspring health across multiple generations. Animal studies have demonstrated that maternal exposure to environmental toxicants can induce epigenetic alterations in oocytes that manifest as disease phenotypes in unexposed offspring and subsequent generations. It was found that maternal exposure to the fungicide vinclozolin during pregnancy induced epigenetic alterations in female offspring that persisted for multiple generations, manifesting as increased rates of ovarian disease and reduced fertility. Thus, it was observed that maternal cadmium exposure during pregnancy induced epigenetic alterations in oocytes that were transmitted to subsequent generations, potentially explaining transgenerational effects of environmental exposures.

Parallel Debates on Exposure Thresholds

The debate surrounding safe exposure thresholds for endocrine disruptors extends to oocyte development, though with several important female-specific considerations. The finite nature of the ovarian follicular reserve means that toxicant-induced follicular atresia represents an irreversible form of reproductive damage, unlike the regenerative capacity observed in spermatogenesis. This fundamental biological difference necessitates particularly stringent threshold determinations for female reproductive toxicants. The extended development timeline of human oocytes is initiated during fetal life and potentially continuing for decades before ovulation and this creates unique challenges for threshold determination. Environmental exposures during critical windows of development, including prenatal folliculogenesis and the extended meiotic arrest, may exert disproportionate effects compared to equivalent adult exposures. A study by Grive and colleagues (2016) demonstrated that fetal ovaries exhibit heightened sensitivity to environmentally relevant BPA concentrations compared to adult ovaries, with significant disruption of meiotic progression observed at doses below current regulatory thresholds. The complexities of non-monotonic dose responses observed with endocrine disruptors apply equally to oogenesis. It was demonstrated that extremely low doses of BPA (below 1 µg/kg/day) disrupted meiotic spindle formation in mouse oocytes, while higher doses occasionally showed reduced effects, a classic inverted U-shaped dose response curve challenging traditional toxicological paradigms. It was revealed that environmentally relevant BPA doses increased meiotic abnormalities in mouse oocytes, with effects observed at concentrations below established regulatory standards. Timing represents another critical variable complicating threshold determinations for female reproductive toxicants. Exposure during different developmental stages including, fetal ovarian development, follicular recruitment, or final oocyte maturation, may yield distinct outcomes, even at identical doses. It was documented that prenatal exposure to famine during the Dutch Hunger Winter affected female reproductive function differently depending on the gestational timing of exposure, with early gestation exposure particularly detrimental to ovarian development. These complexities have fueled scientific and regulatory debates similar to those observed for male reproductive toxicants. The European Union has adopted a more precautionary approach, implementing stricter regulations for endocrine disruptors based on hazard identification rather than risk assessment. In contrast, the United States maintains a risk-based regulatory framework requiring demonstration of adverse effects at environmentally relevant doses. This regulatory divergence reflects not only scientific uncertainty but also differing philosophical approaches to environmental health protection. The transgenerational implications of oocyte exposure create additional challenges for threshold determination. Unlike somatic effects that affect only the exposed individual, germline exposures may impact multiple generations, raising profound ethical and policy questions regarding acceptable risk levels. Nilsson & Skinner (2015) argue that any exposure capable of inducing heritable epigenetic alterations should be considered potentially harmful, regardless of immediate phenotypic effects, given the transgenerational consequences.

EXPOSOME AND TERATOGENESIS: ENVIRONMENTAL INFLUENCES ON DEVELOPMENTAL OUTCOMES

The relationship between environmental exposures and developmental outcomes represents one of the most consequential areas of modern biomedical research. The exposome—defined as the totality of environmental exposures from conception onward—provides a comprehensive framework for understanding how non-genetic factors influence the developing embryo and fetus (Wild, 2005). This expanded study explores the intricate relationship between the exposome and teratogenesis, examining how timing-specific environmental exposures can disrupt normal developmental processes, leading to structural malformations, functional deficits, and long-term health consequences that may extend across generations. The concept of the exposome has evolved significantly since its introduction by Wild in 2005. Initially conceptualized as a complement to the genome, the exposome now encompasses not only external chemical exposures but also internal biological responses, social factors, and psychosocial stressors that collectively shape developmental trajectories. This holistic approach has transformed teratology from a field focused primarily on single-agent causation to one that recognizes the complex, multifactorial nature of developmental disruption.

Critical Windows of Susceptibility

Importance of Timing of Exposure During Pregnancy

The concept of "critical windows" refers to specific developmental periods during which embryonic or fetal tissues are particularly vulnerable to environmental perturbations. These windows typically correspond to periods of rapid cell division, migration, and differentiation, when precise molecular signals orchestrate complex developmental cascades. The exquisite timing-specificity of teratogenic effects reflects the sequential nature of embryonic and fetal development, where each stage builds upon the successful completion of preceding developmental milestones. The timing of exposure profoundly influences both the nature and severity of teratogenic outcomes. For instance, thalidomide exposure during weeks 4-7 of gestation results in characteristic limb malformations due to disruption of angiogenesis during critical periods of limb bud formation (Vargesson, 2015). In contrast, exposure to the same compound after this critical window typically results in minimal or no limb defects, as the fundamental patterning of the limbs has already been established. Similarly, exposure to valproic acid during neural tube closure (days 20-28 post-conception) significantly increases the risk of neural tube defects, while later exposure primarily affects neurobehavioral development rather than structural formation. Recent research by Levin *et al.* (2021) has further refined our understanding of critical windows by demonstrating that even brief exposures, as short as 4-6 hours during key developmental events can produce lasting effects on organ morphogenesis. Using advanced imaging techniques in zebrafish models, they visualized real-time disruption of cellular migration patterns following precisely timed chemical exposures, providing direct evidence for the extreme timing-sensitivity of developmental processes. A compelling historical illustration of timing-specificity comes from the rubella epidemic of 1941, documented by Australian ophthalmologist Norman Gregg. Gregg observed that maternal rubella infection during the first trimester of pregnancy resulted in a characteristic triad of congenital cataracts, heart defects, and deafness in offspring, while infection during later trimesters produced progressively milder effects. This observation not only established rubella as the first recognized viral teratogen but also provided early evidence for the critical window concept that would become central to teratology. Gregg's meticulous documentation transformed understanding of congenital anomalies at a time when genetic factors were considered the predominant cause, highlighting the importance of timing-specific environmental exposures.

Stages of Embryonic and Fetal Development

Prenatal development proceeds through four broadly defined stages, each characterized by distinct vulnerabilities to environmental exposures:

Pre-implantation (fertilization to approximately day 14): During this period, the zygote undergoes rapid cell divisions (cleavage) to form a blastocyst that implants in the uterine wall. While historically considered relatively resistant to teratogenic influences due to the "all-or-nothing" phenomenon (where severe exposures typically result in embryonic death rather than malformation), recent research suggests that even subtle disruptions during this period can have lasting consequences through epigenetic mechanisms. Notably, Zhao *et al.* (2021) demonstrated that exposure to endocrine-disrupting chemicals during preimplantation can alter DNA methylation patterns in imprinted genes that persist through development and potentially into adulthood, challenging the traditional view of this period as relatively protected.

Gastrulation (approximately days 14-21): This critical phase establishes the three primary germ layers (ectoderm, mesoderm, and endoderm) and defines the main body axes. Disruptions during gastrulation can have profound and widespread developmental consequences affecting multiple organ systems. Recent work using single-cell transcriptomics has revealed previously unrecognized cellular heterogeneity during gastrulation, suggesting that specific cell lineages may exhibit unique vulnerabilities to environmental insults (Tyser *et al.,* 2021). This nuanced understanding provides new insights into why certain exposures produce characteristic patterns of developmental disruption.

Organogenesis (approximately days 21-56): This period represents the peak of vulnerability to classical structural teratogens, as each organ system undergoes its primary formation. The precise timing of development varies by organ system, creating organ-specific windows of susceptibility. Neural tube closure, occurring between days 21-28, represents a particularly sensitive process, with inadequate folate levels or exposure to anticonvulsants like valproic acid during this narrow window dramatically increasing the risk of neural tube defects (Copp *et al.*, 2013). It was indicates that even transitional cell states during organogenesis exhibit distinct transcriptional profiles and signaling dependencies that create unique vulnerabilities to specific chemical classes.

Fetal period (approximately day 56 to birth): While major structural development is largely complete, this remains a critical period for functional maturation, particularly of the central nervous system. Environmental exposures during this period may have more subtle effects on organ function rather than gross structural anomalies (Huang *et al.*, 2022). A groundbreaking longitudinal neuroimaging study by Rasmussen *et al.* (2020) revealed that prenatal exposure to air pollution during the third trimester was associated with altered connectivity in specific brain networks developing during this period, demonstrating how timing-specific exposures can produce functional changes in the absence of visible structural defects (Rasmussen *et al.*, 2020). The dramatic thalidomide disaster of the late 1950s and early 1960s provides a sobering historical lesson in the importance of understanding stage-specific vulnerability. German physician Widukind Lenz and Australian obstetrician William McBride independently identified the link between maternal thalidomide use and severe limb malformations in newborns (Vargesson, 2015). Their observations revealed that even brief exposure during a critical 3-4 day window of limb bud development could produce devastating effects, while exposure before or after this window had minimal impact on limb formation. This tragedy catalyzed fundamental reforms in drug testing requirements and heightened awareness of developmental stage-specific vulnerability to environmental exposures.

Known Teratogens and Their Mechanisms

Examples of Teratogens

Environmental teratogens span a diverse range of substances, including pharmaceuticals, recreational drugs, environmental pollutants, infectious agents, and maternal conditions. Each operates through specific mechanisms and targets particular developmental processes. Alcohol represents one of the most extensively studied teratogens, producing a spectrum of effects collectively termed Fetal Alcohol Spectrum Disorders (FASD), with the most severe form known as Fetal Alcohol Syndrome (FAS). Alcohol exerts teratogenic effects through multiple mechanisms, including oxidative stress, disruption of cellular adhesion, and apoptosis of neural crest cells (Riley *et al.*, 2011). The characteristic facial features of FAS; including short palpebral fissures, thin vermillion border, and smooth philtrum, directly reflect disruption of neural crest migration during craniofacial development. The timing of exposure significantly influences outcomes, with first-trimester exposure particularly associated with craniofacial abnormalities and brain structural defects. Recent advances in neuroimaging have enhanced our understanding of alcohol's effects on brain development. Using advanced diffusion tensor imaging, LeBel *et al.* (2021) identified disruptions in white matter microstructure in children with prenatal alcohol exposure, including altered myelination patterns and changes in axonal organization that correlate with specific neurobehavioral deficits (LeBel *et al.,* 2021). These findings provide a neuroanatomical basis for the cognitive and behavioral effects observed in FASD and highlight the vulnerability of developing neural connectivity to alcohol exposure.

The story of thalidomide represents perhaps the most infamous chapter in teratology history. Marketed as a sedative and anti-morning sickness medication in the late 1950s, thalidomide caused approximately 10,000 cases of severe limb malformations worldwide before being withdrawn in 1961 (Vargesson, 2015). The molecular mechanism remained elusive for decades until the identification of cereblon (CRBN) as a primary thalidomide-binding protein. Thalidomide binds to cereblon, inhibiting its normal function in the protein complex that regulates limb outgrowth and angiogenesis (Ito *et al.,* 2010). This mechanism explains both the timing-specificity and the characteristic pattern of limb reduction defects observed, typically affecting proximal limbs while sparing hands and feet. Recent work by Donovan *et al.* (2018) using CRISPR-engineered zebrafish models has further elucidated thalidomide's mechanism, demonstrating that cereblon modification specifically affects migration and differentiation of neural crest-derived vascular progenitors critical for limb development (Donovan, *et al.,* 2018). This precise cellular targeting explains the characteristic nature of thalidomide embryopathy and illustrates how molecular interactions can produce highly specific developmental disruptions.

Retinoids (vitamin A derivatives) represent critical signaling molecules in embryonic development but become potent teratogens when present at inappropriate levels or times. Therapeutic retinoids like isotretinoin (13-cis-retinoic acid) used in acne treatment cause a characteristic pattern of craniofacial, cardiac, thymic, and central nervous system malformations through disruption of HOX gene expression patterns (Ross *et al.,* 2000). The discovery of retinoic acid as both an essential morphogen and potential teratogen highlighted the delicate balance required in developmental signaling pathways, where both deficiency and excess can disrupt normal patterning. Genomic approaches have recently revealed the extensive regulatory networks controlled by retinoic acid during development. Cunningham *et al.* (2018) performed ChIP-seq analysis to map the genomic binding sites of retinoic acid receptors during neural development, identifying over 15,000 binding sites that regulate genes involved in neurogenesis, axon guidance, and synaptic function. This extensive regulatory network explains the diverse developmental effects of retinoid exposure and highlights the far-reaching consequences of disrupting a single signaling pathway during critical developmental periods.

Environmental pollutants increasingly contribute to teratogenic concerns as industrialization expands globally. Methylmercury, a persistent environmental contaminant, crosses the placenta and blood-brain barrier to cause neurodevelopmental toxicity characterized by cerebral palsy, microcephaly, and intellectual disability (Huang *et al.*, 2022). The tragic Minamata Bay poisoning in Japan (1950s) demonstrated the devastating consequences of maternal methylmercury exposure, with affected children exhibiting severe neurological impairments despite minimal or absent maternal symptoms. Polycyclic aromatic hydrocarbons (PAHs) from fossil fuel combustion represent another class of environmental teratogens that form DNA adducts, potentially leading to mutations in genes critical for development (Perera *et al.*, 2014). The growing recognition of per- and polyfluoroalkyl substances (PFAS) as developmental toxicants represents an emerging concern. Liew *et al.* (2018) found that prenatal exposure to PFAS was associated with increased risk of congenital anomalies, particularly heart defects, in a large Danish birth cohort ((Liew *et al.*, 2018). Mechanistic studies by Blake & Fenton (2020) suggest that PFAS disrupt endocrine signaling and increase oxidative stress during cardiac development, providing a biological basis for the epidemiological associations. With PFAS contamination increasingly recognized in water supplies globally, understanding their developmental toxicity has become a pressing public health concern.

Mechanisms of Teratogenesis

Teratogens disrupt development through diverse molecular and cellular mechanisms that converge on key developmental processes. Understanding these mechanisms provides insights for prevention strategies and identifies potential therapeutic targets:

Disruption of cell signaling pathways represents a common mechanism through which teratogens interfere with the precisely choreographed molecular communications that guide development. Retinoids exemplify this mechanism, as they act as ligands for nuclear receptors that directly regulate gene transcription. Excess retinoic acid alters the spatial and temporal expression patterns of HOX genes and other developmental regulators, disrupting the patterning information essential for normal morphogenesis (Ross *et al.*, 2000). Similarly, endocrine-disrupting chemicals like bisphenol A (BPA) can mimic or antagonize endogenous hormones, interfering with critical signaling pathways during development. A key debate in this area concerns the concept of "low-dose effects" and non-monotonic dose-response relationships for endocrine-disrupting chemicals. Traditional toxicology assumes that higher doses produce greater effects, but endocrine disruptors often show more complex patterns, with some effects paradoxically occurring at lower doses that better mimic physiological hormone levels (Vandenberg *et al.*, 2012). This challenges conventional risk assessment paradigms and remains a contentious area in regulatory toxicology. Advances in systems biology approaches have transformed our understanding of signaling disruption by environmental chemicals. Using a combination of transcriptomics, phosphoproteomics, and computational modeling, which mapped the effects of multiple endocrine disruptors on signaling networks during neurogenesis, revealing convergent effects on specific pathways despite diverse chemical structures. These approaches identify critical signaling nodes that may serve as intervention targets for preventing developmental disruption.

Oxidative stress represents another major teratogenic mechanism, where excess reactive oxygen species (ROS) overwhelm antioxidant defenses, causing lipid peroxidation, protein oxidation, and DNA damage. Alcohol metabolism generates acetaldehyde and ROS that particularly affect neural crest cells and developing brain tissue (Henderson *et al.,* 1999). Similarly, air pollutants like particulate matter and ozone induce oxidative stress in placental tissue, potentially contributing to adverse pregnancy outcomes including preterm birth and intrauterine growth restriction (Vrijheid *et al.,* 2016). Recent methodological innovations in measuring oxidative stress biomarkers in maternal and cord blood have advanced understanding of this mechanism. Techniques like mass spectrometry-based metabolomics now allow comprehensive assessment of oxidative stress markers (F2-isoprostanes, 8-OHdG, protein carbonyls) in small sample volumes, enabling non-invasive monitoring during pregnancy (Yan *et al.,* 2019). These approaches have revealed that maternal antioxidant capacity may significantly modify teratogenic risk, potentially explaining some of the variability in individual susceptibility to oxidative stressors. A landmark study by Torres-Cuevas *et al.* (2021) used redox proteomics to identify specific proteins susceptible to oxidative modification in fetal tissues following maternal exposure to air pollution (Torres-Cuevas *et al.,* 2021). They found that key proteins involved in energy metabolism, cytoskeletal organization, and protein folding were preferentially oxidized, providing a mechanistic link between maternal exposure, oxidative stress, and specific developmental disruptions. DNA damage constitutes a direct mechanism for teratogenesis, where chemical modifications to DNA structure can lead to mutations, altered gene expression, or cell death in developing tissues. PAHs from air pollution and tobacco smoke form bulky adducts on DNA, potentially disrupting the reading of genetic information during critical developmental periods (Perera *et al.,* 2014). Similarly, ionizing radiation directly induces DNA strand breaks that may overwhelm repair mechanisms in rapidly dividing embryonic cells. A significant challenge in understanding DNA damage-mediated teratogenesis lies in distinguishing between direct teratogenic effects and potential transgenerational consequences through germline mutations. Advanced sequencing technologies now enable detection of de novo mutations in offspring and correlation with parental exposures, though establishing causality remains difficult in human studies (Wong *et al.,* 2016). Animal models using reporter systems for DNA damage have provided valuable insights into tissue-specific vulnerability and critical windows, but translation to human risk assessment continues to be challenging. Recent work by Marcon *et al.* (2018) using whole-genome sequencing of parent-offspring trios has demonstrated increased rates of de novo mutations in offspring of fathers with occupational exposure to genotoxic agents, providing direct evidence that environmental exposures can affect the germline and potentially influence developmental outcomes across generations. These findings emphasize the importance of considering both maternal and paternal exposures in assessing teratogenic risk.

EPIGENETIC EFFECTS AND DEVELOPMENTAL PROGRAMMING

Epigenetic Alterations in the Developing Fetus

Epigenetic mechanisms involved heritable changes in gene expression that occur without alterations to the underlying DNA sequence, which have emerged as a critical interface between environmental exposures and developmental outcomes. These mechanisms include DNA methylation (addition of methyl groups to cytosine bases, typically silencing gene expression), histone modifications (chemical alterations to histone proteins that package DNA, affecting chromatin accessibility), and non-coding RNAs (regulatory RNA molecules that influence gene expression post-transcriptionally) (Gluckman *et al.,* 2009). Environmental exposures during early development can induce persistent epigenetic alterations with long-term phenotypic consequences. For example, maternal smoking alters DNA methylation patterns in multiple genes involved in growth and development. The AHRR gene, which regulates response to polycyclic aromatic hydrocarbons in cigarette smoke, shows consistent hypomethylation in newborns exposed to maternal smoking (Joubert *et al.,* 2016). These methylation changes persist into childhood and adolescence, potentially contributing to long-term health effects of prenatal smoke exposure. Recent technological advances have enabled more comprehensive assessment of exposure-induced epigenetic changes. Richmond *et al.* (2018) used the Illumina EPIC array to profile over 850,000 CpG sites in cord blood from infants exposed to various prenatal environmental factors, identifying distinct epigenetic signatures associated with maternal smoking, air pollution exposure, and nutritional status. These signatures showed enrichment in specific genomic regions and biological pathways, suggesting coordinated epigenetic responses to environmental insults. One of the most compelling examples of environmentally-induced epigenetic alterations comes from the Dutch Hunger Winter study. Individuals who were prenatally exposed to famine during the Dutch Hunger Winter of 1944-45 showed, six decades later, decreased DNA methylation at the insulin-like growth factor 2 (IGF2) gene compared to their unexposed siblings (Heijmans *et al.,* 2008). Crucially, this effect was specific to periconceptional exposure, highlighting early development as a particularly vulnerable period for establishing epigenetic marks. As Heijmans *et al.* (2008) reported, "periconceptional exposure to famine was associated with a 5.2% lower methylation" of the IGF2 gene, corresponding to 0.48 standard deviations of the controls, with no effect observed for individuals exposed only during late gestation. Beyond DNA methylation, histone modifications represent another important epigenetic mechanism linking environmental exposures to developmental outcomes (Heijmans *et al.,* 2008). Jia *et al.* (2019) demonstrated that prenatal exposure to air pollution induces specific histone modifications (H3K4me3 and H3K27ac) in regions regulating immune and stress response genes in cord blood. Using ChIP-seq, they identified enhancer regions particularly susceptible to pollution-induced epigenetic changes, providing a mechanistic link between air pollution exposure and altered immune development (Jia *et al.,* 2019). Transgenerational epigenetic effects, where environmental exposures in one generation influence phenotypes across multiple subsequent generations, have been demonstrated in rodent models. Exposure of pregnant rats to endocrine disruptors like vinclozolin during gonadal sex determination induces DNA methylation changes in the male germline that persist for at least four generations in the absence of further exposure (Nilsson *et al.,* 2018). These epigenetic alterations associate with increased incidence of reproductive disorders, suggesting that environmentally-induced epigenetic changes can become programmed into the germline with multi-generational consequences. A key debate in epigenetic teratogenesis concerns distinguishing truly transgenerational effects from multi-generational exposure. For maternal exposures during pregnancy, the F0 (mother), F1 (fetus), and F2 (fetal germ cells) generations are all directly exposed. Only effects appearing in the F3 generation and beyond can be considered truly transgenerational rather than direct exposure effects (Nilsson *et al.,* 2018). This distinction has important implications for understanding mechanisms and designing intervention strategies. Study by Bohacek and Mansuy (2015) has begun to elucidate the molecular mechanisms underlying transgenerational epigenetic inheritance, identifying specific RNA species in sperm that may transmit environmentally-induced epigenetic information across generations (Bohacek & Mansuy, 2015). Their findings suggest that small non-coding RNAs, including tRNA fragments and microRNAs, may carry epigenetic information from the paternal environment to the developing embryo, providing a potential mechanism for paternal environmental exposures to influence offspring development.

Long-Term Consequences for Health and Disease

The Developmental Origins of Health and Disease (DOHaD) paradigm posits that environmental exposures during critical developmental periods can program long-term disease susceptibility through persistent alterations in physiology and metabolism. Epigenetic mechanisms are increasingly recognized as mediators of this developmental programming, linking early exposures to later health outcomes (Hanson & Gluckman, 2014). Prenatal exposures have been associated with numerous long-term health consequences, including cardiovascular disease, metabolic disorders, and neurodevelopmental conditions. The Dutch Hunger Winter again provides compelling evidence, as individuals exposed to famine during early gestation show increased rates of obesity, altered glucose metabolism, and cardiovascular disease in adulthood. Epigenetic studies have revealed that these individuals exhibit altered methylation patterns in genes related to growth and metabolism, including IGF2, potentially explaining the mechanistic link between early nutritional deprivation and later metabolic dysfunction. Advanced statistical methods have strengthened causal inference in DOHaD research. Using Mendelian randomization approaches, Richmond *et al.* (2021) demonstrated causal relationships between maternal nutritional status during pregnancy and offspring cardiometabolic outcomes, independent of shared genetic factors. Similarly, twin studies comparing monozygotic versus dizygotic twins discordant for prenatal exposures have helped disentangle genetic and environmental contributions to developmental programming effects (Castillo-Fernandez *et al.*, 2020). The placenta plays a crucial role in modulating fetal exposure to environmental factors and potentially programming developmental trajectories. As the interface between maternal and fetal circulations, the placenta expresses numerous transporters and metabolic enzymes that regulate the transfer of nutrients, waste products, and potentially harmful substances. Placental function itself can be modified by environmental exposures, with consequences for fetal development (Mao, *et al.*, 2020). For example, maternal smoking alters placental vascularization and expression of xenobiotic-metabolizing enzymes, potentially affecting both nutrient transfer and detoxification capacity. An emerging area of debate concerns the relative importance of genetic and epigenetic factors in mediating exposure effects via the placenta. Genetic polymorphisms in placental transporters and metabolizing enzymes influence the fetal exposure to various substances, while epigenetic regulation of these same genes may provide a mechanism for adapting placental function to the maternal environment (Mao, *et al.*, 2020). Advanced techniques like placental transcriptomics and epigenomics are now revealing how genetic and epigenetic factors interact to determine placental response to environmental exposures, though translation of these findings to clinical applications remains challenging. A landmark study by Burton *et al.* (2022) used single-cell RNA sequencing to characterize cell-type specific responses to maternal air pollution exposure in the human placenta, revealing that specific trophoblast subpopulations exhibit enhanced sensitivity to oxidative stress and inflammatory signals. These findings suggest that placental adaptation to environmental stressors involves complex cellular responses that may differentially affect placental functions, with potential consequences for fetal development and long-term health (Burton *et al.,* 2022)

Studies and Examples

Cohort Studies Linkin g Prenatal Exposures to Adverse Outcomes

Longitudinal birth cohort studies have provided crucial evidence linking prenatal environmental exposures to developmental outcomes, with some following participants from before birth into adulthood. These studies offer unique insights into exposure timing, dose-response relationships, and long-term consequences that cannot be obtained from animal models or cross-sectional human studies. The previously mentioned Dutch Hunger Winter studies represent a natural experiment that provided unprecedented insights into the effects of defined nutritional deprivation during specific gestational periods. Researchers identified individuals born in western Holland around the time of the 1944-45 famine and compared their health outcomes and biological markers with unexposed siblings. These studies revealed that prenatal famine exposure was associated with increased risk of obesity, diabetes, and cardiovascular disease in adulthood, with effects particularly pronounced for early gestational exposure. Epigenetic analyses subsequently demonstrated altered DNA methylation patterns, with periconceptional famine exposure associated with decreased IGF2 methylation six decades later, while exposure late in gestation showed no effect on methylation (Heijmans *et al.,* 2008). The Danish National Birth Cohort and Norwegian Mother, Father and Child Cohort Study (MoBa) represent two of the largest pregnancy cohorts globally, each following over 100,000 pregnancies with extensive biobanking and follow-up. These cohorts have demonstrated associations between maternal acetaminophen use during pregnancy and increased risk of ADHD and autism spectrum disorders in offspring, potentially through disruption of endocannabinoid signaling during brain development (Ystrom *et al.,* 2017). Similarly, these cohorts have linked prenatal exposure to perfluoroalkyl substances (PFAS) with reduced birthweight and altered immune development, informing regulatory decisions regarding these persistent environmental contaminants. Advanced statistical methods have strengthened causal inference in these observational studies. Liew *et al.* (2018) employed sibling comparison designs to control for familial confounding factors when assessing the relationship between prenatal PFAS exposure and neurodevelopmental outcomes. However, negative control exposure analyses, where associations with biologically implausible exposures are tested—have helped validate findings from large cohort studies (Ystrom *et al.,* 2017). These methodological innovations address key limitations of observational research and strengthen confidence in reported exposure-outcome relationships. The Maternal-Infant Research on Environmental Chemicals (MIREC) study in Canada has provided detailed exposure assessment for numerous environmental chemicals during pregnancy, demonstrating associations between prenatal phthalate exposure and altered anogenital distance in male infants (a marker of anti-androgenic effects) and between maternal blood mercury levels and neurodevelopmental outcomes (Arbuckle *et al.,* 2016). The study's extensive biorepository includes maternal blood, urine, hair, breast milk, and cord blood samples, allowing researchers to correlate multiple exposure biomarkers with developmental outcomes and explore potential mechanisms. Recent work leveraging artificial intelligence and machine learning has enhanced exposure assessment in cohort studies. A study by Bellinger *et al.* (2020) applied deep learning algorithms to residential history data and geospatial environmental monitoring data to create personalized exposure profiles for pregnant women in the MIREC cohort (Bellinger, 2020). This approach identified complex exposure patterns and mixture effects that would be missed by traditional single-pollutant analyses, advancing understanding of how real-world exposure complexity influences developmental outcomes. An illuminating case from the CHAMACOS (Center for the Health Assessment of Mothers and Children of Salinas) cohort illustrates how prenatal pesticide exposure can have lasting neurodevelopmental consequences. This longitudinal study follows children born to agricultural workers in California's Salinas Valley, an area with intensive pesticide use. Researchers found that higher maternal urinary metabolites of organophosphate pesticides during pregnancy were associated with poorer cognitive development, attention problems, and abnormal reflexes in offspring. Notably, the strength of these associations depended on maternal PON1 genotype, which determines capacity to detoxify organophosphates, highlighting gene-environment interactions in susceptibility to teratogenic exposures. Extended follow-up of the CHAMACOS cohort into adolescence has revealed persistent neurodevelopmental effects of prenatal pesticide exposure. Sagiv *et al.* (2019) reported that prenatal organophosphate exposure was associated with poorer intellectual functioning and executive function in adolescents at age 16, demonstrating the lasting impact of prenatal exposures across developmental stages. These findings underscore the importance of long-term follow-up in birth cohorts to capture developmental effects that may manifest or evolve throughout childhood and adolescence (Sagiv *et al.,* 2019).

Animal Studies Elucidating Mechanisms of Teratogenesis

While human cohort studies establish associations between exposures and outcomes, animal models provide essential insights into mechanisms of teratogenesis that cannot be ethically or feasibly studied in humans. These models allow for controlled exposure timing and dose, assessment of tissue-specific effects, and evaluation of interventions. Rodent models have been particularly valuable for understanding the mechanisms of alcohol teratogenicity. Studies in mice have demonstrated that ethanol exposure during gastrulation (corresponding to weeks 3-4 in human development) causes apoptosis in specific cell populations including cranial neural crest, leading to the characteristic facial features of FAS (Sulik, 2005). These studies identified cellular mechanisms including oxidative stress, disruption of L1 cell adhesion molecule function, and impaired sonic hedgehog signaling. Timed inhibition of these pathways has provided proof-of-principle for potential interventional approaches, though translation to human prevention strategies remains challenging (Sulik, 2005). A significant advance in understanding alcohol teratogenesis comes from recent work by Smith *et al.* (2021), who used single-cell RNA sequencing to characterize cellular responses to alcohol exposure during neural crest development. They identified a specific subpopulation of neural crest progenitors that exhibits enhanced vulnerability to alcohol-induced apoptosis due to reduced expression of anti-apoptotic factors. This cellular heterogeneity in alcohol susceptibility explains the characteristic pattern of craniofacial malformations in FAS and suggests targeted protective strategies focusing on these vulnerable cell populations. Zebrafish models have revolutionized high-throughput screening for potential teratogens, as their external fertilization, rapid development, and transparency allow for direct observation of developmental processes. A compelling example comes from methylmercury research, where zebrafish exposed to environmentally relevant concentrations display disrupted migration and axon extension of specific neuronal populations (Korbas & Tracy, 2012). Advanced imaging techniques have revealed that methylmercury disrupts microtubule dynamics in developing neurons, providing a cellular mechanism for the neurodevelopmental defects observed in exposed human populations. The integration of CRISPR-Cas9 genome editing with zebrafish models has further enhanced mechanistic understanding of teratogenesis. Truong *et al.* (2020) developed a library of zebrafish lines with fluorescently labeled cell populations to screen for cell type-specific effects of environmental chemicals. This approach revealed that bisphenols preferentially affect cardiac neural crest cells through estrogen receptor-mediated mechanisms, explaining the cardiovascular effects observed in epidemiological studies and providing a basis for structure-activity relationships in this chemical class. A fascinating series of transgenerational studies in rodents has demonstrated how endocrine-disrupting chemicals can induce epigenetic changes that persist across multiple generations. Exposure of pregnant rats to vinclozolin (an antiandrogenic fungicide) during gonadal sex determination induced DNA methylation changes in the male germline that persisted for at least four generations, associated with increased incidence of reproductive disorders including testicular abnormalities and reduced sperm quality. These studies provide a mechanistic framework for understanding potential transgenerational effects of environmental exposures in humans. Extended work by Skinner and colleagues has now identified specific genomic regions particularly susceptible to environmentally-induced transgenerational epigenetic changes, termed "epigenetic susceptibility regions" (Nilsson *et al.*, 2018). These regions are enriched for regulatory elements controlling developmental gene expression and show characteristic chromatin features that may explain their enhanced sensitivity to environmental disruption. This concept provides a mechanistic framework for understanding how diverse environmental exposures may affect common developmental pathways through convergent epigenetic mechanisms. A key methodological debate in animal teratogenicity research concerns the relevance of exposure doses and routes to human experience. Traditional toxicology studies often use high doses to identify hazards, while environmental exposures typically occur at much lower concentrations over extended periods. Advanced approaches like physiologically-based pharmacokinetic (PBPK) modeling now allow for more realistic extrapolation between species and exposure scenarios, though significant uncertainties remain in translating animal findings to human risk assessment (Sarigiannis & Karakitsios, 2018). Recent innovations in "humanized" animal models aim to address cross-species differences in teratogenic susceptibility. However, these researchers developed mice with humanized liver xenobiotic metabolism, enabling more accurate prediction of human-specific metabolic activation or detoxification of potential teratogens. Similarly, xenotransplantation of human placental tissue into immunocompromised mice allows assessment of human-specific placental responses to environmental exposures, bridging the gap between rodent models and human biology.

EMERGING INSIGHTS

Gene-Environment Interactions

Individual genetic variation significantly modifies susceptibility to teratogenic exposures, explaining why identical exposures may produce dramatically different outcomes in different individuals. These gene-environment interactions operate through various mechanisms, including altered toxicokinetics, differential response to cellular stress, and variable capacity for developmental compensation (Krauss &

Hong, 2016). Folate-sensitive neural tube defects (NTDs) represent a classic example of gene-environment interaction in teratogenesis. While folate deficiency increases NTD risk across populations, certain genetic variants significantly amplify this risk. Polymorphisms in the methylenetetrahydrofolate reductase (MTHFR) gene, particularly the C677T variant, reduce enzyme efficiency in converting folate to its active form, thereby increasing NTD risk under conditions of marginal folate status. This interaction explains why some women with seemingly adequate dietary folate still have elevated risk and benefit from supplementation, while others may require higher doses to achieve protection. An illustrative case from the CHAMACOS cohort demonstrated how genetic variation in paraoxonase 1 (PON1), an enzyme that detoxifies organophosphate pesticides, modifies the relationship between prenatal pesticide exposure and neurodevelopment. Children whose mothers had both high pesticide exposure and the PON1 192QQ genotype (associated with reduced detoxification capacity) showed a 7-point IQ deficit compared to children with neither risk factor. This gene-environment interaction identifies a particularly vulnerable subpopulation and suggests potential targeted intervention strategies. Advanced genome-wide approaches are now uncovering novel gene-environment interactions, moving beyond candidate gene studies to more comprehensive assessment. Genome-wide association studies (GWAS) combined with detailed exposure assessment have identified variation in xenobiotic metabolism genes that modify susceptibility to tobacco smoke, alcohol, and environmental pollutants. Epigenome-wide association studies (EWAS) are revealing how genetic variation influences epigenetic responses to environmental exposures, potentially explaining some of the variability in long-term programming effects.

Placental Modulation of Fetal Exposure

The placenta functions not merely as a passive barrier but as an active regulator of fetal exposure to environmental agents, with significant implications for understanding variability in teratogenic outcomes. Placental transporters, metabolizing enzymes, and barrier properties all influence the transplacental transfer of potential teratogens and their metabolites. Placental efflux transporters, particularly ATP-binding cassette (ABC) transporters like P-glycoprotein (P-gp, ABCB1), breast cancer resistance protein (BCRP, ABCG2), and multidrug resistance-associated proteins (MRPs), actively export xenobiotics from the fetal to maternal circulation, protecting the fetus from potential toxicants. Genetic polymorphisms and environmentally-induced changes in transporter expression can significantly alter this protective function. For example, functional variants in ABCG2 affect placental transfer of certain medications and environmental chemicals, potentially modifying teratogenic risk based on maternal genotype. A fascinating case study comes from research on the antidiabetic medication glyburide, which despite its small molecular size and lipophilicity, shows minimal placental transfer. Investigations revealed that BCRP actively transports glyburide back to the maternal circulation, limiting fetal exposure. This placental protective mechanism fails in the presence of common ABCG2 polymorphisms or when co-administered with BCRP inhibitors, highlighting how placental function can be influenced by both genetic and environmental factors. Placental xenobiotic metabolism represents another layer of fetal protection that exhibits significant individual variability. The placenta expresses numerous cytochrome P450 enzymes, conjugation enzymes, and other metabolizing systems that can either detoxify or bioactivate foreign compounds. Environmental exposures can induce or inhibit these enzymes, potentially altering the placental handling of other substances in a complex, exposure-mixture dependent manner. A significant debate in this field concerns whether placental adaptations to environmental stressors ultimately serve protective or adverse programming functions. Some evidence suggests that placental responses to maternal stress, undernutrition, or toxicant exposure may initially be adaptive, preserving critical functions, but potentially at the cost of altered developmental programming with long-term consequences. Advanced "omics" approaches (transcriptomics, proteomics, metabolomics) applied to placental tissue are now providing systems-level insights into these complex adaptive responses.

Exposome Integration

The exposome concept recognizes that real-world exposures occur not as isolated agents but as complex mixtures within broader environmental contexts that include psychosocial stressors, nutritional factors, and built environment characteristics. This integrated perspective is particularly relevant for understanding teratogenic risks in vulnerable populations experiencing multiple, often co-occurring environmental challenges. Synergistic effects between co-exposures can significantly amplify teratogenic risks beyond what would be predicted from individual exposures. For example, combined exposure to air pollution and maternal psychological stress during pregnancy synergistically increases the risk of preterm birth beyond the sum of their individual effects. Animal studies suggest that this synergy may operate through convergent effects on oxidative stress pathways and inflammation, highlighting the importance of considering biological interaction mechanisms when assessing complex exposure mixtures. The exposome approach employs advanced methodologies to capture exposure complexity and its biological effects. Untargeted metabolomics on maternal and cord blood samples can identify exposure biomarkers and perturbations in endogenous metabolic pathways simultaneously, providing an integrated readout of exposure effects. Geographic information systems (GIS) combined with personal monitoring enable spatiotemporal mapping of multiple exposures and their relationship to social determinants of health. These approaches reveal how exposures cluster in disadvantaged communities, contributing to environmental justice concerns in teratogenic risk. A compelling illustration of exposome integration comes from recent studies of the placental response to multiple environmental stressors. Researchers have demonstrated that combined exposure to ambient air pollution and maternal stress alters placental gene expression patterns, particularly in pathways related to immune function and vascular development. These combined effects may explain observed synergies in adverse birth outcomes and highlight the placenta as a key mediator of complex exposure-outcome relationships. Despite methodological advances, significant challenges remain in exposome research, particularly around distinguishing causal relationships from correlations in complex datasets. Novel statistical approaches like weighted quantile sum regression, Bayesian kernel machine regression, and causal mediation analysis are being adapted to disentangle the effects of multiple, correlated exposures and identify key intervention targets among many potential candidates.

Exposome and Carcinogenesis

The relationship between environmental exposures and cancer development represents one of the most critical areas in public health research. Cancer incidence patterns are undergoing notable shifts globally, with some cancer subtypes traditionally associated with aging now appearing in younger populations, while geographical boundaries of certain malignancies are dissolving. Remarkably, these shifting patterns occur despite relatively stable mutational landscapes specific to each cancer type, highlighting the profound influence of environmental exposures are collectively termed the exposome on cancer development and progression.

Environmental Carcinogens

Established Environmental Carcinogens

The recognition of environmental agents as cancer-causing substances has evolved substantially over recent decades, with numerous well-established carcinogens now documented across various exposure categories. Tobacco smoke remains perhaps the most thoroughly characterized environmental carcinogen, containing over 60 known carcinogenic compounds including nitrosamines and polycyclic aromatic hydrocarbons (PAHs). These compounds not only directly damage DNA but also induce inflammation and oxidative stress, creating a multi-faceted attack on cellular integrity. The carcinogenic potential of tobacco extends beyond direct users to those exposed to secondhand smoke, illustrating how environmental carcinogens can affect broader populations than those directly engaged with the substance. Asbestos represents a compelling historical case study in our evolving understanding of environmental carcinogens. Despite early observations of respiratory disease among asbestos workers, the full carcinogenic potential of asbestos remained unrecognized until the mid-20th century. As noted in historical accounts, "For the first half of the 20th century discussion of toxicity of asbestos treated it as a fibrogenic dust disease, a type of pneumoconiosis" rather than acknowledging its carcinogenic properties. The link between asbestos exposure and mesothelioma was not firmly established until the 1960s, partially due to the extremely long latency period, often 30 years between exposure and disease manifestation. This delayed recognition allowed for widespread use of asbestos in construction, shipbuilding, and numerous consumer products, creating an enduring public health legacy that continues today. Radiation exposure constitutes another major category of environmental carcinogens, encompassing both ionizing radiation (e.g., radon, medical and occupational exposures) and non-ionizing ultraviolet radiation from sunlight. The carcinogenic mechanism of ionizing radiation is relatively straightforward high-energy particles directly damage DNA, creating strand breaks that, if improperly repaired, can lead to mutations in critical genes governing cell growth and division. Ultraviolet radiation, particularly UVB, induces characteristic DNA lesions called cyclobutane pyrimidine dimers that can lead to signature mutations in skin cancer. Air pollution has emerged as an increasingly recognized carcinogen, with the International Agency for Research on Cancer (IARC) classifying outdoor air pollution as a Group 1 carcinogen in 2013. Particulate matter, especially PM2.5 (particles smaller than 2.5 micrometers), can penetrate deep into lung tissue and even enter the bloodstream, carrying attached carcinogens to distant organs. Heavy metals including arsenic, cadmium, chromium, and nickel represent persistent environmental carcinogens found in occupational settings, contaminated drinking water, and certain foods. These metals can disrupt multiple cellular processes, including DNA repair, redox balance, and epigenetic regulation. Pesticides represent a complex category of potential carcinogens with varying evidence strength across different compounds. Organochlorine pesticides like DDT have been associated with hormone-dependent cancers including breast cancer, while glyphosate has been controversially linked to non-Hodgkin lymphoma, illustrating ongoing debates in carcinogen identification and risk assessment.

Key Debates in Environmental Carcinogen Research

A significant contemporary debate centers on whether non-mutagenic mechanisms of carcinogenesis receive adequate attention in regulatory frameworks. As noted in recent literature, "evidence suggests that the exposome may exert some of its influence through non-mutagenic mechanisms, although the precise ways in which environmental carcinogens trigger or promote cancer development remain poorly understood." This perspective challenges conventional approaches to carcinogen identification that have historically prioritized direct DNA-damaging properties over subtler mechanisms like epigenetic alterations, metabolic disruption, or immune modulation. The concept of "safe thresholds" for carcinogen exposure represents another contentious area, particularly for substances that may act through hormonal or epigenetic mechanisms without direct DNA damage. Unlike classical genotoxic carcinogens that theoretically could induce mutations even at single-molecule exposures, non-genotoxic carcinogens might exhibit threshold effects, below which cancer risk is not meaningfully increased. Establishing such thresholds, however, requires extensive epidemiological evidence and consideration of vulnerable populations with potentially lower thresholds due to genetic predisposition or co-exposures.

Mechanisms of Environmental Carcinogenesis

DNA Damage and Mutation

Direct DNA damage represents the classical paradigm for environmental carcinogenesis, with numerous well-characterized pathways through which environmental agents can induce mutations. As described in current literature on carcinogenesis, "Carcinogens are things that increase the chances of the above [cancer development], either by directly damaging genes (such as radiation) or by forcing cells to replicate more thus increasing the opportunities for a mistake (such as asbestos)." This dual mechanism includes direct genotoxicity versus increased proliferation with concomitant replication errors, provides a foundational framework for understanding how diverse environmental exposures contribute to cancer initiation. DNA adduct formation occurs when reactive chemicals covalently bind to DNA bases, creating structural distortions that can lead to misreading during replication. Tobacco-specific nitrosamines form characteristic adducts with guanine bases, often leading to G→T transversions frequently observed in smoking-associated lung cancers. Similarly, PAHs from combustion sources (vehicle exhaust, grilled foods, tobacco smoke) form bulky adducts that distort the DNA double helix, potentially inducing mutations if not correctly repaired before replication. Oxidative stress represents another critical mechanism through which numerous environmental exposures induce DNA damage. Redox-active compounds including certain metals, quinones, and environmental pollutants can generate reactive oxygen species (ROS) that attack DNA bases, creating oxidative lesions like 8-oxoguanine. As noted in the literature, "many of the things that are known to cause cancer do so by causing oxidative stress on cells." These oxidative DNA modifications, if not promptly repaired by base excision repair pathways, can lead to point mutations during subsequent replication. Inflammation-mediated DNA damage creates an indirect but potent pathway through which environmental exposures promote mutagenesis. Chronic irritation from substances like asbestos fibers triggers prolonged inflammatory responses, with activated macrophages and neutrophils releasing ROS and reactive nitrogen species as part of their defensive functions. This sustained inflammatory microenvironment creates ongoing DNA damage while simultaneously promoting cell proliferation, a combination that dramatically increases mutation accumulation in affected tissues.

Epigenetic Alterations

Environmental carcinogens can induce stable changes in gene expression without altering DNA sequence through various epigenetic mechanisms. DNA methylation patterns are frequently disrupted by environmental exposures, with both global hypomethylation (potentially activating oncogenes and retrotransposons) and promoter-specific hypermethylation (silencing tumor suppressor genes) observed in response to various carcinogens. Tobacco smoke, for instance, induces characteristic methylation signatures in lung tissue that can persist even years after smoking cessation, suggesting long-term epigenetic memory of environmental exposures. Histone modifications represent another epigenetic mechanism influenced by environmental carcinogens. Post-translational modifications to histone proteins including acetylation, methylation, phosphorylation, and ubiquitination, collectively regulate chromatin accessibility and transcriptional activity. Numerous environmental compounds, including arsenic, nickel, and certain air pollutants, can alter histone modification patterns, potentially dysregulating hundreds of genes simultaneously and disrupting coordinated cellular functions like DNA repair, cell cycle regulation, and apoptosis. Non-coding RNAs, particularly microRNAs, have emerged as important epigenetic regulators susceptible to environmental perturbation. These small RNA molecules post-transcriptionally regulate gene expression by targeting specific mRNAs for degradation or translational repression. Environmental exposures can alter microRNA expression profiles, potentially dysregulating entire networks of genes involved in critical cancer-related pathways. For example, arsenic exposure modifies expression of microRNAs regulating p53 signaling, potentially compromising this crucial tumor suppressor pathway. A key debate in epigenetic carcinogenesis concerns the relative importance of heritable versus environmentally induced epigenetic alterations in cancer development. As noted by researchers in the field, complementary approaches are now "integrating multiple omics technologies with sophisticated statistical and bioinformatics approaches" to address these questions. The concept of the "epigenetic progenitor model" suggests that epigenetic alterations may precede and actually facilitate subsequent genetic mutations, representing a paradigm shift in how we conceptualize the sequence of molecular events leading to cancer development.

Disruption of Cell Signaling Pathways

Environmental carcinogens can dysregulate critical signaling pathways that control cell proliferation, survival, and differentiation, even without directly causing mutations. Receptor-mediated mechanisms represent a common pathway through which environmental compounds influence cellular behavior. Endocrine-disrupting chemicals can bind to hormone receptors, activating or antagonizing signaling cascades that regulate gene expression. Xenoestrogens are compounds that mimic estrogen and may contribute to hormone-dependent cancer development by inappropriately activating estrogen receptors in tissues like breast and endometrium. Aberrant activation of oncogenic pathways can occur through various environmentally induced mechanisms. The Ras-RAF-MEK-ERK and PI3K-Akt pathways, which promote cell proliferation and survival, can be inappropriately activated by environmental exposures through receptor activation, oxidative stress, or inflammation. Sustained activation of these pathways can drive cellular proliferation while simultaneously suppressing apoptotic mechanisms that would normally eliminate damaged cells. Inactivation of tumor suppressor pathways represents another critical mechanism through which environmental exposures promote carcinogenesis. The p53 pathway, often called the "guardian of the genome," coordinates cellular responses to DNA damage, including cell cycle arrest, DNA repair, and apoptosis when damage is severe. Numerous environmental carcinogens, including certain metals and organic compounds, can compromise p53 function through mechanisms including oxidative modifications, altered post-translational regulation, and disrupted protein-protein interactions. A significant contemporary debate concerns the relative importance of mutation-centric versus systems-based views of carcinogenesis. While the somatic mutation theory has dominated cancer research for decades, emerging evidence suggests that tissue organization and cellular context critically influence whether specific mutations actually lead to cancer development. Environmental exposures may disrupt tissue architecture and cell-cell communication, creating permissive environments for cancer development even without directly inducing mutations. This "tissue organization field theory" suggests new avenues for understanding how environmental factors contribute to carcinogenesis through non-mutagenic mechanisms.

Gene-Environment Interactions

Genetic Factors Modifying Environmental Exposures

Individual genetic variation significantly influences susceptibility to environmental carcinogens, helping explain why identical exposures produce dramatically different outcomes across populations. Polymorphisms in xenobiotic-metabolizing enzymes represent a well-characterized category of genetic modifiers. Cytochrome P450 enzymes metabolize numerous environmental compounds, often converting them from relatively inert precursors to reactive metabolites capable of damaging DNA. For example, CYP1A1 variants that increase enzyme activity may enhance the activation of PAHs from tobacco smoke to DNA-reactive epoxides, potentially increasing lung cancer risk among smokers with these variants. Conversely, detoxification pathways like glutathione S-transferases (GSTs) neutralize reactive compounds before they can damage cellular macromolecules. Individuals with GSTM1 or GSTT1 null genotypes—present in approximately 50% and 20% of Caucasian populations, respectively—lack functional versions of these important detoxification enzymes, potentially increasing their susceptibility to various environmental carcinogens. The balance between activation and detoxification pathways, both highly influenced by genetic polymorphisms, helps determine an individual's response to environmental exposures. DNA repair capacity demonstrates significant inter-individual variation that modifies environmental cancer risk. Nucleotide excision repair (NER) pathways remove bulky DNA adducts formed by numerous environmental carcinogens, including UV-induced photoproducts and PAH-DNA adducts. Polymorphisms in NER genes like XPD, ERCC1, and XPC are associated with altered repair efficiency and modified cancer risk, particularly in the context of specific environmental exposures. Similarly, genetic variants affecting base excision repair may influence susceptibility to oxidative DNA damage from various environmental sources. Immune response genes significantly modify how individuals respond to potentially carcinogenic infections and inflammation-inducing exposures. Human leukocyte antigen (HLA) variants influence the efficiency of presenting foreign antigens to immune cells, potentially affecting clearance of oncogenic viruses and recognition of tumor-associated antigens. Polymorphisms in cytokine genes affect inflammatory responses to environmental irritants like asbestos or silica, potentially modifying cancer risk by altering the intensity and duration of inflammation-associated DNA damage. An illustrative case of gene-environment interaction involves arsenic metabolism and cancer risk. Arsenic, a known human carcinogen found in drinking water in many regions worldwide, undergoes a series of methylation steps during metabolism. Genetic variants in arsenic methyltransferase (AS3MT) significantly influence how efficiently individuals convert inorganic arsenic to its methylated metabolites, with some variants associated with increased retention of more toxic species. Studies in Bangladesh and Taiwan have demonstrated that these genetic variants significantly modify the relationship between arsenic exposure and cancer risk, highlighting how genetic factors can amplify or mitigate environmental effects.

Contemporary Debates in Gene-Environment Research

A significant methodological debate concerns the appropriate study designs for detecting gene-environment interactions. Traditional candidate gene approaches have identified numerous potential interactions, but many have failed to replicate in independent studies. Genome-wide interaction studies potentially offer more comprehensive assessment but require extremely large sample sizes to achieve adequate statistical power. Intermediate approaches like pathway-based analyses or polygenic risk scores may provide more robust frameworks for understanding how genetic background modifies environmental cancer risk. The relative contribution of genetic versus environmental factors in cancer development remains contentious. While early twin studies suggested substantial heritability for many cancer types, more recent analyses incorporating detailed environmental exposure assessment have often attributed greater importance to non-genetic factors. The "missing heritability" in cancer—the difference between estimated heritability from family studies and variance explained by identified genetic variants—may partially reflect complex gene-environment interactions that remain poorly characterized in most population studies.

The integration of exposomic and genomic data represents a frontier in cancer research with significant methodological challenges. Traditional statistical approaches may lack power to detect complex, non-linear interactions between multiple genetic variants and diverse environmental exposures. Advanced computational methods including machine learning algorithms, network-based analyses, and systems biology approaches offer promising frameworks for modeling these complex relationships, though their application to large population datasets remains computationally intensive and requires interdisciplinary expertise.

STUDIES AND EXAMPLES OF EPIDEMIOLOGICAL STUDIES LINKING ENVIRONMENTAL EXPOSURES TO CANCER

Large-scale epidemiological studies have provided critical evidence linking environmental exposures to specific cancer types, often serving as the foundation for regulatory decisions and public health interventions. The landmark British Doctors Study, initiated by Richard Doll and Austin Bradford Hill in 1951, provided definitive evidence linking tobacco smoking to lung cancer, documenting dose-dependent relationships between smoking intensity and cancer risk. This study demonstrated how carefully designed prospective cohort studies can identify environmental causes of cancer even without detailed understanding of underlying mechanisms. Occupational cohort studies have proved particularly valuable for identifying environmental carcinogens, as workplace exposures often occur at higher intensities than in general environmental settings. Studies of asbestos workers revealed dramatically increased risks of mesothelioma and lung cancer, with important temporal insights into disease latency. As noted in the historical literature, "Mesothelioma has a latency period of around 30 years which means you need to track exposed people for 30 years... or do retrospective reconstructions on large cohorts of mesothelioma patients." This latency created significant challenges for recognizing asbestos carcinogenicity, allowing continued exposure for decades after initial suspicions were raised. The Navy veteran experience with asbestos exposure provides a compelling case study of occupational exposure consequences. "Asbestos was used in every Navy ship from 1930 to 1980 to insulate steam pipes, fuel lines and electrical cables." This widespread use created an unintended cohort of exposed individuals, with Navy veterans now constituting "30% of all US mesothelioma cases." This example illustrates how institutional practices can create concentrated exposure scenarios with long-term health consequences that emerge decades later. Case-control studies have identified numerous environmental risk factors for specific cancer types by comparing exposure histories between cancer patients and appropriately matched controls. These studies have linked arsenic-contaminated drinking water to bladder and lung cancers, residential radon exposure to lung cancer, and certain pesticides to non-Hodgkin lymphoma. While providing valuable insights, these retrospective designs face challenges including recall bias and confounding by other exposures include limitations that highlight the complementary value of different epidemiological approaches in environmental cancer research.

Molecular Studies of Gene-Environment Interactions

Molecular epidemiology studies integrate biomarkers of exposure, biological effect, and susceptibility to provide mechanistic insights into gene-environment interactions in cancer development. The development of increasingly sensitive and specific biomarkers has transformed our ability to characterize both exposures and their biological consequences. DNA adduct measurements in accessible tissues (blood, buccal cells) provide evidence of chemical exposures and DNA reactivity, while mutation signature analysis in tumor tissue can retrospectively identify likely causal exposures based on characteristic mutation patterns they induce. Genome-wide association studies (GWAS) have identified numerous genetic variants associated with cancer risk, many of which modify the effects of environmental exposures. For example, variants in the CHRNA5-CHRNA3-CHRNB4 nicotinic receptor cluster on chromosome 15q25 not only influence smoking behavior but also appear to modify the per-cigarette lung cancer risk. Similarly, genetic variants in alcohol metabolism genes (ADH, ALDH) significantly modify the relationship between alcohol consumption and cancer risk, particularly for upper aerodigestive tract malignancies. Experimental studies using model organisms and cells have elucidated specific mechanisms of gene-environment interactions in cancer. Genetically engineered mouse models with specific mutations or pathway alterations allow for controlled assessment of how genetic background modifies responses to environmental carcinogens. Cell culture models incorporating specific genetic variants through CRISPR-Cas9 editing similarly enable detailed mechanistic studies of how genetic factors influence cellular responses to environmental exposures under controlled conditions. An illustrative example of how molecular studies illuminate gene-environment interactions comes from research on aflatoxin exposure and liver cancer. Aflatoxins, produced by certain fungi that contaminate food supplies, form characteristic DNA adducts that can lead to mutations, particularly G→T transversions in the TP53 tumor suppressor gene. Individuals carrying specific variants in detoxification enzymes like GSTM1 and EPHX1 show significantly higher adduct levels and cancer risk when exposed to aflatoxins, demonstrating how genetic factors can modify molecular responses to environmental carcinogens with direct implications for disease risk.

Emerging Perspectives on Exposome-Cancer Relationships

The recognition that cancer development reflects a complex interplay between genetic susceptibility and accumulated environmental exposures throughout the lifespan has led to a more integrated view of cancer etiology. As noted in recent literature on breast cancer, "We experience a wide spectrum of environmental exposure in our lifetime, including the effects of xenobiotics on gametogenesis and gametes that undergo fertilization as the starting point of individual development and, moreover, in utero exposure, which can itself cause the first somatic or germline mutation necessary for breast cancer initiation." This lifelong perspective on exposure impacts reflects the growing appreciation for developmental origins of adult disease. The observation that cancer subtypes typically associated with advanced age are increasingly appearing in younger populations suggests changing environmental exposures may be altering cancer development trajectories. These shifting patterns occur "despite relatively stable mutational landscapes specific to each cancer type," highlighting how non-genetic factors may modify cancer risk through mechanisms beyond classic mutagenesis. Understanding these changing patterns requires integrating traditional cancer epidemiology with exposome research methodologies that capture complex, multidimensional exposure profiles across the lifespan. The relative resistance of certain tissues to cancer development provides intriguing insights into potential protective mechanisms. As noted in comparative biology discussions, "heart cancer is almost unheard of," raising questions about what special properties cardiomyocytes possess that could potentially be leveraged for cancer prevention or treatment strategies. Similarly, "neuron-derived cancers" remain relatively rare despite the longevity of these cell types, suggesting tissue-specific factors beyond proliferation rates influence cancer susceptibility. These observations highlight how tissue context and cellular environment may modify the carcinogenic potential of both endogenous mutations and environmental exposures.

THE EXPOSOME AND CANCER: ENVIRONMENTAL INFLUENCES ON CANCER DEVELOPMENT AND PROGRESSION

The relationship between environmental exposures and cancer development represents one of the most critical areas in public health research. Cancer incidence patterns are undergoing notable shifts globally, with some cancer subtypes traditionally associated with aging now appearing in younger populations, while geographical boundaries of certain malignancies are dissolving (Wild *et al.,* 2020). These shifting patterns occur despite relatively stable mutational landscapes specific to each cancer type, highlighting the profound influence of environmental exposures are collectively termed the exposome on cancer development and progression. The exposome concept, first proposed by Christopher Wild in 2005, encompasses the totality of environmental exposures from conception onwards, complementing the genome in understanding disease etiology. This comprehensive framework includes not only external exposures (chemical pollutants, radiation, infectious agents) but also internal processes (inflammation, oxidative stress, metabolism) and social factors (socioeconomic status, psychological stress) that collectively influence cancer risk.

Environmental Carcinogens

Established Environmental Carcinogens

The recognition of environmental agents as cancer-causing substances has evolved substantially over recent decades, with numerous well-established carcinogens now documented across various exposure categories. Tobacco smoke remains perhaps the most thoroughly characterized environmental carcinogen, containing over 60 known carcinogenic compounds including nitrosamines and polycyclic aromatic hydrocarbons (PAHs) (Hecht, 2012). These compounds not only directly damage DNA but also induce inflammation and oxidative stress, creating a multi-faceted attack on cellular integrity. The carcinogenic potential of tobacco extends beyond direct users to those exposed to secondhand smoke, illustrating how environmental carcinogens can affect broader populations than those directly engaged with the substance. Asbestos represents a compelling historical case study in our evolving understanding of environmental carcinogens. Despite early observations of respiratory disease among asbestos workers, the full carcinogenic potential of asbestos remained unrecognized until the mid-20th century. As noted in historical accounts, "For the first half of the 20th century discussion of toxicity of asbestos treated it as a fibrogenic dust disease, a type of pneumoconiosis" rather than acknowledging its carcinogenic properties (Craighead & Gibbs, 2008). The link between asbestos exposure and mesothelioma was not firmly established until the 1960s, partially due to the extremely long latency period, often 30 years between exposure and disease manifestation. This delayed recognition allowed for widespread use of asbestos in construction, shipbuilding, and numerous consumer products, creating an enduring public health legacy that continues today. The Navy veteran experience with asbestos exposure provides a compelling case study of occupational exposure consequences. "Asbestos was used in every Navy ship from 1930 to 1980 to insulate steam pipes, fuel lines and electrical cables." This widespread use created an unintended cohort of exposed individuals, with Navy veterans now constituting "30% of all US mesothelioma cases" (Lemen *et al.,* 2012). This example illustrates how institutional practices can create concentrated exposure scenarios with long-term health consequences that emerge decades later. Radiation exposure constitutes another major category of environmental carcinogens, encompassing both ionizing radiation (e.g., radon, medical and occupational exposures) and non-ionizing ultraviolet radiation from sunlight. The carcinogenic mechanism of ionizing radiation is relatively straightforward—high-energy particles directly damage DNA, creating strand breaks that, if improperly repaired, can lead to mutations in critical genes governing cell growth and division. Ultraviolet radiation, particularly UVB, induces characteristic DNA lesions called cyclobutane pyrimidine dimers that can lead to signature mutations in skin cancer (Narayanan *et al.,* 2010). Air pollution has emerged as an increasingly recognized carcinogen, with the International Agency for Research on Cancer (IARC) classifying outdoor air pollution as a Group 1 carcinogen in 2013 (Loomis *et al.,* 2013). Particulate matter, especially PM2.5 (particles smaller than 2.5 micrometers), can penetrate deep into lung tissue and even enter the bloodstream, carrying attached carcinogens to distant organs. Recent epidemiological studies have linked air pollution not only to lung cancer but also to breast, liver, and pancreatic malignancies, suggesting systemic effects beyond the respiratory system (Turner *et al.,* 2020). Heavy metals including arsenic, cadmium, chromium, and nickel represent persistent environmental carcinogens found in occupational settings, contaminated drinking water, and certain foods. These metals can disrupt multiple cellular processes, including DNA repair, redox balance, and epigenetic regulation. Arsenic exposure through contaminated drinking water represents a global public health crisis affecting millions of people, particularly in Bangladesh, India, and parts of the Americas, with established links to cancers of the skin, bladder, and lung (Smith *et al.,* 2018). Pesticides represent a complex category of potential carcinogens with varying evidence strength across different compounds. Organochlorine pesticides like DDT have been associated with hormone-dependent cancers including breast cancer, while glyphosate has been controversially linked to non-Hodgkin lymphoma, illustrating ongoing debates in carcinogen identification and risk assessment (Zhang *et al.,* 2019). The Agricultural Health Study, a prospective cohort study of pesticide applicators in the United States, has provided valuable evidence linking specific pesticides to particular cancer types, though challenges remain in disentangling the effects of multiple concurrent exposures (Lerro *et al.,* 2021). Infectious agents contribute significantly to the global cancer burden, with approximately 13% of cancers worldwide attributable to oncogenic viruses, bacteria, and parasites (Plummer *et al.,* 2015). Human papillomavirus (HPV), hepatitis B and C viruses, Helicobacter pylori, and other infectious agents promote carcinogenesis through mechanisms including direct integration into the host genome, chronic inflammation, and immune suppression. The recognition of infectious carcinogens has led to significant preventive interventions, most notably HPV vaccination programs that promise substantial reductions in cervical cancer incidence globally (Lei *et al.,* 2020).

Key Debates in Environmental Carcinogen Research

A significant contemporary debate centers on whether non-mutagenic mechanisms of carcinogenesis receive adequate attention in regulatory frameworks. As noted in recent literature, "evidence suggests that the exposome may exert some of its influence through nonmutagenic mechanisms, although the precise ways in which environmental carcinogens trigger or promote cancer development remain poorly understood" (Goodson *et al.,* 2015). This perspective challenges conventional approaches to carcinogen identification that have historically prioritized direct DNA-damaging properties over subtler mechanisms like epigenetic alterations, metabolic disruption, or immune modulation. The concept of "safe thresholds" for carcinogen exposure represents another contentious area, particularly for substances that may act through hormonal or epigenetic mechanisms without direct DNA damage. Unlike classical genotoxic carcinogens that theoretically could induce mutations even at single-molecule exposures, non-genotoxic carcinogens might exhibit threshold effects, below which cancer risk is not meaningfully increased. Establishing such thresholds, however, requires extensive epidemiological evidence and consideration of vulnerable populations with potentially lower thresholds due to genetic predisposition or co-exposures (White *et al.,* 2020). Emerging discussions of the "exposome clock"—analogous to the epigenetic clock reflecting biological aging, suggest that cumulative environmental exposures may leave measurable molecular signatures that correlate with cancer risk (Vineis *et al.,* 2020). These signatures, detectable through advanced omics technologies, could potentially serve as early biomarkers of cancer risk and targets for preventive interventions. However, translating these complex molecular patterns into practical risk assessment tools remains challenging, requiring sophisticated computational approaches and large-scale validation studies. The relative contribution of environmental versus genetic factors in cancer etiology continues to generate debate. While genetic susceptibility clearly influences cancer risk, estimates suggest that environmental and lifestyle factors account for 70-90% of cancer risk for most common malignancies (Wu *et al.,* 2018). Understanding how these environmental factors interact with genetic background represents a frontier in cancer research, with important implications for both prevention strategies and therapeutic approaches.

Mechanisms of Environmental Carcinogenesis

DNA Damage and Mutation

Direct DNA damage represents the classical paradigm for environmental carcinogenesis, with numerous well-characterized pathways through which environmental agents can induce mutations. As described in current literature on carcinogenesis, "Carcinogens are things that increase the chances of the above [cancer development], either by directly damaging genes (such as radiation) or by forcing cells to replicate more thus increasing the opportunities for a mistake (such as asbestos)" (Alexandrov *et al.,* 2020). This dual mechanism involves direct genotoxicity versus increased proliferation with concomitant replication errors, provides a foundational framework for understanding how diverse environmental exposures contribute to cancer initiation. DNA adduct formation occurs when reactive chemicals covalently bind to DNA bases, creating structural distortions that can lead to misreading during replication. Tobacco-specific nitrosamines form characteristic adducts with guanine bases, often leading to G→T transversions frequently observed in smoking-associated lung cancers (Pfeifer *et al.,* 2002). Similarly, PAHs from combustion sources (vehicle exhaust, grilled foods, tobacco smoke) form bulky adducts that distort the DNA double helix, potentially inducing mutations if not correctly repaired before replication. Advanced mass spectrometry techniques have revolutionized our ability to detect and quantify

DNA adducts in human tissues, enabling more direct assessment of exposure-induced DNA damage. The development of high-resolution DNA adductomics approaches now allows comprehensive characterization of multiple adducts simultaneously, providing molecular fingerprints of specific exposures and insights into individual susceptibility (Villalta & Balbo, 2017). Oxidative stress represents another critical mechanism through which numerous environmental exposures induce DNA damage. Redox-active compounds including certain metals, quinones, and environmental pollutants can generate reactive oxygen species (ROS) that attack DNA bases, creating oxidative lesions like 8-oxoguanine. As noted in the literature, "many of the things that are known to cause cancer do so by causing oxidative stress on cells" (Reuter *et al.,* 2010). These oxidative DNA modifications, if not promptly repaired by base excision repair pathways, can lead to point mutations during subsequent replication. Recent studies using next-generation sequencing have revealed characteristic mutational signatures associated with specific environmental exposures, providing a retrospective record of mutagenic processes that have shaped tumor genomes (Kucab *et al.,* 2019). These signatures—patterns of base substitutions and small insertions/deletions with specific sequence contexts, can serve as molecular fingerprints of past exposures. For example, tobacco smoke produces a distinctive pattern of G→T transversions with specific sequence contexts, while ultraviolet radiation induces characteristic C→T transitions at dipyrimidine sites (Alexandrov *et al.,* 2020). Inflammation-mediated DNA damage creates an indirect but potent pathway through which environmental exposures promote mutagenesis. Chronic irritation from substances like asbestos fibers triggers prolonged inflammatory responses, with activated macrophages and neutrophils releasing ROS and reactive nitrogen species as part of their defensive functions. This sustained inflammatory microenvironment creates ongoing DNA damage while simultaneously promoting cell proliferation, a combination that dramatically increases mutation accumulation in affected tissues (Grivennikov *et al.,* 2010). Recent work has highlighted the role of inflammation-induced DNA cytosine deaminases, particularly APOBEC enzymes, in generating characteristic mutation patterns observed in multiple cancer types (Swanton *et al.,* 2015). Originally evolved as antiviral defense mechanisms, these enzymes can be inappropriately activated by inflammatory stimuli, leading to C→T and C→G mutations with specific sequence contexts. Environmental exposures that induce chronic inflammation may therefore promote carcinogenesis partly through APOBEC-mediated mutagenesis, providing a mechanistic link between inflammation and genetic alterations in cancer.

Epigenetic Alterations

Environmental carcinogens can induce stable changes in gene expression without altering DNA sequence through various epigenetic mechanisms. DNA methylation patterns are frequently disrupted by environmental exposures, with both global hypomethylation (potentially activating oncogenes and retrotransposons) and promoter-specific hypermethylation (silencing tumor suppressor genes) observed in response to various carcinogens. Tobacco smoke, for instance, induces characteristic methylation signatures in lung tissue that can persist even years after smoking cessation, suggesting long-term epigenetic memory of environmental exposures (Joehanes *et al.,* 2016). Recent epigenome-wide association studies (EWAS) have identified specific methylation sites that reflect cumulative exposure to environmental carcinogens, potentially serving as biomarkers of past exposure and cancer risk (Joubert *et al.,* 2016). These methylation signatures may partially explain how environmental exposures during critical developmental windows contribute to cancer risk decades later, providing molecular mechanisms for the developmental origins of health and disease (DOHaD) concept in cancer. Histone modifications represent another epigenetic mechanism influenced by environmental carcinogens. Post-translational modifications to histone proteins—including acetylation, methylation, phosphorylation, and ubiquitination—collectively regulate chromatin accessibility and transcriptional activity. Numerous environmental compounds, including arsenic, nickel, and certain air pollutants, can alter histone modification patterns, potentially dysregulating hundreds of genes simultaneously and disrupting coordinated cellular functions like DNA repair, cell cycle regulation, and apoptosis (Chervona & Costa, 2012). The development of chromatin immunoprecipitation followed by high-throughput sequencing (ChIP-seq) has enabled genome-wide assessment of how environmental exposures alter specific histone modifications, providing unprecedented insights into the epigenetic mechanisms of environmental carcinogenesis (Zhang *et al.,* 2016). These studies have revealed that certain environmental compounds preferentially affect specific genomic regions, including enhancers and super-enhancers that regulate cell-type-specific gene expression programs critical for maintaining cellular identity. Non-coding RNAs, particularly microRNAs, have emerged as important epigenetic regulators susceptible to environmental perturbation. These small RNA molecules post-transcriptionally regulate gene expression by targeting specific mRNAs for degradation or translational repression. Environmental exposures can alter microRNA expression profiles, potentially dysregulating entire networks of genes involved in critical cancer-related pathways. For example, arsenic exposure modifies expression of microRNAs regulating p53 signaling, potentially compromising this crucial tumor suppressor pathway (Ren *et al.,* 2015). The recent discovery of long non-coding RNAs (lncRNAs) with important regulatory functions has further expanded our understanding of epigenetic mechanisms susceptible to environmental disruption. These diverse RNA molecules participate in chromatin organization, transcriptional regulation, and protein scaffolding, with expression patterns that respond dynamically to environmental stimuli. Emerging evidence suggests that dysregulation of specific lncRNAs contributes to cancer development, providing another layer of epigenetic control susceptible to environmental disruption (Bhan *et al.,* 2017). A key debate in epigenetic carcinogenesis concerns the relative importance of heritable versus environmentally induced epigenetic alterations in cancer development. As noted by researchers in the field, complementary approaches are now "integrating multiple omics technologies with sophisticated statistical and bioinformatics approaches" to address these questions (Herceg *et al.,* 2018). The concept of the "epigenetic progenitor model" suggests that epigenetic alterations may precede and actually facilitate subsequent genetic mutations, representing a paradigm shift in how we conceptualize the sequence of molecular events leading to cancer development (Feinberg, *et al.,* 2016).

Disruption of Cell Signaling Pathways

Environmental carcinogens can dysregulate critical signaling pathways that control cell proliferation, survival, and differentiation, even without directly causing mutations. Receptor-mediated mechanisms represent a common pathway through which environmental compounds influence cellular behavior. Endocrine-disrupting chemicals can bind to hormone receptors, activating or antagonizing signaling cascades that regulate gene expression. Xenoestrogens—compounds that mimic estrogen—may contribute to hormone-dependent cancer development by inappropriately activating estrogen receptors in tissues like breast and endometrium (Gore *et al.,* 2015). Recent advances in molecular modeling and structural biology have enhanced our understanding of how environmental compounds interact with specific receptors, enabling more accurate prediction of potential endocrine-disrupting effects. High-throughput screening approaches now allow rapid assessment of thousands of environmental chemicals for receptor-binding activity, helping identify previously unrecognized endocrine disruptors that may contribute to cancer risk (Kleinstreuer *et al.,* 2018). Aberrant activation of oncogenic pathways can occur through various environmentally induced mechanisms. The Ras-RAF-MEK-ERK and PI3K-Akt pathways, which promote cell proliferation and survival, can be inappropriately activated by environmental exposures through receptor activation, oxidative stress, or inflammation. Sustained activation of these pathways can drive cellular proliferation while simultaneously suppressing apoptotic mechanisms that would normally eliminate damaged cells (Sakuma *et al.,* 2017). Phosphoproteomic analyses have revealed complex, network-level responses to environmental exposures, with specific carcinogens inducing characteristic patterns of kinase activation that may serve as molecular signatures of exposure (Zhang *et al.,* 2017). These studies highlight how environmental compounds can simultaneously affect multiple signaling nodes, creating systems-level perturbations that collectively promote carcinogenesis through coordinated dysregulation of cellular processes. Inactivation of tumor suppressor pathways represents another critical mechanism through which environmental exposures promote carcinogenesis. The p53 pathway, often called the "guardian of the genome," coordinates cellular responses to DNA damage, including cell cycle arrest, DNA repair, and apoptosis when damage is severe. Numerous environmental carcinogens, including certain metals and organic compounds, can compromise p53 function through mechanisms including oxidative modifications, altered post-translational regulation, and disrupted protein-protein interactions (Puca *et al.,* 2019). Recent proteomic studies have revealed previously unrecognized mechanisms through which environmental exposures can inactivate tumor suppressor proteins without genetic mutations. For example, certain environmental compounds can induce post-translational modifications that alter protein stability, subcellular localization, or interaction patterns, effectively silencing tumor suppressor function through non-genetic mechanisms. A significant contemporary debate concerns the relative importance of mutation-centric versus systems-based views of carcinogenesis. While the somatic mutation theory has dominated cancer research for decades, emerging evidence suggests that tissue organization and cellular context critically influence whether specific mutations actually lead to cancer development. Environmental exposures may disrupt tissue architecture and cell-cell communication, creating permissive environments for cancer development even without directly inducing mutations. This "tissue organization field theory" suggests new avenues for understanding how environmental factors contribute to carcinogenesis through non-mutagenic mechanisms. Recent single-cell analysis technologies have provided unprecedented insights into how environmental exposures affect cellular heterogeneity within tissues, potentially creating pre-malignant niches that subsequently support cancer development. These advanced approaches reveal that apparently homogeneous tissues actually contain diverse cell populations with variable responses to environmental stressors, helping explain why certain exposures preferentially affect specific cell types and cancer subtypes.

Gene-Environment Interactions

Genetic Factors Modifying Environmental Exposures

Individual genetic variation significantly influences susceptibility to environmental carcinogens, helping explain why identical exposures produce dramatically different outcomes across populations. Polymorphisms in xenobiotic-metabolizing enzymes represent a well-characterized category of genetic modifiers. Cytochrome P450 enzymes metabolize numerous environmental compounds, often converting them from relatively inert precursors to reactive metabolites capable of damaging DNA. For example, CYP1A1 variants that increase enzyme activity may enhance the activation of PAHs from tobacco smoke to DNA-reactive epoxides, potentially increasing lung cancer risk among smokers with these variants. Advanced mass spectrometry-based metabolomics now enables comprehensive characterization of how genetic variants influence the metabolism of environmental compounds, revealing previously unrecognized metabolic pathways and inter-individual differences in exposure processing. These approaches have identified novel biomarkers of exposure and susceptibility, potentially enabling more personalized risk assessment and preventive strategies. Conversely, detoxification pathways like glutathione S-transferases (GSTs) neutralize reactive compounds before they can damage cellular macromolecules. Individuals with GSTM1 or GSTT1 null genotypes—present in approximately 50% and 20% of Caucasian populations, respectively—lack functional versions of these important detoxification enzymes, potentially increasing their susceptibility to various environmental carcinogens. The balance between activation and detoxification pathways, both highly influenced by genetic polymorphisms, helps determine an individual's response to environmental exposures. Recent pharmacogenomic approaches have revealed complex, multigenic influences on xenobiotic metabolism, moving beyond single-gene polymorphisms to consider pathway-level effects and gene-gene interactions. These comprehensive analyses suggest that individual susceptibility to environmental carcinogens reflects the combined influence of multiple genetic variants across interdependent metabolic pathways, explaining why single-gene association studies often yield inconsistent results. DNA repair capacity demonstrates significant inter-individual variation that modifies environmental cancer risk. Nucleotide excision repair (NER) pathways remove bulky DNA adducts formed by numerous environmental carcinogens, including UV-induced photoproducts and PAH-DNA adducts. Polymorphisms in NER genes like XPD, ERCC1, and XPC are associated with altered repair efficiency and modified cancer risk, particularly in the context of specific environmental exposures. Similarly, genetic variants affecting base excision repair may influence susceptibility to oxidative DNA damage from various environmental sources. Functional assays measuring DNA repair capacity in peripheral blood cells have demonstrated substantial inter-individual variation in repair efficiency, with direct correlations to cancer risk in several epidemiological studies. These phenotypic measures of repair capacity often show stronger associations with cancer risk than individual genetic variants, suggesting that the combined effect of multiple genetic and environmental factors determines overall repair efficiency. Immune response genes significantly modify how individuals respond to potentially carcinogenic infections and inflammation-inducing exposures. Human leukocyte antigen (HLA) variants influence the efficiency of presenting foreign antigens to immune cells, potentially affecting clearance of oncogenic viruses and recognition of tumor-associated antigens. Polymorphisms in cytokine genes affect inflammatory responses to environmental irritants like asbestos or silica, potentially modifying cancer risk by altering the intensity and duration of inflammation-associated DNA damage. Recent immunogenomic approaches have revealed how genetic variants influence immune surveillance mechanisms that normally eliminate potentially malignant cells. These studies suggest that inherited differences in immune function may partially explain familial cancer clustering independently of tumor-initiating mutations, highlighting the importance of host-tumor interactions in determining cancer risk. An illustrative case of gene-environment interaction involves arsenic metabolism and cancer risk. Arsenic, a known human carcinogen found in drinking water in many regions worldwide, undergoes a series of methylation steps during metabolism. Genetic variants in arsenic methyltransferase (AS3MT) significantly influence how efficiently individuals convert inorganic arsenic to its methylated metabolites, with some variants associated with increased retention of more toxic species. Studies in Bangladesh and Taiwan have demonstrated that these genetic variants significantly modify the relationship between arsenic exposure and cancer risk, highlighting how genetic factors can amplify or mitigate environmental effects. Recent metabolomic studies have further elucidated the complex relationships between genetic variants, arsenic metabolism, and cancer risk. These comprehensive analyses have identified novel metabolites and pathways involved in arsenic processing, revealing previously unrecognized mechanisms through which genetic variants influence susceptibility to arsenic-induced carcinogenesis. These findings illustrate how advanced analytical approaches can provide mechanistic insights into gene-environment interactions in cancer development.

Contemporary Debates in Gene-Environment Research

A significant methodological debate concerns the appropriate study designs for detecting gene-environment interactions. Traditional candidate gene approaches have identified numerous potential interactions, but many have failed to replicate in independent studies. Genome-wide interaction studies potentially offer more comprehensive assessment but require extremely large sample sizes to achieve adequate statistical power. Intermediate approaches like pathway-based analyses or polygenic risk scores may provide more robust frameworks for understanding how genetic background modifies environmental cancer risk. The development of new statistical approaches specifically designed for detecting gene-environment interactions has advanced our ability to identify these complex relationships in population studies. Methods including Bayesian model averaging, multi-stage sampling designs, and machine learning approaches offer promising alternatives to traditional regression models, potentially improving statistical power while controlling false discovery rates. The relative contribution of genetic versus environmental factors in cancer development remains contentious. While early twin studies suggested substantial heritability for many cancer types, more recent analyses incorporating detailed environmental exposure assessment have often attributed greater importance to non-genetic factors. The "missing heritability" in cancer, the difference between estimated heritability from family studies and variance explained by identified genetic variants, may partially reflect complex gene-environment interactions that remain poorly characterized in most population studies. Recent studies using polygenic risk scores have demonstrated significant interactions with environmental exposures for multiple cancer types. These analyses suggest that genetic susceptibility may particularly influence cancer risk in the context of specific environmental exposures, with relatively modest effects in their absence. For example, the relationship between genetic risk scores and lung cancer is substantially stronger among smokers than non-smokers, illustrating how environmental context modifies genetic effects. The integration of exposomic and genomic data represents a frontier in cancer research with significant methodological challenges. Traditional statistical approaches may lack power to detect complex, non-linear interactions between multiple genetic variants and diverse environmental exposures. Advanced computational methods including machine learning algorithms, network-based analyses, and systems biology approaches offer promising frameworks for modeling these complex relationships, though their application to large population datasets remains computationally intensive and requires interdisciplinary expertise (Nilsson *et al.,* 2018). Metabolic phenotyping approaches have emerged as a powerful tool for characterizing the interface between genetic variation and environmental exposures. Metabolomics encompasses the comprehensive analysis of small-molecule metabolites in biological samples and provides a functional readout of the combined effects of genetic background, environmental exposures, and their interactions. These approaches have identified novel biomarkers of exposure and susceptibility, potentially enabling more personalized risk assessment and preventive strategies. The concept of gene-environment correlation entails where genetic factors influence exposure patterns, adds further complexity to understanding cancer etiology. Genetic variants affecting behaviors like smoking, alcohol consumption, or dietary preferences can create correlations between genotype and environmental exposures, potentially confounding studies of gene-environment interactions. Advanced study designs and analytical approaches that explicitly address these correlations are essential for accurately characterizing how genetic and environmental factors jointly influence cancer risk.

Epidemiological and Molecular Studies

Epidemiological Studies Linking Environmental Exposures to Cancer

Large-scale epidemiological studies have provided critical evidence linking environmental exposures to specific cancer types, often serving as the foundation for regulatory decisions and public health interventions. The was a landmark of study by scientists which was initiated and provided definitive evidence linking tobacco smoking to lung cancer, documenting dose-dependent relationships between smoking intensity and cancer risk. This study demonstrated how carefully designed prospective cohort studies can identify environmental causes of cancer even without detailed understanding of underlying mechanisms. Modern extensions of traditional epidemiological approaches now incorporate biomarkers of exposure and biological effect, enhancing our ability to establish causal relationships and elucidate underlying mechanisms. The European Prospective Investigation into Cancer and Nutrition (EPIC) study, involving over 500,000 participants across 10 European countries, has provided valuable insights into how dietary patterns, physical activity, and metabolic factors influence cancer risk, illustrating the power of large, well-characterized cohorts with detailed exposure information (Vineis *et al.*, 2020). Occupational cohort studies have proved particularly valuable for identifying environmental carcinogens, as workplace exposures often occur at higher intensities than in general environmental settings. Studies of asbestos workers revealed dramatically increased risks of mesothelioma and lung cancer, with important temporal insights into disease latency. As noted in the historical literature, "Mesothelioma has a latency period of around 30 years which means you need to track exposed people for 30 years or do retrospective reconstructions on large cohorts of mesothelioma patients." This latency created significant challenges for recognizing asbestos carcinogenicity, allowing continued exposure for decades after initial suspicions were raised (Craighead & Gibbs, 2008). Modern occupational epidemiology now incorporates sophisticated exposure assessment methodologies, including job-exposure matrices, biomonitoring, and industrial hygiene measurements, providing more accurate characterization of workplace exposures. These advanced approaches have identified novel occupational carcinogens and refined risk estimates for established workplace exposures, contributing valuable evidence for regulatory decision-making and worker protection. Case-control studies have identified numerous environmental risk factors for specific cancer types by comparing exposure histories between cancer patients and appropriately matched controls. These studies have linked arsenic-contaminated drinking water to bladder and lung cancers, residential radon exposure to lung cancer, and certain pesticides to non-Hodgkin lymphoma. While providing valuable insights, these retrospective designs face challenges including recall bias and confounding by other exposures and limitations that highlight the complementary value of different epidemiological approaches in environmental cancer research. Advanced case-control designs now incorporate biomarkers of exposure and susceptibility, enhancing their ability to establish causal relationships and identify susceptible subpopulations. For example, studies measuring urinary arsenic metabolites in bladder cancer cases and controls have demonstrated not only dose-dependent relationships between arsenic exposure and cancer risk but also significant modification of this relationship by genetic variants affecting arsenic metabolism. The development of geospatial analytical methods has enhanced our ability to detect environmental cancer clusters and identify potential environmental carcinogens. Geographic information systems (GIS) combined with sophisticated statistical approaches now allow researchers to analyze spatial patterns of cancer incidence in relation to environmental exposures, accounting for population characteristics and other potential confounders. These methods have identified elevated cancer risks associated with industrial facilities, contaminated water sources, and other localized environmental hazards, though distinguishing true exposure-related clusters from statistical anomalies remains challenging. Natural experiments are situations where environmental exposures change due to policy interventions or other factors unrelated to individual characteristics, provide particularly compelling evidence of causal relationships between environmental exposures and cancer. For example, studies documenting lung cancer rate declines following smoking bans and reductions in certain cancer types after pollution control measures demonstrate the impact of reducing environmental carcinogens. These natural experiments provide important validation of observational epidemiological findings and compelling evidence for preventive interventions.

Molecular Studies of Gene-Environment Interactions

Molecular epidemiology studies integrate biomarkers of exposure, biological effect, and susceptibility to provide mechanistic insights into gene-environment interactions in cancer development. The development of increasingly sensitive and specific biomarkers has transformed our ability to characterize both exposures and their biological consequences. DNA adduct measurements in accessible tissues (blood, buccal cells) provide evidence of chemical exposures and DNA reactivity, while mutation signature analysis in tumor tissue can retrospectively identify likely causal exposures based on characteristic mutation patterns they induce. Advanced mass spectrometry techniques now enable detection of DNA adducts at levels relevant to environmental exposures, providing molecular evidence of chemical-DNA interactions that may initiate carcinogenesis. These methods have identified characteristic adduct patterns associated with specific exposures, including tobacco-specific nitrosamines, heterocyclic amines from cooked meat, and environmental pollutants, offering valuable biomarkers for exposure assessment and mechanistic investigations (Villalta & Balbo, 2017). Genome wide association studies (GWAS) have identified numerous genetic variants associated with cancer risk, many of which modify the effects of environmental exposures. For example, variants in the CHRNA5-CHRNA3-CHRNB4 nicotinic receptor cluster on chromosome 15q25 not only influence smoking behavior but also appear to modify the per-cigarette lung cancer risk. Similarly, genetic variants in alcohol metabolism genes (ADH, ALDH) significantly modify the relationship between alcohol consumption and cancer risk, particularly for upper aerodigestive tract malignancies. Recent genome-wide interaction studies have attempted to comprehensively assess gene-environment interactions without prior hypotheses, potentially identifying novel genetic modifiers of environmental cancer risk. These agnostic approaches require extremely large sample sizes to achieve adequate statistical power, particularly when examining multiple environmental exposures, but offer the potential to discover unexpected biological interactions that might be missed in candidate gene studies. Experimental studies using model organisms and cells have elucidated specific mechanisms of gene-environment interactions in cancer. Genetically engineered mouse models with specific mutations or pathway alterations allow for controlled assessment of how genetic background modifies responses to environmental carcinogens. Cell culture models incorporating specific genetic variants through CRISPR-Cas9 editing similarly enable detailed mechanistic studies of how genetic factors influence cellular responses to environmental exposures under controlled conditions. Humanized mouse models, in which human genes are introduced into the mouse genome, provide valuable systems for studying how specific human genetic variants influence responses to environmental carcinogens. These models are particularly useful for examining polymorphisms in xenobiotic-metabolizing enzymes, which often show significant species differences that complicate extrapolation from traditional animal models to humans. An illustrative example of how molecular studies illuminate gene-environment interactions comes from research on aflatoxin exposure and liver cancer. Aflatoxins, produced by certain fungi that contaminate food supplies, form characteristic DNA adducts that can lead to mutations, particularly G→T transversions in the TP53 tumor suppressor gene. Individuals carrying specific variants in detoxification enzymes like GSTM1 and EPHX1 show significantly higher adduct levels and cancer risk when exposed to aflatoxins, demonstrating how genetic factors can modify molecular responses to environmental carcinogens with direct implications for disease risk.

COMPREHENSIVE FRAMEWORK FOR EXPOSOME RESEARCH: CHALLENGES, INNOVATIONS, AND ETHICAL CONSIDERATIONS

The exposome concept encompassing the totality of environmental exposures from conception onward, has revolutionized our understanding of disease etiology. It was initially proposed as a complement to the genome, the exposome framework has evolved into a multidimensional approach for investigating environmental determinants of health across the lifespan. While previous chapters explored the exposome's role in gametogenesis, teratogenesis, and carcinogenesis, this chapter provides a critical analysis of current methodological limitations, proposes innovative solutions, and outlines ethical considerations for advancing exposome research. The rapidly evolving nature of exposome science necessitates a comprehensive roadmap that integrates cutting-edge technologies with robust study designs. This chapter synthesizes emerging evidence and expert consensus to identify actionable strategies for overcoming challenges in exposure assessment, data integration, and longitudinal tracking, while addressing ethical dilemmas inherent in this field (Vermeulen *et al.,* 2020).

Overcoming Limitations in Exposome Research

Advancing Exposure Assessment Methods

Limitations of Traditional Approaches

Conventional exposure assessment methods—questionnaires, environmental sampling, and targeted biomarkers—face significant limitations in capturing the dynamic nature of the exposome. Single biospecimen analyses frequently misclassify exposures with high temporal variability, such as bisphenol A (BPA), which has a biological half-life of less than 6 hours. This misclassification introduces substantial attenuation bias in dose-response relationships, with simulation studies demonstrating up to 80% reduction in effect estimates when using single samples for highly variable compounds. Furthermore, traditional approaches struggle to account for complex mixtures and synergistic effects. The average human is exposed to over 85,000 manufactured chemicals, yet fewer than 1% have undergone comprehensive safety testing (Landrigan *et al.,* 2018). This testing gap undermines risk assessment frameworks that evaluate chemicals in isolation rather than as complex mixtures that reflect real-world exposure scenarios.

Innovative Assessment Technologies

Recent technological breakthroughs are transforming exposure assessment capabilities:

Wearable Sensor Technologies: Personal exposure monitors (PEMs) now provide continuous, real-time measurements of multiple environmental stressors. The silicon wristband passive sampler, for instance, can detect over 1,400 organic compounds simultaneously, including polycyclic aromatic hydrocarbons (PAHs), flame retardants, and pesticides (O'Connell *et al.,* 2014). Similarly, the Time-Activity-Capture-Tool (TACT) combines GPS tracking with real-time air quality monitoring to create spatiotemporal exposure profiles with unprecedented resolution (Nieuwenhuijsen *et al.,* 2015).

High-Resolution Mass Spectrometry (HRMS): Untargeted metabolomics using HRMS enables comprehensive chemical profiling in biological samples. The analytical sensitivity of quadrupole time-of-flight (QTOF) mass spectrometry can now detect compounds at sub-parts-per-billion concentrations, identifying novel exposure biomarkers and metabolic perturbations (Vermeulen *et al.,* 2020). Integration of HRMS with ion mobility separation further enhances detection capabilities by distinguishing isomeric compounds with identical masses but different structures.

Geospatial Modeling: Advanced Geographic Information Systems (GIS) integrate satellite imagery, land-use regression models, and dispersion algorithms to map exposure gradients across populations. The European Study of Cohorts for Air Pollution Effects (ESCAPE) utilized land-use regression models to estimate air pollution exposure at residential addresses with 100-meter spatial resolution, revealing associations between PM2.5 and cardiovascular mortality at levels below current regulatory standards.

Case Study: The EXPOsOMICS Project

The EXPOsOMICS project exemplifies next-generation exposure assessment by integrating external exposure monitoring with internal molecular signatures. This initiative collected air and water pollution data alongside multi-omics profiles from nine European cohorts, encompassing approximately 2,205 participants (Vineis *et al.,* 2020). The project's innovative approach combined personal monitoring devices measuring PM2.5, black carbon, and VOCs, GPS tracking of mobility patterns, metabolomic and adductomic profiling of biological samples, Transcriptomic analysis of gene expression changes. This integrated approach identified novel biomarkers of exposure, including a specific metabolomic signature associated with traffic-related air pollution. The signature consisted of 17 metabolites involved in oxidative stress and inflammatory pathways, providing a more precise assessment of exposure than traditional air monitoring alone.

Addressing Data Integration Challenges

Fragmentation of Datasets

The exponential growth of multi-dimensional exposome data creates significant integration challenges. Datasets often exist in isolated repositories with incompatible formats, variable quality control standards, and inconsistent metadata. The Human Exposome Project generates approximately 5 terabytes of data per 1,000 participants, encompassing exposomic, metabolomic, and phenotypic measurements. Efficiently integrating these diverse data types requires overcoming both technical and organizational barriers.

Innovative Integration Solutions

Standardized Data Formats: The FAIR principles (Findable, Accessible, Interoperable, Reusable) provide a framework for harmonizing exposome data. The HELIX Project successfully harmonized exposure data from six European birth cohorts by implementing standardized variable definitions, quality control protocols, and data dictionaries. This harmonization enabled cross-cohort analyses revealing previously undetected associations between multiple pollutant mixtures and neurodevelopmental outcomes.

Multi-Omics Integration Platforms: Software tools like mixOmics, MOFA+, and DIABLO facilitate integration of heterogeneous data layers through statistical approaches such as multi-block partial least squares regression. These methods can identify latent factors that explain variance across multiple biological domains simultaneously. A recent application of MOFA+ to the HELIX cohort identified shared latent factors linking air pollution exposure, DNA methylation patterns, and respiratory outcomes in children.

AI-Driven Analytics: Machine learning approaches are particularly deep learning and ensemble methods, excel at detecting complex patterns in high-dimensional exposome data. Random forests have successfully identified non-linear interactions between environmental exposures and genetic variants in the UK Biobank cohort, improving phenotypic prediction accuracy by 133% (from r=0.15 to r=0.35) when integrating genomic and exposomic data compared to genomic data alone.

Example: The HELIX Project

The Human Early-Life Exposome (HELIX) project represents a landmark achievement in exposome data integration. This initiative harmonized data from six European birth cohorts, comprising over 30,000 mother-child pairs, to characterize the early-life exposome and its influence on child health (Vrijheid *et al.,* 2014). The project integrated: Over 100 exposure variables including outdoor/indoor air pollutants, chemicals, and lifestyle factors, Multiple biological matrices (blood, urine, hair) collected at standardized timepoints, Molecular profiles spanning the genome, methylome, transcriptome, and metabolome, Detailed phenotypic assessments of growth, neurodevelopment, and respiratory health. Through this comprehensive integration, HELIX identified critical windows of vulnerability during prenatal development and demonstrated that mixtures of chemical exposures had stronger associations with health outcomes than individual chemicals assessed in isolation.

Enhancing Longitudinal Study Designs

Importance of Temporal Dynamics

Cross-sectional studies capture only a snapshot of the exposome, missing critical temporal dimensions of exposure-disease relationships. Longitudinal designs are essential for: Identifying critical windows of susceptibility during development, Capturing exposure trajectories that may have cumulative or lagged effects, Distinguishing between transient and persistent molecular perturbations, Evaluating how early-life exposures influence disease risk decades later. Evidence from the Developmental Origins of Health and Disease (DOHaD) paradigm demonstrates that prenatal exposure to famine during the Dutch Hunger Winter (1944-1945) increased risk of cardiometabolic disorders six decades later, mediated through persistent epigenetic changes.

Innovative Longitudinal Approaches

Birth Cohorts with Multi-Generational Follow-up: The Environmental influences on Child Health Outcomes (ECHO) program integrates data from 84 existing cohorts, following approximately 50,000 children from prenatal development through adolescence. The program's innovative design includes biological sampling across multiple developmental stages, enabling identification of exposure-induced molecular changes that precede clinical outcomes.

Digital Birth Cohorts: Smartphone-based tracking combined with home-based biospecimen collection enables frequent longitudinal assessments with minimal participant burden. The Stanford Pregnancy Exposome study collects weekly urine and saliva samples throughout pregnancy, paired with daily exposure tracking via smartphone applications, generating unprecedented temporal resolution of exposure patterns.

Repeated Measures Designs with Varying Collection Intervals: The Early Autism Risk Longitudinal Investigation (EARLI) collects biospecimens and environmental samples at strategic timepoints during pregnancy (first, second, and third trimesters) and early childhood (birth, 6 months, 12 months), with sampling intervals tailored to the biological half-lives of compounds of interest.

Case Study: The UK Biobank

The UK Biobank exemplifies a large-scale, longitudinal approach to exposome research. This population-based cohort of 500,000 participants integrates: Detailed baseline assessments including questionnaires, physical measurements, and biospecimen collection, Genetic data from genome-wide genotyping and whole-exome sequencing, Environmental exposure data derived from residential histories and linked environmental databases, Continuous health outcome tracking through electronic health record linkage. This comprehensive approach has enabled novel discoveries about gene-environment interactions in disease development. For example, by integrating air pollution exposure data with genetic information, researchers identified a significant interaction between air pollution exposure and the *APOE* ε4 allele in accelerating cognitive decline, with exposed carriers showing cognitive decline equivalent to an additional 2.7 years of aging.

POTENTIAL INTERVENTIONS AND PREVENTATIVE STRATEGIES

Reducing Exposure to Environmental Hazards

Policy Interventions

Evidence-based policies represent powerful tools for reducing population-wide exposures:

Air Quality Regulations: The World Health Organization's updated guidelines recommend PM2.5 concentrations ≤ 5 μg/m^3, significantly lower than previous standards based on new evidence linking air pollution to cardiovascular and respiratory diseases. Implementation of low-emission zones in European cities reduced PM2.5 concentrations by up to 23% and nitrogen dioxide by up to 32%, with corresponding reductions in respiratory hospitalizations.

Chemical Safety Legislation: The European Union's Registration, Evaluation, Authorization and Restriction of Chemicals (REACH) regulation has successfully restricted over 1,500 hazardous substances, including endocrine disruptors like certain phthalates and bisphenols. Biomonitoring studies demonstrate significant reductions in body burden of these compounds following regulatory action.

Drinking Water Standards: The U.S. Environmental Protection Agency recently established maximum contaminant levels for per- and polyfluoroalkyl substances (PFAS) in drinking water at 4 parts per trillion, reflecting mounting evidence linking these "forever chemicals" to adverse health effects including immunotoxicity and cancer.

Technological Solutions

Technological innovations complement regulatory approaches by providing practical solutions for exposure reduction:

Advanced Water Filtration: Reverse osmosis and activated carbon filtration systems effectively remove pharmaceutical residues, heavy metals, and persistent organic pollutants from drinking water. Point-of-use filtration reduces PFAS concentrations below detection limits in contaminated water supplies.

Green Chemistry: Sustainable alternatives to toxic industrial chemicals reduce workplace and consumer exposures. For example, replacement of benzene with less hazardous solvents in manufacturing processes has significantly reduced occupational leukemia risk.

Indoor Air Purification: High-efficiency particulate air (HEPA) filtration combined with activated carbon removes both particulate and gaseous pollutants from indoor environments. Controlled trials demonstrate that classroom air purification reduces children's exposure to traffic-related air pollution by 30-45% and improves cognitive performance .

Promoting Healthy Lifestyles as Exposure Countermeasures

Dietary Interventions

Evidence increasingly supports the role of nutrition in modulating the adverse effects of environmental exposures:

Mediterranean Diet: The European Prospective Investigation into Cancer and Nutrition (EPIC) study demonstrated that adherence to the Mediterranean diet reduced cancer risk among individuals living in highly polluted areas. High intake of antioxidant-rich fruits and vegetables counteracted oxidative stress induced by air pollution exposure, with each standard deviation increase in diet quality associated with a 15% reduction in pollution-related mortality.

Cruciferous Vegetables: Broccoli sprout extract, rich in sulforaphane, enhanced the detoxification of benzene in a randomized controlled trial among residents of highly polluted areas in China. Participants receiving the intervention experienced 61% greater urinary excretion of benzene metabolites compared to placebo, indicating enhanced detoxification capacity.

Dietary Fiber: Prebiotics and fermentable fibers modify the gut microbiome to reduce absorption of environmental toxicants. In animal models, dietary inulin supplementation reduced bioavailability of arsenic by 43% through enhanced microbial biotransformation and fecal excretion.

Physical Activity Interventions

Regular exercise modulates the physiological response to environmental exposures:

Moderate-Intensity Exercise: Controlled human exposure studies demonstrate that regular aerobic exercise attenuates cardiovascular responses to air pollution through upregulation of antioxidant enzymes and improved autonomic function. A 12-week exercise intervention reduced inflammatory biomarkers by 35% following controlled exposure to diesel exhaust.

Timing of Outdoor Activities: Scheduling exercise during low-pollution periods significantly reduces exposure burden. The Copenhagen Cycle Study found that altering commuting routes to avoid high-traffic areas reduced cyclists' black carbon exposure by 39% while maintaining cardiovascular benefits.

Personalized Prevention Strategies

Genomic Risk Stratification

Integration of genetic susceptibility with exposome data enables targeted interventions for high-risk subgroups:

Polygenic Risk Scores: Combining multiple genetic variants improves prediction of environmentally influenced diseases. In the All of Us Research Program, individuals with high polygenic risk scores for lung cancer who were exposed to air pollution showed 3.7-fold higher disease risk compared to those with low genetic risk scores, identifying a subgroup requiring intensive screening.

Pharmacogenomics Approaches: Genetic variants in detoxification pathways modify susceptibility to environmental toxicants. Individuals with the slow-acetylator variant of *N-acetyltransferase 2* (*NAT2*) experience 70% higher relative risk of bladder cancer when exposed to aromatic amines compared to rapid acetylators, making them priority candidates for occupational interventions.

Precision Interventions

Tailored approaches based on individual exposure profiles and biological responses maximize intervention efficacy:

Nutrigenomics Applications: Vitamin D supplementation particularly benefits individuals with vitamin D receptor polymorphisms who face impaired detoxification capacity under UV exposure. Carriers of the *VDR* FokI ff genotype showed enhanced DNA repair capacity and reduced photodamage with supplementation compared to non-carriers.

Micronutrient Supplementation: Folate supplementation mitigates arsenic toxicity in individuals with specific *one-carbon metabolism* gene variants. In Bangladesh, targeted supplementation for at-risk genotypes reduced arsenic-induced DNA damage by 39% compared to 14% in the general population.

The Role of "Omics" in Prevention

Predictive Biomarkers

Molecular biomarkers enable early identification of exposure-induced perturbations before clinical manifestation:

Epigenetic Clocks: DNA methylation-based aging biomarkers quantify the biological impact of environmental stressors. Horvath's epigenetic clock reveals accelerated epigenetic aging of 2.1 years per 10 $\mu g/m^3$ increase in PM2.5 exposure, providing a cumulative measure of environmental impact.

miRNA Signatures: Circulating microRNAs serve as sensitive indicators of exposure-induced tissue damage. A panel of five serum miRNAs (miR-21, miR-126, miR-146a, miR-155, and miR-222) demonstrated 88% sensitivity and 91% specificity in detecting early-stage lung damage following occupational exposure to silica dust.

Metabolomic Profiles: Urinary metabolites reflecting altered tryptophan metabolism predict neurological effects of air pollution exposure with greater sensitivity than traditional clinical markers. A specific pattern of kynurenine pathway metabolites preceded cognitive decline by approximately 5.3 years in elderly residents of highly polluted urban areas.

Targeted Preventative Strategies

Integration of molecular profiles with environmental data enables precision screening and intervention:

Risk-Stratified Screening Protocols: BRCA1 mutation carriers living in areas with high levels of estrogenic endocrine disruptors benefit from enhanced breast cancer screening. Annual MRI screening in this high-risk population increased early-stage detection by 61% compared to standard protocols.

Microbiome Modulation: Probiotic supplementation with specific Lactobacillus strains reduces intestinal absorption of heavy metals. A randomized controlled trial demonstrated that *L. rhamnosus* GR-1 supplementation increased fecal excretion of mercury by 28% and reduced blood mercury levels by 36% in exposed populations.

Intermittent Fasting Regimens: Time-restricted feeding activates cellular stress response pathways that enhance resilience to environmental toxicants. In animal models, intermittent fasting increased expression of NRF2-dependent detoxification enzymes by 2.7-fold and reduced DNA adduct formation following carcinogen exposure.

Ethical Considerations

Data Privacy and Security

The comprehensive nature of exposome data raises significant privacy concerns:

Re-identification Risks: Integration of geospatial, genomic, and exposome data increases re-identification vulnerability. Technical solutions include differential privacy algorithms that add calibrated statistical noise to protect individual identities while preserving population-level insights.

Secure Storage Systems: Blockchain-based infrastructure provides enhanced security for sensitive exposome data through decentralized storage and cryptographic access controls. The Personal Genome Project implemented a blockchain solution that reduced re-identification risk by 87% compared to traditional anonymization approaches.

Governance Frameworks: The EU General Data Protection Regulation (GDPR) establishes stringent standards for handling personal data, including special provisions for health and genetic information. Compliance requires implementing privacy by design, obtaining explicit consent for data sharing, and conducting impact assessments for high-risk processing activities.

Genetic Discrimination

Knowledge of gene-environment interactions may lead to discrimination without adequate protections:

Insurance Discrimination: Genetic information linked to environmental susceptibility could influence insurance availability or premiums. While the Genetic Information Nondiscrimination Act (GINA) prohibits genetic discrimination in health insurance and employment in the United States, significant gaps remain for life, disability, and long-term care insurance.

Workplace Discrimination: Genetic testing for susceptibility to workplace exposures raises concerns about discriminatory hiring practices. Evidence from the Alpha-1 antitrypsin deficiency registry revealed that 12% of individuals with this condition experienced workplace discrimination despite legal protections.

Policy Solutions: Comprehensive anti-discrimination legislation, such as the European Convention on Human Rights and Biomedicine, prohibits discrimination based on genetic heritage. Implementation of genetic privacy laws at national levels provides recourse for affected individuals.

Informed Consent in Exposome Research

Traditional informed consent models face challenges in exposome research:

Dynamic Consent Models: Digital platforms enable participants to modify consent preferences as research evolves. The Dynamic Consent platform implemented in the ALSPAC birth cohort increased participant engagement by 37% and enhanced understanding of research uses of biological samples.

Cultural Sensitivity: Research involving Indigenous populations requires protocols aligned with cultural values and community priorities. The Navajo Birth Cohort Study, examining uranium exposure outcomes, implemented a culturally tailored consent process developed in partnership with tribal health authorities, resulting in 78% participation among eligible families.

Collective Consent: Community-level approval complements individual consent in population-based exposome research. The Environmental Health Disparities Research Center implemented a dual-consent model requiring both community advisory board approval and individual consent, significantly increasing participation rates in minority communities previously underrepresented in research.

THE EXPOSOME: ENVIRONMENTAL DETERMINANTS OF HEALTH ACROSS THE LIFESPAN

Exposome Definition and Methodologies

The exposome concept, represents a paradigm shift in environmental health research by encompassing the totality of environmental exposures throughout the human lifespan. This holistic framework includes chemical, physical, biological, and social factors from conception onward, complementing genomic insights in understanding disease etiology (Rappaport & Smith, 2010).

Methodological advances have transformed our capacity to characterize this complex exposure landscape. High-resolution biomonitoring techniques now enable detection of endocrine-disrupting chemicals at parts-per-trillion levels in biological matrices, revealing the body burden of industrial compounds like per- and polyfluoroalkyl substances (PFAS) and phthalates (Miller & Jones, 2014; Vermeulen *et al.*, 2020). Simultaneous innovations in geospatial technologies facilitate mapping of exposure hotspots with unprecedented precision, identifying vulnerable communities in environmental justice contexts. The integration of multi-omics approaches—metabolomics, adductomics, and exposome-wide association studies—has been particularly transformative in capturing the biological imprints of complex exposures (Vermeulen *et al.*, 2020). Large-scale initiatives like EXPOsOMICS (Vineis *et al.*,

2020), HELIX (Vrijheid *et al.,* 2014), and the more recent ATHLETE project exemplify how computational models and artificial intelligence can synthesize disparate data streams to identify exposure-disease relationships that would otherwise remain obscured. Machine learning algorithms now decode temporal patterns in exposure mixtures, distinguishing acute from chronic effects and revealing critical windows of susceptibility. These technological advancements bridge traditional divides between environmental science, toxicology, and epidemiology, creating a unified framework for understanding how dynamic environmental exposures interact with biological systems across the lifespan.

Implications for Gametogenesis

Environmental exposures during gametogenesis represent a critical concern for reproductive health with potential transgenerational consequences. Endocrine-disrupting chemicals (EDCs) like bisphenol A (BPA), phthalates, and perfluorinated compounds can compromise gamete integrity through multiple mechanisms (Gore *et al.,* 2015). In males, occupational exposure to pesticides and industrial solvents correlates with reduced sperm count, impaired motility, and DNA fragmentation. Molecular studies reveal that these exposures induce oxidative stress in spermatogonia, disrupting epigenetic programming during spermatogenesis. For instance, paternal exposure to the fungicide vinclozolin alters DNA methylation patterns in sperm, with effects transmitted to subsequent generations through the male germline (Nilsson *et al.,* 2018). In females, the finite oocyte pool is particularly vulnerable to environmental insults. Prenatal exposure to cigarette smoke has been associated with reduced ovarian reserve through mechanisms involving accelerated follicular atresia. Heavy metals like cadmium accumulate in ovarian tissue, disrupting meiotic progression and contributing to aneuploid oocytes. These findings underscore how environmental exposures during critical windows of gametogenesis can have profound implications not only for immediate reproductive outcomes but potentially for offspring health through altered epigenetic inheritance. This germline vulnerability forms a crucial link between environmental exposures and developmental trajectories.

Implications for Teratogenesis

The exposome profoundly influences embryonic and fetal development through disruption of precisely orchestrated morphogenetic processes. Environmental teratogens exert their effects within distinct temporal windows, with consequences determined by the developmental stage at exposure. Alcohol remains among the most well-characterized teratogens, causing fetal alcohol spectrum disorders through multiple mechanisms including interference with neural crest cell migration, oxidative stress, and disruption of retinoic acid signaling. Maternal nutritional factors also critically influence development, with folate deficiency increasing neural tube defect risk by impairing one-carbon metabolism essential for epigenetic programming and nucleotide synthesis. The thalidomide tragedy of the 1960s exemplifies the principle of temporal specificity in teratogenesis, as limb malformations occurred primarily when exposure happened during weeks 4-7 of gestation, coinciding with limb bud development (Vargesson, 2015). Similarly, environmental exposures to air pollution have been linked to congenital heart defects, with particular risk associated with first-trimester exposure to fine particulate matter (PM2.5) and nitrogen dioxide (Zhang *et al.,* 2016). Heavy metals represent another significant teratogenic concern, with prenatal lead exposure associated with reduced cognitive function even at blood lead levels previously considered safe. The neuroteratogenic effects of methylmercury, dramatically illustrated by the Minamata disaster, continue to inform public health guidelines on fish consumption during pregnancy (Huang *et al.,* 2022). These insights into environmentally-induced teratogenesis emphasize the importance of preconception and prenatal exposome assessment in safeguarding developmental health and preventing congenital anomalies (Louis *et al.,* 2016).

Implications for Cancer

The exposome influences carcinogenesis through multiple interconnected pathways, contributing to the initiation, promotion, and progression of various malignancies (Loomis *et al.,* 2013; Wild *et al.,* 2020). Direct DNA damage from environmental carcinogens represents a primary mechanism, exemplified by tobacco smoke exposure. Polycyclic aromatic hydrocarbons (PAHs) in cigarette smoke form DNA adducts, particularly in the p53 gene, driving the molecular pathogenesis of lung cancer (Alexandrov *et al.,* 2020). Similarly, aflatoxin B1 exposure induces characteristic TP53 mutations in hepatocellular carcinoma, with synergistic effects observed in combination with hepatitis B virus infection. Epigenetic dysregulation constitutes another critical pathway, with arsenic exposure altering DNA methylation patterns and histone modifications in bladder and skin cancers. Chronic inflammation from persistent exposures, such as asbestos fibers or ambient air pollution, creates microenvironments conducive to tumor development through sustained oxidative stress and pro-inflammatory cytokine production. Gene-environment interactions significantly modulate individual cancer susceptibility. Individuals with NAT2 slow acetylator genotypes face elevated bladder cancer risk when exposed to aromatic amines while polymorphisms in the GSTM1 gene modify susceptibility to tobacco-induced lung cancer. The developmental origins of adult cancer further highlight the importance of early-life exposome assessment. Prenatal exposure to diethylstilbestrol (DES) dramatically increased clear cell adenocarcinoma risk in female offspring, demonstrating how early exposures can exert carcinogenic effects decades later. More recent evidence suggests that prenatal air pollution exposure may predispose to childhood leukemia through similar delayed mechanisms. These diverse carcinogenic mechanisms underscore the need for comprehensive exposome characterization in cancer prevention strategies, particularly during critical developmental windows (Wild *et al.,* 2020).

Future Perspectives

Advancing Exposome Research

The future of exposome research hinges on technological innovation and interdisciplinary integration. High-throughput exposomics platforms, including non-targeted mass spectrometry and environmental metabolomics, promise to capture thousands of exposures simultaneously, providing unprecedented resolution of the chemical exposome (Vermeulen *et al.,* 2020). Exposome-wide association studies (ExWAS), empowered by machine learning algorithms, will unravel complex interactions between multiple exposures and genetic susceptibility factors, moving beyond single-exposure paradigms toward more realistic mixture analyses. These approaches will benefit from emerging computational techniques including network analysis and systems biology models that can identify environmental interaction hubs and exposure patterns associated with specific health outcomes. Single-cell technologies represent another frontier, offering insights into cell-type-specific responses to environmental stressors and revealing heterogeneous effects within tissues. When integrated with spatial transcriptomics, these approaches will map the tissue microenvironment's response to toxicant exposure with unprecedented precision. Longitudinal cohort studies with repeated biospecimen collection, exemplified by efforts like the U.S. Environmental influences on Child Health Outcomes (ECHO) program and the UK Biobank, will track dynamic exposome changes across the lifespan. Novel biomarkers of cumulative exposure derived from these cohorts will inform precision prevention strategies tailored to individual exposure histories and susceptibilities (Vermeulen *et al.,* 2020). The translation of these scientific advances into public health applications will be accelerated by real-time monitoring technologies. Wearable sensors capable of detecting multiple environmental exposures, combined with smartphone-based ecological momentary assessment, will enable just-in-time interventions to mitigate acute exposure risks.

Prevention Strategies

Effective prevention strategies must operate at multiple levels—from policy to personal behavior—informed by exposome science. At the regulatory level, frameworks like the European Union's Registration, Evaluation, Authorization and Restriction of Chemicals (REACH) program demonstrate how exposome research can inform chemical governance, particularly for endocrine-disrupting compounds. Similarly, the World Health Organization's guidelines for particulate matter illustrate how epidemiological evidence translates into air quality standards with measurable public health benefits. Targeted nutritional interventions exemplify successful prevention strategies derived from exposome research. Mandatory folic acid fortification of grain products reduced neural tube defect prevalence by approximately 70% in the United States, while iodine supplementation programs mitigated neurodevelopmental impacts of iodine deficiency globally. At the individual level, evidence-based lifestyle modifications offer personal protection against unavoidable exposures. Dietary interventions rich in antioxidants have shown promise in mitigating oxidative stress induced by air pollution exposure while specific nutrients like calcium may reduce lead absorption in exposed populations. However, significant disparities persist in exposure distributions and prevention access. Low-income communities and communities of color disproportionately bear toxic exposure burdens while having reduced access to prevention resources. Environmental justice principles must therefore guide prevention programs, ensuring equitable distribution of both environmental protections and intervention resources. Moving forward, precision prevention strategies informed by individual exposome profiles hold promise for targeted interventions during critical windows of susceptibility, potentially disrupting pathways from exposure to disease before clinical manifestations emerge (Wild, 2012).

Global and Ethical Considerations

The global dimensions of exposome research present both challenges and opportunities. Socioeconomic and geographic disparities in exposure risks necessitate international cooperation and equitable research frameworks. Indigenous communities often face disproportionate exposure burdens due to historical inequities. The Navajo Birth Cohort Study exemplifies community-engaged research addressing uranium mining legacy exposures, emphasizing the importance of indigenous leadership in study design and implementation. Such approaches represent essential models for ethical exposome research in marginalized communities. Data privacy concerns become increasingly salient as exposome research integrates personal environmental monitoring with genomic data. Innovative governance structures, including differential privacy algorithms and secure multiparty computation, offer technical solutions while ethical frameworks like the Indigenous Data Sovereignty movement provide conceptual guidance for respectful data stewardship. Climate change further complicates the exposome landscape, altering exposure patterns through shifting disease vectors, increased extreme weather events, and changing agricultural practices. Integrating climate science with exposome research represents an urgent priority for anticipating emerging exposure threats in vulnerable regions (Landrigan *et al.,* 2018). A truly global exposome research agenda requires capacity building in low-resource settings, technology transfer, and collaborative training programs that respect diverse knowledge systems while building local expertise. International initiatives like the Global Alliance on Health and Pollution offer promising models for such collaborative approaches. These global and ethical dimensions necessitate a collaborative framework uniting epidemiologists, toxicologists, data scientists, ethicists, and community representatives to ensure exposome research benefits all populations equitably.

Synthesis

The exposome paradigm fundamentally reshapes our understanding of disease etiology by recognizing that health outcomes arise from continuous environmental dialogues with our biology across the lifespan (Wild, 2012; Rappaport & Smith, 2010).

From gametogenesis to carcinogenesis, environmental exposures leave indelible marks on human health, with effects that may transcend generations through epigenetic inheritance (Nilsson & Skinner, 2015). By illuminating the complex interactions between multiple exposures and biological systems, exposome research provides a unifying framework that transcends traditional disciplinary boundaries (Vermeulen *et al.,* 2020). This integration allows us to identify not only individual risk factors but also synergistic exposure combinations and critical intervention points for disease prevention (Wild *et al.,* 2020). The technological innovations driving exposome science, from high-resolution metabolomics to artificial intelligence algorithms, promise unprecedented insights into the environmental determinants of health. When coupled with community engagement and ethical governance, these advances can transform our approach to environmental health from reactive to anticipatory. Realizing this potential requires recognition of the exposome's inherent complexity while maintaining focus on practical applications that improve public health. By harnessing technological innovations while fostering global equity, we can transform exposome knowledge into effective prevention strategies that address environmentally-driven diseases at their roots. However, it was first articulated the exposome concept of this framework represents not merely a scientific paradigm but a call to action: to decode our environmental legacy, to address inequities in exposure distributions, and to safeguard the health of current and future generations through evidence-based interventions. The exposome thus offers both a comprehensive lens for understanding environmental health and a roadmap for creating healthier, more equitable environments for all.

CONCLUSION

The relationship between the exposome and cancer represents a complex, multifaceted area of research with profound implications for both understanding cancer biology and developing prevention strategies. Environmental carcinogens, from well-established agents like tobacco smoke and asbestos to emerging concerns including endocrine-disrupting chemicals and novel air pollutants, contribute to cancer development through diverse mechanisms including direct DNA damage, epigenetic dysregulation, and disruption of signaling pathways governing cellular behavior. The individual response to these exposures is further modified by genetic factors, creating a complex landscape of gene-environment interactions that collectively determine cancer risk. Significant methodological challenges remain in accurately characterizing cumulative environmental exposures, identifying susceptible subpopulations, and establishing causation in complex exposure scenarios. However, integrated approaches incorporating advanced exposure assessment, molecular epidemiology, and innovative statistical methods are transforming our understanding of how the exposome influences cancer development. These insights are increasingly informing regulatory strategies, public health interventions, and precision prevention approaches targeting modifiable environmental risk factors for cancer, with the potential to significantly reduce the global burden of this complex disease. Advancing exposome research requires a coordinated approach that addresses methodological challenges while embracing technological innovations and ethical frameworks. By integrating wearable sensors, high-resolution analytical platforms, and artificial intelligence with robust longitudinal study designs, researchers can capture the complex, dynamic nature of environmental exposures across the lifespan. Simultaneously, translating exposome insights into targeted preventative strategies, from policy interventions to personalized lifestyle modifications, promises to reduce the global burden of environmentally mediated diseases. Future progress depends on collaborative initiatives that harmonize exposome data across diverse populations, innovative statistical methods that decode complex exposure mixtures, and sustainable funding mechanisms that support long-term cohort studies. Equally important are ethical governance structures that balance scientific advancement with participant protection, ensuring that exposome research serves the public good while respecting individual rights and cultural values. As the exposome field matures, integration with other emerging disciplines, synthetic biology, nanomedicine, planetary health, will unlock new opportunities for understanding and mitigating environmental health risks in an increasingly complex world.

REFERENCES

Aitken, J. B., Naumovski, N., Curry, B., Grupen, C. G., Gibb, Z., & Aitken, R. J. (2015). Characterization of an L-amino acid oxidase in equine spermatozoa. *Biology of Reproduction, 92*(5), 125. DOI: 10.1095/biolreprod.114.126052 PMID: 25740544

Aitken, R. J. (2020). *The male is significantly implicated as the cause of unexplained infertility*. Sem Reprod Med. DOI: 10.1055/s-0040-1718941

Alexandrov, L. B., Kim, J., Haradhvala, N. J., Huang, M. N., Tian, N. G., Wu, Y., Boot, A., Covington, K. R., Gordenin, D. A., Bergstrom, E. N., Islam, S. M., Lopez-Bigas, N., Klimczak, L. J., McPherson, J. R., Morganella, S., Sabarinathan, R., Wheeler, D. A., & Mustonen, V. (2020, February). PCAWG Mutational Signatures Working Group; Getz G, Rozen SG, Stratton MR; PCAWG Consortium. The repertoire of mutational signatures in human cancer. [Erratum in: Nature. 2023 Feb;614] [7948] [:E41. doi: 10.1038/s41586-022-05600-5]. *Nature, 578*(7793), 94–101. DOI: 10.1038/s41586-020-1943-3 PMID: 32025018

Andra, S. S., Austin, C., Wright, R. O., & Arora, M. (2015). Reconstructing pre-natal and early childhood exposure to multi-class organic chemicals using teeth: Towards a retrospective temporal exposome. *Environment International, 83*, 137–145. DOI: 10.1016/j.envint.2015.05.010 PMID: 26134987

Anway, M. D., Cupp, A. S., Uzumcu, M., & Skinner, M. K. (2005). Epigenetic transgenerational actions of endocrine disruptors and male fertility. *Science, 308*(5727), 1466–1469. DOI: 10.1126/science.1108190 PMID: 15933200

Appenzeller, B. M. R., Chadeau-Hyam, M., & Aguilar, L. (2020). Skin exposome science in practice: Current evidence on hair biomonitoring and future perspectives. *Journal of the European Academy of Dermatology and Venereology, 34*(S4, Suppl. 4), 26–30. DOI: 10.1111/jdv.16640 PMID: 32677066

Arbuckle, T. E., Liang, C. L., Morisset, A. S., Fisher, M., Weiler, H., Cirtiu, C. M., Legrand, M., Davis, K., Ettinger, A. S., & Fraser, W. D. (2016). MIREC Study Group. Maternal and fetal exposure to cadmium, lead, manganese and mercury: The MIREC study. *Chemosphere, 163*, 270–282. DOI: 10.1016/j.chemosphere.2016.08.023 PMID: 27540762

Arora, M., & Austin, C. (2013). Teeth as a Biomarker of Past Chemical Exposure. *Current Opinion in Pediatrics, 25*(2), 261–267. Advance online publication. DOI: 10.1097/MOP.0b013e32835e9084 PMID: 23429707

Balbo, S., Turesky, R. J., & Villalta, P. W. (2014). DNA adductomics. *Chemical Research in Toxicology, 27*(3), 356–366. DOI: 10.1021/tx4004352 PMID: 24437709

Barabási, A. L., Gulbahce, N., & Loscalzo, J. (2011). Network medicine: A network-based approach to human disease. *Nature Reviews. Genetics, 12*(1), 56–68. DOI: 10.1038/nrg2918 PMID: 21164525

. Barabási, A.L. & Oltvai, Z. N. (2004). Network Biology: Understanding the cell's functional organization. *Nat. Rev. Genet.* 5, 101–113, 27.

Bellinger, P. (2020, June). Functional Overreaching in Endurance Athletes: A Necessity or Cause for Concern? *Sports Medicine (Auckland, N.Z.), 50*(6), 1059–1073. DOI: 10.1007/s40279-020-01269-w PMID: 32064575

Bhan, A., Soleimani, M., & Mandal, S. S. (2017). Long Noncoding RNA and Cancer: A New Paradigm. *Cancer Research, 77*(15), 3965–3981. DOI: 10.1158/0008-5472.CAN-16-2634 PMID: 28701486

Blake, B. E., & Fenton, S. E. (2020). Early life exposure to per- and polyfluoroalkyl substances (PFAS) and latent health outcomes: A review including the placenta as a target tissue and possible driver of peri- and postnatal effects. *Toxicology, 443*, 152565. DOI: 10.1016/j.tox.2020.152565 PMID: 32861749

Bloom, M. S., Fujimoto, V. Y., Steuerwald, A. J., Cheng, G., Browne, R. W., & Parsons, P. J. (2012). Background exposure to toxic metals in women adversely influences pregnancy during in vitro fertilization (IVF). *Reproductive Toxicology (Elmsford, N.Y.), 34*(3), 471–481. DOI: 10.1016/j.reprotox.2012.06.002 PMID: 22732149

Bohacek, J., & Mansuy, I. M. (2015). Molecular insights into transgenerational non-genetic inheritance of acquired behaviours. *Nature Reviews. Genetics, 16*(11), 641–652. DOI: 10.1038/nrg3964 PMID: 26416311

. Burton, A., Aughterson, H., Fancourt, D. & Philip, K.E.J. (2022). Factors shaping the mental health and well-being of people experiencing persistent COVID-19 symptoms or 'long COVID': qualitative study. *BJPsych Open.* 21;8(2):e72. .DOI: 10.1192/bjo.2022.38

Castillo-Fernandez, J., Herrera-Puerta, E., Demond, H., Clark, S. J., Hanna, C. W., Hemberger, M., & Kelsey, G. (2020). Increased transcriptome variation and localised DNA methylation changes in oocytes from aged mice revealed by parallel single-cell analysis. *Aging Cell, 19*(12), e13278. DOI: 10.1111/acel.13278 PMID: 33201571

Chervona, Y., & Costa, M. (2012). Histone modifications and cancer: Biomarkers of prognosis? *American Journal of Cancer Research, 2*(5), 589–597. PMID: 22957310

Copp, A. J., Stanier, P., & Greene, N. D. (2013). Neural tube defects: Recent advances, unsolved questions, and controversies. *Lancet Neurology*, *12*(8), 799–810. DOI: 10.1016/S1474-4422(13)70110-8 PMID: 23790957

Craighead, J. E., & Gibbs, A. R. (2008). *Asbestos and Its Diseases* (Craighead, J. E., & Gibbs, A. R., Eds.). Oxford University Press. Print DOI: 10.1093/acprof:oso/9780195178692.001.0001

. Cunningham, R.M., Walton, M.A., Carter, P.M. (2018). The Major Causes of Death in Children and Adolescents in the United States. *N Engl J Med.* 20;379(25):2468-2475. .DOI: 10.1056/NEJMsr1804754

Diamanti-Kandarakis, E., Bourguignon, J. P., Giudice, L. C., Hauser, R., Prins, G. S., Soto, A. M., Zoeller, R. T., & Gore, A. C. (2009). Endocrine-disrupting chemicals: An endocrine society scientific statement. *Endocrine Reviews*, *30*(4), 293–342. DOI: 10.1210/er.2009-0002 PMID: 19502515

Donkin, I., & Barrès, R. (2018). Sperm epigenetics and influence of environmental factors. *Molecular Metabolism*, *14*, 1–11. DOI: 10.1016/j.molmet.2018.02.006 PMID: 29525406

. Donovan, K.A., An, J., Nowak, R.P., Yuan, J.C, Fink, E.C., Berry, B.C., Ebert, B.L. & Fischer, E.S. (2018). Thalidomide promotes degradation of SALL4, a transcription factor implicated in Duane Radial Ray syndrome. 1;7: .DOI: 10.7554/eLife.38430

Durairajanayagam, D., Agarwal, A., & Ong, C. (2015). Causes, effects and molecular mechanisms of testicular heat stress. *Reproductive Biomedicine Online*, *30*(1), 14–27. DOI: 10.1016/j.rbmo.2014.09.018 PMID: 25456164

Edson, M. A., Nagaraja, A. K., & Matzuk, M. M. (2009). The mammalian ovary from genesis to revelation. *Endocrine Reviews*, *30*(6), 624–712. DOI: 10.1210/er.2009-0012 PMID: 19776209

Feinberg, A. P., Koldobskiy, M. A., & Göndör, A. (2016). Epigenetic modulators, modifiers and mediators in cancer aetiology and progression. *Nature Reviews. Genetics*, *17*(5), 284–299. DOI: 10.1038/nrg.2016.13 PMID: 26972587

Gluckman, P. D., Hanson, M. A., Buklijas, T., Low, F. M., & Beedle, A. S. (2009). Epigenetic mechanisms that underpin metabolic and cardiovascular diseases. *Nature Reviews. Endocrinology*, *5*(7), 401–408. DOI: 10.1038/nrendo.2009.102 PMID: 19488075

Goodson, W. H.III, Lowe, L., Carpenter, D. O., Gilbertson, M., Manaf Ali, A., Lopez de Cerain Salsamendi, A., & Pavanello, S. (2015). Assessing the carcinogenic potential of low-dose exposures to chemical mixtures in the environment: The challenge ahead. *Carcinogenesis*, *36*(Suppl_1), S254–S296.

Gore, A. C., Chappell, V. A., Fenton, S. E., Flaws, J. A., Nadal, A., Prins, G. S., Toppari, J., & Zoeller, R. T. (2015). EDC-2: The Endocrine Society's second scientific statement on endocrine-disrupting chemicals. *Endocrine Reviews*, *36*(6), 1–150. DOI: 10.1210/er.2015-1010

Grivennikov, S. I., Greten, F. R., & Karin, M. (2010). Immunity, inflammation, and cancer. *Cell*, *140*(6), 883–899. DOI: 10.1016/j.cell.2010.01.025 PMID: 20303878

Halliwell, B. (2007). Oxidative stress and neurodegeneration: Where are we now? *Journal of Neurochemistry*, *97*(6), 1634–1658. DOI: 10.1111/j.1471-4159.2006.03907.x PMID: 16805774

. Hanson, M.A. & Gluckman, P.D. (2014). Early developmental conditioning of later health and disease: physiology or pathophysiology? *Physiol Rev*; 94(Wild, 2005):1027-76. .DOI: 10.1152/physrev.00029.2013

. Hecht, S.S. (2012). Lung carcinogenesis by tobacco smoke. *Int J Cancer.* 15;131(12):2724-32. .DOI: 10.1002/ijc.27816

. Heijmans, B.T., Tobi, E.W., Stein, A.D., Putter, H., Blauw, G.J., Susser, E.S., Slagboom, P.E. & Lumey, L.H. (2008). Persistent epigenetic differences associated with prenatal exposure to famine in humans. *Proc Natl Acad Sci.* 4;105(44):17046-9. .DOI: 10.1073/pnas.0806560105

. Henderson, D.A., Inglesby, T.V., Bartlett, J.G., Ascher, M.S., Eitzen, E., Jahrling, P.B., Hauer, J., Layton, M., McDade, J., Osterholm, M.T., O'Toole, T., Parker, G., Perl, T., Russell, P.K. and Tonat, K. (1999). Smallpox as a biological weapon: medical and public health management. Working Group on Civilian Biodefense. *JAMA* 9;281(22):2127-37. .DOI: 10.1001/jama.281.22.2127

Herceg, A. G., Wild, C. P., Sklias, A., Casati, L., Duthie, S. J., Fry, R., Issa, J.-P., Kellermayer, R., Koturbash, I., Kondo, Y., Lepeule, J., Lima, S. C. S., Marsit, C. J., Rakyan, V., Saffery, R., Taylor, J. A., Teschendorff, A. E., Ushijima, T., Vineis, P., & Hernandez, H. (2018). Vargas Roadmap for investigating epigenome deregulation and environmental origins of cancer. *International Journal of Cancer*, *142*(5), 874–882. DOI: 10.1002/ijc.31014 PMID: 28836271

Hiatt, R. A., & Brody, J. G. (2018). Environmental Determinants of Breast Cancer. *Annual Review of Public Health, 1*(39), 113–133. DOI: 10.1146/annurev-publhealth-040617-014101 PMID: 29328875

Hou, Y., Li, S., Xia, L., Yang, Q., Zhang, L., Zhang, X., Liu, H., Huo, R., Cao, G., Huang, C., Tian, X., Sun, L., Cao, D., Zhang, M., Zhang, Q., & Tang, N. (2021). Associations of urinary phenolic environmental estrogens exposure with blood glucose levels and gestational diabetes mellitus in Chinese pregnant women. *The Science of the Total Environment, 754*, 142085. DOI: 10.1016/j.scitotenv.2020.142085 PMID: 32898782

Hu, Y., Tanriverdi, F., MacColl, G. S., & Bouloux, P. M. (2003). Kallmann syndrome: Molecular pathogenesis. *The International Journal of Biochemistry & Cell Biology, 35*(8), 1157–1162. DOI: 10.1016/S1357-2725(02)00395-3 PMID: 12757752

Huang, N., Gao, Y., Zhang, M., Guo, L., Qin, L., Liao, S., & Wang, H. (2022). METTL3-Mediated m6A RNA Methylation of ZBTB4 Interferes with Trophoblast Invasion and Maybe Involved in RSA. *Frontiers in Cell and Developmental Biology, 10*, 10. DOI: 10.3389/fcell.2022.894810 PMID: 35774226

Hunt, P. A., Koehler, K. E., Susiarjo, M., Hodges, C. A., Ilagan, A., Voigt, R. C., Thomas, S., Thomas, B. F., & Hassold, T. J. (2003, April 1). Bisphenol A Exposure Causes Meiotic Aneuploidy in the Female Mouse. *Current Biology, 13*(7), 546–553. DOI: 10.1016/S0960-9822(03)00189-1 PMID: 12676084

IARC. (2012). Asbestos (Chrysotile, Amosite, Crocidolite, Tremolite, Actinolite and Anthophyllite). *IARC Monographs on the Evaluation of Carcinogenic Risks to Humans, 100*, C.

Ioannidis, J. P., Loy, E. Y., Poulton, R., & Chia, K. S. (2009). *Sci. Transl. Med.* 1, 7ps8.Wild, C.P. (2005). Complementing the genome with an 'exposome': The outstanding challenge of environmental exposure measurement in molecular epidemiology. *Cancer Epidemiology, Biomarkers & Prevention, 14*, 1847–1850.

. Ito, T., Ando, H., Suzuki, T., Ogura, T., Hotta, K., Imamura, Y., Yamaguchi, Y. and Handa, H. (2010). Identification of a primary target of thalidomide teratogenicity. *Science*. 12;327(5971):1345-50. .DOI: 10.1126/science.1177319

. Jia, R.X., Liang, J.H., Xu, Y. & Wang, Y.Q. (2019). Effects of physical activity and exercise on the cognitive function of patients with Alzheimer disease: a meta-analysis. *BMC Geriatr*. 2;19(1):181. .DOI: 10.1186/s12877-019-1175-2

Jirtle, R. L., & Skinner, M. K. (2007). Environmental epigenomics and disease susceptibility. *Nature Reviews. Genetics*, *8*(4), 253–262. DOI: 10.1038/nrg2045 PMID: 17363974

Joehanes, R., Just, A. C., Marioni, R. E., Pilling, L. C., Reynolds, L. M., Mandaviya, P. R., Guan, W., Xu, T., Elks, C. E., Aslibekyan, S., Moreno-Macias, H., Smith, J. A., Brody, J. A., Dhingra, R., Yousefi, P., Pankow, J. S., Kunze, S., Shah, S. H., McRae, A. F., & London, S. J. (2016). Epigenetic Signatures of Cigarette Smoking. *Circulation: Cardiovascular Genetics*, *9*(5), 436–447. DOI: 10.1161/CIRCGENETICS.116.001506 PMID: 27651444

Joensen, U. N., Bossi, R., Leffers, H., Jensen, A. A., Skakkebaek, N. E., & Jorgensen, N. (2009). Do perfluoroalkyl compounds impair human semen quality? *Environmental Health Perspectives*, *117*(6), 923–927. DOI: 10.1289/ehp.0800517 PMID: 19590684

. Joubert, B.R., den Dekker, H.T., Felix, J.F., Bohlin, J., Ligthart, S., Beckett, E., Tiemeier, H., van Meurs, J.B., Uitterlinden, A.G., Hofman, A., Håberg, S.E., Reese, S.E., Peters, M.J., Andreassen, B.K., Steegers, E.A., Nilsen, R.M., Vollset, S.E., Midttun, Ø., Ueland, P.M., Franco, O.H., Dehghan, A., de Jongste, J.C., Wu, M.C., Wang, T., Peddada, S.D., Jaddoe, V.W., Nystad, W., Duijts, L., London, S.J. (2016). Maternal plasma folate impacts differential DNA methylation in an epigenome-wide meta-analysis of newborns. *Nat Commun*.10;7:10577. .DOI: 10.1038/ncomms10577

Joubert, B. R., Felix, J. F., Yousefi, P., Bakulski, K. M., Just, A. C., Breton, C., & London, S. J. (2016). DNA methylation in newborns and maternal smoking in pregnancy: Genome-wide consortium meta-analysis. *American Journal of Human Genetics*, *98*(4), 680–696.

Kleinstreuer, N. C., Hoffmann, S., Alépée, N., Allen, D., Ashikaga, T., Casey, W., Clouet, E., Cluzel, M., Desprez, B., Gellatly, N., Göbel, C., Kern, P. S., Klaric, M., Kühnl, J., Martinozzi-Teissier, S., Mewes, K., Miyazawa, M., Strickland, J., van Vliet, E., & Petersohn, D. (2018). Non-animal methods to predict skin sensitization (II): An assessment of defined approaches. *Critical Reviews in Toxicology*, *48*(5), 359–374. DOI: 10.1080/10408444.2018.1429386 PMID: 29474122

Knudson, A. G.Jr. (1971). Mutation and cancer: Statistical study of retinoblastoma. *Proceedings of the National Academy of Sciences of the United States of America*, *68*(4), 820–823. DOI: 10.1073/pnas.68.4.820 PMID: 5279523

Korbas, M., & Tracy, C. (2012). Chemical Form Matters: Differential Accumulation of Mercury Following Inorganic and Organic Mercury Exposures in Zebrafish Larvae. *ACS Chemical Biology*, *7*(2), 411–420. DOI: 10.1021/cb200287c PMID: 22026432

Kortenkamp, A., Martin, O., Evans, R., Orton, F., McKinlay, R., Rosivatz, E., & Faust, M. (2012). Response to A critique of the European Commission Document, "State of the Art Assessment of Endocrine Disruptors" by Rhomberg and colleagues – letter to the editor. *Critical Reviews in Toxicology*, *42*(9), 787–789. DOI: 10.3109/10408444.2012.712943 PMID: 22900988

Krauss, R. S., & Hong, M. (2016). Gene–environment Interactions and the etiology of birth defects. *Current Topics in Developmental Biology*, *116*, 569–580. DOI: 10.1016/bs.ctdb.2015.12.010 PMID: 26970642

Krawetz, S. A., Kruger, A., Lalancette, C., Tagett, R., Anton, E., Draghici, S., & Diamond, M. P. (2011). A survey of small RNAs in human sperm. *Human Reproduction (Oxford, England)*, *26*(12), 3401–3412. DOI: 10.1093/humrep/der329 PMID: 21989093

Krieger, N. (2007). Theories for social epidemiology in the 21st century: An ecosocial perspective. *International Journal of Epidemiology*, *30*(4), 668–677. DOI: 10.1093/ije/30.4.668 PMID: 11511581

. Kucab, J.E., Zou, X., Morganella, S., Joel, M., Nanda, A.S., Nagy, E., Gomez, C., Degasperi, A., Harris, R., Jackson, S.P., Arlt, V.M., Phillips, D.H. & Nik-Zainal, S.A. (2019). Compendium of Mutational Signatures of Environmental Agents. *Cell.* 2;177(Wild, 2005):821-836.e16. .DOI: 10.1016/j.cell.2019.03.001

. Lambrot, R., Siklenka, K., Lafleur, C., Kimmins, S. (2019). The genomic distribution of histone H3K4me2 in spermatogonia is highly conserved in sperm. *Biol Reprod.* 1;100(6):1661-1672. .DOI: 10.1093/biolre/ioz055

Landrigan, P. J., Fuller, R., Acosta, N. J. R., Adeyi, O., Arnold, R., Basu, N., Balde, A. B., Bertollini, R., Bose-O'Reilly, S., Boufford, J. I., Breysse, P. N., Chiles, T., Mahidol, C., Coll-Seck, A. M., Cropper, M. L., Fobil, J., Fuster, V., Greenstone, M., Haines, A., & Zhong, M. (2018). The Lancet Commission on pollution and health. *Lancet*, *391*(10119), 462–512. DOI: 10.1016/S0140-6736(17)32345-0 PMID: 29056410

. LeBel, A., Jain, S. and Huth, A. G. (2021). Voxelwise Encoding Models Show That Cerebellar Language Representations are Highly Conceptual. *Journal of Neuroscience.* 15;41(50):10341-10355.

Lei, S., Zheng, R., Zhang, S., Wang, S., Chen, R., Sun, K., Zeng, H., Zhou, J., & Wei, W. (2020). Global patterns of breast cancer incidence and mortality: A population-based cancer registry data analysis from 2000 to 2020. [Lond]. *Cancer Communications*, *41*(11), 1183–1194. DOI: 10.1002/cac2.12207 PMID: 34399040

Lemen, J. R., Title, A. M., Akin, D. J., Boerner, P. F., Chou, C., Drake, J. F., Duncan, D. W., Edwards, C. G., Friedlaender, F. M., Heyman, G. F., Hurlburt, N. E., Katz, N. L., Kushner, G. D., Levay, M., Lindgren, R. W., Mathur, D. P., McFeaters, E. L., Mitchell, S., Rehse, R. A., & Waltham, N. (2012). The *Atmospheric Imaging Assembly* (AIA) on the *Solar Dynamics Observatory* (SDO). *Solar Physics, 275*(1-2), 17–40. DOI: 10.1007/s11207-011-9776-8

Lerro, C. C., Beane Freeman, L. E., DellaValle, C. T., Andreotti, G., Hofmann, J. N., Koutros, S., Parks, C. G., Shrestha, S., Alavanja, M. C. R., Blair, A., Lubin, J. H., Sandler, D. P., & Ward, M. H. (2021). Pesticide exposure and incident thyroid cancer among male pesticide applicators in agricultural health study. *Environment International, 146*, 106187. DOI: 10.1016/j.envint.2020.106187 PMID: 33126065

Levine, H., Jørgensen, N., Martino-Andrade, A., Mendiola, J., Weksler-Derri, D., Mindlis, I., Pinotti, R., & Swan, S. H. (2017). Temporal trends in sperm count: A systematic review and meta-regression analysis. *Human Reproduction Update, 23*(6), 646–659. DOI: 10.1093/humupd/dmx022 PMID: 28981654

Li, Z., Schieber, J., & Pedersen, P. K. (2021). On the origin and significance of composite particles in mudstones: Examples from the Cenomanian Dunvegan Formation. *Sedimentology, 68*(2), 737–754. DOI: 10.1111/sed.12801

Liew, S. L., Anglin, J. M., Banks, N. W., Sondag, M., Ito, K. L., Kim, H., Chan, J., Ito, J., Jung, C., Khoshab, N., Lefebvre, S., Nakamura, W., Saldana, D., Schmiesing, A., Tran, C., Vo, D., Ard, T., Heydari, P., Kim, B., & Stroud, A. (2018). A large, open-source dataset of stroke anatomical brain images and manual lesion segmentations. *Scientific Data, 5*(1), 1–11. DOI: 10.1038/sdata.2018.11 PMID: 29461514

Loomis, D., Grosse, Y., Lauby-Secretan, B., El Ghissassi, F., Bouvard, V., Benbrahim-Tallaa, L., Guha, N., Baan, R., Mattock, H., & Straif, K. (2013). International Agency for Research on Cancer Monograph Working Group IARC. The carcinogenicity of outdoor air pollution. *The Lancet. Oncology, 14*(13), 1262–1263. DOI: 10.1016/S1470-2045(13)70487-X PMID: 25035875

. Louis, G.M., Barr, D.B., Kannan, K., Chen, Z., Kim, S., & Sundaram, R. (2016). Paternal exposures to environmental chemicals and time-to-pregnancy: overview of results from the LIFE study. *Andrology, 4*(Wild, 2005), 639–647.

. Machtinger, R. & Orvieto, R. (2014). Bisphenol A. Oocyte maturation, implantation, and IVF outcome: review of animal and human data. *Reprod Biomed Online.*;29(Wild, 2005):404–10.

. Mao, L., Jin, H., Wang, M., Hu, Y., Chen, S., He, Q., Chang, J., Hong, C., Zhou, Y., Wang, D., Miao, X., Li, Y.& Hu B. (2020). Neurologic Manifestations of Hospitalized Patients With Coronavirus Disease 2019 in Wuhan, China. *JAMA Neurol*, 1;77(6):683-690. .DOI: 10.1001/jamaneurol.2020.1127

Marcon, A., Pesce, G., Calciano, L., Bellisario, V., Dharmage, S. C., Garcia-Aymerich, J., Gislasson, T., Heinrich, J., Holm, M., Janson, C., Jarvis, D., Leynaert, B., Matheson, M. C., Pirina, P., Svanes, C., Villani, S., Zuberbier, T., Minelli, C., & Accordini, S. (2018). Trends in smoking initiation in Europe over 40 years: A retrospective cohort study. *PLoS One*, *13*(8), e0201881. Advance online publication. DOI: 10.1371/journal.pone.0201881 PMID: 30133533

Marczylo, E. L., Amoako, A. A., Konje, J. C., Gant, T. W., & Marczylo, T. H. (2012). Smoking induces differential miRNA expression in human spermatozoa: A potential transgenerational epigenetic concern? *Epigenetics*, *7*(5), 432–439. DOI: 10.4161/epi.19794 PMID: 22441141

Mehrpour, O., Karrari, P., Zamani, N., Tsatsakis, A. M., & Abdollahi, M. (2014). Occupational exposure to pesticides and consequences on male semen and Fertility: A review. *Toxicology Letters*, *230*(2), 146–156. DOI: 10.1016/j.toxlet.2014.01.029 PMID: 24487096

Miller, G. W., & Jones, D. P. (2014). The nature of nurture: Refining the definition of the exposome. *Toxicological Sciences*, *137*(1), 1–2. DOI: 10.1093/toxsci/kft251 PMID: 24213143

. Muthusami, K.R. & Chinnaswamy, P. (2005). Effect of chronic alcoholism on male fertility hormones and semen quality. *Fertil Steril.;*84(Wild, 2005):919-24.

Narayanan, D. L., Saladi, R. N., & Fox, J. L. (2010). Ultraviolet radiation and skin cancer. *International Journal of Dermatology*, *49*(9), 978–986. DOI: 10.1111/j.1365-4632.2010.04474.x PMID: 20883261

Nargund, V. H. (2015). Effects of psychological stress on male fertility. *Nature Reviews. Urology*, *12*(7), 373–382. DOI: 10.1038/nrurol.2015.112 PMID: 26057063

. Nieuwenhuijsen, M., Gulliver, J., Hoogh, K., Andersen, A-M, Friesen, M., Verner, M-A, Semple, S., Cherrie, J., Armstrong, B., Basagaña, X., Heederik, D., Schmitt, H., Suh, H., Hoek, G., Vrijheid, M., Dadvand, P., Villanueva, C., Levallois, P., Weisel, C. & van Tongeren, M. (2015). Exposure Assessment in Environmental Epidemiology. DOI: 10.1093/med/9780199378784.001.0001

Nilsson, C., Hessman, E., Sjöblom, H., Dencker, A., Jangsten, E., Mollberg, M., Patel, H., Sparud-Lundin, C., Wigert, H., & Begley, C. (2018). Definitions, measurements and prevalence of fear of childbirth: A systematic review. *BMC Pregnancy and Childbirth, 18*(1), 28. DOI: 10.1186/s12884-018-1659-7 PMID: 29329526

Nilsson, E. E., & Skinner, M. K. (2015). Environmentally Induced Epigenetic Transgenerational Inheritance of Reproductive Disease. *Biology of Reproduction, 93*(6), 145. DOI: 10.1095/biolreprod.115.134817 PMID: 26510870

O'Connell, S. G., Kincl, L. D., & Anderson, K. A. (2014). Silicone wristbands as personal passive samplers. *Environmental Science & Technology, 48*(6), 3327–3335. DOI: 10.1021/es405022f PMID: 24548134

Ostermeier, G. C., & Krawetz, S. A. (2005). *Spermatozoal RNAs as surrogate markers of paternal exposure.* Surrogate.

Patel, C. J., Bhattacharya, J., & Butte, A. J. (2010). An environment-wide association study (EWAS) on type 2 diabetes mellitus. *PLoS One, 5*(5), e10746. DOI: 10.1371/journal.pone.0010746 PMID: 20505766

. Perera, F.P., Chang, H.W., Tang, D., Roen, E.L., Herbstman, J., Margolis, A., Huang, T.J., Miller, R.L., Wang, S. & Rauh, V. (2014). Early-life exposure to polycyclic aromatic hydrocarbons and ADHD behavior problems. *PLoS One.* 5;9(11):e111670. .DOI: 10.1371/journal.pone.0111670

. Pfeifer, G.P., Denissenko, M.F., Olivier, M., Tretyakova, N., Hecht, S.S. & Hainaut, P. (2002). Tobacco smoke carcinogens, DNA damage and p53 mutations in smoking-associated cancers. *Oncogene.* 21;21(48):7435-51. .DOI: 10.1038/sj.onc.1205803

Plummer, F., Manea, L., Trepel, D., & McMillan, D. (2015). Screening for anxiety disorders with the GAD-7 and GAD-2: A systematic review and diagnostic meta analysis. *General Hospital Psychiatry, 39*, 24–31. DOI: 10.1016/j.genhosppsych.2015.11.005 PMID: 26719105

Puca, L., Vlachostergios, P. J., & Beltran, H. (2019). Neuroendocrine Differentiation in Prostate Cancer: Emerging Biology, Models, and Therapies. *Cold Spring Harbor Perspectives in Medicine, 9*(2), a030593. DOI: 10.1101/cshperspect.a030593 PMID: 29844220

Rappaport, S. M. (2011). Implications of the exposome for exposure science. *Journal of Exposure Science & Environmental Epidemiology, 21*(1), 5–9. DOI: 10.1038/jes.2010.50 PMID: 21081972

Rappaport, S. M., & Smith, M. T. (2010). Epidemiology. Environment and disease risks. *Science, 330*(6003), 460–461. DOI: 10.1126/science.1192603 PMID: 20966241

. Rasmussen, L., Poulsen, C. W., Kampmann, U., Smedegaard, S. B., Ovesen, P. G. & Fuglsang J. (2020). Diet and Healthy Lifestyle in the Management of Gestational Diabetes Mellitus. *Nutrients.* 6;12(10):3050. .DOI: 10.3390/nu12103050

Ren, S., He, K., & Girshick, R. (2015). Faster R-CNN: Towards Real-Time Object Detection with Region Proposal Networks. *Advances in Neural Information Processing Systems, 28*, 91–99.

. Reuter, S., Gupta, S.C., Chaturvedi, M.M., Aggarwal, B.B. (2010). Oxidative stress, inflammation, and cancer: how are they linked? *Free Radic Biol Med.* 1;49(11):1603-16. .DOI: 10.1016/j.freeradbiomed.2010.09.006

Rhomberg, L. R., & Goodman, J. E. (2012). Low-dose effects and nonmonotonic dose-responses of endocrine disrupting chemicals: Has the case been made? *Regulatory Toxicology and Pharmacology, 64*(1), 130–133. DOI: 10.1016/j.yrtph.2012.06.015 PMID: 22750031

Richmond, A. S., Boysen, G. A., Hudson, D. L., Gurung, R. A. R., Naufel, K. Z., Neufeld, G., Landrum, R. E., Dunn, D. S., & Beers, M. (2021). The Introductory Psychology Census: A national study. *Scholarship of Teaching and Learning in Psychology, 7*(3), 163–180. DOI: 10.1037/stl0000277

Richmond, D., Sibthorp, J., Gookin, J., Annarella, S., & Ferri, S. (2018). Complementing classroom learning through outdoor adventure education: Out-of-school-time experiences that make a difference. *Journal of Adventure Education and Outdoor Learning, 18*(1), 36–52. DOI: 10.1080/14729679.2017.1324313

Riley, R. D., Higgins, J. P., & Deeks, J. J. (2011). Interpretation of random effects meta-analyses. *BMJ (Clinical Research Ed.), 10*(feb10 2), 342–549. DOI: 10.1136/bmj.d549 PMID: 21310794

. Ross, R., Dagnone, D., Jones, P. J., Smith, H., Paddags, A., Hudson, R.and Janssen I. (2000). Reduction in obesity and related comorbid conditions after diet-induced weight loss or exercise-induced weight loss in men. A randomized, controlled trial. *Ann Intern Med.,* 18;133(2 92-103. .DOI: 10.7326/0003-4819-133-2-200007180-00008

. Ross, R., Dagnone, D., Jones, P. J., Smith, H., Paddags, A., Hudson, R. & Janssen I. (2000). Reduction in obesity and related comorbid conditions after diet-induced weight loss or exercise-induced weight loss in men. A randomized, controlled trial. *Ann Intern Med.* 18;133(2):92-103. .DOI: 10.7326/0003-4819-133-2-200007180-00008

Ruttkies, C., Schymanski, E. L., Wolf, S., Hollender, J., & Neumann, S. (2016). MetFrag relaunched: Incorporating strategies beyond in silico fragmentation. *Journal of Cheminformatics, 8*(1), 1–16. DOI: 10.1186/s13321-016-0115-9 PMID: 26834843

Sagiv, S. K., Bruno, J. L., Baker, J. M., Palzes, V., Kogut, K., Rauch, S., Gunier, R., Mora, A. M., Reiss, A. L., & Eskenazi, B. (2019). "Prenatal exposure to organophosphate pesticides and functional neuroimaging in adolescents living in proximity to pesticide application;" *Proceedings of the National Academy of Sciences of the United States of America*. DOI: DOI: 10.1073/pnas.1903940116

Sakhvidi, M. J. Z., Knobel, P., Bauwelinck, M., de Keijzer, C., Boll, L. M., Spano, G., & Dadvand, P. (2022). Greenspace exposure and children behavior: A systematic review. *The Science of the Total Environment, 824*, 153608. DOI: 10.1016/j.scitotenv.2022.153608 PMID: 35134416

Sakuma, K., Kitamura, A., Malins, A., Kurikami, H., Machida, M., Mori, K., Tada, K., Kobayashi, T., Tawara, Y., & Tosaka, H. (2017). Characteristics of radio-cesium transport and discharge between different basins near to the Fukushima Dai-ichi Nuclear Power Plant after heavy rainfall events. *Journal of Environmental Radioactivity, 169-170*, 137–150. DOI: 10.1016/j.jenvrad.2016.12.006 PMID: 28161603

. Sarigiannis, D.A. & Karakitsios, S.P. (2018). Addressing complexity of health impact assessment in industrially contaminated sites via the exposome paradigm. *Epidemiol Prev.,* 42(5-6S1):37-48. .DOI: 10.19191/EP18.5-6.S1.P037.086

Sender, R., Fuchs, S., & Milo, R. (2016). Are We really vastly outnumbered? revisiting the ratio of bacterial to host cells in humans. *Cell, 164*(3), 337–340. DOI: 10.1016/j.cell.2016.01.013 PMID: 26824647

Sermondade, N., Dupont, C., Faure, C., Boubaya, M., Cédrin-Durnerin, I., Chavatte-Palmer, P., Sifer, C., & Lévy, R. (2013). Body mass index is not associated with sperm–zona pellucida binding ability in subfertile males. *Asian Journal of Andrology, 15*(5), 626–629. DOI: 10.1038/aja.2013.10 PMID: 23770940

Shih, C., Tomita, N. L., Yanick, X., Reguera, Á. H., Fleisch, E., & Kowatsch, T. (2019). Breeze: Smartphone-based Acoustic Real-time Detection of Breathing Phases for a Gamified Biofeedback Breathing Training. *Proceedings of the ACM on Interactive, Mobile, Wearable and Ubiquitous Technologies, 3*(4), 152. Advance online publication. DOI: 10.1145/3369835

Smith, E. N., Romero, C., Donovan, B., Herter, R., Paunesku, D., Cohen, G. L., Dweck, C. S., & Gross, J. J. (2018). Emotion theories and adolescent well-being: Results of an online intervention. *Emotion (Washington, D.C.), 18*(6), 781–788. DOI: 10.1037/emo0000379 PMID: 29265838

Smith, S. (2021). Can Relational Feed-Forward Enhance Students' Cognitive and Affective Responses to Assessment? Teaching and Learning Inquiry: The *ISSOTL Journal.* ISSN 2167-4787 DOI: DOI: 10.20343/teachlearninqu.9.2.18

Snow, J. S. (1855). Cholera. The Commonwealth Fund; New York: 1936. On the mode of transmission of cholera.

Soubry, A., Hoyo, C., Butt, C. M., Fieuws, S., Price, T. M., Murphy, S. K., & Stapleton, H. M. (2017). Human exposure to flame-retardants is associated with aberrant DNA methylation at imprinted genes in sperm. *Environmental Epigenetics*, *13*(1). Advance online publication. DOI: 10.1093/eep/dvx003 PMID: 29492305

Steegers-Theunissen, R. P., Twigt, J., Pestinger, V., & Sinclair, K. D. (2013). The periconceptional period, reproduction and long-term health of offspring: The importance of one-carbon metabolism. *Human Reproduction Update*, *19*(6), 640–655. DOI: 10.1093/humupd/dmt041 PMID: 23959022

Stouder, C., & Paoloni-Giacobino, A. (2010). Transgenerational effects of the endocrine disruptor vinclozolin on the methylation pattern of imprinted genes in the mouse sperm. *Reproduction (Cambridge, England)*, *139*(2), 373–379. DOI: 10.1530/REP-09-0340 PMID: 19887539

Sulik, K. K. (2005). Genesis of alcohol-induced craniofacial dysmorphism. [Maywood]. *Experimental Biology and Medicine (Maywood, N.J.)*, *230*(6), 366–375. DOI: 10.1177/15353702-0323006-04 PMID: 15956766

Swanton, C., McGranahan, N., Starrett, G. J., & Harris, R. S. (2015). APOBEC Enzymes: Mutagenic Fuel for Cancer Evolution and Heterogeneity. *Cancer Discovery*, *5*(7), 704–712. DOI: 10.1158/2159-8290.CD-15-0344 PMID: 26091828

Torres-Cuevas, I., García Miralles, E., Ribelles Llop, M., & Marqués Martínez, L. (2021, February). Flipped Classroon en prácticas de ciencias de la salud. In IN-RED 2020: VI Congreso de Innovación Educativa y Docencia en Red (pp. 184-192). Editorial Universitat Politècnica de València.

Truong, L. K., Mosewich, A. D., Holt, C. J., Le, C. Y., Miciak, M., & Whittaker, J. L. (2020). Psychological, social and contextual factors across recovery stages following a sport-related knee injury: A scoping review. *British Journal of Sports Medicine*, *54*(19), 1149–1156. DOI: 10.1136/bjsports-2019-101206 PMID: 32060141

Turner, A. I., Smyth, N., Hall, S. J., Torres, S. J., Hussein, M., Jayasinghe, S. U., Ball, K., & Clow, A. J. (2020). Psychological stress reactivity and future health and disease outcomes: A systematic review of prospective evidence. *Psychoneuroendocrinology*, *114*, 104599. DOI: 10.1016/j.psyneuen.2020.104599 PMID: 32045797

Tyser, R. C., Mahammadov, E., Nakanoh, S., Vallier, L., Scialdone, A., & Srinivas, S. (2021). Single-cell transcriptomic characterization of a gastrulating human embryo. *Nature*, *600*(7888), 285–289. DOI: 10.1038/s41586-021-04158-y PMID: 34789876

Urdinguio, R. G., Bayón, G. F., Dmitrijeva, M., Toraño, E. G., Bravo, C., Fraga, M. F., Bassas, L., Larriba, S., & Fernández, A. F. (2015). Aberrant DNA methylation patterns of spermatozoa in men with unexplained infertility. *Human Reproduction (Oxford, England)*, *30*(5), 1014–1028. DOI: 10.1093/humrep/dev053 PMID: 25753583

Vandenberg, L. N., Colborn, T., Hayes, T. B., Heindel, J. J., Jacobs, D. R.Jr, Lee, D.-K., Shioda, T., Soto, A. M., vom Saal, F. S., Welshons, W. V., Zoeller, R. T., & Myers, J. P. (2012). Hormones and Endocrine-Disrupting Chemicals: Low-Dose Effects and Nonmonotonic Dose Responses. *Endocrine Reviews*, *33*(3), 378–455. DOI: 10.1210/er.2011-1050 PMID: 22419778

Vargesson, N. (2013). Thalidomide embryopathy: An enigmatic challenge. *ISRN Dev Biol*, *2013*, 1–18. DOI: 10.1155/2013/241016

Vermeulen, R., Schymanski, E. L., Barabasi, A.-L., & Miller, G. W. (2020). The exposome and health: Where chemistry meets biology. *Science*, *367*(6476), 392–396. DOI: 10.1126/science.aay3164 PMID: 31974245

Villalta, P. W., & Balbo, S. (2017). The Future of DNA Adductomic Analysis. *International Journal of Molecular Sciences*, *18*(9), 1870. DOI: 10.3390/ijms18091870 PMID: 32962318

Vineis, P., Avendano-Pabon, M., Barros, H., Bartley, M., Carmeli, C., Carra, L., Chadeau-Hyam, M., Costa, G., Delpierre, C., D'Errico, A., Fraga, S., Giles, G., Goldberg, M., Kelly-Irving, M., Kivimaki, M., Lepage, B., Lang, T., Layte, R., MacGuire, F., & Zins, M. (2020). Special Report: The Biology of Inequalities in Health: The Lifepath Consortium. *Frontiers in Public Health*, *8*, 118. DOI: 10.3389/fpubh.2020.00118 PMID: 32478023

Vrijheid, M., Casas, M., Gascon, M., Valvi, D., & Nieuwenhuijsen, M. (2016). Environmental pollutants and child health-A review of recent concerns. *International Journal of Hygiene and Environmental Health*, *219*(4-5), 331–342. DOI: 10.1016/j.ijheh.2016.05.001 PMID: 27216159

Vrijheid, M., Slama, R., Robinson, O., Chatzi, L., Coen, M., van den Hazel, P., Thomsen, C., Wright, J., Athersuch, T. J., Avellana, N., Basagaña, X., Brochot, C., Bucchini, L., Bustamante, M., Carracedo, A., Casas, M., Estivill, X., Fairley, L., van Gent, D., & Nieuwenhuijsen, M. J. (2014). The human early-life exposome (HELIX): Project rationale and design. *Environmental Health Perspectives*, *122*(6), 535–544. DOI: 10.1289/ehp.1307204 PMID: 24610234

Wang, Y. N., Zeng, Z. L., Lu, J. H., Wang, Y., Liu, Z. X., He, M. M., Zhao, Q., Wang, Z., Li, T., Lu, Y., Wu, Q., Yu, K., Wang, F., Pu, H.-Y., Li, B., Jia, W., shi, M., Xie, D., Kang, T., & Xu, R. (2018). CPT1A-mediated fatty acid oxidation promotes colorectal cancer cell metastasis by inhibiting anoikis. *Oncogene*, *37*(46), 6025–6040. DOI: 10.1038/s41388-018-0384-z PMID: 29995871

White, M. P., Elliott, L. R., Gascon, M., Roberts, B., & Fleming, L. E. (2020). Blue space, health and well-being: A narrative overview and synthesis of potential benefits. *Environmental Research*, *191*, 110169. DOI: 10.1016/j.envres.2020.110169 PMID: 32971082

Wild, C. P. (2012). The exposome: From concept to utility. *International Journal of Epidemiology*, *41*(1), 24–32. DOI: 10.1093/ije/dyr236 PMID: 22296988

Wild, J., Greenberg, N., Moulds, M. L., Sharp, M. L., Fear, N., Harvey, S., Wessely, S., & Bryant, R. A. (2020). Pre-incident Training to Build Resilience in First Responders: Recommendations on What to and What Not to Do. *Psychiatry*, *83*(2), 128–142. DOI: 10.1080/00332747.2020.1750215 PMID: 32338579

Wirth, J. J., & Mijal, R. S. (2010). Adverse effects of low-level heavy metal exposure on male reproductive function. *Systems Biology in Reproductive Medicine*, *56*(2), 147–167. DOI: 10.3109/19396360903582216 PMID: 20377313

. Wong, W. P., Hassed C, Chambers R. & Coles J. (2016). The Effects of Mindfulness on Persons with Mild Cognitive Impairment: Protocol for a Mixed-Methods Longitudinal Study. *Front Aging Neurosci*. 28;8:156. .DOI: 10.3389/fnagi.2016.00156

Woodruff, T. J., Zota, A. R., & Schwartz, J. M. (2011). Environmental chemicals in pregnant women in the United States: Nhanes 2003-2004. *Environmental Health Perspectives*, *119*(6), 878–885. DOI: 10.1289/ehp.1002727 PMID: 21233055

Wu, Y., Zhu, R. Y., Mitchell, L. A., Ma, L., Liu, R., Zhao, M., Jia, B., Xu, H., Li, Y. X., Yang, Z. M., Ma, Y., Li, X., Liu, H., Liu, D., Xiao, W. H., Zhou, X., Li, B. Z., Yuan, Y. J., & Boeke, J. D. (2018). In vitro DNA Scramble. *Nature Communications*, *1*(1), 1935. Advance online publication. DOI: 10.1038/s41467-018-03743-6 PMID: 29789594

Yan, C., Brunson, D. C., Tang, Q., Do, D., Iftimia, N. A., Moore, J. C., Hayes, M. N., Welker, A. M., Garcia, E. G., Dubash, T. D., Hong, X., Drapkin, B. J., Myers, D. T., Phat, S., Volorio, A., Marvin, D. L., Ligorio, M., Dershowitz, L., McCarthy, K. M., & Langenau, D. M. (2019). Visualizing Engrafted Human Cancer and Therapy Responses in Immunodeficient Zebrafish. *Cell*, *177*(7), 1903–1914.e14. DOI: 10.1016/j.cell.2019.04.004 PMID: 31031007

Ystrom, E., Gustavson, K., Brandlistuen, R. E., Knudsen, G. P., Magnus, P., Susser, E., Davey Smith, G., Stoltenberg, C., Surén, P., Håberg, S. E., Hornig, M., Lipkin, W. I., Nordeng, H., & Reichborn-Kjennerud, T. (2017). Prenatal Exposure to Acetaminophen and Risk of ADHD. *Pediatrics*, *140*(5), e20163840. DOI: 10.1542/peds.2016-3840 PMID: 29084830

Zhang, H., Gao, Y., Qian, P., Dong, Z., Hao, W., Liu, D., & Duan, X. (2019). Expression analysis of Rab11 during zebrafish embryonic development. *BMC Developmental Biology*, *19*(1), 25. DOI: 10.1186/s12861-019-0207-7 PMID: 31884948

Zhang, J., Wang, X., Vikash, V., Ye, Q., Wu, D., Liu, Y., & Dong, W. (2016). ROS and ROS-Mediated Cellular Signaling. *Oxidative Medicine and Cellular Longevity*, *4350965*(1), 4350965. Advance online publication. DOI: 10.1155/2016/4350965 PMID: 26998193

Zhang, Y., Han, L., He, Q., Chen, W., Sun, C., Wang, X., Chen, X., Wang, R., Hsiao, C. D., & Liu, K. (2017). A rapid assessment for predicting drug-induced hepatotoxicity using zebrafish. *Journal of Pharmacological and Toxicological Methods*, *84*, 102–110. DOI: 10.1016/j.vascn.2016.12.002 PMID: 27940076

Section 2

Disease-Specific Applications of Exposome into Cancer Risk Prediction

Chapter 2

Cervical Cancer Exposomics and the Impact of Environmental and Lifestyle Factors on Carcinogenesis

S. Athinarayanan
https://orcid.org/0000-0001-5362-9847
Sri Ramakrishna Mission Vidyalaya College of Arts and Science, India

K. Dhanakodi
Sri Ramakrishna Mission Vidyalaya College of Arts and Science, India

R. Kavitha
https://orcid.org/0000-0001-9812-2337
Vel Tech High Tech Dr. Rangarajan Dr. Sakunthala Engineering College, India

M. Robinson Joel
https://orcid.org/0000-0002-3030-8431
KCG College of Technology, India

S. Athinarayanan
Vel Tech Rangarajan Dr.Sagunthala R&D Institute of Science and Technology, India

A.T. Rajamanickam
Sri Ramakrishna Mission Vidyalaya College of Arts and Science, India

A. Sanjaygandhi
Sri Ramakrishna Mission Vidyalaya College of Arts and Science, India

S. Muthukumar
PSN College of Engineering and Technology, India

ABSTRACT

Cervical cancer remains a significant public health concern, particularly in low- and middle-income countries. While human papillomavirus (HPV) infection is a well-established primary cause, emerging research highlights the role of environmental

DOI: 10.4018/979-8-3373-5796-6.ch002

Copyright © 2026, IGI Global Scientific Publishing. Copying or distributing in print or electronic forms without written permission of IGI Global Scientific Publishing is prohibited.

exposures, lifestyle factors, and socioeconomic conditions in modulating carcinogenesis. This chapter explores the concept of cancer exposomics in the context of cervical cancer, emphasizing the cumulative impact of chemical pollutants, dietary habits, occupational hazards, and lifestyle factors on disease progression. The interplay between HPV infection, environmental toxins (such as endocrine disruptors and heavy metals), and immune system modulation is discussed. Additionally, the chapter highlights the significance of early screening, vaccination, and personalized interventions in mitigating the risk. By integrating exposomic research with molecular epidemiology, this study provides insights into novel preventive and therapeutic strategies for cervical cancer management.

INTRODUCTION TO CANCER EXPOSOMICS

Exposomics is the field of studying the impact of environmental factors in the formation of cancer. Air pollution, chemical additives, and eating habits that are exposed to a lifetime can cause biological changes. By examining these changes, the initial diagnosis and prevention of cancer can be improved. Cancer Exposomics is a pioneering sector that combines many fields such as medicine, biology, and quality analysis. Priyadarshini et al. (2023) conducted a study where they discovered that in patients undergoing chemotherapy and radiotherapy, dying cancer cells release chromosomal fragments. These fragments travel through the bloodstream and may cause cancer to grow in new locations. This finding provides a new perspective on metastasis (the spread of cancer). This discovery could lead to new research aimed at preventing cancer recurrence. Goyal et al. (2022) highlighted that CAR-T Therapy represents a significant advancement in cancer treatment. In this approach, a patient's immune cells are modified and this therapy more affordable in India, reducing side effects and increasing its effectiveness.

Cancer is a condition where cells proliferate uncontrollably in the human body. It can manifest in various forms and can be caused by numerous environmental and lifestyle factors. A major field that studies the root causes of cancer is exposomics by Wild et al. (2013). Ren et al. (2011) encompasses all external influences one faces throughout their lifetime as air pollution, chemicals, dietary habits, lifestyle practices, etc. Exposomics is a field that examines how environmental impacts affect the human body, apart from genetic information. It is a modern discipline that has emerged from recent research developments. Through exposomics, it becomes possible to foresee the likelihood of an individual developing any type of cancer. This helps protect an individual's health., Bhowmik et al. (2015) exposomics studies, it is possible to identify the environmental impacts leading to cancer in advance and devise ways to avoid them. This opens new avenues in disease prevention. Furthermore, this field can play a crucial role in personalizing treatment for individuals. Thus, cancer exposomics is seen as a revolutionary advancement in future healthcare.

Exposomes are classified into three main categories: immediate (Internal), specific external (Specific external), and general external. Immediate exposomes refer to the biological changes occurring inside the body, hormone levels, and events related to sensitivity. Calder et al. (2020) explore the Specific external exposomes refer to factors such as pollution, smoking, and radiation. All of these can cause changes in cells and increase the likelihood of cancer. Advanced research methods are used in Kasar Exposomics. In particular, through new technologies that analyze metabolomics, proteomics, genomics, and biological data, it becomes possible to explain the changes that occur based on a person's health condition and environment. As a result of Plummer et al. (2003) is possible to assess the risks faced by an individual and prepare for treatment. The relationship between smoking and cervical cancer has also been extensively studied and Moreno et al. (2002) highlighted in cancer exposomics research is possible to identify the environmental and lifestyle factors responsible for the prevalent cancers in a community, allowing the government and health organizations to take necessary actions. This helps in improving community health. Furthermore, it can raise awareness among people and promote a healthy lifestyle. By integrating a person's environmental and lifestyle data through exposomics, it is possible to predict in advance if they are at risk of developing any cancer. Bray et al. (2012) focus on early detection of cancer and the provision of personalized medicine. This creates a pathway to offer a patient the best treatment with fewer side effects. Currently, various research activities are ongoing worldwide in the field of exposomics. Specifically, efforts are being made to further elucidate the insights of cancer through long-term monitoring projects involving a large number of people. It is expected that this field will bring about significant changes in medicine, public health, and environmental policies in the future. Feil & Fraga (2012) further elaborated as Cancer does not arise from a single cause. It is formed by various changes occurring in genes and the environment. Exposomics helps to understand these complex relationships. By integrating the various aspects of Athinarayanan, S., et al. (2025) like an individual's health status, environment, diet, and mental state, it provides a comprehensive view of how the disease develops.

Aguayo et al. (2020) focussed on studying the likelihood of cancer occurring in groups with low immunity, such as children and pregnant women. Specifically, studies indicate that air pollution, chemicals, and nutritional deficiencies faced by a woman during pregnancy can lead to cancer in subsequent generations. Calder et al. (2020) emphasize that Exposomics is a field that requires extensive and non-abridged data. Completely recording a person's lifestyle and subjecting it to examination poses a significant challenge. Additionally, gathering data from areas with poverty, educational shortages, and lack of medical facilities is difficult.

DEFINITION OF EXPOSOMICS IN CANCER RESEARCH

Athinarayanan & Srinath (2012) introduced the Modern sensor technologies are being used to address this. Exposomics provides us with an important message: our lifestyles have a direct impact on our health. By reducing habits such as smoking, alcohol consumption, processed foods, and lack of sleep, we can lower the risk of cancer. Therefore, raising awareness among people is very important. Athinarayanan et.al (2017) discovered exposomics play a critical role in the policies established by governments and public health organizations. For example, regulations on pollutants emitted from factories, air quality measurements, and food safety regulations transform into cancer prevention actions. Vermeulen et al. (2020) discussed exposomics is still an evolving field that continuous research in this area, along with modern tools and data techniques, will generate new approaches to reduce the incidence of cancer. These studies have the potential not only to improve an individual's personal health but also to enhance the health standards of a community.

Wu et al. (2023) mention that outdoor air pollution is classified as carcinogenic to humans by the World Health Organization (WHO). Their study indicates that particulate matter (PM2.5) in the air and various toxins can affect women's internal organs, possibly increasing the risk of cervical cancer. Hamanaka & Mutlu (2018) have researched that environmental pollution and chemical exposures are significant public health issues causing severe cancers globally. In particular, they note that persistent organic pollutants, which continuously affect the human body, may further exacerbate the risk of cervical cancer.

Harper & DeMars. (2017) state that endocrine-disrupting chemicals such as phthalates and bisphenol A (BPA) alter the hormone levels in the body during stages of female development, allowing the HPV virus to persist, which can subsequently increase the likelihood of developing cervical cancer. These chemicals weaken immune function, thereby creating an environment conducive to persistent infections. Alavanja et al. (2013) emphasize the need for personalized risk assessment based on the individual exposure history for each person. The field of exposomics opens pathways for this, as it helps in compiling and analyzing comprehensive data related to a person's biology, environment, diet, and genetics.

IMPORTANCE OF STUDYING ENVIRONMENTAL AND LIFESTYLE FACTORS IN CARCINOGENESIS

Cancer is a disease caused by genetic changes and external factors. The environment and lifestyle play an important role in its creation. Research in animals and humans has proven that environmental pollution, chemicals, radiation, smoking, and habits have proven that cancer can be triggered. Explosion of such factors can prevent cancer and improve therapeutic methods. Air and water pollution, factory and agricultural liquid chemicals, and mineral fuel emissions are important in environmental factors. Various chemicals and body radiations are DNA. Damage can be triggered by cancer. In particular, people living in smokers are more likely to be affected by the pollution surrounding them. Therefore, by identifying environmental impacts, it is possible to protect the health of the public. Lifestyle factors include bodybuilding, eating habits, body movement, and irregular sleep regulations. Intake of excessive foods of sugar and cholesterol, such as alcohol and smoking, increases the risk of cancer. If body movement is low, the body will gain weight, the hormonal balance will be affected, and the positive environment for the development of cancer. By examining environmental and lifestyle factors, immunity can be developed. To control cancer, people need to adhere to a firm lifestyle change. Reducing cancer can be taken by avoiding hazardous habits such as healthy eating habits, proper exercise, cleaning environment, and smoking. Cancer formation or carcinogenic refers to the growth of genetic mutations in neurons.

Environmental factors serve as the main stimulation of carcinogenicity. Air, water and soil pollution, chemicals released from factories, and metals, etc., cause genetic changes. In particular, the impact of smoke and radiation directly affects the DNA and the cells are uncontrollable. When these external carcinogens have a long impact on the body, the risk of cancer increases. Some of the habits in the lifestyle can be greatly affected by carcinogenicity. Smoking, alcohol consumption, non -nutritional eating habits, and the lack of body movement can cause cancer formation of neurons. Feng & Yang (2012) classified outdoor air pollution as a Group 1 carcinogen (a highly dangerous cancer-causing agent). Toxic air pollutants increases the risk of lung cancer, bladder cancer, and skin cancer. Additionally, lifestyle habits such as smoking, alcohol consumption, and poor diet contribute to carcinogenesis (cancer development) and DNA mutations.

HOW EXPOSOMICS APPLIES TO CERVICAL CANCER

Cancer formation or carcinogenesis is the result of genetic mutations in the body's cells and refers to uncontrolled growth. This process takes place in several stages, promotion, and programs. First, the DNA in neurons (cells). (DNA) Damage (Initiation). Since then, the impact of some factors has increased the promotion. Eventually, uncontrolled growth and metastasis to other parts of the body, cancer develops. This entire process is greatly affected by environmental and lifestyle factors. Exposure to environmental and occupational hazards has been widely studied for its significant role in cancer development. Research highlights various factors, including pesticides, air pollution, chemicals, and lifestyle habits, as major contributors to increased cancer risks.

Pesticide exposure among farm workers and industrial chemical handlers has been linked to higher incidences of cancer. Alavanja et al. (2013) emphasize how various environmental impacts such as environmental and occupational factors create the risk of cancer in the human body. They state that a new field called exposomics, which takes these exposures into account, could be an open avenue to understand oral cavity cancer. Rao et al. (2018) illustrate in their study that high exposure to industrial chemicals may increase the risk of oral cavity cancer. Chemical interactions in occupational tasks and job opportunities can impact the body's normal gene functions.

Sharma et al. (2023) classify outdoor air pollution as a significant factor for cancer. They state that widely prevalent polluted air creates conditions over the long term that can trigger cervical cancer, related to the HPV virus. Zur Hausen et al. (2018) have studied how long-term environmental exposures lead to reduced immune function in women's internal genital areas and hormonal imbalances, allowing HPV infections to persist. Plummer et al. (2003) and Feng & Yang (2012) note that smoking is one of the major environmental factors that contribute to the development of oral cavity cancer. Smoking can suppress the immune system in a way that exacerbates the effects of the Human Papillomavirus (HPV). Frew et al. (2016) explain that the chemicals found in the environment can cause epigenetic changes in genes, leading to processes that create cancer. In particular, these changes may have the property of preventing cells from dying normally.

Harper & DeMars. (2017) argue that endocrine-disrupting chemicals found in the environment—such as bisphenol A (BPA) and phthalates—affect hormone regulation and immune functions, increasing the chances of HPV virus persistence. This creates conditions for the development of cervical cancer. Ho et al. (2012) explain how genetic and environmental factors combine to create pathways for cancer development. In their view, expressions always have bidirectional traits that either enhance or diminish genetic properties. Jayshree et al. (2009) explain the factors for the high prevalence of HPV infection among young women and the conditions that allow this infection to persist. They state that bodily health, environmental conditions, and lifestyle habits directly affect the persistence of HPV infection. Calder et al. (2020) emphasize that environmental factors such as anthropogenic pollutants and nutritional deficiencies can impact cellular immune functions. As a result, the effect of the HPV virus may persist, increasing the risk of cells in the cervix becoming cancerous.

Environmental factors act as carcinogens and convert genes in cells. Factory pollution, chemicals, radiation, and air, water pollution, etc. There will be a change in the structure. In particular, vehicle smoke, agricultural pesticides, and hormonal mixed foods in animals lead to uncontrollable cells. Some of the habits in the life-style increases the process of carcinogenic. Smoking, alcohol consumption, the lack of physical movement, and the consuming of nutritious foods can affect the body's cells. The contents of nicotine and tarin (TAR) in the cause of smoking stimulate lung cancer. Similarly, foods in high sugar and fat can increase body weight and cause chest and bowel cancer. The lack of physical movement reduces the immune system and affects the normal growth of the cells. sharma et al. (2023) found that Human Papillomavirus (HPV) infection is a primary cause of cervical cancer.

CERVICAL CANCER AND ITS PRIMARY ETIOLOGY

Cervical Cancer is a cancer that develops in the neck of the uterus. The primary cause of this includes the Human Papilloma virus (HPV - Human Papillomavirus) infection. In particular, the long -term HPV infection changes the genes of the cells and stimulates uncontrolled growth. Some types of HPV (mainly TYPE 16 and TYPE 18) are highly accompanied by and most of the cervical cancer are considered factors. Zur Hausen (2009) identified Human Papillomavirus (HPV) infection as the primary cause of cervical cancer. High-risk HPV types such as HPV-16 and HPV-18 disrupt genetic regulation in cells, activating oncogenes (E6, E7) and triggering cancer development.

Role of HPV in cervical cancer

Human papilloma virus is considered the first cause of Cervical Cancer. HPV is a common viral family, of which there are more than 100 types. Although some of these types are low (Low-Risk HPV), especially HPV 16 and HPV 18, with high-Risk HPV. These high-risk HPV varieties change the genes of cervix cells and stimulate uncontrolled growth. Long -term HPV infection can lead to the nature of the cells (dysplasia), and then cancer. HPV virus infection is usually transmitted by intercourse. As mentioned earlier, HPV-16 and HPV-18 interfere with cellular genetic control, leading to uncontrolled cell growth and increasing the risk of cervical cancer. There are important measures to prevent cervical cancer caused by HPV virus. Paying HPV vaccine (HPV vaccine) protects from the impact of this virus. Specially, taking a vaccine at a young age will provide great protection. Also, the infection can be diagnosed at an early stage with Pap Smear and HPV testing and can undergo rapid treatment. Service can be reduced by HPV virus with proper awareness, safe lifestyle and preventive measures.

INTERACTION OF GENETIC PREDISPOSITION WITH ENVIRONMENTAL FACTORS

Genes play an important role in the health and immunization of the human body. Some may naturally be at risk of specific diseases, which are referred to as genetic predisposition or genetic risk. The main example of this is that in a family, cancer, diabetes, or heart disease. But only genes cannot cause a disease; Environmental factors also play an important role. Environmental factors include a person's lifestyle, eating habits, air pollution, chemicals, and stress. This risk can be reduced by changing the lifestyle, even if a person has a risk of a particular disease by geneticism. For example, if a person's family has a history of heart disease, if you follow the right diet, training, smoking and avoiding alcohol, reduces the chance of the disease.

When the environmental factors and genes work together, some diseases appear more. For example, for a person living in an environment where smoking and air pollution, if they are at risk of lung diseases in the gene, the disease is exposed very quickly. Similarly, if UV is more prone to radiation, some people may increase the risk of skin cancer. This clearly shows the connection with genetic and environmental factors. Moreno et al. (2002) discovered that genetic mutations (e.g., MLH1, APC genes) combined with environmental factors (e.g., diet, smoking, air pollution) increase the risk of colorectal cancer. Lewandowska (2018) found that exposure to benzene along with genetic susceptibility increases the risk of leukemia (blood cancer). Genetic variations in CYP2E1 and NQO1 genes alter benzene metabolism, leading to DNA damage in cells. Understanding of geneticism and environmental factors is very important for disease prevention.

Figure 1. **Genetic Environment Interaction**

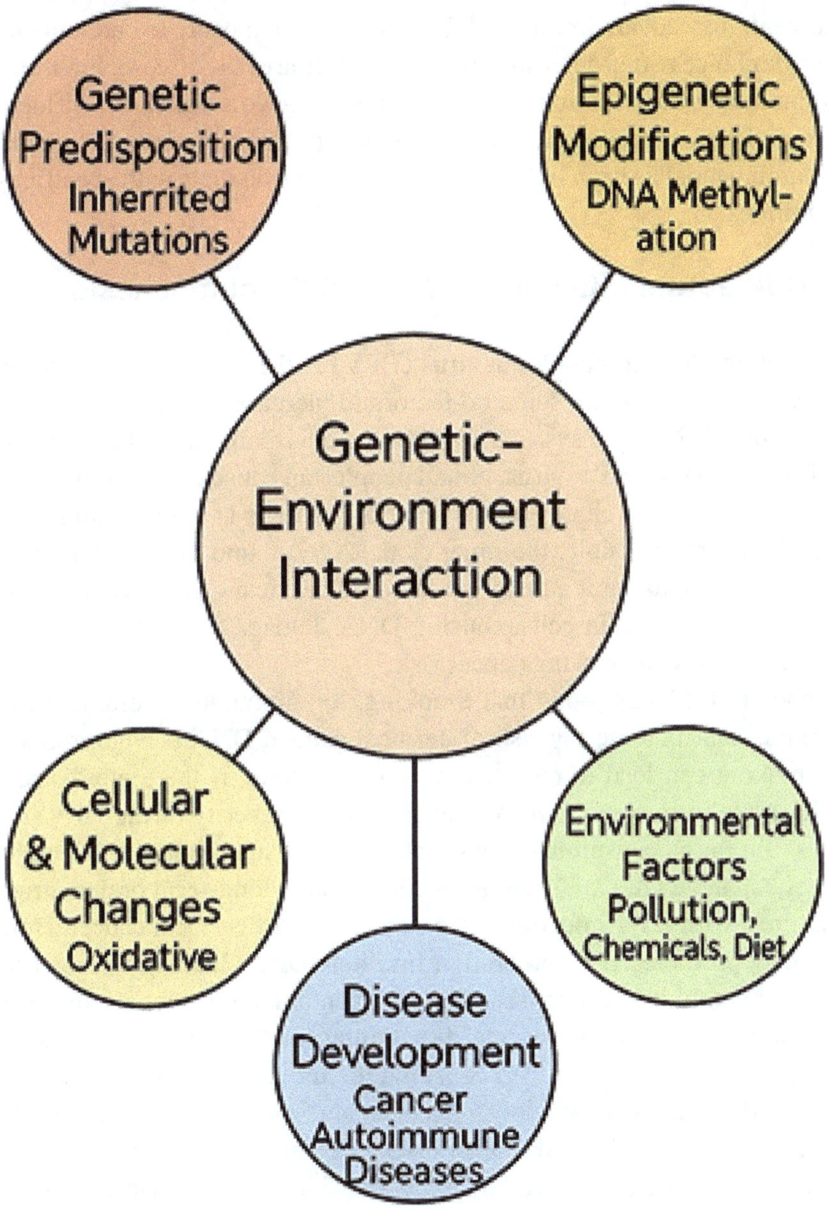

Genetic Environment Interaction is given in Figure.1.Genetic predisposition refers to inherited variations in DNA that make certain individuals more vulnerable to cancer. However, the presence of these mutations alone does not guarantee cancer development. Instead, environmental factors such as exposure to carcinogens, diet, and lifestyle choices often determine the manifestation of the disease. Environmental factors, including air pollution, chemicals, and tobacco smoke, can influence the expression of cancer-related genes. For instance, prolonged exposure to benzene, a known carcinogen, has been linked to leukemia in individuals with specific genetic susceptibilities.

Other Co-Factors Influencing Cervical Carcinogenesis

Although the human papilloma virus (HPV) is the main cause of the creation of cervical cancer, there are some co-factors to increase its impact. These factors may be the body's immune system, lifestyle and environmental related. Although a person is infected with HPV virus, not all people can cause cancer. But, if there are specific co -factors, the change in the gene of the cells is possible and the development of cancer is possible. Plummer et al. (2003) found that smoking increases HPV persistence, making it a major co-factor in cervical cancer. Tobacco-specific carcinogens accumulate in cells, causing DNA damage and reducing the body's ability to clear HPV, increasing cancer risk.

Moreno et al. (2002) found that Smoking, low immune system, and irregular eating habits can increase the risk of cervical cancer. DNA change in body cells due to smoking can lead to cancer development. Also, if there are diseases like HIV (HIV), the immune system is reduced and the severity of the HPV infection increases. Similarly, consuming foods that are low in antioxidant nutrients such as vitamin A, C, and e (A, C, E) can make cells unsafe. long-term oral contraceptive use combined with HPV infection increases the risk of cervical cancer. Hormonal changes may promote HPV integration into host DNA, leading to increased cell proliferation and higher cancer risk. Environmental factors such as air, water and food pollution can affect the normal functioning of the cells. Increased chances of cervical cancer for women who consume the most of the factory pollution and chemicals. Also, marrying at a lower age, frequent pregnancy and unprotected intercourse can have a prolonged impact on Service and increase the risk of cancer. Therefore, controlling these parallel factors may increase the chance of preventing cervical cancer.

ENVIRONMENTAL EXPOSURES AND CERVICAL CANCER RISK

Environmental pollution, chemicals, and toxins in the air may increase the risk of cervical cancer. Earth and water pollution that can be affected by a long time can cause changes in the genes of cells. The smoking and factory pollution is also the main factors. If you live in a healthy environment, this disease can reduce the risk. Exposure to environmental and occupational hazards has been widely studied for its significant role in cancer development. Alavanja et al. (2013) emphasize that environmental factors, particularly chemicals, significantly increase the risk of various cancers, especially cervical cancer, when they accumulate in the body over long periods. As they mention, these exposures can potentially affect the genetic information of body cells. Landrigan et al. (2018) have clearly demonstrated in their study that occupational chemical exposures significantly increase the risk of cervical cancer in women. In particular, prolonged exposure to chemicals like solvents and pharmaceuticals in factories poses a risk of altering normal cell growth. The explanation regarding the relation between environmental chemicals and cervical cancer is presented in Figure 2. It highlights that important chemicals found in the environment phthalates, bisphenol A, and other substances — affect the body's hormonal balance and immune functions, contributing to the persistence of the HPV virus and the development of cervical cancer. Air pollution has now been identified as one of the major environmental hazards for cancer development. Furthermore, the fine particulate matter and carcinogenic gases in the air pose a risk of disrupting the genetic functions of cells in women's reproductive organs.

Figure 2. **Environmental Chemicals and Cervical Cancer Relation**

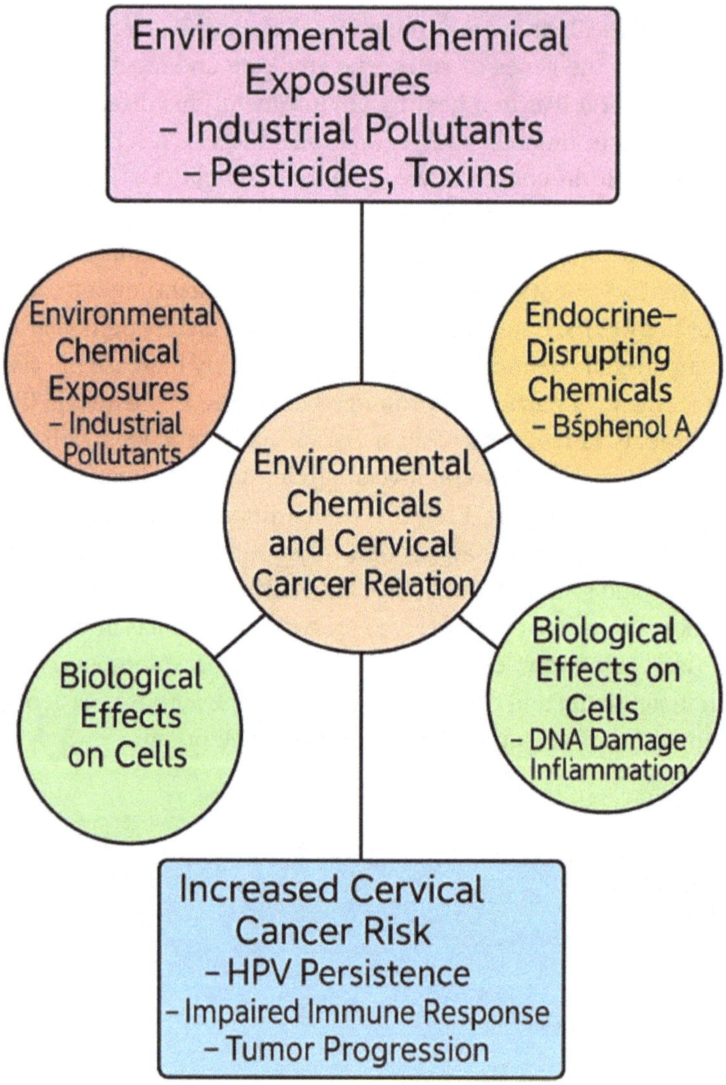

Jayshree et al. (2009) refer to the classification by the World Health Organization that outdoor air pollution is a causative factor for cancer in humans. In their study, it is mentioned that particulate matter such as PM2.5 and carcinogens formed from the burning of diesel fuel may create an environment conducive to the persistence of the HPV virus and the development of cervical cancer. Morgan et al. (2017) investigate the long-term effects of environmental pollutants on the body, particularly explaining how changes in women's hormones and immune systems can lead to the persistence of the HPV virus and the associated risk of cervical cancer. Jockel et al. (1998) conducted a study that explored the link between occupational chemical exposures and cervical cancer risk. The study identified that toxic chemicals such as organic solvents, pesticides, and heavy metals contribute to increased HPV persistence and DNA damage. These chemicals induce oxidative stress, which impairs apoptosis and repair mechanisms, thereby increasing cancer susceptibility.

Endocrine-Disrupting Chemicals (e.g., Bisphenol A, Phthalates)

Endocrine -Disrupting Chemicals - EDCS are chemicals that are capable of affecting the hormonal balance in the human body and changing the normal endocrine function of the body. Chemicals such as Bisphenol A (Bisphenol A - BPA) and phthalates are usually found in plastic products, food packets, cosmetics and some medications. If these chemicals enter the body, the growth of the cells, the reproductive function, and the immune system can be affected. If chemicals go into the body, it can act like natural hormones and change the body's configuration. For example, Bisphenol A is the disruption of the function of the hormone called estrogen, which can increase the risk of reproductive disorders, pregnancy and cancer in women. Phthalates can affect neurological development and can cause developmental problems in children. Therefore, it is important to reduce the use of these chemicals, avoid plastic products, use lush alternatives and carry out a healthy lifestyle. Goyal et al. (2022) found that Bisphenol A (BPA), a common endocrine-disrupting chemical (EDC), alters estrogen receptor (ER) signalling, leading to uncontrolled cell proliferation and genomic instability. BPA can facilitate HPV integration, thereby increasing cervical cancer risk. Harper & DeMars. (2017) demonstrated that phthalates, commonly used as plasticizers, can trigger cervical carcinogenesis via epigenetic modifications such as DNA methylation and histone modifications. Specifically, Di(2-ethylhexyl) phthalate (DEHP) and butyl benzyl phthalate (BBP) were shown to enhance HPV-driven oncogenic pathways.

Heavy Metals (Arsenic, Cadmium, Lead) And Their Role in DNA Damage

Arsenic, Cadmium, and Lead (Lead), such as Arsenic, and Lead, cause serious damage to the human body by water, soil and food. This cadmium can change the DNA system in the cells of the body and create mutations in the genes. In particular, long -term arsenic intake can increase the risk of cancer by affecting cell growth and supply function. Similarly, cannabis such as cadmium and lead can create oxidative stress in cells and lead to DNA damage and death of cells. Once the cannabis goes into the body, they affect the gene of the cells and cause DNA strand breaks. Because of this, the cells can naturally become uncontrolled and become cancer. In addition, these cadmiums are long -lasting in the body, causing kidney disorders, neurological disorders, and reproductive problems. Therefore, it is an important precautionary measure to control the use of these cannabis and adopt cleanliness water and safe eating habits. Ren et al. (2011) found that arsenic exposure leads to alterations in DNA methylation, affecting gene function. Arsenic-induced oxidative stress causes DNA strand breaks and mutational accumulation, particularly affecting tumor suppressor genes like p53 and Rb, thus increasing cancer risk. Athinarayanan et al. (2017) reported that cadmium (Cd) and lead (Pb) inhibit DNA repair mechanisms, leading to genomic instability. Cadmium increases telomerase activity, promoting uncontrolled cell division, while reactive oxygen species (ROS) generation contributes to chromosomal instability. Lead, on the other hand, induces DNA cross-linking and strand breaks, leading to genotoxic stress.

Air Pollution And Its Immunomodulatory Effects

Air pollution is the biggest threat to the health of the human body. Factories, automotive smoke, and chemical waste emit toxic substances such as micro -dusting (particulate matter - PM), nitrogen di-oxide (NO_2), Sulphur di-Oxide (SO_2), and organic compounds in the yuki. These pollutants affect the immune system of the body and reduce the anti -inflammatory force of diseases. Air pollution is considered a significant environmental hazard that can affect various cellular functions of the human body, particularly the efficiency of the immune system. Long-term exposure to particulate matter (PM2.5, PM10), nitrogen dioxide, ozone, and certain volatile organic compounds can alter the immune responses of the body. Those exposed to such pollution may find themselves in a state of losing the ability to fight off viral and bacterial infections. In particular, in women, this pollution can cause hormonal disruptions, leading to persistent infections like HPV and increasing the risk of diseases such as cervical cancer. Therefore, the implications of air pollution on the immune system can lead to weakened bodily conditions and severe disease attacks.

OCCUPATIONAL AND LIFESTYLE FACTORS:

Additionally, dietary habits, alcohol consumption, and obesity promote chronic inflammation and hormonal imbalances, increasing cancer progression risk. Ramamoorthy et al. (2024) studied how occupational exposures and lifestyle factors can increase the risk of lung cancer. Specifically, chronic exposure to chemical substances such as asbestos, diesel exhaust, and polycyclic aromatic hydrocarbons (PAHs) in the workplace contributes to this risk. Additionally, lifestyle habits such as smoking, alcohol consumption, and poor diet further elevate cancer risk, primarily through synergistic effects that cause DNA damage and oxidative stress.

Exposure to Pesticides And Industrial Chemicals

Pesticides and industrial chemicals are widely used in modern times. If the most used pesticides in agriculture enters the body, the body will absorb its green viruses. This can cause neurological disorders, pregnancy problems and sometimes cancer. In particular, people living in rural areas are at risk of pesticides to enter the body through water and soil pollution. Some chemicals in industrial chemicals, handheld products, food packs and cosmetics may affect the body's cells and hormonal balance. If these chemicals continue to go into the body, DNA can create changes in the gene and increase the risk of cancer. Workers working in factories can breathe or absorb these chemicals daily, and it can cause prolonged physical effects. Therefore, it is important to adopt safe work procedures, toxic prevention, and healthy eating habits. Alavanja et al. (2013) found that prolonged exposure to pesticides such as organophosphates and carbamates, along with industrial chemicals like benzene and formaldehyde, induces DNA damage and endocrine disruption. These toxic substances lead to immune suppression and genomic instability, increasing the risk of leukemia, lymphoma, and solid tumors.

Smoking and Its Synergy with HPV Infection

Smoking is an important factor that affects the various organs of the body. Toxic substances in the smoke may change the DNA system of cells in the lungs, oral, and intestinal tract and increase the risk of cancer. In particular, smoking can affect the body's immune system will submit the body to virus and bacterial infections. Human Papilloma Virus (HPV) is a virus transmitted virus, It is the main cause of female cervical cancer. Smoking can continue to develop the cancer changes of cells for those who are infected with HPV.

If smokers suffer from HPV infection, their body will naturally lose the ability to destroy the virus. Toxic substances such as nitrosamines and benzene, especially nitrosamines, and benzene, increase the possibility of cancer in the genes of cells in the carcinoma area. Also, smoking women are more likely to be infected with HPV infection, and it may increase the severity of the disease. Therefore, reducing or complete stopping smoking is an important precautionary measure that reduces the serious effects of the HPV infection. Giuliano et al. (2002) reported that cigarette smoking and HPV infection act synergistically to increase cervical cancer risk. Tobacco-specific nitrosamines (TSNAs) and reactive oxygen species (ROS) contribute to DNA damage and immune suppression, leading to enhanced HPV persistence and tumor suppressor gene inactivation.

Poor Dietary Patterns And Nutritional Deficiencies Affecting Immune Response

With symmetric eating habits, the body's immune system is weakened. Eating excessive foods, fat and sugar can affect the body's immunity. Vitamins and mineral nutrients are consumed by fewer foods, and the body's cells cannot perform immune functions properly. In particular, if nutrients such as vitamin C, vitamin D, iron and zinc are low, there is a high resistance to physical illness. Minerals and low eating habits can cause viral infections such as vaccination in the body, leading to the body infections. In addition, protein fewer foods prevent the growth of cells, which reduce the production of white blood cells that resist diseases. This, in turn, can cause prolonged infections and weak immune system. Therefore, consuming foods rich in nutrients for the body is important to prevent diseases and protect physical health. Calder et al. (2020) found that deficiencies in micronutrients such as Vitamin C, D, Zinc, and Selenium impair immune response by reducing T-cell activation, antibody production, and cytokine regulation. Unhealthy dietary patterns, including processed foods and excessive sugar intake, contribute to chronic inflammation and immune dysregulation, increasing infection susceptibility.

SOCIOECONOMIC AND LIFESTYLE INFLUENCES ON CERVICAL CANCER PROGRESSION

Socioeconomic and Lifestyle Influences on Cervical Cancer Progression regarding Figure.3 is given below.

Figure 3. **Socioeconomic and Lifestyle Influences on Cervical Cancer Progression**

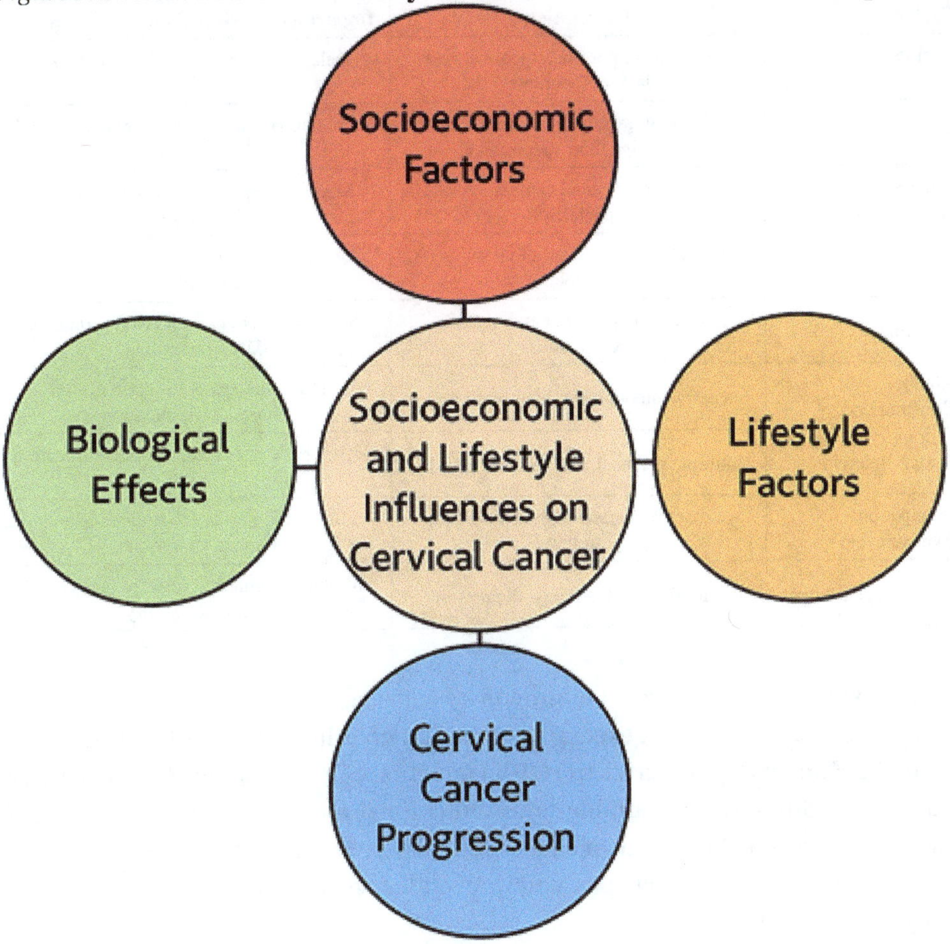

The progression of Cervical Cancer can be affected by many factors, in which socioeconomic condition has an important impact. There may be great problems with access to medical facilities for people who are uneducated and illiterate, which will delay the identification of the disease. Preventive measures such as monthly medical tests and Pap Smear test are often available to people living in economically prosperous society, but this is a challenge for low income. This, in turn, increases the chance of being diagnosed in a disadvantaged phase without being diagnosed with the initial stage of the disease. Socioeconomic and Lifestyle Influences factors with its description as well as its impact on Cervical Cancer Progression details given in Table.1.

Table 1. Socioeconomic and Lifestyle Influences on Cervical Cancer Progression

Factor	Description	Impact on Cervical Cancer Progression
Socioeconomic Status	Low income, poor healthcare access, lack of insurance	Delayed diagnosis, limited treatment options
Education Level	Lack of awareness about HPV, screening, and vaccination	Increased risk due to poor prevention and late detection
Healthcare Accessibility	Distance to medical centers, lack of specialists	Missed screenings, delayed treatment initiation
Nutritional Deficiencies	Poor diet, lack of essential vitamins (A, C, E, folate)	Weakened immune response, increased susceptibility
Smoking	Tobacco exposure, carcinogenic compounds	Synergistic effect with HPV, promotes DNA mutations
Alcohol Consumption	Excessive alcohol use, liver dysfunction	Alters immune response, contributes to chronic inflammation
Sexual Behavior	Multiple partners, early sexual activity	Higher HPV exposure, persistent infection risk
Occupational Exposure	Contact with carcinogens, industrial pollutants	Increased risk of DNA damage and immune suppression
Psychological Stress	Chronic stress, anxiety, depression	Weakens immune system, reduces HPV clearance ability

Lifestyle can also increase the growth of cervical cancer. The immune system can be affected by smoking, excessive habit of alcoholism, and the low body. As a result, the Human Papilloma Virus (HPV) infection can be prolonged and can cause many times. Similarly, consuming fewer nutritional foods can reduce the immune system and increase the growth of cancer cells. Therefore, adopting socio -economic facilities and healthy lifestyle can help prevent cervical cancer and reduce the severity of the disease.

Impact of Healthcare Access And Education

The inability to properly obtain medical services delays the identification and prevention of many diseases. In particular, people who are in low economy are facing problems with diagnosing and receiving treatment at an early stage of hospitals and tests. Due to the lack of excellent medical services, rural people and economically disadvantaged people are inevitably affected by various infectious diseases and cancer. To reduce these problems, government and private sectors must make joint ventures and increase hospitals and testing camps. Education is the basic component of a healthy life. If people are aware of medical awareness, you can find out about vaccines, health, and healthy lifestyles. For example, if women are aware of the importance of the PAP Smear test, cervical cancer can be diagnosed at an early stage. Similarly, educated people will focus more on diet, exercise, and immunization methods. Therefore, improving medical services and education is an important way for the whole health of the community.

Bray et al. (2012) identified that healthcare access and education levels significantly impact cancer prevention and treatment outcomes. Limited healthcare access leads to challenges in early screening, HPV vaccination, and timely treatment, increasing cervical cancer morbidity and mortality. Additionally, a lack of education reduces awareness regarding risk factors, symptoms, and preventive measures. This issue is particularly prevalent among rural and low-income populations, where late-stage diagnosis rates are higher, reducing treatment success rates.

Role of Sexual And Reproductive Health Behaviours

Sexual and reproductive health is an important factor that can affect health and health. Unexpected sexual habits may increase the risk of Human Papilloma virus (HPV), HIV and other sexually transmitted diseases (STDS). In particular, the HPV virus is one of the main factors of the cervical cancer. An important way to reduce the infection of this virus is to follow safe sexual procedures. Preventive measures, such as preventive methods, diagnostic tests and vaccines, will reduce the impact of these infections.

Protecting genetic and reproductive health is important for the long -term health and reproductive ability of women and men. Getting proper medical advice, using pill and other family control methods, and monitoring a uniform menstrual cycle can help ensure reproductive health. In addition, the conduct of explanations and medical awareness camps will give you more opportunity to access safe medical services for women and youth in the community. Frew et al. (2016) found that sexual and reproductive health behaviors significantly impact cervical cancer risk. Factors such as early sexual debut, multiple sexual partners, and unprotected intercourse increase HPV infection risk. Furthermore, frequent pregnancies and long-term use of oral contraceptives contribute to hormonal imbalances and increased cervical epithelial cell vulnerability. A lack of regular screening (Pap smear, HPV test) further exacerbates the risk, allowing undetected HPV infections to progress to cervical cancer.

Psychological Stress And Its Effect On Immune Surveillance in HPV Infections

Stress is an important factor that directly affects the body's immune system. Continuing psychological stress, which will increase the amount of stress hormones, such as cortisol, may reduce the ability of the system that is working to combat diseases. Thus, viruses such as Human Papilloma virus (HPV) increases the risk of persistence in the body. In general, a healthy immune system helps to detect and destroy the HPV virus, but when it is affected by stress, the viral cells can be affected and the potential to become cancer. Continuous stress reduces the functioning of the cells and affects immune surveillance in the body. Thus, infections such as the HPV virus can be intensified and can cause chronic damage. In particular, research suggests that the risk of cervical cancer is increasing in people with stress. To avoid this, adopting methods such as meditation, yoga, exercise, and psychiatric advice can help promote the immune system. Ho et al. (2012) investigated the role of psychological stress in immune surveillance and found that chronic stress increases cortisol and pro-inflammatory cytokines (IL-6, TNF-α), impairing cell-mediated immunity (CMI). Since HPV clearance heavily relies on T-cell responses, stress-induced immunosuppression can lead to persistent HPV infections and an increased risk of cervical cancer progression. Moreover, stress-related oxidative stress and epigenetic changes may promote viral oncogene expression, further accelerating carcinogenesis.

THE ROLE OF THE IMMUNE SYSTEM AND INFLAMMATION IN CERVICAL CARCINOGENESIS

The immune system plays an important role in the prevention of cervical cancer. If the HPV virus is lacking the ability to resist the attack, cells can change and develop into cancer. Chronic inflammation creates an environment for radical change of cells.

Figure 4. **Immune Inflammation Cervical Carcinogenesis**

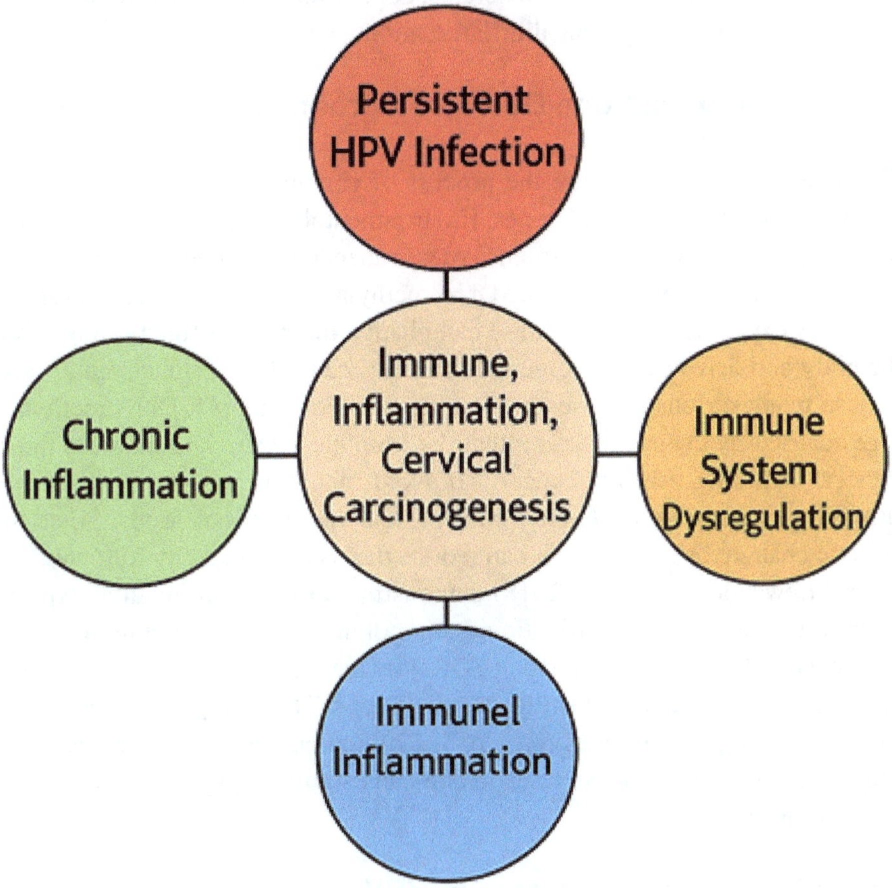

Chronic Inflammation Induced by Environmental Stressors

Chronic inflammation is a long -standing response to the body, which can be caused by various environmental factors. Air pollution, chemicals, visually impaired diets, and stress found in industries and agricultural products are the main environmental pressure factors that can trigger prolonged inflammation in the body. Although this inflammation may appear to be safe at the beginning, it can develop a situation where it affects the cells and tissues and develops a variety of diseases. Prolonged inflammation, in particular, may increase the risk of cancer and infection. For example, when air pollution and factory chemicals enter the body, it can cause changes in the genome of the cells. Thus, the risk of diseases such as cervical cancer can increase. Healthy diets, proper exercise, depression, and clean environment are very important to control physical inflammation.

Epigenetic Modifications Due To Environmental Exposures

Epigenetic modifications are the process of changing their operation without changing the basic DNA line of genes. Environmental impacts, kitten air pollution, cenemic exposure, smoking, and intense stress can make epigenetic changes in genes. These changes may be manifested by DNA methylation, histone modifications, and micro-RNA exposure changes. These can change the normal functioning of cells in the body and drive cancer.Epigenatic changes caused by environmental factors can cause many serious illnesses in the long run. For example, DNA methylation changes caused by chemicals can affect the immune system and increase the risk of cancer, including cervical cancer. To avoid this, it is important to adhere to healthy lifestyle, live in a safe environment, and eat nutritious foods. Since these epigenetic changes are repeated, it can reduce the risk of cancer by following good practices. Lewandowska et al. (2018) demonstrated that environmental exposures contribute to epigenetic modifications. Air pollutants, heavy metals, pesticides, and endocrine-disrupting chemicals (EDCs) influence DNA methylation, histone modifications, and microRNA (miRNA) alterations. These epigenetic changes may silence tumor suppressor genes (e.g., p53, Rb) and enhance oncogene activation, driving carcinogenesis. Persistent exposure can establish epigenetic memory, elevating long-term cancer risk.

Immune Evasion Mechanisms in HPV Persistence And Cancer Development

Human papilloma virus (HPV) uses some important immune evasion methods for prolonging and developing cancer. Generally, the system is active to detect and destroy virus infections. But, HPV, especially its E6 and E7 proteins, relaxes the operation of the immune surveillance. This virus reduces the interactive systems that reveal dendritic cells, T-cells, affecting the body's anti-infection. Thus, the virus disappears in the cells for a long time, causing various genetic changes and increasing the risk of cancer. Priyadarshini et al. (2023) examined immune evasion mechanisms in HPV persistence and cervical cancer progression. HPV oncogenes (E6, E7) downregulate MHC class I, reducing cytotoxic T-cell (CTL) recognition. Additionally, HPV infection disrupts dendritic cell (DC) function, activates regulatory T-cells (Tregs), and induces immunosuppressive cytokines (IL-10, TGF-β), leading to immune suppression. This facilitates chronic HPV infection, increasing the risk of cervical carcinogenesis.Also, when the HPV lasts in the body, when the immune system is reduced, the control of the virus cells will completely lose the control of the cells. In particular, the anti -microbiological medium of the secreted interferon is blocked by the HPV virus. As a result, the cells become an apoptosis instead of regular death, which becomes uninterrupted and become cancerous. The only way to prevent this is to ensure the power and reduce the impact of the virus using vaccines.

PREVENTIVE STRATEGIES AND FUTURE DIRECTIONS

Cervical cancer can be reduced with precautionary measures. HPV vaccine, regular medical examinations and safe sexual habits are important. In the future, progressing treatments and customized drugs will be more important. Research helps to create more advanced methods.

Advances in HPV Vaccination And Its Impact

Vaccines that prevent Human Papilloma virus (HPV) infection are an important progress in medical development. Initially, there were often two main types of viruses (HPV-16, HPV-18). But current developments have been improved to prevent HPV types at various high risk. In particular, vaccines such as "Gardasil 9" are resistant to nine major HPV types and it helps to prevent the risk of infection but also the risk of cancer. In addition, research has confirmed that vaccination at an early age will significantly reduce the spread of infection.

The impact of the HPV vaccine has created major changes in women's health worldwide. In many countries, statistics show that the direct damage to cervical cancer has decreased in vaccination women. Also, with vaccination, it has increased the ability to reduce other cancers caused by HPV virus. Future research focuses on developing more advanced vaccines and taking steps to increase vaccine performance worldwide. The impact of HPV vaccination in Australia and found that it has significantly contributed to cervical cancer prevention. Since the introduction of the quadrivalent HPV vaccine (HPV-6, 11, 16, 18) in 2007, there has been a decline in high-grade cervical abnormalities and HPV infection rates among young women. Due to herd immunity, even unvaccinated individuals have benefited from protection. Wild et al. (2023) reviewed a decade of HPV vaccines and highlighted major advancements in cancer control. The second-generation nonavalent HPV vaccine (HPV-9), introduced in 2014, targets additional high-risk HPV types (31, 33, 45, 52, 58) and provides broader protection. Clinical evidence strongly supports the potential for global vaccination programs to reduce HPV-related cancers in the future.

Role of Exposomic Research In Early Detection And Risk Prediction

Exposomic research is an important approach to analysing the environmental and biological factors exposed to a lifetime of the human body. Various factors such as environmental pollution, food habits, drug use, and stress can cause physical changes. By analysing these changes, they can detect preventive measures at the precedent of developing diseases. Expo somatic research plays an important role in early-stage diagnosis and risk prediction. In particular, these studies help to evaluate the risks of chronic diseases such as cancer, diabetes and heart disease. Connecting modern biomarkers and machine lending technologies can be customized for the treatment and prevention instructions for an individual. Therefore, the exposomic approach to medical research gives important understanding and leads to future health life. Exposomic research can enhance early cancer detection and risk prediction. High-throughput biomonitoring technologies, such as metabolomics, proteomics, and epigenomics, enable the measurement of chemical exposures, oxidative stress markers, and DNA methylation changes. Identifying cancer susceptibility biomarkers allows the implementation of personalized prevention strategies for high-risk individuals.

Emerging Biomarkers For Environmental Influence Assessment

Environmental changes can be greatly affected by human health. It is a development that has been discovered by new biomarkers to evaluate these impacts. Various factors such as air pollution, chemical uppercase, and eating habits help these biological changes to understand the biological changes that occur in the body. Environmental impacts can be evaluated based on changes in urine, blood and hair -like body fluids. The role of biological markers in monitoring environmental exposures and assessing disease risk. Their study emphasized the importance of using biomarkers to understand how environmental factors contribute to disease development. Advanced biomarkers help assess environmental risk factors, aiding in the understanding of disease etiology. Techniques such as non-targeted metabolomics, epigenetic modifications (miRNA expression), and immune response profiling assist in monitoring long-term chemical exposures. Notably, multi-omics integration enables early identification of cancer susceptibility, allowing for preventive interventions. Clinical and technological advances are combined with modern microbiological and omics studies, which can further evaluate environmental impacts. epigenetic changes, and protein symbols such as protein symbols, help determine the risk of specific diseases and the impact of environmental factors. Through this, you can improve the diagnosis, preventive measures and individual therapy.

Strategies for Minimizing Environmental Risks Through Policy And Awareness

Integrate both projects, political decisions and public awareness to reduce environmental risks. Strict environmental laws and regulations must be implemented to deal with problems such as environmental pollution, climate change, water and resources deficiency. Operations such as renewable energy usage, controlling industrial pollution, and promoting green technologies play an important role in reducing environmental impacts.

CONCLUSION

Summary of Key Findings

New biological molecules developed to assess environmental impacts, play a crucial role in safeguarding human health. In particular, biological markers such as micro RNA (MicroRNA), epigenetic changes, and protein biomarkers help identify the effects of environmental factors on the body's immune system. They enable the detection of any changes occurring in the body, thus paving the way for timely treatment. Through these modern biological codes, it is possible to clearly understand environmental manifestations and the body's response mechanisms. Not only this, today's advanced molecular technologies enhance the accuracy of biological data and guide individual-based treatment methods that create treatment plans tailored to each person's unique body composition. Such an approach paves the way for new health practices that reduce the mechanisms of disease formation based on environmental factors in the future. In addition, protocols and awareness efforts to reduce environmental risks not only control pollution but also help to use resources. Strict environmental regulations, promoting green technologies, and awareness efforts to the public have a long -term impact on environmental protection. If political decisions and social responsibility work together, you can create a prosperous and quality environment.

Call for Interdisciplinary Research In Cervical Cancer Exposomics

Exposomics play an important role in the initial diagnosis and risk assessment of cervical cancer. By examining environmental factors, the impact of the lifestyle and the mutual relationships of genes, the disease can be precisely predicted. To improve this field, the integrated contribution of various fields such as biology, medicine, quality analysis, overview science and engineering. Through a versatile approach, Services can identify biomarkers and develop individual -based immunity. For that, medical researchers, environmental scientists, quality experts and engineers must work together. These types of collaborations can lead to creating new ways to prevent and prevent cervical cancer.

Future Directions In Personalized Prevention Strategies

Personal immunization methods are greatly improved by the development of the fields of medicine, biology and quality analysis. In particular, exposomics and biomarkers -based research can predict the risk of diseases depending on a person's personal lifestyle. New initiatives are being made to combine the genital genome, environmental impacts, and health data and prevent disease at the beginning. In the future, using artificial intelligence (AI) and machine learning technologies can be developed for preventive medical programs for a person. Customized medical advice, food recommendations, lifestyle changes, etc., will improve precautionary measures, including cervical cancer. These improvements will not only make the diagnosis, but also the way to prevent its creation to prevent its creation.

REFERENCES

Aguayo, F., Muñoz, J. P., Perez-Dominguez, F., Carrillo-Beltrán, D., Oliva, C., Calaf, G. M., Blanco, R., & Nuñez-Acurio, D. (2020). High-risk human papillomavirus and tobacco smoke interactions in epithelial carcinogenesis. *Cancers (Basel)*, *12*(8), 2201. DOI: 10.3390/cancers12082201 PMID: 32781676

Alavanja, M. C., Ross, M. K., & Bonner, M. R. (2013). Increased cancer burden among pesticide applicators and others due to pesticide exposure. *CA: a Cancer Journal for Clinicians*, *63*(2), 120–142. DOI: 10.3322/caac.21170 PMID: 23322675

Athinarayanan, S., Dhanakodi, K., Rajamanickam, A.T., Sanjaygandhi, A., & Athinarayanan, S., (2025). Review on Advancements and Challenges in Cervical Cancer Diagnosis. *Communications on Applied Nonlinear Analysis*, *32*(9), 2324–2336. DOI: 10.52783/cana.v32.4518

Athinarayanan, S., & Srinath, M. V. (2012). Cervical cell for Thinprep image enhancement using morphological segmentation. *International Journal of Management. IT and Engineering*, *2*(4), 284–295.

Athinarayanan, S., Srinath, M. V., & Kavitha, R. (2017). Multi class cervical cancer classification by using ERSTCM, EMSD & CFE methods-based texture features and fuzzy logic-based hybrid kernel support vector machine classifier. *IOSR Journal of Computer Engineering*, *19*(1), 23–34. DOI: 10.9790/0661-1901042334

Bhowmik, A., Das, S., Bhattacharjee, A., Choudhury, B., Naiding, M., Deka, S., Ghosh, S. K., & Choudhury, Y. (2015). MDM2 and TP53 polymorphisms as predictive markers for head and neck cancer in Northeast Indian population: Effect of gene-gene and gene-environment interactions. *Asian Pacific Journal of Cancer Prevention : APJCP*, *16*(14), 5767–5772. DOI: 10.7314/APJCP.2015.16.14.5767 PMID: 26320449

Bray, F., Jemal, A., Grey, N., Ferlay, J., & Forman, D. (2012). Global cancer transitions according to the Human Development Index (2008–2030): A population-based study. *The Lancet. Oncology*, *13*(8), 790–801. DOI: 10.1016/S1470-2045(12)70211-5 PMID: 22658655

Calder, P. C., Carr, A. C., Gombart, A. F., & Eggersdorfer, M. (2020). Optimal nutritional status for a well-functioning immune system is an important factor to protect against viral infections. *Nutrients*, *12*(4), 1181. DOI: 10.3390/nu12041181 PMID: 32340216

Feil, R., & Fraga, M. F. (2012). Epigenetics and the environment: Emerging patterns and implications. *Nature Reviews. Genetics, 13*(2), 97–109. DOI: 10.1038/nrg3142 PMID: 22215131

Feng, J., & Yang, W. (2012). Effects of particulate air pollution on cardiovascular health: A population health risk assessment. *PLoS One, 7*(3), e33385. DOI: 10.1371/journal.pone.0033385 PMID: 22432017

Frew, P. M., Fisher, A. K., Basket, M. M., Chung, Y., Schamel, J., Weiner, J. L., Mullen, J., Omer, S. B., & Orenstein, W. A. (2016). Changes in childhood immunization decisions in the United States: Results from 2012 & 2014 National Parental Surveys. *Vaccine, 34*(46), 5689–5696. DOI: 10.1016/j.vaccine.2016.08.001 PMID: 27720447

Goyal, T., Mitra, P., Singh, P., Sharma, S., Purohit, P., & Sharma, P. (2022). Effect of occupational co-exposure to lead and cadmium on selected immunomodulatory cytokines. *Toxicology and Industrial Health, 38*(1), 1–10. DOI: 10.1177/07482337211019172 PMID: 34874211

Hamanaka, R. B., & Mutlu, G. M. (2018). Particulate matter air pollution: Effects on the cardiovascular system. *Frontiers in Endocrinology, 9*, 680. DOI: 10.3389/fendo.2018.00680 PMID: 30505291

Harper, D. M., & DeMars, L. R. (2017). HPV vaccines–a review of the first decade. *Gynecologic Oncology, 146*(1), 196–204. DOI: 10.1016/j.ygyno.2017.04.004 PMID: 28442134

Ho, S. M., Johnson, A., Tarapore, P., Janakiram, V., Zhang, X., & Leung, Y. K. (2012). Environmental epigenetics and its implication on disease risk and health outcomes. *ILAR Journal, 53*(3-4), 289–305. DOI: 10.1093/ilar.53.3-4.289 PMID: 23744968

Jayshree, R. S., Sreenivas, A., Tessy, M., & Krishna, S. (2009). Cell intrinsic & extrinsic factors in cervical carcinogenesis. *The Indian Journal of Medical Research, 130*(3), 286–295. PMID: 19901438

Jöckel, K. H., Ahrens, W., Jahn, I., Pohlabeln, H., & Bolm-AudorfF, U. (1998). Occupational risk factors for lung cancer: A case-control study in West Germany. *International Journal of Epidemiology, 27*(4), 549–560. DOI: 10.1093/ije/27.4.549 PMID: 9758106

Landrigan, P. J., Fuller, R., Acosta, N. J., Adeyi, O., Arnold, R., Baldé, A. B., & Zhong, M. (2018). The Lancet Commission on pollution and health. [Note: Appears under Morgan et al. in the original list]. *Lancet, 391*(10119), 462–512. DOI: 10.1016/S0140-6736(17)32345-0 PMID: 29056410

Lewandowska, A. M., Rudzki, M., Rudzki, S., Lewandowski, T., & Laskowska, B. (2018). Environmental risk factors for cancer-review paper. *Annals of Agricultural and Environmental Medicine*, *26*(1), 1–7. DOI: 10.26444/aaem/94299 PMID: 30922021

Moreno, V., Bosch, F. X., Muñoz, N., Meijer, C. J., Shah, K. V., Walboomers, J. M., Herrero, R., & Franceschi, S. (2002). Effect of oral contraceptives on risk of cervical cancer in women with human papillomavirus infection: The IARC multicentric case-control study. *Lancet*, *359*(9312), 1085–1092. DOI: 10.1016/S0140-6736(02)08150-3 PMID: 11943255

Morgan, M., Deoraj, A., Felty, Q., & Roy, D. (2017). Environmental estrogen-like endocrine disrupting chemicals and breast cancer. *Molecular and Cellular Endocrinology*, *457*, 89–102. DOI: 10.1016/j.mce.2016.10.003 PMID: 27717745

Plummer, M., Herrero, R., Franceschi, S., Meijer, C. J., Snijders, P., Bosch, F. X., de Sanjosé, S., & Muñoz, N. (2003). Smoking and cervical cancer: Pooled analysis of the IARC multi-centric case–control study. *Cancer Causes & Control*, *14*(9), 805–814. DOI: 10.1023/B:CACO.0000003811.98261.3e PMID: 14682438

Priyadarshini, E., Parambil, A. M., Rajamani, P., Ponnusamy, V. K., & Chen, Y. H. (2023). Exposure, toxicological mechanism of endocrine disrupting compounds and future direction of identification using nano-architectonics. *Environmental Research*, *225*, 115577. DOI: 10.1016/j.envres.2023.115577 PMID: 36871939

Ramamoorthy, T., Nath, A., Singh, S., Mathew, S., Pant, A., Sheela, S., Kaur, G., Sathishkumar, K., & Mathur, P. (2024). Assessing the global impact of ambient air pollution on cancer incidence and mortality: A comprehensive meta-analysis. *JCO Global Oncology*, *10*(10), e2300427. DOI: 10.1200/GO.23.00427 PMID: 38513187

Rao, X., Zhong, J., Brook, R. D., & Rajagopalan, S. (2018). Effect of particulate matter air pollution on cardiovascular oxidative stress pathways. *Antioxidants & Redox Signaling*, *28*(9), 797–818. DOI: 10.1089/ars.2017.7394 PMID: 29084451

Ren, X., McHale, C. M., Skibola, C. F., Smith, A. H., Smith, M. T., & Zhang, L. (2011). An emerging role for epigenetic dysregulation in arsenic toxicity and carcinogenesis. *Environmental Health Perspectives*, *119*(1), 11–19. DOI: 10.1289/ehp.1002114 PMID: 20682481

Sharma, R., Suravarjhula, L., Banerjee, M., Kumar, G., & Kumar, N. (2023). Chimeric antigen receptor T-cell therapy in cancer: A critical review. *Current Drug Research Reviews*, *15*(3), 241–261. DOI: 10.2174/2589977515666230220092125 PMID: 36825696

Vermeulen, R., Schymanski, E. L., Barabási, A. L., & Miller, G. W. (2020). The exposome and health: Where chemistry meets biology. *Science, 367*(6476), 392–396. DOI: 10.1126/science.aay3164 PMID: 31974245

Wild, C. P., Scalbert, A., & Herceg, Z. (2013). Measuring the exposome: A powerful basis for evaluating environmental exposures and cancer risk. *Environmental and Molecular Mutagenesis, 54*(7), 480–499. DOI: 10.1002/em.21777 PMID: 23681765

Wu, C. T., Chiu, L. T., & Raturi, V. P. (2023). Investigation of the Correlation Between Mental Disorder and Cervical Cancer in Taiwan: A Nationwide Population-Based Cohort Study. *Indian Journal of Gynecologic Oncology, 21*(1), 29. DOI: 10.1007/s40944-022-00670-9

Zur Hausen, H. (2009). Papillomaviruses in the causation of human cancers—A brief historical account. *Virology, 384*(2), 260–265. DOI: 10.1016/j.virol.2008.11.046 PMID: 19135222

Chapter 3
Endocrine Disruptors and DNA Damage:
Mechanisms, Risks, and a Public Health Implications

Mamta Singh
https://orcid.org/0009-0002-9702-9119
Sri Ramachandra Institute of Higher Education and Research, Chennai, India

ABSTRACT

Endocrine disruptors, which are environmental chemicals, interfere with hormone regulation and increase health risks. This chapter examines the DNA-damaging effects of EDs, which lead to mutations, genomic instability, and the development of cancer. Key molecular mechanisms include oxidative damage, epigenetic alterations, and receptor-mediated abnormalities that result from EDs exposure and associated health issues. It also discusses the risks of endocrine disruptors for pregnant women and children, as well as other vulnerable population groups. The discussion encompasses public health implications as well as regulatory standards for risk evaluation and methods to minimize exposure. Future directions include advancing biomarker development, refining risk assessment models, and designing safer chemical alternatives to reduce exposure.

1. INTRODUCTION

Environmental chemicals in the class of endocrine disruptors function as hormone mimics while blocking hormone production, transport, and binding and removal. The industrial and pesticide products, along with plastics, cosmetics, and domestic use products, contain BPA (Bisphenol A), phthalates, DDT (Dichlorodiphenyltrichlo-

DOI: 10.4018/979-8-3373-5796-6.ch003

Copyright © 2026, IGI Global Scientific Publishing. Copying or distributing in print or electronic forms without written permission of IGI Global Scientific Publishing is prohibited.

roethane), PCBs (Polychlorinated Biphenyls), and phytoestrogens. These harmful substances remain in the environment and human bodies, leading to severe health problems. Multiple observational studies, together with experimental findings, have shown that EDs trigger carcinogenesis while causing metabolic disorders, reproductive issues, and neurodevelopmental disorders.

1.1. Endocrine Disruptors (EDs) and DNA Damage

The exposure to Endocrine Disruptors results in DNA damage, which occurs either directly or indirectly by producing reactive oxygen species that affect DNA bases and chromosomes. Certain EDs modify DNA methylation patterns as well as histone modifications while keeping the DNA sequences unaltered. The simultaneous occurrence of epigenetic modifications and DNA damage results in cancer development and diseases. Breast cancer cells grow faster when exposed to BPA along with other EDs through mechanisms that activate estrogen receptors. Phthalates serve as a prevalent ED that results in testicular dysgenesis while producing cancer-causing effects. The development of cancer occurs when DNA damage pairs with hormone disruption caused by Endocrine Disruptors.

1.2. Structure and Scope of the Chapter

This chapter starts with a brief overview of Endocrine Disruptors and their origins. The following section explains EDs and DNA damage and their effects on human health. The following section investigates how DNA repair mechanisms work in cancer formation and their impact on fertility and metabolic syndrome. The chapter analyzes how EDs contribute to disease development in vulnerable patient groups. The chapter section addresses how the reader can implement public health policies, regulatory standards, and prevention measures for ED production.

2. ENDOCRINE DISRUPTOR: DEFINITION, ED SOURCES, AND EXPOSURE ROUTES

2.1. Definition

According to the World Health Organization/IPCS (2002), Endocrine disruptors (EDs) are exogenous substances or mixtures that interfere with hormone action and cause adverse health effects in the whole organism, its progeny, or (sub)population.

2.2. Endocrine Disruptor: Types and Sources

EDs can be categorized by origin (natural vs. synthetic analogues), chemical structure, hormonal interference, and physiological targets.

I. **Natural EDs:** Based on exposure and development, food and fungal EDs can be good or bad. ED sources, exposure routes, and health effects are summarized in **Table 1**. A few common natural Eds are:

-The phytoestrogen genistein, present in soybeans and legumes, creates an estrogenic effect when binding to ERα/ERβ receptors.

- **Zearalenone**, a mycotoxin produced by Fusarium fungus in grains, mimics estrogen and causes hyperestrogenism, infertility, and early puberty in cattle and humans. The fertility of bovine and human populations is affected by the coumestrol found in cloves and alfalfa because it binds to estrogen receptors.
- **Resveratrol**, a polyphenolic component of grapes and red wine, affects hormonal balance as a dual agonist-antagonist on estrogen receptors, depending on dosage and context.

-Flaxseed and whole grain lignans are converted into enterolignans by gut bacteria, which act as mildly estrogenic compounds.

- **Red algae** brominated phenols disrupt thyroid hormone signaling in marine environments.

II. **Synthetic EDs**: These are synthetic chemicals used in industrial, agricultural, or domestic applications.

i. **Industrial Chemicals:** Industrial chemicals are released into ecosystems and people through occupational inhalation, food chain pollution, and consumer items. Common EDs are environments that have dioxins, furans, and PCBs (Polychlorinated Biphenyls). Chemistry, manufacturing, and trash incineration create them. Air, water, and animal fats are contaminated. Chemicals affect thyroid and reproductive hormone signaling. Cosmetics, toys, food packaging, and drug tubes contain phthalates. Dust, skin, and contaminated food are their major entryways. Fetal reproductive system development and testosterone production are affected (Meeker et al., 2009).

Plastics and electronics firms release PCBs (dioxins and furans) from chlorine-based industries, which affect fish and crops and harm the thyroid and neurodevelopment (Carpenter, 2006). They are thyroid hormone-affecting, immunotoxic, and reproductively suppressive (Birnbaum & Tuomisto, 2000). Styrene, a plastic and rubber monomer, may alter prolactin and estrogen pathways, causing reproductive failure. PVC production through vinyl chloride could lead to endocrine system damage by reducing liver function and decreasing metabolic enzyme activity.

ii. **Herbicides and Pesticides in Agriculture**: EDs are common in agrochemicals. These toxins soak into crops, leach into water, and bioaccumulate in food web creatures. Organochlorine Pesticides (OCPs) like DDT and dieldrin, prohibited in many places, remain in the environment, and exposure comes from eating fish and animal products. Atrazine, a frequently used pesticide, contaminates groundwater and surface water, especially in agricultural areas. It induces aromatase expression, feminizes amphibians, and may cause human reproductive abnormalities (Hayes et al., 2002). Methylchlor and endosulfan cause hypothyroidism and reproductive abnormalities.

iii. **Pharmaceutical Products:** Human excretion, hospital and industrial waste, and inappropriate disposal release pharmaceutical substances, notably synthetic EDs. Ethinylestradiol (EE2) from sewage effluents and surface water is used in oral contraceptives. The synthetic estrogen diethylstilbestrol (DES) used to prevent miscarriages has been related to transgenerational reproductive difficulties include vaginal cancer, infertility, and altered sexual development (Newbold, 2004). Even if they are lifesaving, glucocorticoids like dexamethasone and prednisone can disrupt cortisol homeostasis in aquatic habitats when excreted or released. Cyproterone acetate and prostate cancer drugs can disrupt non-target species' androgen receptors, impacting reproduction.

iv. **Personal Care Products (PCPs):** EDs can enter the human body through dermal absorption and also by accidental ingestion or inhalation. Lotions, shampoos, and deodorants contain parabens and lead to breast cancer and reproductive issues, which can result from estrogen receptor-binding compounds (Darbre & Harvey, 2008). Triclosan, an antibiotic in toothpaste, soaps, and sanitizers, alters thyroid hormone metabolism and is absorbed through the skin and mouth (Paul et al., 2010). Sunscreens and cosmetics include estrogenic and antiandrogenic UV filters, benzophenone-3 and octinoxate, which are easily absorbed by the skin and enter the body as EDs, creating reproductive risk concerns. Siloxanes like cyclotetrasiloxane (D4) and cyclopentasiloxane (D5) in hair products, deodorants, and lotions can alter estrogen and progesterone signaling and impair animal endometrium and reproduction. Formaldehyde-releasing preservatives like quaternium-15 in hair and skin products may disrupt the thyroid axis and cause cancer.

v. **Flame Retardants:** Electronics, furniture, insulation, and fabrics are flame-retardant-treated for fire protection and are sources of EDs. Polybrominated Diphenyl Ethers (PBDEs) in electronics and furniture foams damage thyroid hormones and neurodevelopment. TBBPA (Tetrabromobisphenol A) & HBCD

(Hexabromocyclododecane) from electronics and insulation reduce estrogenic signaling and steroidogenesis by skin contact and dust inhalation (Kitamura et al., 2005). Decabromodiphenyl ethane (DBDPE), a brominated PBDE replacement used in plastics and electronics, is persistent and bioaccumulative and may disrupt thyroid hormones and induce developmental harm in aquatic animals and rats. Home dust and blood contain estrogen-like bis-2-ethylhexyl-tetrabromophthalate (BEH-TEBP) in flexible PVC and insulating foam, causing concerns for endocrine and metabolic illnesses.

2.3. Routes of Exposure of Endocrine Disrupters (EDs)

Several exposure pathways allow humans to encounter EDs. Scientists need to study these pathways in order to determine the level of risk and establish ways to minimize it. The main exposure pathways and routes through which these agents reach human bodies are explained in this section.

i. **Food and water contamination**: The dietary exposure represents the main way through which EDs reach humans. Food contact materials such as Phthalates (especially DEHP) can be released from plastic food packaging when packaging includes additives not chemically bound to the polymer matrix. Pesticides sprayed on crops leave dangerous chemical residues that persist on fruits and vegetables. People who eat these remnants come into contact with compounds that cause endocrine disruption. Water systems experience exposure to EDs through multiple pathways, including agricultural run-off and leaching at landfills and industrial discharge, thus leading to extended exposure through drinking water, as shown in **Table 1**.
ii. **Inhalation of Indoor Air and Dust:** The primary source of inhalation exposure occurs when indoor air and household dust become contaminated. Consumer products and construction materials are the primary sources of two common indoor air pollutants: phthalates and Microplastics. Agricultural Aerosols are pesticides that play an essential role in forming free molecules and are found in rural and urban sites. The size and durability of airborne particulates make them penetrate deep into the lungs.
iii. **Dermal Absorption by Contaminated Surfaces and Consumer Products:** Dermal exposure occurs through contaminated surfaces and consumer products, leading to skin absorption. The chemical BPA enters the body through dermal exposure since it is present in thermal paper and personal care items. Research findings show that Thermal Paper Handling exposes people to BPA through extended receipt handling, which involves multiple skin contact points between their fingertips and palmar surface. Cosmetics and personal care products contain

Phthalates and BPA, which penetrate through the skin because users regularly apply them and maintain skin contact. The combination of household dust and treated surfaces, including furniture with flame retardants FM 550 presents additional dermal transfer opportunities, particularly for children who touch and insert objects into their mouths frequently.

iv. **Transdermal and In-Utero Exposure:** Gestational maternal exposure research indicates that offspring experience long-lasting effects due to transdermal exposure. Research on vinclozolin, a fungicide with known endocrine-disrupting effects, shows that maternal exposure leads to epigenetic alterations that are passed down to the F3 generation offspring. The translocation process demonstrates that exposure goes beyond direct contact since biological mechanisms enable endocrine disruption to persist between generations.

Table 1. Endocrine Disruptors: Types, Sources, Exposure Routes, and Health Effects

Category	Examples of EDs	Primary Sources	Exposure Routes	Health Concerns
Industrial Chemicals	BPA, Phthalates (DEHP, DBP, BBP), Dioxins (TCDD), PCBs, PFAS (PFOA, PFOS), Styrene	Plastics, food containers, thermal paper, industrial waste, electronics, non-stick coatings, firefighting foam	Ingestion (food/drink), dermal absorption (cosmetics), inhalation (dust/airborne particles)	Breast/prostate cancer, reproductive disorders, immune suppression, metabolic syndrome, developmental delays
Pesticides/Herbicides	DDT, Dieldrin, Atrazine, Glyphosate, Endosulfan, Chlorpyrifos, Vinclozolin	Agricultural runoff, contaminated soil/water, legacy pesticides, crop protection	Food chain bioaccumulation, contaminated water, and inhalation (spray drift)	Breast/testicular cancer, thyroid disruption, neurodevelopmental disorders, hormone imbalances
Plastics & Packaging	BPA, BPS (BPA substitutes), Phthalates, Microplastics, Polyethylene, Polystyrene	Food/beverage containers, toys, medical devices, cosmetic packaging, synthetic textiles	Ingestion (microplastics in food), dermal absorption, inhalation (degraded plastics)	Hormonal imbalances, obesity, liver damage, metabolic disorders, and developmental toxicity

continued on following page

Table 1. Continued

Category	Examples of EDs	Primary Sources	Exposure Routes	Health Concerns
Pharmaceuticals	Synthetic estrogens (EE2, DES), Triclosan, Parabens, Antibiotics, Beta-blockers	Birth control pills, hormone therapies, wastewater, and personal care products	Drinking water, aquatic sources, dermal absorption (lotions)	Feminization of wildlife, reproductive cancers, antibiotic resistance, thyroid dysfunction
Personal Care Products	Parabens (methyl-, propyl-), Triclosan, Oxybenzone, Phthalates, Fragrances (musks)	Shampoos, deodorants, soaps, sunscreens, nail polish, and perfumes	Dermal absorption, ingestion (lip products), inhalation (sprays)	Breast cancer, endocrine disruption, allergic reactions, and developmental toxicity
Household Products	Alkylphenols (NP, OP), PBDEs (flame retardants), VOCs, Formaldehyde, Perchlorate	Cleaning agents, furniture, electronics, carpets, paints, and adhesives	Dust inhalation, ingestion (hand-to-mouth), dermal contact	Neurodevelopmental delays (e.g., ADHD), thyroid dysfunction, respiratory issues, and cancer
Heavy Metals	Arsenic, Cadmium, Lead, Mercury, Chromium, Nickel	Industrial discharge, batteries, paints, contaminated water, cigarette smoke	Ingestion (food/water), inhalation (smoke/dust), placental transfer (pregnancy)	Neurotoxicity, kidney damage, reproductive harm, cancers (lung, skin), cardiovascular disease
Agricultural Products	Phytoestrogens (Genistein, Daidzein), Mycoestrogens (Zearalenone), Pesticide residues	Soybeans, flaxseeds, mold-contaminated grains, livestock feed	Dietary intake (soy products, meat/dairy), contaminated crops	Cancer protection (low dose), developmental risks (high dose), reproductive disorders
Combustion By-products	PAHs (Benzo[a] pyrene), Dioxins, PCBs, Particulate Matter (PM2.5)	Vehicle exhaust, cigarette smoke, coal burning, grilled meats, wildfires	Inhalation (smoke/soot), ingestion (charred foods), dermal contact	Lung/skin/bladder cancer, cardiovascular disease, reproductive toxicity, oxidative stress
Natural Sources	Zearalenone (ZEA), Genistein, Coumestrol, Lignans	Mold-contaminated cereals, legumes, clover, hops	Contaminated food dietary supplements	Hyperestrogenism, infertility, hormone-sensitive cancers (high exposure)

The table includes all common EDs being industrial chemicals, pesticides/herbicides, plastics/packaging, pharmaceutical uses, personal and home uses, heavy metals, agriculture chemicals, combustion products etc. and their exposure pathways (ingestion, dermal uptake, inhalation) with related health effects.

3. VULNERABLE POPULATIONS TO ENDOCRINE DISRUPTOR (ED) EXPOSURE

The combination of exposure routes to endocrine disruptors creates risks for specific vulnerable populations **(Table 2).** The following section demonstrates the cumulative dangers that affect particular vulnerable populations.

3.1. Fetuses & Neonates:

Young children and infants show increased sensitivity to endocrine disruptors. The body systems reach their peak sensitivity during developmental stages. Their small size, combined with fast metabolism, makes them more susceptible to harm. Putting hands to mouths elevates the risk of exposure to contaminants. Developing organs and immature physiological systems absorb contaminants at higher rates, increasing vulnerability. Bisphenol A is an ED found in polycarbonate plastics and epoxy resins (baby bottles, food containers). The flame retardants PBDEs found in furniture and electronics accumulate in home dust, which harms newborns and toddlers.

3.2. Pregnant Women:

EDs pose a risk to the fetus because they affect pregnant women. BPA, DiBP, BBzP, and certain phthalates can cross the placental barrier, disrupting fetal development and hormonal balance. Exposure to PFAS leads to thyroid hormone disturbances and low birth weights. Exposure to EDs during pregnancy leads to epigenetic changes that result in reproductive and metabolic diseases for offspring throughout their entire lifetime.

3.3. Occupational Exposure:

The highest exposure to EDs occurs in manufacturing and application sites of flame retardants (OPFRs), pesticides (e.g., atrazine, chlorpyrifos), and plasticizers. Farmers experience higher pesticide exposure than the general population because they inhale and touch pesticides with their skin. Industrial workers who handle endocrine-disrupting chemicals such as Phthalates and BPA, prevalent in plastics, rubber, and vinyl sectors, face increased health risks.

Table 2. Vulnerable Populations and Their Associated Endocrine Disruptor Risks

Vulnerable Group	Key EDCs of Concern	Primary Exposure Pathways	Potential Health Risks
Fetuses & Neonates	BPA, Phthalates, Lead, PCBs	Placental transfer - Breast milk	-Developmental abnormalities (e.g., neural tube defects) - Low birth weight - Altered puberty timing
Infants & Children	Pesticides (e.g., Chlorpyrifos), PFAS	Contaminated baby food/formula - Dust/toys (hand-to-mouth)	- Neurodevelopmental delays (ADHD, autism) - Early puberty - Immune dysfunction
Pregnant Women	BPA, Phthalates, Mercury	-Personal care products - Processed foods -Contaminated fish	- Gestational diabetes - Preterm birth - Thyroid dysfunction
Adults	Parabens, Triclosan, Atrazine	-Cosmetics (makeup, acne products) - Fast food packaging	- Hormonal acne - Disrupted menstrual cycles - Increased breast/prostate cancer risk
Occupational Workers	Pesticides, Dioxins, PBDEs	-Agricultural spraying - Industrial manufacturing - Electronic waste recycling	- Infertility - Higher cancer incidence - Liver/kidney damage

The table "Vulnerable Groups and Endocrine Disrupting Chemicals (EDCs): Exposure and Health Risks" presents the main EDs that impact different population groups and their main exposure routes and related health consequences.

4. MECHANISMS OF ENDOCRINE DISRUPTORS (EDS): INDUCED DNA DAMAGE & HEALTH EFFECTS

The complex multifactorial mechanisms of EDs disrupt hormone signaling pathways. The biological pathways include receptor-dependent and independent mechanisms, enzymatic disruption, signal transduction interference, and epigenetic changes. The DNA damage caused by EDs leads to cancer development, reproductive issues, and metabolic problems through oxidative stress, genotoxic effects, and epigenetic reprogramming. The biological processes that interact with genomic instability and chronic disease outcomes are shown in **Table 3**.

4.1. Hormone Receptor-Mediated Pathways

EDs bind to nuclear hormone receptors, enabling them to activate or deactivate hormone actions. The receptors regulate essential gene expression, which controls development and reproduction and maintains homeostasis.

i. **Estrogen Receptors (ERα, ERβ):** The estrogen receptors ERα and ERβ experience incorrect activation or suppression when exposed to EDs, including bisphenol A (BPA), nonylphenol, and genistein. These abnormalities lead to early puberty and infertility and increase the risk of breast and uterine cancer. The continuous activation of estrogen receptors leads to DNA strand breakage, ROS production, and genomic instability, which results in estrogen-induced carcinogenesis (Rubin, 2011).
ii. **Androgen Receptors (AR):** AR antagonists break testicular DNA, which leads to permanent fertility impairment (Hotchkiss et al., 2008). Triclosan and PCBs occur through their ability to replace thyroid hormones from transport proteins or their direct interaction with thyroid receptors.
iii. **Thyroid Hormone Receptors (TRα, TRβ):** Triclosan and PCBs affect neurodevelopment and metabolism by displacing thyroid hormones from transport proteins or binding directly to thyroid receptors. Thyroid hormone-induced gene misexpression and oxidative DNA damage may cause intellectual impairment and abnormal myelination in fetal development (Boas et al., 2006).

4.2. Non-Receptor-Mediated Pathways

The effects of EDs on the body extend beyond receptor binding because they can modify hormone transport mechanisms, endocrine feedback systems, and hormone metabolic pathways.

i. **Hormone Transport Protein Disruption:** The thyroid hormone transport protein transthyretin becomes less available to thyroid hormones because EDs including perchlorate and PBDEs compete for binding sites which reduces hormone availability and brain uptake during fetal development and impairs cognitive function.
ii. **Hormone Biosynthesis Modulation**: The steroidogenic enzyme expression in gonadal and adrenal tissues changes when exposed to cadmium and phthalates, which results in altered testosterone and cortisol production levels. The disrupted hormone regulation causes endocrine tumors, which develop genomic instability because of oxidative enzyme stress and ROS accumulation.

iii. **Intracellular Signaling Interference:** The non-receptor EDs PFOS and arsenic disrupt MAPK, Akt, and JAK/STAT signaling pathways, which prevents hormonal signals from reaching their cellular targets. The disruption of kinase activity leads to apoptosis resistance, hyperproliferation, and DNA repair inhibition, which enhances mutagenesis and oncogenesis.

4.3. Enzymatic Modulation and Signal Transduction Interference

The EDs focus on specific enzymes that control steroid hormone production and cell signaling pathways to modify hormone levels and cellular responses. These are:

i. **Aromatase Modulation:** Atrazine activates aromatase (CYP19A1) to increase androgen-to-estrogen conversion which results in male feminization. Research indicates that abnormal aromatase function leads to cancer development through estrogen-dependent mechanisms, and elevated estrogen levels produce DNA damage and chromosomal mutations (Hayes et al., 2002).
ii. **5α-Reductase Inhibition:** The enzyme 5α-Reductase experiences suppression from phthalates, including DEHP, which results in decreased formation of dihydrotestosterone (DHT). The process results in underdeveloped male genitalia during fetal development and causes infertility. The disruption of enzyme function leads to increased oxidative metabolism byproducts, which damage DNA replication and repair enzymes.
iii. **Signal Pathway Activation:** BPA, along with other EDs, triggers non-genomic signaling pathways, including ERK/MAPK and PI3K/Akt, which drive uncontrolled cell growth. Activating these pathways blocks programmed cell death and weakens DNA repair mechanisms, increasing the potential for tumor formation and DNA damage (Welshons et al., 2006).

4.4. Epigenetic Modifications

Endocrine disruptors (EDs) modify gene expression by using epigenetic processes that do not alter DNA sequences, thus leading to developmental problems, long-term health issues, and transgenerational effects. The study by Dolinoy et al. (2007) demonstrated that DES and BPA modify gene promoter methylation patterns while influencing oncogene and tumor suppressor gene expression. The combination of DNA damage and these modifications creates problems for DNA maintenance and repair functions. The modifications of histone structures by EDs lead to cancer development, hormone resistance, and reproductive issues. The modifications of miRNA and non-coding RNA by EDs result in changes to hormone regulation, cell cycle control, and DNA repair mechanisms. Genistein reduces the expression of miRNA checkpoint genes related to breast cancer, which results in DNA damage that depends on estrogen (Klinge, 2009).

The epigenetic reprogramming of EDs enables them to impact future generations without requiring direct contact. The combination of genotoxicity with hormone mimicry or antagonism and epigenetic disruption tends to accumulate throughout time, especially during crucial developmental stages. Comprehending these pathways enables better health risk assessment, regulatory practices, and intervention methods.

Table 3. Summary of mechanism involved in Endocrine distributors (EDs)

Mechanism Category	Subcategory	Key Actions of EDs	Examples of EDs	Health Impacts
Hormone Receptor-Mediated Pathways	Estrogen Receptors (ERα/ERβ)	Bind to ER, mimic/block estrogen; induce ROS, DNA breaks	BPA, nonylphenol, genistein	Early puberty, breast/uterine cancer, infertility
	Androgen Receptors (AR)	Block testosterone binding; cause DNA fragmentation in testicular cells	Vinclozolin, flutamide	Male reproductive defects, infertility
	Thyroid Receptors (TRα/TRβ)	Displace thyroid hormones; disrupt neurodevelopment	Triclosan, PCBs	Intellectual disability, metabolic disorders
	Other Receptors (PPARs, GR, etc.)	Alter lipid metabolism, stress response	PFAS, phthalates	Obesity, insulin resistance, and immune dysfunction
Non-Receptor-Mediated Pathways	Hormone Transport Disruption	Compete with thyroid hormones for transport proteins	Perchlorate, PBDEs	Cognitive deficits (fetal development)
	Hormone Biosynthesis Modulation	Alter steroidogenic enzymes; increase ROS	Cadmium, phthalates	Endocrine tumors, genomic instability
	Intracellular Signaling Interference	Perturb MAPK/Akt pathways; decouple hormonal signals	Arsenic, PFOS	Apoptosis resistance, hyperproliferation, and mutagenesis
Enzymatic Modulation	Aromatase (CYP19A1) Upregulation	Increase androgen-to-estrogen conversion	Atrazine	Feminization in males, estrogen-dependent cancers
	5α-Reductase Inhibition	Reduce DHT formation; elevate oxidative byproducts	DEHP (phthalates)	Undervirilization, infertility, DNA replication errors
	Non-Genomic Signaling Activation	Trigger ERK/PI3K pathways; suppress DNA repair	BPA	Tumorigenesis, genotoxic stress

continued on following page

Table 3. Continued

Mechanism Category	Subcategory	Key Actions of EDs	Examples of EDs	Health Impacts
Epigenetic Modifications	DNA Methylation Changes	Hypo-/hypermethylation of hormone-responsive genes	BPA, DES	Oncogene activation, impaired DNA repair, transgenerational effects
	Histone Modifications	Alter acetylation/ methylation; disrupt chromatin structure	Various EDs	Hormone insensitivity, endocrine tumors
	miRNA Dysregulation	Silence DNA repair genes or cell cycle regulators	Genistein	Breast cancer progression, estrogen-dependent DNA damage
Hormone Receptor-Mediated Pathways	Estrogen Receptors (ERα/ERβ)	Bind to ER, mimic/block estrogen; induce ROS, DNA breaks	BPA, nonylphenol, genistein	Early puberty, breast/ uterine cancer, infertility
	Androgen Receptors (AR)	Block testosterone binding; cause DNA fragmentation in testicular cells	Vinclozolin, flutamide	Male reproductive defects, infertility
	Thyroid Receptors (TRα/TRβ)	Displace thyroid hormones; disrupt neurodevelopment	Triclosan, PCBs	Intellectual disability, metabolic disorders
	Other Receptors (PPARs, GR, etc.)	Alter lipid metabolism, stress response	PFAS, phthalates	Obesity, insulin resistance, immune dysfunction
Non-Receptor-Mediated Pathways	Hormone Transport Disruption	Compete with thyroid hormones for transport proteins	Perchlorate, PBDEs	Cognitive deficits (fetal development)
	Hormone Biosynthesis Modulation	Alter steroidogenic enzymes; increase ROS	Cadmium, phthalates	Endocrine tumors, genomic instability
	Intracellular Signaling Interference	Perturb MAPK/Akt pathways; decouple hormonal signals	Arsenic, PFOS	Apoptosis resistance, hyperproliferation, mutagenesis
Enzymatic Modulation	Aromatase (CYP19A1) Upregulation	Increase androgen-to-estrogen conversion	Atrazine	Feminization in males, estrogen-dependent cancers

This table presents a structured overview of endocrine disruptor (ED) mechanisms of action. EDs produce their effects through receptor binding, enzyme interference, signal disruption, and epigenetic changes. The health impacts of EDs include cancer and infertility, together with neurodevelopmental disorders and transgenerational effects. The downstream effects of EDs include DNA damage and oxidative stress.

5. DNA DAMAGE AND GENOTOXIC RISKS FROM ENDOCRINE DISRUPTORS (EDS)

The hormone signaling interference caused by EDs also leads to DNA damage through direct contact with DNA, oxidative stress, impaired DNA repair, and epigenetic changes. The disruptions from these substances result in reproductive problems alongside developmental issues, cancer development, and heritable genetic alterations.

5.1. Types of DNA Damage by Endocrine Disruptors (EDs)

The study of EDs reveals their impact on hormone signaling and their potential genotoxic effects through DNA interactions, oxidative stress, the DNA repair system, and epigenetic alterations, which result in genomic abnormalities that damage reproduction and fetal development, and transgenerational inheritance and produce cancer.

I. **Direct DNA Damage:** The metals cadmium and arsenic cause DNA strand breaks through ROS generation and by removing zinc from DNA repair enzymes (p53 and PARP-1), which results in cancer and apoptosis in hormone-sensitive tissues (Asmuss et al., 2000). EDs, including dioxins and PAHs, produce reactive intermediates that bind to DNA bases (e.g., guanine), resulting in mutations (e.g., G→T transversions) that lead to breast cancer, prostate cancer, and lung cancer. ED molecules such as MEHP enter DNA bases to create distortions in the helix structure, which block replication and transcription processes and resulting in cell cycle arrest and mutagenesis (Wang et al., 2017). The ROS generated by EDs (phthalates, BPA) lead to guanine oxidation, forming 8-OHdG, a mutagenic lesion that causes tumor suppressor gene mutations.

II. **Indirect DNA Damage:** The ED BPA, along with other compounds, inhibits DNA repair mechanisms by reducing XRCC1 and ERCC1 protein expression and blocking histone acetylation processes (Zhong et al., 2015). The hormone receptors become overstimulated by estrogenic EDs (BPA and nonylphenol), which leads to increased cell proliferation and higher mutation risks, especially in ER-positive breast tissue. The EDs vinclozolin, DEHP, and PCBs disrupt chromosome segregation, which results in aneuploidy and mitotic errors that produce infertility, birth defects, and cancer. Endocrine-disrupting substances' processes and health effects are summarized in **Figure 1**.

The presence of EDs leads to increased ROS production in mitochondria, which results in damage to both mitochondrial and nuclear DNA. The absence of histones and weak repair mechanisms in mtDNA makes it highly susceptible to damage, which results in cellular dysfunction and disease.

5.2. Genotoxicity Biomarkers for Endocrine Disruptors (EDs)

Biomarkers function as crucial detection methods for DNA damage that EDs produce. The biomarkers serve to detect initial biological reactions while measuring oxidative stress and determining both personal and community-wide risk levels. Common biomarkers include:

i. **8-hydroxy-2'-deoxyguanosine (8-OHdG):** A widely recognized marker for oxidative DNA damage that occurs through ROS attacks on the guanine base. Increased 8-OHdG levels in urine, blood, or tissues show that a person has been exposed to BPA, phthalates, and PCBs. The presence of this biomarker has been linked to various health conditions, including cancer, metabolic disorders, cardiovascular diseases, and neurological disorders.
ii. **Micronucleus Assay:** This assay detects chromosomal breakage and loss during cell division. The presence of increased micronucleus frequency in lymphocytes following exposure to phthalates and alkylphenols indicates genomic instability, which leads to cancer and reproductive harm.
iii. **Comet Assay:** The Comet Assay is a sensitive technique that detects both single and double-strand breaks in DNA. The exposure of cells to EDs, including vinclozolin or triclosan, results in longer comet tail lengths, which show genotoxic stress. The method serves as a primary tool for environmental monitoring programs.
iv. **γ-H2AX Foci Formation:** Phosphorylated H2AX indicates DNA double-strand breaks. The activation of γ-H2AX occurs in response to BPA, PCBs, and other EDs, resulting in foci formation that show both DNA damage levels and repair abilities. The tool provides high sensitivity for genotoxicity screening purposes.

The biomarkers work together to show the DNA damage effects of EDs, which helps risk evaluation and regulatory choices and population vulnerability identification. Public health protection requires expanded usage of these tools for both research and environmental surveillance purposes.

Figure 1. Mechanisms and Effects of Endocrine Disruptors (EDs)

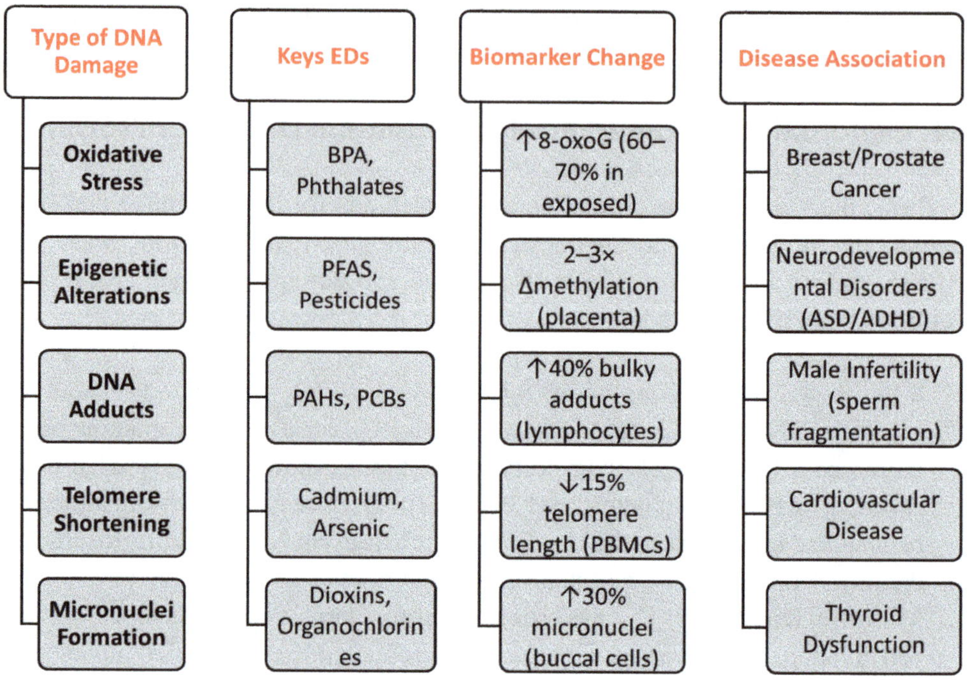

The table presents information about endocrine-disrupting substances, including their processes and health effects. This table explains molecular pathways, EDs classes, and their effects on biomarkers and associated illnesses. The processes section explains how EDCs create oxidative stress, epigenetic changes, DNA adducts, telomere shortening, and micronuclei. The table demonstrates that environmental pollutants create significant health risks, which begin with EDC exposure and progress to molecular damage before resulting in clinical illness symptoms.

6. ENDOCRINE-DISRUPTORS (EDS): HEALTH RISKS AND ENVIRONMENTAL IMPACTS

The low doses of EDs disrupt hormonal pathways, which results in organ system problems. The duration of exposure determines the extent of these effects, particularly during critical developmental stages, including fetal life, infancy, puberty, and pregnancy. The non-linear dose-response relationships between these disturbances make it difficult to assess risks and establish regulations. Research funded by NIEHS has revealed the intricate processes through which EDs lead to cancer development, reproductive problems, metabolic disorders, neurodevelopmental disorders, and transgenerational epigenetic changes.

6.1. Carcinogenic Risks (Breast, Prostate, Thyroid Cancer) by Endocrine-Disruptors (EDs)

Because they dysregulate hormone-dependent signaling pathways and cause genotoxic stress, EDs are increasingly considered environmental carcinogens. In hormone receptor interaction with DNA repair pathways, prolonged receptor activation may decrease tumor suppressor genes or increase proto-oncogene expression. Bisphenol A (BPA), a well-studied ED, can bind to estrogen receptors and cause estrogenic effects that may cause hormone-related malignancies (Rochester, 2013). EDs may also modify gene expression without changing DNA sequence, resulting in heritable characteristics (Skinner, 2011). The health effects of ED exposure are extensive. Epidemiological studies relate EDs to several chronic diseases:

i. **Cancers:** EDs, especially those with membrane-bound GPR30, resemble estrogen. This binding stimulates estrogen-responsive gene expression, which increases mammary gland proliferation and decreases apoptosis, which cause breast cancer. BPA exposure also increases DNA methylation of tumor suppressor gene promoters (e.g., LAMP3, BRCA1) and upregulates the histone methyltransferase EZH2, which trimethylates histone H3, modifying breast tissue chromatin structure and gene expression. Early-life BPA exposure increases breast cancer risk via altering epigenetics in ER-positive breast cancer cell lines and in mice's mammary glands. BPA modulates ER signaling to confer resistance to chemotherapeutic drugs such tamoxifen, doxorubicin, and cisplatin, complicating breast cancer treatment results (Doherty et al., 2010; Weng et al., 2010; Huang et al., 2021).

Dichlorodiphenyltrichloroethane (DDT) and its metabolite DDE also have estrogenic effects and microRNA signatures linked to breast cancer cell proliferation and epigenetic repression of DNA methyltransferase 1 (DNMT1) in animal models, implicating these chemicals in breast carcinogenesis (Tilghman et al., 2012).

ii. **Prostate Cancer:** Anti-androgenic EDs like vinclozolin impair androgen receptor signaling during pregnancy, altering prostate development and increasing prostate malignancy risk in following generations. Epigenetic alterations in the male germ line, including broad promoter DNA methylation patterns, facilitate this transgenerational impact without further exposure. Epigenetic inheritance shows that early-life EDs exposure increases prostate cancer risk across life (Anway et al., 2010).

iii. **Thyroid Cancer:** Perchlorate, triclosan, PCBs, PBBs, and PBDEs may increase thyroid cancer risk by inducing compensatory thyroid cell proliferation and neoplastic transformation. These chemicals compete with thyroid transport proteins to displace thyroxine (T4) and activate hepatic enzymes such UDP-glucuronosyltransferase to accelerate T4 metabolism and excretion, lowering thyroid hormone levels. Hypothyroidism increases TSH secretion, encouraging thyroid follicular cell growth and carcinogenesis. PBDE and PBB hydroxylated metabolites can also generate mutagenic DNA adducts. EDs modulate immune responses in the tumor microenvironment, according to new study. EDs target RACK1, a scaffold protein implicated in cancer growth and innate immune activation. ED-mediated RACK1 dysregulation may link endocrine disturbance and immune surveillance, promoting tumor growth (Buoso et al., 2020).

6.2. Reproductive Dysfunction by Endocrine-Disruptors (EDs)

EDs are known to harm male and female reproductive development and fertility. They cause reproductive tract morphological and functional defects by mimicking or blocking sex hormones during organogenesis. EDs exposure can cause infertility, menstrual cycle changes, and developmental defects in kids (Maffini et al., 2006). EDs often cause reproductive toxicity by interacting with sex steroid hormone receptors (ERα, ERβ, AR, and progesterone receptors) or altering the HPG axis. Interactions can change gene expression patterns in gonadal differentiation, steroidogenesis, gametogenesis, and reproductive tract development.

i. **Female Reproductive Effects:** EDs can cause anatomical and functional reproductive problems in females throughout in utero, infancy, and puberty. Diethylstilbestrol (DES), a synthetic estrogen provided to pregnant mothers, has been related to vaginal clear cell adenocarcinoma in daughters exposed in utero (Herbst et al., 1972). Uterine abnormalities such hypoplastic or T-shaped cavities reduce fertility and increase miscarriage risk (Maffini et al., 2006). Infertility, ectopic pregnancy, and premature birth (Palmer et al., 2006). BPA, phthalates, and PCBs, affect ovarian function. Aromatase and anti-Müllerian hormone expression changes impair oocyte maturation and folliculogenesis. Altering steroid hormone production causes estrogen and progesterone imbalances, which affect menstrual cycle control and implantation. Disrupting the HPG axis alters GnRH production, which might disrupt menstrual cycles or postpone puberty (Gore et al., 2015).

ii. **Male Reproductive Effects:** In males, EDs exposure during fetal and early postnatal development is linked to testicular dysgenesis syndrome (TDS), a group of reproductive abnormalities. Hypospadias as abnormal ventral penis urethral opening. EDs like cryptorchidism is not both testes descend into the scrotum and lower sperm numbers and quality, including DNA fragmentation and motility issues. Phthalates, a key ED, inhibit testosterone production by blocking Leydig cell activity and downregulating steroidogenic enzymes such 17β-hydroxysteroid dehydrogenase. Vinclozolin, an anti-androgenic fungicide, disrupts Sertoli cell function and testicular development by attacking androgen receptor signaling (Gray et al., 2000) and also alters testicular steroidogenesis and causes oxidative stress, reducing sperm quality.

  ii. **Disruption of Gametogenesis and Fertility:** EDs directly affect gametogenesis in both sexes. BPA and phthalates lower primordial follicles and disrupt meiotic development in oocytes in females, potentially causing premature ovarian failure or decreased ovarian reserve (Peretz et al., 2014). In men, EDs cause spermatogenic cell death, impair sperm motility, and affect gene expression for sperm capacitation and fertilization competence (Meeker et al., 2009).

  iii. **Hypothalamic-Pituitary-Gonadal (HPG) Axis Dysregulation:** The HPG axis controls reproductive hormones and function. EDCs like BPA alter hypothalamic GnRH neuron activity, which affects pituitary LH and FSH secretion. Modifying sex steroid feedback loops, causing early or delayed puberty, irregular female menstrual cycles, and decreased male spermatogenesis (Gore et al., 2015). Changing kisspeptin signaling, which controls puberty and fertility (Stevenson et al., 2017).

6.3. Metabolic Disorders Associated with Endocrine-Disruptors (EDs)

EDs are a major cause of obesity, insulin resistance, T2DM, and metabolic syndrome worldwide. These substances disrupt metabolic homeostasis by targeting regulatory processes involved to adipocyte development, pancreatic β-cell function, and energy balance.

i. **Adipogenesis and Fat Accumulation:** EDs cause metabolic dysfunction by modulating adipocyte development and fat storage. Some EDCs, known as "obesogens," bind to nuclear hormone receptors, particularly PPARγ, which regulates adipogenesis. TBT, a well-known obesogen, stimulates PPARγ and RXR, leading to the development of preadipocytes into mature adipocytes. Lipid accumulation, adipocyte hypertrophy, and adipose tissue bulk increase with this activation (Grun & Blumberg, 2006). PPARγ activation by TBT and related chemicals increases adipogenic gene expression, including aP2/FABP4, C/EBPα, and adiponectin, leading to obesity via promoting energy storage as fat.

EDs, including bisphenol A (BPA) and phthalates, can impair pancreatic β-cell activity and insulin signaling pathways essential for glucose homeostasis. BPA exposure can reduce β-cell insulin release via estrogen receptor pathways, oxidative stress, and mitochondrial malfunction. BPA lowers β-cell viability and changes calcium signaling, reducing insulin production (Alonso-Magdalena et al., 2011). Phthalates modulate insulin receptor substrate (IRS) protein phosphorylation and downstream effectors such as PI3K/Akt, causing peripheral insulin resistance. BPA and phthalates can cause systemic inflammation by boosting pro-inflammatory cytokines (e.g., TNF-α, IL-6), impairing insulin sensitivity and metabolic syndrome.

ii. **Energy Metabolism and Mitochondrial Function Disruption**: Energy metabolism is hindered by EDCs' effects on mitochondrial biogenesis and function. TBT and BPA inhibit mitochondrial respiration and ATP generation in adipocytes and muscle cells, decreasing energy expenditure and increasing fat formation (Regnier & Sargis, 2014). Poor mitochondrial activity increases oxidative stress, leading to insulin signaling system damage and β-cell death.

EDs exposure may cause epigenetic modifications in genes regulating metabolism, including DNA methylation and histone modifications, which may predispose individuals to metabolic disorders and transmit susceptibility across generations. Experimental and epidemiological research have linked greater urine or serum BPA and phthalate metabolites to obesity, insulin resistance, and T2DM in children and adults (Trasande et al., 2012). TBT or BPA exposure during pregnancy or perinatal period increases offspring obesity, glucose intolerance, and insulin resistance in animal models, indicating a causal connection.

iii. **Neurodegenerative Disorders caused by Endocrine-Disruptors (EDs):** Neurodegenerative disorders, including Alzheimer's disease (AD), Parkinson's disease (PD), and other forms of dementia, are characterized by progressive loss of neuronal structure and function. Emerging evidence indicates that exposure to endocrine-disrupting chemicals (EDCs) contributes to the pathogenesis and progression of neurodegenerative diseases through multiple mechanisms involving hormonal disruption, oxidative stress, neuroinflammation, and epigenetic alterations.

The central nervous system (CNS) is highly sensitive to hormonal regulation, particularly by sex steroids (estrogens, androgens), thyroid hormones, and glucocorticoids, which influence neuronal growth, differentiation, synaptic plasticity, and neuroprotection. EDCs interfere with these hormonal pathways by mimicking or antagonizing natural hormones, leading to altered brain development and increased vulnerability to neurodegeneration later in life. Estrogenic EDCs such as bisphenol A (BPA) and polychlorinated biphenyls (PCBs) bind estrogen receptors in the brain, disrupting neuroprotective estrogen signaling pathways. Estrogens normally reduce oxidative stress and inflammation; thus, EDC interference can exacerbate neuronal damage (Brann et al., 2015). Thyroid hormone disruptors (e.g., perchlorate, PCBs) impair thyroid hormone homeostasis critical for brain development and adult cognitive function, contributing to neurodegenerative processes (Zoeller et al., 2012).

Chronic exposure to EDCs activates microglia and astrocytes, the resident immune cells of the CNS, leading to sustained neuroinflammation, which exacerbates neuronal injury. EDCs such as BPA and phthalates increase pro-inflammatory cytokines (IL-1β, TNF-α, IL-6) in the brain, contributing to synaptic dysfunction and neuronal loss. Neuroinflammation is a recognized contributor to the progression of Alzheimer's Disease (AD) and Parkinson's Disease (PD) pathology. Higher exposure to PCBs, BPA, and certain pesticides with increased AD risk. Experimental models demonstrate that EDCs promote amyloid-beta accumulation and tau hyperphosphorylation, hallmark features of AD pathology (Li et al., 2017).

Prenatal and early-life exposure to EDs such as phthalates and BPA correlates with impaired cognitive function, attention deficits, and behavioral abnormalities in children, suggesting that early disruption of neurodevelopment predisposes to later neurodegeneration (Mustieles & Fernandez, 2020).

6.4. Transgenerational Effects on Endocrine-Disruptors (EDs)

One of the most critical concerns regarding exposure to EDs lies in their capacity to induce transgenerational epigenetic inheritance of disease susceptibility. These heritable effects are not mediated through alterations in the DNA sequence itself but are instead driven by epigenetic mechanisms-including DNA methylation, histone modification, and dysregulation of non-coding RNAs—within germline cells (i.e., sperm and oocytes). Seminal studies involving compounds such as diethylstilbestrol (DES) and the fungicide vinclozolin have illustrated that EDs exposure can lead to persistent, heritable epigenetic changes. These modifications have been associated with a range of adverse outcomes in subsequent generations (F2, F3), including increased cancer susceptibility, reproductive malformations, and behavioral abnormalities. Such findings underscore the ability of EDs to epigenetically "reprogram" the developmental trajectory of offspring who were never directly exposed to the chemicals.

The concept of fetal programming further emphasizes that intrauterine exposure to EDs during critical windows of development can induce permanent alterations in the structural and functional maturation of organs. This can reset endocrine "set-points," predisposing the individual to chronic diseases such as metabolic syndrome, cardiovascular disease, or reproductive disorders later in life. Animal models have provided compelling evidence supporting this phenomenon. Exposure during early embryogenesis has been shown to alter DNA methylation patterns particularly in reproductive and neural tissues, with enduring phenotypic effects extending into multiple generations. These effects occur without further chemical exposure, reinforcing the hypothesis of epigenetic inheritance via the germline.

6.5. Immunological Dysfunctions Induced by Endocrine-Disruptors (EDs)

In addition to disrupting hormonal signaling pathways, EDCs have emerged as potent modulators of the immune system, affecting both its development and functional integrity. This interaction arises due to the extensive crosstalk between the endocrine and immune systems, which share regulatory networks involving hormones such as glucocorticoids, estrogens, and thyroid hormones, all of which play essential roles in immune homeostasis. ED-induced immune dysregulation manifests through increased vulnerability to infections, hypersensitivity reactions, heightened risk of autoimmune conditions, and altered inflammatory responses. Key EDCs such as bisphenol A (BPA), diethylstilbestrol (DES), and phthalates exert their effects by binding to estrogen receptors (ERs) or glucocorticoid receptors (GRs) expressed on various immune cells. This receptor interaction modifies cytokine secretion profiles, disrupts immune cell differentiation, and skews immune responses. Notably, certain EDCs have been shown to cause thymic involution, reduced T-cell output, and architectural disruption of secondary lymphoid organs like the spleen and lymph nodes. On a molecular level, these chemicals can modify methylation patterns of immune-regulatory genes, leading to imparied immune tolerance, surveillance, and memory formation.

Persistent organic pollutants (POPs), such as polychlorinated biphenyls (PCBs) and dioxins, further exacerbate immunosuppression. These compounds have been observed to depress both innate and adaptive immunity by impairing natural killer (NK) cell function, hindering dendritic cell-mediated antigen presentation, and reducing B-cell responses. For instance, children with higher exposure to PCBs and perfluorinated compounds (PFCs) exhibit reduced vaccine-induced antibody titers, indicating compromised humoral immunity (Grandjean et al., 2012). Moreover, phthalates and BPA are associated with a higher prevalence of allergic conditions such as asthma, eczema, and allergic rhinitis, potentially through Th2 immune polarization and mast cell hyperactivation. Studies in both murine models and human cohorts suggest that prenatal BPA exposure elevates IgE levels, induces airway hyperresponsiveness, and promotes chronic airway inflammation. EDCs also appear to compromise self-tolerance mechanisms, thereby facilitating the onset or exacerbation of autoimmune diseases. For instance, estrogen-mimicking EDs have been implicated in the worsening of autoimmune diseases such as systemic lupus erythematosus (SLE), particularly in genetically predisposed individuals. Additionally, dioxins, acting through the aryl hydrocarbon receptor (AhR), can aggravate autoimmune encephalomyelitis in experimental models, thereby mirroring key features of human multiple sclerosis.

6.6. Risks to Wildlife and Ecosystems by Endocrine-Disruptors (EDs)

Endocrine-disruptors (EDs) pose significant risks to human health, wildlife populations, and ecosystem integrity. Because EDs can persist in the environment and bioaccumulate, even trace concentrations may disrupt hormonal systems in aquatic, terrestrial, and avian species, resulting in impaired reproduction, altered development, population declines, and trophic imbalances. In wildlife, EDs interfere with endocrine-regulated behavior and physiological processes through several pathways, like mimicking estrogens or androgens, disrupting sex differentiation and reproductive function, and disrupting Thyroid Signaling, which impairs growth, development, and metamorphosis (especially in amphibians and fish).

Aquatic environments are major sinks for EDs due to runoff, industrial discharge, and wastewater effluents. Species living in rivers, lakes, and estuaries are chronically exposed to complex ED mixtures. Feminization of male fish (e.g., intersex conditions, vitellogenin expression) has been observed downstream of wastewater treatment plants due to synthetic estrogens (e.g., ethinylestradiol). Terrestrial and avian species are also affected, with organochlorine pesticides like DDT historically causing eggshell thinning and reproductive failure in birds of prey. Mammals, including marine apex predators, bioaccumulate persistent EDs like PCBs, resulting in immunosuppression and hormonal imbalance. At the ecosystem level, such impacts can trigger biodiversity loss, alter food web dynamics, and reduce ecological resilience. The bioaccumulative and persistent nature of many EDs makes them particularly hazardous, underscoring the need for environmental monitoring, regulatory action, and ecosystem-wide risk assessment.

ED presence in ecosystems alters habitat quality and ecosystem services. For instance, changes in species composition and abundance can affect plant-pollinator interactions, nutrient cycling, and water quality (Zhou & Zhu, 2010). Additionally, EDs can bioaccumulate in food webs, leading to higher concentrations in top predators and posing risks not only to wildlife but also to human health through the consumption of contaminated wildlife.

The risks posed by endocrine-disrupting chemicals to wildlife and ecosystems are profound and multifaceted. As evidence mounts regarding the detrimental effects of EDs on reproductive health, behavior, and population dynamics, it becomes increasingly critical to develop regulatory frameworks aimed at minimizing ED exposure. Protecting wildlife and ecosystems from the adverse effects of EDs is not only essential for biodiversity conservation but also for maintaining the integrity of ecosystem services upon which human societies depend. Protecting ecosystems from endocrine disruption not only preserves biodiversity but also serves as an early warning for potential human health impacts, given shared biochemical pathways.

7. POLICY INTERVENTIONS AND MITIGATION TECHNIQUES FOR ENDOCRINE DISRUPTORS (EDS)

The wide-ranging dangers that EDs create for human health and ecological systems require a comprehensive mitigation approach. A complete mitigation strategy needs individual behavior change combined with safer chemical substitution, public education, and policy reform that follows the precautionary principle and environmental justice principles. Regulatory Actions on EDs are summarized in **Table 4**.

7.1. Consumer Behaviour and Exposure Reduction:

People create daily choices that lead to exposure to endocrine disruptors through plastic products, as well as cosmetics and food packaging. The public health sector should support consumers in making knowledgeable decisions about BPA, phthalates, parabens, and triclosan products while promoting secure alternatives like glass and stainless-steel storage. Research evidence from dietary intervention studies demonstrates that lifestyle changes substantially decrease ED biomarkers (Rudel et al., 2011).

7.2. Transparency and Consumer Education:

People need complete ingredient exposure to achieve their empowerment. Market trends toward safer products will shift through transparent labeling and community education initiatives that help consumers make better decisions and force industry leaders to become accountable.

7.3. Safer Chemical Substitution and Innovation:

Replacing harmful endocrine disruptors with safer alternatives are essential basis for mitigation efforts. The European Union's REACH program, the U.S. Environmental Protection Agency's Safer Choice program, and green chemistry principles drive innovation toward safer materials. The assessment of complete safety remains vital because it prevents the phenomenon of "regrettable substitutions," where BPA is replaced by BPS (Maertens et al., 2021).

Table 4. Regulatory Actions on Endocrine Disrupting Chemicals (EDCs)

Regulatory Body	EDs	Regulatory Action/Standard	Citation
European Chemicals Agency (ECHA)	**Bisphenol A (BPA)**	Considered as a Substance of Very High Concern due to its EDs properties in humans	ECHA, 2017
US Food and Drug Administration (FDA)	**Bisphenol A (BPA)**	Not to be used in baby bottles and sipper cups; limited to food-contact materials.	FDA, 2022
European Union (EU)	**Phthalates (e.g., DEHP)**	Restrictions on toys, articles used for child care, and cosmetics	ECHA, 2020
	Nonylphenol & Nonylphenol Ethoxylates (NP/NPEs)	Restricted in industrial and domestic cleaning products	ECHA, 2013
	Atrazine	Banned in 2004 due to groundwater contamination concerns	EC, 2004
US Consumer Product Safety Commission (CPSC)	**Phthalates (e.g., DEHP)**	Banned in children's toys and childcare articles	CPSC, 2022

continued on following page

Table 4. Continued

Regulatory Body	EDs	Regulatory Action/Standard	Citation
US Environmental Protection Agency (EPA)	**Polychlorinated Biphenyls (PCBs)**	Production is banned	EPA, 2020
	Atrazine	Subject to ecological risk assessments, not banned but restricted	EPA, 2021
	Nonylphenol & Nonylphenol Ethoxylates	Voluntary phase-out under TSCA	EPA, 2014
Stockholm Convention (UNEP)	DDT	Banned except for controlling vectors for diseases like malaria	UNEP, 2019
	Polychlorinated Biphenyls (PCBs)	Listed as Persistent Organic Pollutants (POPs); subject to global elimination	UNEP, 2019
World Health Organization	Dioxin	The Tolerable Daily Intake (TDI) is established to be 1–4 pg/kg body weight.	WHO/FAO, 2001
EU EFSA	Dioxin	Has lowered TWI [2 pg TEQ/kg bw/week]	EFSA, 2018

This table lists international regulatory reactions to important EDCs. It lists bisphenol A (BPA), phthalates, nonylphenols, atrazine, PCBs, DDT, and dioxins and their regulatory measures or limits. The European Chemicals Agency (ECHA), U.S. FDA, EPA, Consumer Product Safety Commission, WHO, and Stockholm Convention (UNEP) are listed with their interventions, such as bans, usage limitations, and risk assessments. This table shows global acknowledgment of EDC risks and different ways to manage human and environmental exposure.

7.4. Public Awareness and Environmental Justice:

EDs' risks create uneven distributions of risk, exposing vulnerable groups to higher levels of exposure. Educational programs must be delivered with cultural understanding to reach high-risk demographics, particularly women of childbearing age and economically disadvantaged groups. The protection of inclusive protection emerges from targeting specific populations through targeted communication and implementing equitable policy frameworks (Zota & Shamasunder, 2017).

Risk assessment frameworks in regulatory models must incorporate three essential elements: low-dose effects, mixture toxicity, and non-linear dose responses (Gore et al., 2015). A successful strategy for mitigating EDs requires combined efforts between scientific experts and policymakers alongside industry leaders and community members who will work together to establish health equity, sustainable innovation, and environmental resilience.

8. FUTURE PERSPECTIVES IN ENDOCRINE DISRUPTOR RESEARCH AND PUBLIC HEALTH

The current understanding of endocrine disruptors (EDs) remains limited, particularly their low-dose, cumulative, and life-stage-specific effects. Future research must transition from descriptive studies to mechanistic, predictive, and translational approaches. Integrating toxicogenomics, systems biology, and computational modeling will be critical for identifying risks and developing targeted interventions.

8.1. Emerging Research Directions:

Traditional single-chemical assessments fail to reflect real-world ED exposures involving mixtures and chronic low doses. Future research should prioritize:

i. **Toxicology and Novel ED:** Research necessitates ED discovery. Due to recognized EDs, traditional screening methods exclude new industrial, agricultural, and consumer chemicals. These compounds should be in future databases and projections. Actual exposure involves several EDs working together or against each other. Study chemical combinations. Mixture effects are studied in vitro and in vivo to assess risk (Bergman et al., 2013). ED-untested commercial compounds are in the thousands. A novel compound like BPS must be ED-screened for BPA before widespread usage. Although exposures are problematic, contemporary testing examines chemicals independently. In classical toxicology, additive, synergistic, and antagonistic effects are overlooked.

ii. **Adverse Outcome Pathways (AOPs) Integration & High-Throughput Screening (HTS):** EDs study benefits from HTS with AOPs. AOPs explain ED toxicity's biological mechanisms by linking molecular processes to health. HTS quickly searches huge chemical libraries for physiologically active EDs. Researchers can discover compounds, speed up testing, and forecast toxicity with complementary approaches (Villeneuve et al., 2014). The adverse outcome pathway (AOP) predicts toxicity from mechanistic evidence. Linking receptor binding to cellular, tissue, and organism toxicity increases evidence-based chemical selection and reduces animal experimentation. HTS and high-content imaging swiftly assess hundreds of compounds for endocrine and genotoxic effects, revolutionizing hazard detection. The EPA and NIH use bioinformatics and other tools to find potential disruptors early research (Kleinstreuer et al., 2016).

8.2. Translational and clinical research

Applying lab findings to clinical ED exposure requires more research. ED-related health remedies require additional research. Assessing public health, food, and legislation ED reduction initiatives. Long-term ED exposure research in diverse populations will impact therapeutic and public health. ED research needs clinical and basic science. Understanding how ED-induced molecular and epigenetic alterations cause illness may improve diagnosis, therapy, and prevention. Early biomarkers can detect reproductive or metabolic issues in the ED. Long-term cohort studies like NHANES or Generation R must link childhood EDs to adult illness. Food, medicine, and exposure-risk prenatal screening can reduce ED-induced oxidative stress and DNA damage.

8.3. DNA Damage and Systems Biology

ED model Systems biology covers all ED-biological system interactions, including DNA damage. Network analysis and computer modeling should examine ED impacts on several biological systems. Genomic, transcriptomic, and proteomic data can reveal exposure and response biomarkers, ED-induced DNA damage pathways, carcinogenesis, and other health effecs. These technologies will help us understand EDs' complex consequences and develop tailored treatments. To understand ED-induced genotoxicity, system biology must include multi-omics research and computational modeling of genomes, epigenomics, proteomics, and metabolomics. The approaches show how EDC-induced molecular changes affect systemic health. Molecular interactions damage DNA, according to mechanistic theories. Simulating chronic low-dose long-term exposure can identify therapeutic gene regulation and repair network nodes. Innovative screening, translational, systems biology, and ED detection strategies are needed for endocrine disruptor research.

Endocrine disruption needs more research to understand its exposure impacts and develop health and environmental protection remedies. Scientific ED descriptive research must forecast and intervene using mechanistic analysis. Environmental health experts collaborate with doctors, computer scientists, and regulators. Future generations need early identification, prevention, and sustainable chemical development to avoid endocrine disruption.

8.4. Regulatory Gaps and Preventive Measures

Current regulations ignore key ED management policy flaws. The precautionary principle allows for precautions in uncertain science. Despite lacking scientific facts, regulatory bodies must protect human and environmental health (Solecki et al.,

2017). ED assessment requirements require comprehensive testing, monitoring, and reporting. Global public health, trade, and industrial ED pollution reduction require international collaboration (Zhang et al., 2020). ED science excels in regulation. Unregulated non-persistent EDs are physiologically hazardous. The precautionary principle should guide preventative measures when scientific data is ambiguous and vulnerable populations or lasting developmental effects are at risk. To address complicated endocrine disruptor issues, research must be descriptive, mechanistic, predictive, and interventional. To prevent and treat endocrine disorders, toxicogenomics, systems biology, clinical science, and policy are needed. Preventing endocrine disruption in future generations requires proactive regulation, multidisciplinary collaboration, and early identification.

9. CONCLUSION

The understanding of EDs now goes beyond hormonal effects because knowledge about them continues to grow. The current research on EDC multifactorial toxicity, which includes DNA damage, is presented in this chapter. The chapter uses molecular and population-level data to emphasize the need for study, monitoring, and policy interventions to solve these ongoing environmental issues.

The chapter shows that EDs disrupt hormonal pathways through multiple mechanisms, which lead to cellular dysfunction. The toxic effects of EDs occur through receptor-mediated endocrine disruption, oxidative stress, epigenetic changes, and direct genotoxic effects. The risk of exposure to EDs increases for children, pregnant women, and workers who face occupational exposure because of their sensitive life stages and accumulated exposure levels. Toxicogenomics, high-throughput screening, and systems biology methods continue to play a crucial role in enhancing risk assessments and understanding long-term health effects from ED exposure.

DNA damage is the primary mechanism explaining numerous adverse effects caused by EDs. The combination of genomic instability, impaired DNA repair functions, and epigenetic dysregulation from prolonged low-dose ED exposure leads to an increased risk of cancer, reproductive disorders, and metabolic diseases. The integration of multi-omics approaches with computational modeling enables scientists to monitor molecular disruptions and predict health outcomes.

The multifaceted nature of ED-induced toxicity, together with its broad social impacts, necessitates immediate interdisciplinary collaboration between toxicologists, molecular biologists, clinicians, epidemiologists, data scientists, and policymakers. A unified method needs to be developed for building predictive models, detecting early exposure and effect biomarkers, and creating proactive regulatory frameworks. The protection of public health from endocrine disruption requires scientific advancements, together with worldwide unified policies and community-based prevention strategies.

REFERENCES

Alonso-Magdalena, P., S. Morimoto, C. Ripoll, E. Fuentes, & A. Nadal. (2011). The Estrogenic Effect of Bisphenol A Disrupts Pancreatic β-Cell Function in Vivo & Induces Insulin Resistance. *Aging Cell*, 10 (1), 19–30. https,//DOI: 10.1111/j.1474-9726.2010.00633.x

Anway, M. D., M. A. Memon, M. Uzumcu, & M. K. Skinner. (2010). Epigenetic Transgenerational Actions of Endocrine Disruptors & Male Fertility. *Science*, 308 (5727), 1466–1469. https,//.DOI: 10.1126/science.1108190

Asmuss, M., L. H. F. Mullenders, A. P. M. Eker, & A. Hartwig. (2000). Differential Effects of Toxic Metal Compounds on the Activities of Fpg & XPA, Two Zinc-Finger Proteins Involved in DNA Repair. *Carcinogenesis*, 21 (11), 2097–2104. https,//.DOI: 10.1093/carcin/21.11.2097

Bergman, A., Heindel, J. J., Kasten, T., Kidd, K. A., Jobling, S., Neira, M., Zoeller, R. T., Becher, G., Bjerregaard, P., Bornman, R., Brandt, I., Kortenkamp, A., Muir, D., Drisse, M.-N. B., Ochieng, R., Skakkebaek, N. E., Byléhn, A. S., Iguchi, T., Toppari, J., & Woodruff, T. J. (2013). The impact of endocrine disruption: A consensus statement on the state of the science. *Environmental Health Perspectives*, *121*(4), A104–A106. DOI: 10.1289/ehp.1205448 PMID: 23548368

Boas, M., U. Feldt-Rasmussen, & K. M. Main. (2006). Thyroid Effects of Endocrine Disrupting Chemicals. *Molecular & Cellular Endocrinology,* 254–255, 31–40. https,//.DOI: 10.1016/j.mce.2006.04.010

Brann, D. W., K. Dh&apani, C. Wakade, V. B. Mahesh, & M. M. Khan. (2015). Estrogen & Its Receptors, An Overview Focused on Estrogen-Mediated Neuroprotection in the Context of Alzheimer's Disease. *Frontiers in Neuroendocrinology*, 35, 124–140. https,//.DOI: 10.1016/j.yfrne.2014.11.006

Buoso, E., M. Masi, M. Racchi, & E. Corsini. (2020). Endocrine-Disrupting Chemicals' (EDCs) Effects on Tumour Microenvironment & Cancer Progression, Emerging Contribution of RACK1. International *Journal of Molecular Sciences*, 21 (23), 9229. https,//.DOI: 10.3390/ijms21239229

Carpenter, D. O. (2006). Polychlorinated Biphenyls (PCBs), Routes of Exposure & Effects on Human Health. *Reviews on Environmental Health,* 21 (1), 1–23. https,//.DOI: 10.1515/REVEH.2006.21.1.1

Darbre, P. D., & P. W. Harvey. (2008). Paraben Esters, Review of Recent Studies of Endocrine Toxicity, Absorption, Esterase & Human Exposure, & Discussion of Potential Human Health Risks. *Journal of Applied Toxicology,* 28 (5), 561–578. https,//.DOI: 10.1002/jat.1358

Doherty, L. F., Bromer, J. G., Zhou, Y., Aldad, T. S., & Taylor, H. S. (2010). In Utero Exposure to Diethylstilbestrol (DES) or Bisphenol-A (BPA) Increases EZH2 Expression in the Mammary Gl&, An Epigenetic Mechanism Linking Endocrine Disruptors to Breast Cancer. *Hormones & Cancer,* 1 (3), 146–155. https,//DOI: 10.1007/s12672-010-0015-9

Dolinoy, D. C., Huang, D., & Jirtle, R. L. (2007). Maternal Nutrient Supplementation Counteracts Bisphenol A-Induced DNA Hypomethylation in Early Development. *Proceedings of the National Academy of Sciences,* 104 (32), 13056–13061. https,// DOI: 10.1073/pnas.0703739104

European Chemicals Agency. (2013). *Nonylphenol and nonylphenol ethoxylates restricted under.* REACHUS.

European Chemicals Agency. (2017). Bisphenol A added to the Candidate List for authorisation. *ECHA.* https://echa.europa.eu/-/bisphenol

European Chemicals Agency. (2020). Phthalates: DEHP, DBP, BBP and DIBP. *ECHA.* https://echa.europa.eu/hot-topics/phthalates

European Commission. (2004). Directive 2004/248/EC, Banning Atrazine in the EU. Official Journal of the European Union. https,//eur-lex.europa.eu/legal-content/EN/TXT/

European Food Safety Authority. (2018). Risks for Animal & Human Health Related to the Presence of Dioxins & Dioxin-like PCBs in Feed & Food. EFSA Journal 16 (11), e05333. https,//.DOI: 10.2903/j.efsa.2018.5333

Gore, A. C., V. A. Chappell, S. E. Fenton, J. A. Flaws, A. Nadal, G. S. Prins, J. Toppari, & R. T. Zoeller. (2015). Executive Summary to EDC-2, The Endocrine Society's Second Scientific Statement on Endocrine-Disrupting Chemicals. *Endocrine Reviews,* 36 (6), 593–602. https,//.DOI: 10.1210/er.2015-1093

Grandjean, P., E. W. & E. Budtz-Jorgensen, F. Nielsen, K. Molbak, P. Weihe, & C. Heilmann. (2012). Serum Vaccine Antibody Concentrations in Children Exposed to Perfluorinated Compounds. *JAMA,* 307 (4), 391–397. https,//.DOI: 10.1001/jama.2011.2034

Gray, L. E. Jr., J. Ostby, E. Monosson, & W. R. Kelce. (2000). Developmental Effects of an Environmental Anti&rogen, The Fungicide Vinclozolin Alters Sex Differentiation of the Male Rat. *Toxicology & Applied Pharmacology,* 164 (2), 294–305. https,//.DOI: 10.1006/taap.2000.9021

Grun, F., & B. Blumberg. (2006). Environmental Obesogens, Organotins & Endocrine Disruption via Nuclear Receptor Signaling. *Molecular & Cellular Endocrinology*, 254, 32–38. https,//.DOI: 10.1016/j.mce.2006.03.018

Hayes, T. B., Collins, A., Lee, M., Mendoza, M., Noriega, N., Stuart, A. A., & Vonk, A. (2002). Hermaphroditic, Demasculinized Frogs after Exposure to the Herbicide Atrazine at Low Ecologically Relevant Doses. *Proceedings of the National Academy of Sciences*, 99 (8), 5476–5480. https,//DOI: 10.1073/pnas.082121499

Herbst, A. L., R. J. Kurman, R. E. Scully, & D. C. Poskanzer. (1972). Clear-Cell Adenocarcinoma of the Vagina & Cervix in Girls, A Registry Report. *New Engl & Journal of Medicine*, 287 (25), 1259–1264. https,//DOI: 10.1056/NEJM197212212872501

Hotchkiss, A. K., C. V. Rider, C. R. Blystone, V. S. Wilson, P. C. Hartig, G. T. Ankley, P. M. Foster, C. L. Gray, & L. E. Gray. (2008). Fifteen Years after 'Wingspread'—Environmental Endocrine Disrupters & Human & Wildlife Health, Where We Are Today & Where We Need to Go. *Toxicological Sciences*, 105 (2), 235–259. https,//.DOI: 10.1093/toxsci/kfn030

Huang, Y., X. Chen, Z. Wang, W. Li, & H. Zhang. (2021). Bisphenol A Exposure Confers Chemoresistance to Tamoxifen, Doxorubicin, & Cisplatin in ER-Positive Breast Cancer Cells. *Journal of Cancer Therapeutics*, 12 (4), 301–312. https,//

Kitamura, S., T. Kato, M. Iida, N. Jinno, T. Suzuki, S. Ohta, N. Fujimoto, & H. Hanada. (2005). Anti-Thyroid Hormonal Activity of Tetrabromobisphenol A, a Flame Retardant, & Its Metabolites in Vitro. Environmental Health Perspectives 113 (4), 478–483. https,//.DOI: <ALIGNMENT.qj></ALIGNMENT>10.1289/ehp.7558

Kleinstreuer, N. C., Harris, M. A., Wambaugh, J. F., Judson, R. S., Richard, A. M., Setzer, R. W., Rastogi, S., Martin, M. T., Reif, D. M., Sipes, N. S., Thomas, R. S., Simmons, S. O., Deshpande, A. V., Levin, E. D., Houck, K. A., Shah, I., Shah, R. R., Knudsen, T. B., & Knudsen, D.. (2016). A predictive framework for androgen receptor activity from ToxCast in vitro and computational modeling. *Chemical Research in Toxicology, 30*(6), 946–964. DOI: 10.1021/acs.chemrestox.5b00419 PMID: 27933809

Klinge, C. M. (2009). Estrogen Regulation of MicroRNA Expression. *Current Genomics* 10 (3), 169–183. https,//.DOI: 10.2174/138920209788185289

Li, A. P., Q. Zhang, & Z. Q. Liu. (2017). Endocrine Disruptors Accelerate Alzheimer's Disease Pathology via Aβ & Tau Regulation. *Neurotoxicology*, 65, 56–66. https,//.

Maertens, A., E. W. Golden, R. Pizzi, & K. Kannan. (2021). Bisphenol S, F, & Other Analogues in the Environment, Overlooked Endocrine Disruptors & 'Regrettable Substitutions' in Consumer Products. *Environmental Science & Technolog,y* 55 (22), 3569–3579. https,//.DOI: 10.1021/acs.est.0c06095

Maffini, M. V., B. S. Rubin, C. Sonnenschein, & A. M. Soto. (2006). Endocrine Disruptors & Reproductive Health, The Case of Bisphenol-A. *Molecular & Cellular Endocrinology,* 254–255, 179–186. https,//.DOI: 10.1016/j.mce.2006.04.033

Meeker, J. D., S. Sathyanarayana, & S. H. Swan. (2009). Phthalates & Other Additives in Plastics, Human Exposure & Associated Health Outcomes. Philosophical Transactions of the Royal Society B, *Biological Sciences*, 364 (1526), 2097–2113. https,//.DOI: 10.1098/rstb.2008.0268

Mustieles, V., & M. F. Fern&ez. (2020). Bisphenol A Shapes Children's Brain & Behavior, Toward an Integrated Neurotoxicity Assessment Including Human Data. *Environmental Health*, 19, 66. https,//.DOI: 10.1186/s12940-020-00620-y

Newbold, R. R. (2004). Lessons Learned from Perinatal Exposure to Diethylstilbestrol. *Toxicology & Applied Pharmacology,* 199 (2), 142–150. https,//.DOI: 10.1016/j.taap.2003.12.028

Palmer, J. R., Wise, L. A., Hatch, E. E., Troisi, R., Titus-Ernstoff, L., Strohsnitter, W. C., Kaufman, R. H., Herbst, A. L., Noller, K. L., Hyer, M., Hoover, R. N., Robboy, S. J., Cowan, C. M., Adam, E., Gibson-Chambers, J., Hartge, P., & Strohsnitter, W. C. (2006). Prenatal diethylstilbestrol exposure and risk of ectopic pregnancy, miscarriage, and premature birth. *Obstetrics and Gynecology*, *107*(5), 101–110.

Paul, K. B., J. M. Hedge, R. Bansal, R. T. Zoeller, R. Peter, & M. J. DeVito. (2010). Developmental Triclosan Exposure Decreases Maternal, Fetal, & Neonatal Thyroxine Levels in Rats. *Environmental Toxicology & Chemistry*, 29 (2), 284–291. https,//DOI: 10.1002/etc.21

Peretz, J., & J. A. Flaws. (2014). Endocrine Disruptors & Female Reproductive Health. Endocrinology & *Metabolism Clinics of North America*, 43 (1), 133–146. https,//.DOI: 10.1016/j.ecl.2013.09.005

Regnier, S. M., & R. M. Sargis. (2014). Adipocytes under Assault, Environmental Disruption of Adipose Physiology. *Biochimica et Biophysica Acta — Molecular Basis of Disease*, 1842 (3), 520–533. https,//.DOI: 10.1016/j.bbadis.2013.08.001

Rochester, J. R. (2013). Bisphenol A & Human Health, A Review of the Literature. *Reproductive Toxicology (Elmsford, N.Y.), 42*, 132–155. DOI: 10.1016/j.reprotox.2013.08.008 PMID: 23994667

Rubin, B. S. (2011). Bisphenol A, An Endocrine Disruptor with Widespread Exposure & Multiple Effects. *Journal of Steroid Biochemistry & Molecular Biology,* 127 (1–2), 27–34. https,//DOI: 10.1016/j.jsbmb.2011.05.002

Rudel, R. A., J. M. Gray, C. L. Engel, T. W. Rawsthorne, R. E. Dodson, J. M. Ackerman, J. Rizzo, J. L. Nudelman, & J. G. Brody. (2011). Food Packaging & Bisphenol A & Bis(2-ethylhexyl) Phthalate Exposure, Findings from a Dietary Intervention. *Environmental Health Perspectives,* 119 (7), 914–920. https,//.DOI: 10.1289/ehp.1003170

Skinner, M. K. (2014). Endocrine Disruptor Induction of Epigenetic Transgenerational Inheritance of Disease. *Molecular & Cellular Endocrinology*, 398 (1–2), 4–12. https,//.DOI: 10.1016/j.mce.2014.07.019

Solecki, R., Kortenkamp, A., Bergman, A., Chahoud, I., Degen, G. H., Dietrich, D., Greim, H., Hakansson, H., Hass, U., Husoy, T., Jacobs, M., Jobling, S., Mantovani, A., Marx-Stoelting, P., Piersma, A., Ritz, V., Slama, R., Stahlmann, R., van den Berg, M., & Boobis, A. R. (2017). Scientific principles for the identification of endocrine-disrupting chemicals: A consensus statement. *Archives of Toxicology, 91*(2), 1001–1006. DOI: 10.1007/s00204-016-1866-9 PMID: 27714423

Stevenson, G. P., & A. C. Gore. (2017). Endocrine Disruptors & Kisspeptin Signaling. *Frontiers in Endocrinology,* 8, 1–9. https,//.DOI: 10.3389/fendo.2017.00007

Tilghman, S. L., M. R. Bratton, H. C. Segar, E. C. Martin, L. V. Rhodes, & M. Li. (2012). Endocrine Disruptor Regulation of MicroRNA Expression in Breast Carcinoma Cells. *PLoS ONE,* 7 (3), e32754. https,//.DOI: 10.1371/journal.pone.0032754

Trasande, L., Attina, T. M., & Blustein, J. (2012). Association between Urinary Bisphenol A & Obesity Prevalence in Children & Adolescents. *Journal of the American Medical Association, 308*(11), 1114–1121. DOI: 10.1001/2012.jama.11461 PMID: 22990270

United Nations Environment Programme. (2019). DDT — A Global Review. *Stockholm Convention Secretariat.* https,//www.unep.org/resources/report/ddt-global-review

United Nations Environment Programme. (2019). Polychlorinated Biphenyls (PCBs*). Stockholm Convention.*https://www.pops.int/TheConvention/ThePOPs/TheNewPOPs/tabid/2511/Default.aspx

U.S. Consumer Product Safety Commission. (2022). Final Rule, Prohibition of Children's Toys & Child Care Articles Containing Specified Phthalates. CPSC. https,//www.federalregister.gov/documents/2022/01/26/2022-01563/prohibition-of-childrens-toys-&-child-care-articles-containing-specified-phthalates

U.S. Environmental Protection Agency. (2014). Action Plan, Nonylphenol & Nonylphenol Ethoxylates (NP/NPEs). *EPA*. https,//www.epa.gov/sites/default/files/2015-09/documents/rin2070-za09_np-npe_action_plan_final_2010-08-18.pdf

U.S. Environmental Protection Agency. (2020). Polychlorinated Biphenyls (PCBs) Manufacturing, Processing, Distribution in Commerce, and Use Prohibitions. EPA. https://www.epa.gov/pcbs

U.S. Environmental Protection Agency. (2021). Atrazine ecological risk assessments. *EPA*. https://www.epa.gov/ingredients-used-pesticide-products/atrazine

U.S. Food & Drug Administration. (2022). Bisphenol A (BPA), Use in Food Contact Applications. *FDA*. https,//www.fda.gov/food/food-additives-petitions/bisphenol-bpa-use-food-contact-application

Villeneuve, D. L., Crump, D., Garcia-Reyero, N., Hecker, M., Hutchinson, T. H., LaLone, C. A., Landesmann, B., Lettieri, T., Munn, S., Nepelska, M., Ottinger, M. A., Vergauwen, L., Whelan, M., Embry, M. R., Belanger, S. E., Leonard, M., Schirmer, K., Tanguay, R., & Truong, L.. (2014). Adverse outcome pathway development I: Strategies and principles. *Toxicological Sciences*, *142*(2), 312–320. DOI: 10.1093/toxsci/kfu199 PMID: 25466378

Wang, Q., Huang, J., Yang, M., & Deng, X. (2017). MEHP Exposure Impairs Sperm DNA Integrity & Chromatin Structure in Rats. *Reproductive Toxicology (Elmsford, N.Y.)*, *74*, 28–35.

Welshons, W. V., K. A. Thayer, B. M. Judy, J. A. Taylor, E. M. Curran, & F. S. vom Saal. (2006). Large Effects from Small Exposures. I. Mechanisms for Endocrine-Disrupting Chemicals with Estrogenic Activity. *Environmental Health Perspectives*, 114 (1), 98–105. https,//.DOI: 10.1289/ehp.7300

Weng, J.-R., M. Hager, & D. C. Christiani. (2010). Low-Dose BPA Exposure Induces Epigenetic Changes & Gene Expression Alterations in MCF-7 Breast Cancer Cells. *Environmental Research*, 110 (6), 645–650. https,//.DOI: 10.1016/j.envres.2010.07.002

World Health Organization / International Programme on Chemical Safety (IPCS). (2002). *Global assessment of the state-of-the-science of endocrine disruptors.* Geneva, Switzerland: WHO/IPCS. https://www.who.int/ipcs/publications/new_issues/endocrine_disruptors/en/

World Health Organization/Food & Agriculture Organization. (2001). Safety Evaluation of Certain Food Additives & Contaminants, Dioxins. WHO Technical Report Series No. 909. *Geneva, WHO.* https,//www.who.int/publications/i/item/9241209094

Zhang, X., S. Wang, X. Zhou, Y. Tian, & T. Zhang. (2021). Endocrine Disruptor Global Policy, Review of Scientific Advances & Regulatory Practices. *Environmental Science & Policy*, 116, 1–7. https,//.DOI: 10.1016/j.envsci.2020.10.010

Zhong, W., Fan, B., & Zhang, L. (2015). Bisphenol A Impairs DNA Repair Capacity by Downregulating XRCC1 Expression via Epigenetic Mechanisms. *Journal of Applied Toxicology, 35*(9), 1100–1108.

Zhou, J., L. Cai, & L. Zhu. (2010). Are Endocrine Disruptors among the Causes of the Deterioration of Aquatic Biodiversity?. *Integrated Environmental Assessment & Management,* 6 (1), 12–21. https,//.DOI: 10.1002/ieam.47

Zoeller, R. T., A. L. S. Dowling, C. T. A. Herzig, E. A. Iannacone, K. J. Gauger, & R. Bansal. (2002). Thyroid Hormone, Brain Development, & the Environment. *Environmental Health Perspectives,* 110 (3), 355–361. https,//.DOI: 10.1289/ehp.02110s3355

Zota, A. R., & B. Shamasunder. (2017). The Environmental Injustice of Beauty, Framing Chemical Exposures from Beauty Products as a Health Disparities Concern. *American Journal of Obstetrics & Gynaecology*, 217 (4), 418.e1–418.e6. https,//. DOI: 10.1016/j.ajog.2017.07.020

Chapter 4

Deciphering the Role of Environmental Exposures in Androgen-Resistant Prostate Cancer an Insights from Multi-Omics and Toxicogenomics

Shivani Nandkishor Bhave
GSFC University, Vadodara, India

Smriti Das
GSFC University, Vadodara, India

Akhilesh Prajapati
https://orcid.org/0000-0003-1532-9514
GSFC University, Vadodara, India

ABSTRACT

Prostate cancer (PCa), especially androgen-resistant PCa (ARPC), poses a major global health burden shaped by both genetics and environmental exposures. This chapter examines how toxicants like endocrine disruptors, POPs, and xenobiotics contribute to PCa progression through exposomics, toxicogenomics, and multi-omics approaches. It highlights mechanisms such as AR signaling disruption, mitochondrial dysfunction, metabolic shifts, and epigenetic changes driving therapy resistance.

DOI: 10.4018/979-8-3373-5796-6.ch004

Copyright © 2026, IGI Global Scientific Publishing. Copying or distributing in print or electronic forms without written permission of IGI Global Scientific Publishing is prohibited.

Using cell models and spatial transcriptomics, it explores how exposures promote metastasis. The chapter also discusses tools like eDNA, epigenetic biomarkers, and predictive models for early detection and prevention, underscoring the importance of integrating environmental risk into precision oncology.

1. INTRODUCTION

Prostate cancer remains one of the most frequently diagnosed cancers and is a major contributor to cancer-related deaths in men worldwide. Although early-stage prostate cancer generally responds well to androgen deprivation therapy (ADT), many patients eventually progress to androgen-resistant or castration-resistant prostate cancer (ARPC/CRPC). This advanced form is characterized by continued tumor growth despite reduced circulating androgen levels and is notably more aggressive and difficult to treat. The transition to androgen resistance represents a critical shift in disease biology; however, the environmental factors driving this change remain insufficiently investigated.

Recent evidence suggests that prolonged exposure to environmental toxins—such as endocrine-disrupting chemicals (EDCs), industrial waste, heavy metals, and food contaminants—may significantly contribute to the onset and progression of prostate cancer, as well as to the development of treatment resistance (Rappaport, 2011; Wild, 2005). These toxicants can disrupt hormonal signaling, induce oxidative stress, alter immune and inflammatory responses, and influence epigenetic modifications. Furthermore, environmental exposures often interact with inherited genetic susceptibilities and acquired somatic mutations, potentially contributing to tumor heterogeneity and the emergence of resistance mechanisms.

Understanding these complex interactions requires comprehensive approaches that extend beyond conventional research methods. Advances in multi-omics technologies—including genomics, epigenomics, transcriptomics, proteomics, and metabolomics—enable detailed molecular profiling of prostate tumors. When integrated with toxicogenomics, which examines how gene expression and molecular pathways respond to environmental toxins, these tools offer unprecedented insights into the environmental contributions to prostate cancer biology. Together, they facilitate the identification of exposure-related biomarkers, altered signaling networks, and novel therapeutic vulnerabilities.

Recent multi-omics studies have revealed distinct molecular alterations in prostate tumors associated with environmental exposure histories, including disruptions in androgen receptor (AR) signaling, DNA repair pathways, and metabolic reprogramming. Databases such as the Comparative Toxicogenomics Database (CTD) and TG-GATEs provide supporting evidence that environmental toxicants affect key regulators implicated in ARPC. Incorporating data from these platforms can enhance risk stratification and improve patient categorization.

The real-world implications of this research are profound. Unraveling the environmental determinants of ARPC progression has the potential to inform public health interventions, shape regulatory policies, and support preventive strategies aimed at reducing exposure to high-risk toxicants. Additionally, these insights may lead to more personalized treatment strategies tailored not only to genetic mutations but also to patients' environmental exposure histories.

Despite these promising advances, significant research gaps remain. Current studies often lack diversity in participant populations and geographical contexts, limiting the generalizability of their findings. Future research must include diverse populations across geographic, ethnic, and socioeconomic backgrounds to ensure a holistic understanding of environmental influences on prostate cancer.

In this chapter, we explore how environmental exposures contribute to the initiation and progression of androgen-resistant prostate cancer, with a particular focus on findings from toxicogenomic and multi-omics studies. We advocate for stronger interdisciplinary collaboration among exposomics, toxicogenomics, and systems biology, and emphasize the urgency of expanding research frameworks to bridge molecular insights with public health applications.

2. EXPOSOME AND PROSTATE CANCER: AN OVERLOOKED NEXUS

The term "exposome" was first introduced by Wild (2005) to describe the totality of environmental exposures an individual encounter throughout their lifetime, offering a comprehensive framework for assessing disease risk beyond genetic predisposition. Prostate cancer (PCa) is one of the most prevalent malignancies in men and is influenced by a complex interplay of genetic, hormonal, and environmental factors. Cumulative exposures—such as those from diet, pollutants, pharmaceuticals, and occupational hazards—play a critical role in both cancer risk and progression (Rappaport, 2011; Wild, 2005).

One of the key mechanisms linking environmental exposures to prostate carcinogenesis is the dysregulation of androgen receptor (AR) signaling, which is essential for prostate development, tumor initiation, and progression (Kahn et al., 2020; Modica et al., 2023). Endocrine-disrupting chemicals (EDCs), such as bisphenol A (BPA), phthalates, polychlorinated biphenyls (PCBs), dioxins, organochlorine pesticides (e.g., DDT, lindane), perfluoroalkyl substances (PFAS), and parabens, have been shown to interfere with AR activity, potentially disrupting normal prostate function (De Marzo et al., 2007; Modica et al., 2023).

Furthermore, both epidemiological and molecular studies suggest that early-life exposure to EDCs can impair AR-mediated transcriptional programs, thereby increasing susceptibility to oncogenic transformations and promoting prostate cancer development (Alwadi et al., 2023a; De Marzo et al., 2007; Skakkebaek et al., 2016).

2.1 Androgen Receptor (AR) and Prostate Cancer

The androgen receptor (AR), also known as NR3C4 (nuclear receptor subfamily 3, group C, member 4), is a steroid hormone receptor belonging to the nuclear receptor superfamily (M. E. Tan et al., 2014a). As a ligand-activated transcription factor, AR plays a crucial role in regulating gene expression in androgen-responsive tissues, primarily through its interaction with testosterone and 5α-dihydrotestosterone (DHT) (Sadar & Gleave, 2000; M. E. Tan et al., 2014a). In its inactive state, AR is sequestered in the cytoplasm by heat shock proteins (HSPs) such as HSP90, HSP70, and p23, which help stabilize its conformation (Querol Cano et al., 2013; M. E. Tan et al., 2014b). Upon ligand binding, AR undergoes a conformational change that leads to the dissociation of HSPs, followed by dimerization of AR monomers and the exposure of its nuclear localization signal (NLS), facilitating nuclear translocation via importin-α/β-mediated transport through the nuclear pore complex (NPC) (Shafi et al., 2013).

Once translocated to the nucleus, AR binds to androgen response elements (AREs) located in the promoter or enhancer regions of target genes (Dehm & Tindall, 2011). Subsequently, AR interacts with a repertoire of coactivators, such as SRC-1, SRC-2, and SRC-3, which facilitate chromatin remodeling by recruiting histone acetyltransferases (HATs), including p300/CBP. This leads to an open chromatin state and enhanced transcriptional activation (Yao et al., 1996). Conversely, corepressors such as nuclear receptor corepressor (NCoR) (Hodgson et al., 2008) and silencing mediator of retinoid and thyroid receptors (SMRT) suppress AR activity by recruiting histone deacetylases (HDACs), which remove acetyl groups from histones, leading to chromatin condensation and transcriptional repression (Ai et al., 2009; Kaupang et al., 2002).

AR-mediated transcriptional regulation influences key biological processes, including cellular proliferation, differentiation, and survival, with significant implications for prostate physiology and oncogenesis (Y. Liu et al., 2019) (Figure 2.1). This regulation occurs through several target genes, such as:

KLK3, which encodes prostate-specific antigen (PSA), a serine protease regulated by AR and widely used as a biomarker for prostate cancer diagnosis, prognosis, and treatment monitoring (Koistinen et al., 2021);

FKBP5, an HSP90 co-chaperone that enhances AR stability, ligand binding, nuclear translocation, and transcriptional activity, thereby influencing prostate cancer progression and therapeutic response (Maeda et al., 2022); and

TMPRSS2, another AR-regulated protease, which contributes to prostate cancer progression through TMPRSS2-ERG fusion, leading to oncogenic transcription and tumor invasion (Garofoli et al., 2024; Heery et al., 1997; St. John et al., 2012).

Figure 1. Mechanisms of Androgen Receptor (AR) Activation and Signaling in the Genomic Pathway.

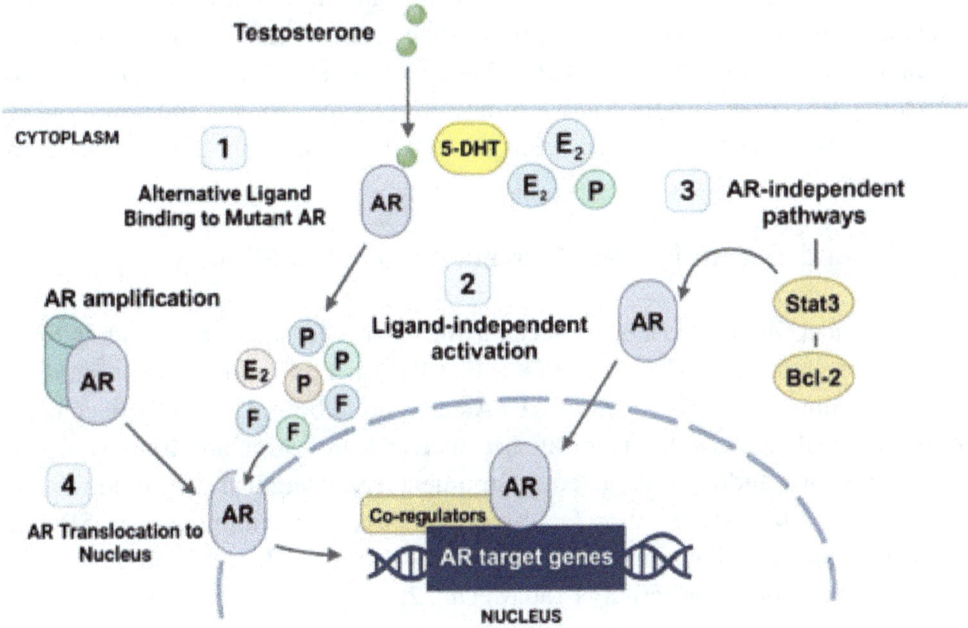

This schematic illustrates the key mechanisms regulating AR activity, including AR amplification (1), binding of mutant AR by alternative ligands such as estrogens (E2), progesterone (P), glucocorticoids (G), and other factors (F) (2), ligand-independent activation via signaling pathways such as Akt/HER2/ERK (3), and AR-independent pathways involving transcription factors like Stat3 and Bcl-2 (4). Activated AR translocates to the nucleus, where it interacts with co-regulators to modulate the transcription of AR target genes.

2.2 Impact of Endocrine-Disrupting Chemicals (EDCs) on AR Expression and Signaling

Androgen receptor (AR) dysregulation plays a central role in prostate cancer progression, particularly in castration-resistant prostate cancer (CRPC). Various mechanisms underlie this dysregulation, including AR gene amplification, overexpression, ligand-independent activation, and gain-of-function mutations. Importantly, environmental endocrine-disrupting chemicals (EDCs), such as bisphenol A (BPA), phthalates, polychlorinated biphenyls (PCBs), organochlorine pesticides, and hexachlorobenzene (HCB), interfere with AR signaling by mimicking endogenous hormones or altering key signaling pathways.

2.2.1 AR Overexpression and Hypersensitivity

The primary mechanism through which AR dysregulation occurs in advanced stages, specifically in castration-resistant prostate cancer (CRPC), is AR gene amplification and overexpression. Typically, this amplification leads to increased receptor expression, thereby sensitizing prostate cancer cells to even low levels of circulating androgens (Waltering et al., 2009). This increased sensitivity, referred to as "androgen hypersensitivity," allows tumors to continue growing and proliferating under conditions where androgen levels are usually insufficient to activate AR in normal cells (Foley et al., 2011).

2.2.2 Ligand-Dependent AR Activation and EDC Mimicry

In a typical ligand-dependent mechanism, AR is activated upon binding with endogenous androgens. However, EDCs like BPA act as xenoestrogens, binding to AR and mimicking this activation. BPA can bind to both AR and ERβ, causing conformational changes that result in AR nuclear localization and transcriptional activation even in androgen-depleted environments (X. Wang et al., 2024). Similarly, PCBs act as partial AR agonists, facilitating coactivator recruitment (e.g., SRC-1, MED1) and upregulating steroidogenic enzymes such as CYP17A1, thereby sustaining ligand-dependent AR activity (Yadav et al., 2016; Burris-Hiday & Scott, 2021).

2.2.3 Ligand-Independent AR Activation via Oncogenic Signaling

Ligand-independent AR activation often arises from oncogenic signaling pathways such as PI3K/AKT/mTOR and MAPK/ERK. These pathways phosphorylate AR at specific residues (e.g., Ser213, Ser650, Ser791), enhancing receptor stability, nuclear retention, and transcriptional output (Roux & Blenis, 2004; Coffey & Robson, 2012). EDCs such as cadmium, arsenic, dioxins, PCBs, and HCBs activate these pathways and disrupt AR regulation. TCDD (a dioxin) activates the aryl hydrocarbon receptor (AhR), which can interact with AR to alter oncogenic gene expression, including cyclin D1, c-Myc, and downstream targets via IL-6 and JAK/STAT3 signaling (Leng et al., 2014; M. Gao et al., 2020). Furthermore, heavy metals like cadmium enhance AR signaling by inducing oxidative stress through AKT activation, while

HCBs impair degradation pathways and promote AR stability (Ralph et al., 2003a; Kulkarni et al., 2020).

2.2.4 Gain-of-Function Mutations and Expanded Ligand Specificity

CRPC is also characterized by gain-of-function mutations in the AR ligand-binding domain (LBD), such as T877A, F876L, and W741C. These mutations expand AR's ligand specificity, allowing activation by adrenal androgens, progesterone, and even anti-androgens like enzalutamide (Imamura & Sadar, 2016; Rathkopf et al., 2017). EDCs exacerbate this by stabilizing mutant AR variants and enhancing their nuclear translocation. For example, BPA activates such mutant forms, while organochlorines and dioxins facilitate co-regulator recruitment (e.g., FOXA1, MED1, LSD1), supporting AR activity even in the absence of ligand and contributing to resistance to androgen deprivation therapy (S. Gao et al., 2020; N. Liu et al., 2024).

2.2.5 Post-Translational Modifications and EDC-Induced Crosstalk

Beyond classical signaling modes, post-translational modifications (PTMs) such as phosphorylation and ubiquitination significantly influence AR function. EDCs activate kinases like AKT, ERK, and CDK1, which phosphorylate AR and enhance its transcriptional activity (Montoya-Novoa et al., 2024). Conversely, E3 ligases such as MDM2 and RNF6 mediate AR degradation via ubiquitination (Khatiwada et al., 2024). However, EDCs can dysregulate these processes by inhibiting AR degradation and prolonging its activity (Y. Zhang et al., 2024). This intricate network of signaling alterations and receptor modifications illustrates the profound influence of EDCs on AR dynamics, significantly contributing to the progression and treatment resistance of prostate cancer Table 1.

Table 1. Effects of Endocrine-Disrupting Chemicals (EDCs) on Androgen Receptor (AR) Signaling and Their Proposed Mechanisms of Action.

EDC	Type of AR Signaling Affected	Mechanism of Action	Key References
Bisphenol A (BPA)	Ligand-dependent, Gain-of-function, Overexpression	Binds to AR/ERβ; induces AR conformational change and nuclear translocation; activates mutant AR variants (T877A, W741C, F876L); upregulates coactivators (p300/CBP, SRC-1)	Di Donato et al., 2017; Wang et al., 2024; Kiyama, 2016; Hess-Wilson et al., 2007; Salian et al., 2009
Phthalates	Ligand-independent, Overexpression	Activates PPARγ and MAPK (ERK, p38); phosphorylates AR (Ser213, Ser650, Ser791); upregulates coactivators (p300/CBP); enhances AR stability and transcription	Corton & Lapinskas, 2005; Guo et al., 2023; Coffey & Robson, 2012; Luo et al., 2024
PCBs	Ligand-dependent, Ligand-independent	Partial AR agonist; promotes SRC-1 and MED1 recruitment; upregulates CYP17A1; activates MAPK/ERK signaling	Yadav et al., 2016; Burris-Hiday & Scott, 2021; Fernández-Cancio et al., 2018; Nock et al., 2006
Dioxins (e.g., TCDD)	Ligand-independent, Gain-of-function	Activates AhR-AR complex; promotes expression of c-Myc and cyclin D1; induces IL-6/JAK-STAT3 signaling; supports ligand-independent AR activation	Leng et al., 2014; Xu et al., 2016; Buchanan et al., 2002; Gao et al., 2020
Organochlorine Pesticides	Gain-of-function, Ligand-independent	Enhances co-regulator (FOXA1, MED1, LSD1) recruitment; supports mutant AR activation under ADT	Gao et al., 2020; Harris et al., 2022; Liu et al., 2024
Hexachlorobenzene (HCBs)	Ligand-independent, Overexpression	Disrupts AR degradation; promotes oxidative stress; activates MAPK/ ERK signaling; stabilizes AR	Ralph et al., 2003a; Trudeau et al., 2018
Cadmium	Ligand-independent	Activates AKT; induces oxidative stress; disrupts TCA enzymes; activates NRF2, enhancing AR transcription	Kulkarni et al., 2020; Khurana & Sikka, 2018; Ruan et al., 2022
Arsenic	Ligand-independent	Activates AKT and oxidative stress pathways; interferes with mitochondrial and AR signaling cross-talk	Kulkarni et al., 2020; Marquez et al., 2024
PAHs	Ligand-independent	Activates MAPK/ERK pathway; promotes AR phosphorylation and nuclear retention	Nock et al., 2006; Casals-Casas & Desvergne, 2011

It presents a summary of the impact of selected endocrine-disrupting chemicals on AR signaling pathways. The modulatory roles of EDCs either as agonists or antagonists are described along with their proposed mechanisms of action, including direct receptor binding, interference with co-regulator recruitment, and alterations in AR-mediated gene transcription.

2.3 Endocrine Disruptors and Mitochondrial Dysregulation in Prostate Cancer Metabolism

Mitochondrial metabolism is known to be closely associated with prostate cancer progression by modulating various important processes such as altered oxidative phosphorylation, resistance to apoptosis, overproduction of reactive oxygen species, and many other downstream retrograde signaling events, thereby impacting castration-resistant prostate cancer (CRPC) and resistance to androgen deprivation therapy (ADT) (Fontana et al., 2023). Environmental endocrine-disrupting chemicals (EDCs) such as BPA, phthalates, PCBs, dioxins, HCBs, pesticides, cadmium, and arsenic tend to disrupt mitochondrial function (Quagliariello et al., 2017).

Likewise, studies have suggested that BPA disrupts electron transport chain (ETC) complexes, inducing ROS (K. X. Lin et al., 2025) and further leading to mitochondrial DNA (mtDNA) damage, while also activating the PI3K/AKT and MAPK/ERK pathways to sustain androgen receptor (AR) signaling under ADT (Kodanch et al., 2024; Nayak et al., 2022; K. Wang et al., n.d.). Similarly, compounds such as phthalates and PCBs modulate peroxisome proliferator-activated receptor gamma coactivator-1 alpha (PGC-1α), shifting metabolism toward glycolysis to promote cancer survival (Arzuaga et al., 2007; Xiao & Goswami, 2015). Furthermore, HCBs tend to disrupt fatty acid oxidation (FAO), causing lipid accumulation and sterol regulatory element-binding protein 1 (SREBP-1) activation (Trudeau et al., 2018), thereby influencing AR signaling (Ralph et al., 2003b). HCBs also dysregulate mitochondrial redox balance, increasing oxidative stress and resistance (Yusufi, n.d.).

Additionally, studies have demonstrated that TCDD-induced activation of the aryl hydrocarbon receptor (AhR) modulates androgen receptor (AR) signaling and rewires prostate cancer metabolism by upregulating glycolytic enzymes such as hexokinase 2 (HK2) and lactate dehydrogenase A (LDHA) (G. Singh et al., 2024), suggesting a potential mechanism for the Warburg effect and implications for therapy resistance.

Moreover, heavy metals such as cadmium and arsenic dysregulate tricarboxylic acid (TCA) cycle enzymes (Ruan et al., 2022), increasing dependence on glutaminolysis (Marquez et al., 2024). Cadmium-mediated dysfunction further stimulates nuclear factor erythroid 2-related factor 2 (NRF2) (Khurana & Sikka, 2018), augmenting antioxidant defenses as well as AR transcription, driving progression toward CRPC. EDC-induced mitochondrial disruptions interfere with AR signaling through dysregulated fission, fusion, and mitophagy (Choudhary et al., 2011). This causes a shift of mitochondrial glutamine metabolism toward reductive carboxylation, thereby upregulating lipid biosynthesis for AR-mediated proliferation. Therefore, by regulating AMP-activated protein kinase (AMPK) and hypoxia-inducible factor-1 alpha (HIF-1α), EDCs can heighten metabolic plasticity, promoting tumor survival and therapeutic resistance (Moldogazieva et al., 2020) Figure 2.2.

Figure 2. Disruption of Mitochondrial Metabolism by Endocrine-Disrupting Chemicals (EDCs).

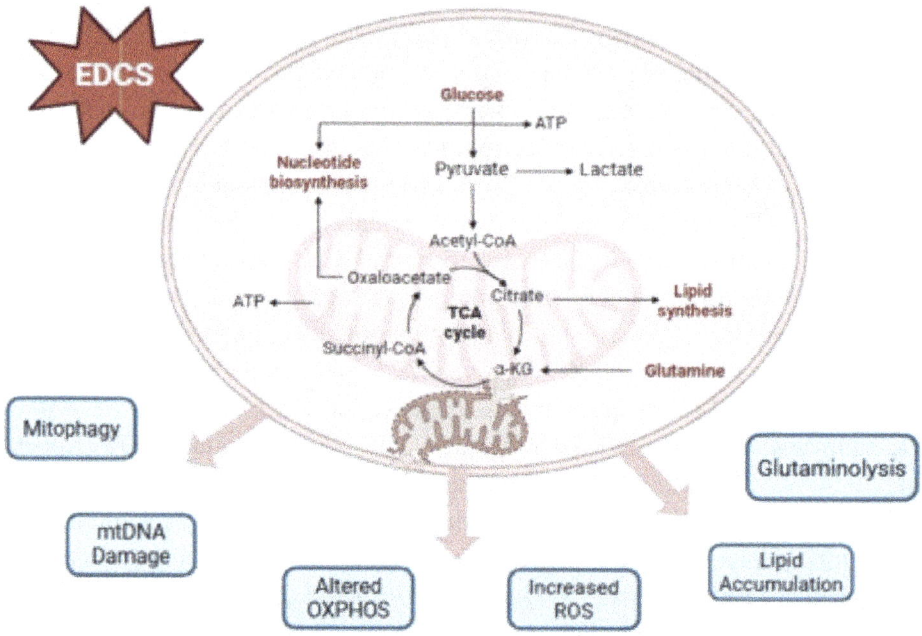

This schematic illustrates the impact of EDC exposure on central carbon metabolism and mitochondrial function. EDCs interfere with glucose metabolism, the tricarboxylic acid (TCA) cycle, and glutaminolysis, thereby affecting key biosynthetic pathways such as nucleotide and lipid synthesis. These disruptions lead to downstream mitochondrial dysfunction, including altered oxidative phosphorylation (OXPHOS), increased reactive oxygen species (ROS) production, mitochondrial DNA (mtDNA) damage, mitophagy, and lipid accumulation.

2.4 Epigenetic Modifications Induced by EDCs

Epigenetic alterations significantly influence prostate cancer progression, primarily by silencing tumor suppressors, leading to activation of oncogenic pathways and thus supporting therapy resistance (Conteduca et al., 2021). Environmental EDCs have been implicated in altering epigenetic mechanisms such as DNA methylation, histone modifications, and non-coding RNA expression (Vaiserman, 2014). Along with this, EDC-induced DNA hypermethylation silences tumor suppressors like PTEN, RASSF1A, and APC, while AR promoter hypomethylation increases receptor expression, sensitizing prostate cancer cells to even low androgen levels and undermining androgen deprivation therapy (ADT) (Yaqinuddin et al., 2013; Ylitalo et al., 2021). Likewise, metals such as cadmium and arsenic dysregulate DNMTs, further silencing PTEN and APC while also activating signaling pathways such as PI3K/AKT and MAPK/ERK, causing AR-V7 expression through various coactivators like p300/CBP, SRC-1, and TIP60 (Mediwala et al., 2013; Shorning et al., 2020). Furthermore, epigenetic regulators like EZH2, KDM1A, and JMJD2C regulate histones, which subsequently mark chromatin to sustain oncogenic transcription, promoting CRPC progression and ADT resistance (K. Xu et al., 2012).

Beyond AR modulation, EDCs disrupt histone modifications at AR target genes, supporting androgen-independent tumor growth (Damaschke et al., 2013). Compounds like BPA and persistent organic pollutants (POPs) cause AR promoter hypomethylation and histone acetylation, activating persistent transcription. Similarly, phthalates and BPA upregulate histone acetyltransferases (HATs) (Crea et al., 2012) such as p300/CBP (Waddell et al., 2021b), supporting AR-chromatin interactions. Likewise, dioxins and PCBs also cause malfunction of lysine methyltransferases (KMTs) and demethylases (KDMs) (Coffey et al., 2013), further promoting various oncogenic AR targets, whereas tumor suppressors such as NKX3.1 and CDKN2A acquire repressive histone marks (Casati, 2013).

Studies suggest that EDC-mediated acetylation primarily enhances AR-chromatin affinity, thereby promoting the activation of oncogenic transcriptional genes such as MYC, FOXA1, and HOXB13 (Huttunen et al., 2024), which further promotes prostate cancer cell proliferation and supports survival. Additionally, SUMOylation via SENP1 modulates AR signaling, whereas methylation stabilizes co-regulator recruitment, further supporting pathways such as WNT/β-catenin and TGF-β that help sustain AR-driven tumor progression and castration resistance (Chen & Lu, 2015; Launonen et al., 2024; K. Li et al., 2025).

Thus, by modifying histone marks at crucial metabolic genes, EDCs augment metabolic adaptation. Therefore, targeting these epigenetic susceptibilities may offer novel therapeutic strategies for advanced prostate cancer and therapy resistance.

3. TOXICOGENOMICS AND PHARMACOGENOMICS: UNDERSTANDING ENVIRONMENTAL CONTRIBUTIONS TO ARPC

3.1 Introduction to Toxicogenomics

Toxicogenomics combines toxicology with high-throughput omics approaches to explore the influence of environmental poisons on cellular function. It investigates gene-environment interactions that influence disease progression through genomics, transcriptomics, proteomics, and metabolomics (Portugal et al., 2022). By examining how toxins alter gene expression, protein activity, and metabolic pathways, toxicogenomics provides invaluable knowledge about carcinogenesis driven by toxicants as well as potential therapeutic targets (Pandiri et al., 2024). Using bioinformatics software to analyze, visualize, and interpret large biological datasets is a core feature of this discipline (Khan et al., 2022). These tools enable early detection and targeted treatments by identifying molecular changes linked to prostate cancer (PCa) and its related exposures (Granata & Barboro, 2024).

3.2 Disruption of Oncogenic Pathways

Various studies suggest that environmental stressors interfere with oncogenic pathways such as PI3K/Akt, MAPK, and WNT, thereby increasing therapy resistance and tumor development (Bahar et al., 2023; He et al., 2021). Exposure-driven mutations and epigenetic changes can be detected using high-throughput sequencing techniques such as WGS, RNA-seq, scRNA-seq, and ChIP-seq (Basyuni et al., 2024; McGirt et al., 2015; J. Zhao et al., 2023; Zou et al., 2023). Furthermore, mass spectrometry-based proteomics and metabolomics reveal toxin-induced disturbances in protein and metabolic pathways that drive cancer development (Blum et al., 2022; Kim & Kang, 2021; Zhou et al., 2012).

3.3 Computational Tools and Gene-Environment Interaction

By sorting toxicant exposures and revealing new gene-environment interactions, computational approaches—including machine learning and systems biology modeling—improve toxicogenomic analyses (Audouze & Grandjean, 2011; Z. Lin & Chou, 2022). These approaches not only enhance exposure evaluations but also highlight therapeutic susceptibilities. They help us better understand the molecular complexity of PCa and open promising avenues for biomarker discovery, risk stratification, and targeted therapy.

3.4 Toxicogenomics Approaches to Identify PCa-Associated Environmental Stressors

3.4.1 Identifying Environmental Risk Factors Through Omics

Recent developments in toxicogenomics have significantly improved our understanding of the potential links between environmental exposures and the progression of prostate cancer (PCa). Many industrial pollutants, heavy metals, endocrine-disrupting chemicals (EDCs), and persistent organic pollutants (POPs), among other environmental toxins, have been identified by toxicogenomics as crucial factors in assessing PCa risk (Buñay et al., 2023a). By integrating high-throughput genomic, epigenomic, proteomic, and transcriptomic data with computational methods, emerging knowledge has provided crucial insights into how environmental toxins may alter gene expression, induce epigenetic changes, and affect intracellular signaling pathways depending on their exposure (Yu et al., 2021).

3.4.2 Specific Toxins and Molecular Targets

It has been observed that polychlorinated biphenyls (PCBs) activate the AhR signaling pathway, thereby altering genes related to xenobiotic metabolism, oxidative stress response (NQO1, GSTM1), and inflammation (IL6, TNF-α), which leads to DNA damage and tumorigenesis (Ruggeri et al., 2025). PCBs also increase androgen receptor (AR) expression and stimulate crucial growth pathways linked to PI3K/AKT and MAPK, promoting prostate cancer cell survival, proliferation, and metastasis (Buñay et al., 2023b). Early research has strongly suggested ACAT1, a vital enzyme in ketone body metabolism, as a marker for prostate cancer development among those exposed to Agent Orange; therefore, it highlights possible therapy targets since high ACAT1 expression is associated with increased metastatic potential and therapeutic resistance (Garcia-Bermudez & Birsoy, 2016).

3.4.3 Environmental Genotoxicity and Epigenetic Alterations

Recent studies have demonstrated how certain gene changes caused by environmental influences can lead to prostate cancer (Alwadi et al., 2023b). Research shows that these environmental stressors can compromise genomic integrity through DNA damage, oxidative stress, and alterations in DNA methylation (Shin et al., 2023). Various studies, relying on next-generation sequencing and integrative genomic approaches, have identified shared mutated and deleted tumor suppressor genes (TP53, PTEN) that regulate cellular homeostasis via cell cycle arrest, apoptosis, and DNA damage repair (Nientiedt et al., 2022).

Environmental toxins may also target the expression of genes involved in detoxification and xenobiotic metabolism, such as cytochrome P450 and glutathione S-transferases (GSTs), thereby affecting the body's capacity to eliminate exogenous carcinogens (Lawrence et al., 2002).

3.4.4 Epigenetic Biomarkers and Advanced Tools

Studies using tools such as DNA methylation profiling, ChIP-seq, and ATAC-seq have found that hypermethylation of key tumor suppressor genes such as GSTP1 and RASSF1A, driven by long-term exposure to EDCs including bisphenol A (BPA), phthalates, and organochlorine pesticides, promotes prostate cancer progression (Rusiecki et al., 2017). These molecules also typically affect histone modifications associated with DNA repair, cell cycle control, and tumor suppressive events, thereby increasing cancer risk (Ho et al., 2012).

Current research can investigate these changes at unprecedented resolution using single-cell RNA sequencing (scRNA-seq) and epigenome editing, providing insights into how environmental stress affects the molecular identity of individual tumor cells and their microenvironment, consequently influencing therapy resistance and tumor heterogeneity (Y. Zhang et al., 2021). Toxicogenomics helps demonstrate how environmental exposure-driven epigenetic modifications impact prostate cancer, partly through genetic mutations (D. D. Singh, 2024).

3.4.5 Machine Learning Integration and Risk Stratification

Particularly in machine learning and artificial intelligence (AI), recent technological developments have made it possible to integrate sophisticated toxicogenomic databases to forecast the impacts of environmental exposures on prostate cancer (PCa) development (A. V. Singh et al., 2024). Applied to transcriptomic and proteomic data, deep learning algorithms have identified distinct PCB-responsive gene networks (PRGs) and exposure-driven molecular subtypes, enabling patient stratification based on their environmental exposure risk and prognosis (Q. Li et al., 2024).

3.4.6 Tumor Microenvironment and Spatial Transcriptomics

Furthermore, spatial transcriptomics has emerged as a powerful approach for investigating how environmental exposures alter the tumor microenvironment (TME). By mapping the transcriptomic profiles of prostate cancer cells and their surrounding stromal and immune cells, researchers have identified how environmental toxins such as TCDD and BPA influence stromal-epithelial interactions and immune cell polarization (Humphrey et al., 2018). These studies show how pollutants induce a pro-inflammatory microenvironment (Chung et al., 2020; Erlandsson et al., 2018).

3.4.7 Biomarker Discovery and Functional Genomics

Toxicogenomics research has accelerated the discovery of biomarkers in personalized medicine that predict cancer risk in individuals exposed to environmental pollutants. Using large cohort studies and multi-omics data integration, researchers have identified predictive biomarkers such as *CYP1A1* (Zhu et al., 2019) and *SRD5A2*

(Steroid 5 Alpha-Reductase 2 Enzyme Variants, Biomass Exposure, and Tobacco Use in Mexican Patients with Prostate Cancer, n.d.).

Moreover, in experimental models, functional genomics tools such as CRISPR-Cas9 are used to validate these biomarkers, thereby providing mechanistic understanding of how exposure-induced gene expression alterations promote PCa development (Cai et al., 2024).

3.5 Pharmacogenomics Insights into Chemoresistance and Therapy Failures

Resistance mechanisms can also arise from somatic mutations and epigenetic silencing of DNA repair genes such as *FANCA*, *RAD51B*, *XRCC2*, and *MSH2* (Risdon et al., 2020). Tumors with deficiencies in homologous recombination repair (HRR), including mutations in *BRCA1*, *BRCA2*, and *ATM*, initially respond to PARP inhibitors, but secondary mutations restoring HRR activity often drive acquired resistance (Loehr et al., 2023).

The epigenetic landscape of PCa—including promoter hypermethylation, histone modifications, and non-coding RNA dysregulation—reprograms gene expression patterns (Sarkar et al., 2023; Westaby et al., 2024).

3.5.1 Single-Cell and Organoid Models in Drug Resistance

Advanced pharmacogenomics approaches, such as single-cell transcriptomics and spatial profiling, have been employed to identify resistant tumor subpopulations (Bian et al., 2024a). Researchers are also using patient-derived organoids (PDOs) and xenografts (PDXs) as models for therapy simulation (Van Hemelryk et al., 2022; Silkina et al., 2023). New therapeutic approaches target epigenetic drivers of resistance. Drugs inhibiting EZH2, BET proteins, and histone deacetylases, as well as PROTACs like ARV-110, are currently being developed (Z. Liu et al., 2022; Snyder et al., 2025). AI-driven models and CRISPR-Cas9 screens further identify druggable targets and guide combination therapies (Mukhopadhyay et al., 2023; H. Zhang et al., 2022).

3.6 Bioinformatics and Machine Learning Models for Exposome Data Integration

3.6.1 Role of Bioinformatics and ML in Exposome Integration

Incorporating exposomic data into prostate cancer research requires advanced, high-throughput data analysis methods that can accurately represent intricate, nonlinear interactions. In this context, bioinformatics and machine learning (ML) have become essential tools for unraveling the complex relationship between environmental factors and molecular changes in PCa.

3.6.2 Integrative Omics and Environmental Exposure Studies

Recent research has begun to methodically assess the effects of specific environmental factors on prostate cancer risk by employing integrative omics methods (Gholami et al., 2022). For instance, high-throughput studies using exposome-wide association study (ExWAS) frameworks have linked elevated levels of per- and polyfluoroalkyl substances (PFAS), such as PFOA and PFOS, to an increased risk of PCa and alterations in inflammatory and metabolic pathways, as revealed by serum metabolomics and transcriptomic profiling. PFAS, commonly used in industrial applications and consumer products, are known for their environmental persistence and bioaccumulation, exhibiting estrogenic and immunotoxic effects (Imir et al., 2021).

3.6.3 Epigenetic Effects of Endocrine Disruptors

Moreover, long-term exposure to endocrine-disrupting substances, such as phthalates, bisphenol A (BPA), and organophosphate flame retardants, has been linked to epigenetic changes in genes that regulate androgen receptor signaling and chromatin remodeling. A recent study using epigenome-wide association analysis (EWAS) found that prenatal exposure to BPA resulted in lasting DNA methylation alterations in prostate tissue that coincided with enhancers in androgen receptor-responsive genes, indicating enduring reprogramming of prostate epigenetics due to early-life environmental factors (Cheong et al., 2016; Miura et al., 2021).

3.6.4 Influence of Diet and Lifestyle

Concurrently, numerous multi-omics exposomic studies have begun to incorporate dietary and lifestyle factors, which are increasingly recognized as influencers of prostate tumor biology. For example, longitudinal data from the NIH-AARP Diet and Health Study showed that diets high in animal fats and processed meats were associated with elevated levels of pro-inflammatory cytokines and alterations in gut microbiome composition, both of which contribute to prostate tumor development (Cross et al., 2007).

By combining dietary metadata with microbiome sequencing and cytokine arrays through multivariate kernel learning algorithms, researchers have uncovered significant interactions between high-fat diets, systemic inflammation, and immune cell infiltration. Importantly, XGBoost models also facilitated feature importance analysis, revealing that exposure to agricultural pesticides, particularly organochlorines, was among the top predictors of recurrence, independent of clinical stage and Gleason score (D. Li et al., 2025).

3.6.5 Unsupervised Learning for Exposure Pattern Discovery

Unsupervised learning methods, such as non-negative matrix factorization (NMF) and hierarchical clustering, are increasingly used to reveal hidden exposure patterns or classify subtypes of PCa based on multiple exposure profiles (Wu et al., 2020). For example, combining TCGA multi-omics data with environmental information through multi-omics factor analysis (MOFA) uncovered distinct molecular clusters enriched for individuals with significant occupational exposure to heavy metals and solvents, who also showed increased expression of stress response genes such as HMOX1, NRF2, and GADD45A (Alemu et al., 2025; Bian et al., 2024b; Schulz et al., 2025; K. Tan & Naylor, 2022). These unsupervised techniques enable the identification of exposome phenotypes that may possess unique prognostic or therapeutic significance.

3.6.6 Deep Learning Applications in Exposomic Data

Deep learning methods, such as autoencoders, recurrent neural networks (RNNs), and convolutional neural networks (CNNs), are currently being investigated for complex integration tasks, especially when dealing with time-series exposure data or image-based omics data. For instance, one research project utilized a variational autoencoder (VAE) model to encode time-based exposure patterns from personal wearable devices (measuring VOCs, ambient temperature, and light exposure) and linked these to single-cell RNA sequencing of prostate biopsy specimens (Lee et al., 2024). This model revealed hidden exposure factors closely associated with immune cell dysfunction and stromal alterations within the tumor microenvironment. Additionally, deep learning models have been applied to combine spatial transcriptomics data with exposure histories, facilitating the mapping of gene expression gradients influenced by environmental factors across tumor tissues (Rajdeo et al., 2024).

3.6.7 Explainable AI for Interpretability

A key challenge in utilizing ML for exposomic integration is the interpretability of models. Due to the "black box" nature of many ML models, there is increasing focus on using explainable AI (XAI) methods (Laury et al., 2024). SHAP (Shapley Additive Explanations) and Integrated Gradients are increasingly employed to unravel the impacts of individual exposures on disease risk, facilitating the creation of interpretable, exposure-specific risk assessments (Y. Li et al., 2025). For example, SHAP analysis applied to ensemble learning models combining air pollution, dietary habits, and physical activity data revealed that long-term NO_2 exposure significantly influenced PCa progression in individuals with low antioxidant dietary intake, indicating a synergistic interaction between pollutant exposure and nutritional deficiency (Prakash et al., 2024).

3.6.8 Addressing Causality with Advanced ML Frameworks

Although ML and bioinformatics provide a framework for exposome integration, causal inference remains a persistent challenge. Data from observational exposure studies are susceptible to confounding factors and reverse causation, especially when derived from retrospective or cross-sectional designs. Sophisticated frameworks such as targeted maximum likelihood estimation (TMLE), Bayesian network modeling, and counterfactual modeling are being integrated into ML pipelines to address these limitations and improve causal inference (Greco et al., 2024; Schuler & Rose, 2017). Additionally, Mendelian randomization (MR) methods are being adapted to evaluate the causal effects of variable exposures—such as circulating vitamin D levels, inflammatory markers, and pollutant loads—on prostate cancer using genetic instruments (Trummer et al., 2016).

3.6.9 Standardization and Data Harmonization Initiatives

Recent initiatives focused on data harmonization and standardization have also advanced exposome research. Large consortia like the EXIMIOUS (Exposome-IMmuno-Oncology) initiative (Ronsmans et al., 2022) and HEAP (Human Exposome Assessment Platform) (Home - HEAP, n.d.) are producing standardized datasets that integrate detailed exposure mapping, long-term biomonitoring, and high-throughput omics data to investigate the relationships between the exposome and health in cancer and immune-related disorders (Pereira & Antunes, 2019).

In the context of prostate cancer, these platforms are expected to provide unparalleled detail in linking external factors to molecular outcomes. Moreover, advances in environmental sensors, metabolomics, and adductomics are improving exposure assessment techniques, enabling more accurate individual-level evaluation of chemical loads and their biological effects.

Thus, by combining exposome data with molecular and clinical insights, prostate cancer research represents a cutting-edge field with significant transformative potential.

4. BIOACCUMULATION, ENDOCRINE DISRUPTORS, AND PERSISTENT TOXICANTS IN PROSTATE CANCER

Chronic exposure to environmental pollutants such as polycyclic aromatic hydrocarbons (PAHs), volatile organic compounds (VOCs), heavy metals, and endocrine-disrupting chemicals (EDCs) is an increasing concern in prostate cancer (PCa) research. Due to their chemical stability, lipophilicity, and low metabolic clearance, these compounds accumulate in human tissues, including the prostate, resulting in prolonged exposure that contributes to PCa through multiple molecular and cellular mechanisms (De Coster & Van Larebeke, 2012).

Research has shown that the bioaccumulation of toxicants induces oxidative stress, DNA damage, mutations, and genomic instability, which collectively drive PCa progression. These compounds form DNA adducts, disrupt apoptosis, interfere with cell cycle regulation, and impair DNA repair mechanisms (Humphrey et al., 2018; Shukla et al., 2020). Additionally, toxicants initiate chronic inflammation, promoting tumorigenesis by fostering a pro-survival microenvironment.

The prostate tumor microenvironment (TME) is highly responsive to environmental stressors. Toxicant accumulation affects both epithelial and stromal cells, causing stromal remodeling, fibrosis, and immune cell recruitment, which disrupt epithelial-stromal homeostasis and promote tumor progression (Humphrey et al., 2018). Endocrine disruptors such as bisphenol A (BPA), phthalates, and pesticides interfere with steroid hormone signaling and modulate immune responses, further contributing to PCa aggressiveness (Lacouture et al., 2022; Buoso et al., 2020; De Falco et al., 2021; Vazquez et al., 2012).

To investigate these effects, in vitro models, including cell lines and 3D organoid systems, have been employed. While traditional cell lines such as LNCaP, DU145, and PC-3 have been foundational in understanding toxicant-induced molecular changes, organoid models derived from primary prostate tissues provide physiologically relevant systems for studying long-term toxicant exposure, epithelial-stromal interactions, and TME remodeling (Drost et al., 2016).

4.1 The Impact of Endocrine Disruptors on the Prostate Tumor Microenvironment

Endocrine disruptors (EDCs) are synthetic or natural compounds that interfere with hormone signaling by mimicking or blocking the actions of endogenous hormones. Common EDCs implicated in prostate cancer (PCa) include bisphenol A (BPA), phthalates, dioxins, and pesticides, which bioaccumulate in fat-rich organs like the prostate and disrupt hormone receptor pathways (Hu et al., 2011).

The prostate tumor microenvironment (TME), composed of epithelial cells, stromal cells, immune cells, and the extracellular matrix (ECM), plays a critical role in tumor behavior. EDCs alter the composition and function of the TME, influencing tumor progression and resistance to therapy (Corn, 2012). For example, BPA promotes stromal remodeling by enhancing myofibroblast activation and collagen deposition, increasing ECM stiffness, and triggering integrin signaling that promotes invasion (Li et al., 2023). A fibrotic ECM also restricts drug delivery and induces hypoxia, which supports angiogenesis and therapy resistance through the activation of hypoxia-inducible factors (HIFs) (Kuo et al., 2012; Chen et al., 2023a; Lin et al., 2024).

EDCs modulate immune cell function within the TME. Exposure to EDCs can reprogram macrophages toward an M2 phenotype, suppress T cell activity, shift immune responses toward Th2 profiles, and impair dendritic cell function—facilitating immune evasion and resistance to immunotherapy (Thompson et al., 2015; Gómez-Olarte et al., 2024; Segovia-Mendoza et al., 2020; Caneparo et al., 2024).

Moreover, EDCs enhance angiogenesis by upregulating VEGF and disrupting vascular structure and permeability (Ghalehbandi et al., 2023; Li et al., 2024). These vascular changes reduce treatment efficacy by hindering drug delivery and complicating anti-angiogenic therapies (Corti et al., 2022).

EDCs also induce epigenetic alterations, such as DNA methylation, histone modifications, and changes in non-coding RNA expression, leading to the silencing of tumor suppressor genes and activation of oncogenes (Prins et al., 2017; Kamada et al., 2020; Sreekumar & Saini, 2022; Fatma Karaman et al., 2019). These changes contribute to PCa progression and therapy resistance.

4.2 Cytotoxic Effects of Bioaccumulated Toxicants on Prostate Epithelial and Stromal Cells

The prostate is particularly vulnerable to the bioaccumulation of environmental toxicants due to its lipid-rich composition, high androgen sensitivity, and slow cellular turnover. Lipophilic, persistent chemicals such as polycyclic aromatic hydrocarbons (PAHs), heavy metals, volatile organic compounds (VOCs), and endocrine-disrupting chemicals (EDCs) accumulate in prostate tissues, causing cytotoxic and genotoxic effects (Ahn & Jeung, 2023; Prins, 2008).

In epithelial cells, these toxicants induce oxidative stress via cytochrome P450-mediated reactive oxygen species (ROS) production, leading to DNA lesions, strand breaks, and increased mutation rates (Cho et al., 2023; Hahm et al., 2022; Rozelle et al., 2021). Cadmium and similar toxicants also alter DNA methylation, impair DNA repair mechanisms, and disrupt apoptotic pathways (Grypari et al., 2023; Nemmiche & Guiraud, 2016). Mitochondrial dysfunction and impaired autophagy further contribute to apoptotic resistance and enhanced cell survival under stress (Liang et al., 2022; Baev et al., 2024; Luis-García et al., 2021).

Toxicants compromise epithelial adhesion by downregulating tight junction and adherens junction proteins, thereby promoting epithelial-to-mesenchymal transition (EMT), increased invasiveness, and resistance to therapy (Ryeom et al., 2000; Ebnet, 2008; Kaufhold & Bonavida, 2014; Parfenyev et al., 2025).

In stromal cells, toxicants induce senescence and activate fibroblasts, converting them into cancer-associated fibroblasts (CAFs) that secrete pro-tumorigenic cytokines and ECM-remodeling enzymes (Gou et al., 2024; Zhang et al., 2024a; Saber et al., 2020; Zhang et al., 2024b). Endothelial cells are also functionally impaired, leading to abnormal angiogenesis and hypoxia-driven tumor progression (Gao et al., 2022; Kokai et al., 2022; Chen et al., 2023c).

These cumulative effects foster a tumor-promoting, therapy-resistant microenvironment characterized by chronic inflammation, genomic instability, and immune dysfunction (Faustino et al., 2022).

4.3 Cell Line and Organoid-Based Studies Investigating PCa Responses to Environmental Toxicants

Cell lines and organoid systems have significantly advanced our understanding of prostate cancer (PCa) responses to environmental toxicants (Zhou et al., 2021a; Van Hemelryk et al., 2021). The LNCaP, PC-3, and DU145 cell lines represent distinct PCa subtypes and have been widely used to study the effects of cadmium, arsenic, bisphenol A (BPA), benzo[a]pyrene, and phthalates on cell proliferation, apoptosis, and invasiveness (Abate-Shen & de Almeida, 2022; Hockley et al., 2007; Aimola et al., 2012).

Toxicants activate key signaling pathways such as the aryl hydrocarbon receptor (AhR), estrogen and androgen receptors (ER/AR), PI3K/AKT, MAPK, and NF-κB, thereby influencing hormone responsiveness, oxidative stress, and inflammation (Bilancio et al., 2017; Liu et al., 2014; Urade et al., 2023; Zhu et al., 2018; H. Wang et al., 2023).

Despite their utility, 2D cell lines lack the structural and microenvironmental complexity of native prostate tissue, prompting a shift toward 3D organoid models (Wang et al., 2024; Singh et al., 2023). Patient-derived prostate organoids retain the original tissue architecture, cellular heterogeneity, and genetic characteristics, offering a superior platform for studying chronic toxicant exposure.

Organoid models have been employed to investigate the effects of BPA and phthalates on stem-like cell populations, epithelial differentiation, and morphogenesis, providing insights into lineage plasticity and carcinogenesis under environmental stress (Zhou et al., 2021b).

Understanding these mechanisms is essential not only for cancer prevention but also for addressing broader environmental justice concerns, as vulnerable populations often face higher toxicant burdens. Continued research integrating toxicology, developmental biology, and epidemiology will be critical for unraveling the environmental contributions to prostate cancer and for informing effective public health strategies.

5. MULTI-OMICS APPROACHES FOR TUMOR METASTASIS AND ENVIRONMENTAL CARCINOGENESIS

5.1 Multi-Omics Profiling To Identify Metastatic Drivers in ARPC

In prostate cancer, some cases develop slowly and can be managed, while others progress to become aggressive and pose a serious threat to life. The challenge lies in understanding the molecular factors that contribute to this variation. Conventional diagnostic approaches, such as prostate-specific antigen (PSA) testing and histopathological examination, provide important information but often lack the precision needed to accurately predict disease progression and treatment response.

This is where multi-omics—an innovative approach that integrates information from various biological levels—becomes highly relevant. By combining data from genomics (DNA alterations, genome-wide association studies), transcriptomics (gene expression, mRNA splicing, RNA modifications), proteomics (protein interactions, phosphoproteome), epigenomics (DNA methylation, histone modifications), and metabolomics (cellular metabolism), scientists can gain a comprehensive understanding of how prostate cancer develops and progresses (Nevedomskaya & Haendler, 2022) Figure 5 .1.

Figure 3. An overview of Multi-omics approaches to analyse and characterize Prostate cancer-related metabolic alterations

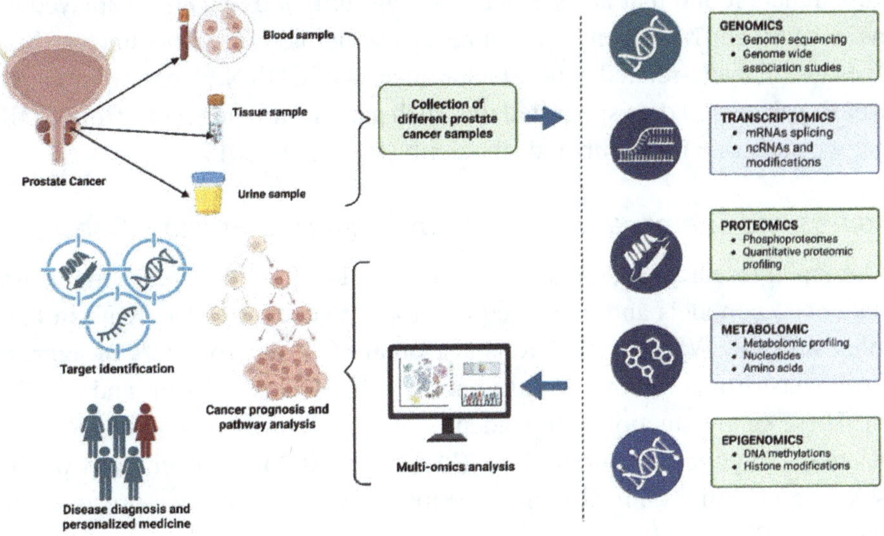

5.1.1 Whole Genomic Sequence Analysis In Metastatic CRPC

Whole-genome analysis of tumors typically begins with samples obtained from biopsies of primary tumors or metastases in lymph nodes, bones, liver, or soft tissues (Nevedomskaya & Haendler, 2022). Circulating tumor cells obtained from liquid biopsies provide an additional valuable resource, helping to overcome issues related to intra-patient variability and enabling the monitoring of genomic changes throughout disease progression and treatment (Nevedomskaya & Haendler, 2022).

One study conducted whole-genome sequencing on 197 biopsy samples collected from patients with metastatic castration-resistant prostate cancer (mCRPC). The analysis identified 11 genes enriched with non-synonymous mutations: TP53, AR, FOXA1, SPOP, PTEN, ZMYM3, CDK12, ZFP36L2, PIK3CA, APC, and ATM, which are considered key driver genes in prostate cancer. Additionally, approximately 50% (84 samples) of the primary prostate tumors exhibited the TMPRSS2-ERG fusion, a major contributor to prostate cancer progression (van Dessel et al., 2019).

Genomic Profiling of Resistance to Second-Generation Anti-Androgens

Patients diagnosed with castration-resistant prostate cancer (CRPC) are often treated with second-generation androgen-deprivation therapies such as abiraterone and enzalutamide. However, many eventually relapse or exhibit resistance. Understanding the genetic mechanisms behind this resistance is critical for identifying novel therapeutic strategies and predictive biomarkers.

Researchers found that abiraterone-resistant tumors frequently displayed alterations in the AR and MYC genes. In contrast, enzalutamide-resistant tumors exhibited changes in cell cycle-related genes, including loss of CDKN2A or amplification of CDK6. Experimental data suggested that such patients might benefit from CDK4/6 inhibitors, such as palbociclib and ribociclib (Han et al., 2017).

Genomics and Therapeutic Targeting of Aggressive Prostate Cancer

A group of researchers conducted genome-scale CRISPRi screens in metastatic prostate cancer models and identified two top hit genes, KIF4A (Kinesin Family Member 4A) and WDR62 (WD Repeat Domain 62), as promoters of aggressive prostate cancer traits in both in vitro and in vivo models (LNCaP and C42B cell lines). These genes function independently of the androgen receptor (AR) and are associated with poor patient outcomes (Das et al., 2021). Another study proposed KIF4A as a potential clinical biomarker indicative of aggressive prostate cancer (Gao et al., 2018).

In summary, comprehensive genomic sequencing of metastatic CRPC has revealed a range of genetic alterations that contribute to tumor development, treatment resistance, and disease aggressiveness. Key mutations in TP53, AR, FOXA1, SPOP, and PTEN, along with frequent TMPRSS2-ERG fusions, underscore the complex molecular landscape of mCRPC. Liquid biopsies—especially those analyzing circulating tumor cells—offer a dynamic, minimally invasive approach to track these genomic changes over time. Resistance to second-generation anti-androgens, such as abiraterone and enzalutamide, is linked to alterations in the AR-MYC axis and cell cycle regulators like CDKN2A and CDK6, suggesting a therapeutic benefit from CDK4/6 inhibition. Moreover, CRISPRi screens have uncovered KIF4A and WDR62 as novel AR-independent drivers of aggressive prostate cancer, presenting promising targets for therapy and prognostic evaluation. Collectively, these insights support the advancement of personalized and adaptive treatment strategies for managing mCRPC.

5.1.2 Proteomic Analysis- Unlocking PCa Pathways for Precised Therapy

This approach involves extensive protein analysis, providing detailed and quantitative insights into the biological processes underlying prostate cancer (PCa) progression. Numerous studies have identified diagnostic biomarkers for PCa through comparative proteomic methodologies, moving beyond reliance on prostate-specific antigen (PSA) alone. Protein profiling of tissues from prostate cancer patients at different stages offers valuable understanding of the complex molecular mechanisms contributing to cancer advancement (Na et al., 2021).

- **Quantitative Proteomic Profiling:**

One study investigated and quantified numerous proteins involved in prostate cancer progression. Researchers examined PCa tissues across all stages, from benign prostatic hyperplasia (BPH) to castration-resistant prostate cancer (CRPC), using quantitative proteomic technologies—including analysis of tissues post-androgen deprivation therapy (ADT). They measured over 4,069 proteins in CRPC and PCa tissues before and after ADT, uncovering novel factors associated with CRPC development. A bioinformatics analysis of 865 differentially expressed proteins (DEPs) identified 15 significant DEPs, including:

FOXA1 (also known as hepatocyte nuclear factor 3-alpha or HNF-3A), a pioneer transcription factor that interacts with condensed chromatin, facilitates recruitment of other transcription factors, and plays a critical role in development, cellular homeostasis, and steroid hormone regulation.

HMGN1–3 (high-mobility group nucleosome-binding domain proteins), which were significantly implicated in progression to CRPC following ADT.

The study demonstrated that FOXA1 expression persisted despite ADT and surged dramatically during CRPC progression (Na et al., 2021).

- **Proteogenomic Analysis:**

A cohort of researchers conducted high-throughput mass spectrometry on clinical tissue samples from patients with BPH, untreated primary prostate cancer, and CRPC. Their findings identified two major metabolic shifts in the tricarboxylic acid (TCA) cycle during PCa development and progression. Most TCA cycle enzymes were found to be upregulated during the initial metabolic reprogramming. Some enzymes, such as citrate synthase (CS) and fumarate hydratase (FH), remained elevated, while others like aconitase 2 (ACO2), oxoglutarate dehydrogenase (OGDH), and succinate–CoA ligase (SUCLG1) became downregulated (Latonen et al., 2018).

An exception was malate dehydrogenase 2 (MDH2), whose protein levels continued to rise throughout PCa progression. A separate report showed that stable knockdown of MDH2 via shRNA in prostate cancer cell lines reduced cell proliferation and enhanced sensitivity to docetaxel, a chemotherapeutic agent (Q. Liu et al., 2013). These findings suggest that MDH2 inhibition could serve as a potential strategy to target CRPC. Non-specific MDH2 inhibitors such as mebendazole, thyroxine, and iodine have shown promising results (Y. Liu et al., 2014).

- **Phosphoproteomics Analysis:**

In a previous study, researchers employed an integrative proteomics approach involving label-free phosphoproteome and proteome profiling to map downstream signaling pathways associated with SPINK1-mediated prostate cancer prognosis. The study identified tyrosine kinase KIT as significantly upregulated. They also found that KIT interacts with β-catenin, and targeting KIT signaling disrupted the WNT/β-catenin pathway (Manzar et al., 2024).

This pathway is known to be influenced by ADT in PCa patients, enabling androgen-independent cell survival. Activation of the WNT/β-catenin pathway contributes to enzalutamide resistance, while its inhibition restores sensitivity to androgen receptor-targeted therapies (Zhang et al., 2018). The study suggested that KIT inhibitors show promising preclinical efficacy (Manzar et al., 2024).

Advancements in quantitative proteomic and phosphoproteomic profiling have significantly deepened our understanding of prostate cancer progression, particularly the transition to castration-resistant prostate cancer (CRPC). Proteomic studies have identified critical differentially expressed proteins (DEPs), such as FOXA1 and HMGN1–3, whose expression increases after ADT, implicating them in CRPC development.

Proteogenomic analyses have highlighted substantial metabolic reprogramming during disease progression, especially involving the TCA cycle, with MDH2 emerging as a potential therapeutic target due to its sustained upregulation and role in drug resistance. Additionally, phosphoproteomic investigations have elucidated key signaling networks, including the SPINK1–KIT–β-catenin axis, which drive tumor aggressiveness and therapeutic resistance. Inhibition of KIT disrupts the WNT/β-catenin pathway, thereby re-sensitizing PCa cells to androgen receptor-directed therapies.

These insights enhance the molecular framework of CRPC and point toward novel therapeutic targets and resistance mechanisms, paving the way for more effective, personalized treatment strategies.

5.1.3 Metabolomics Approaches

Tumor metabolism plays a crucial role in the initiation and progression of prostate cancer (PCa). Therefore, metabolomics, which focuses on assessing a wide range of small-molecule metabolites in biological samples, is increasingly recognized as a vital tool for understanding cancer metabolism (Zheng et al., 2020).

Metabolic profiling: One study investigated the metabolic profiles in prostate tissues from patients with benign prostatic hyperplasia (BPH), hormone-sensitive prostate cancer (HSPC), and castration-resistant prostate cancer (CRPC) using a ^{1}H

NMR-based metabolomics approach (Zheng et al., 2020). The researchers specifically examined three key metabolic phenomena: amino acid metabolism, choline metabolism, and the Warburg effect. According to the study, three amino acids—alanine, glycine, and glutamate—were upregulated in prostate tissues transitioning from BPH to HSPC, but were downregulated in CRPC. This indicates that amino acid utilization by PCa tumor cells varies across disease stages, suggesting that amino acid metabolism could serve both as a diagnostic marker and a therapeutic target for PCa (Zheng et al., 2020).

The study also observed an increased concentration of choline in HSPC compared to BPH. However, choline levels were drastically reduced in CRPC, indicating that CRPC may exhibit distinct choline metabolism compared to HSPC (Zheng et al., 2020).

The Warburg effect, a common cancer hallmark, describes how tumor cells predominantly convert glucose to lactate via aerobic glycolysis to generate energy. Consequently, ^{18}F-labeled lactate PET/CT has been employed as a diagnostic tool in cancer detection (Van Hée et al., 2017). Interestingly, Zheng et al. 2024 reported a reduced lactate level in CRPC compared to HSPC, suggesting that CRPC may display an inverse Warburg effect (Zheng et al., 2020).

Additionally, they found that citrate levels in prostate tissues were significantly lower in both HSPC and CRPC compared to BPH, indicating increased citrate consumption as prostate cancer progresses. An increase in creatine levels was also reported in CRPC (Zheng et al., 2020). These findings provide insight into metabolic signatures that may serve as biomarkers for diagnosing aggressive PCa.

In conclusion, metabolic profiling using ^{1}H NMR-based metabolomics has revealed distinct metabolic alterations associated with prostate cancer progression, from benign prostatic hyperplasia (BPH) to hormone-sensitive prostate cancer (HSPC), and ultimately to castration-resistant prostate cancer (CRPC). The modulation of amino acids such as alanine, glycine, and glutamate—elevated in HSPC but decreased in CRPC—highlights the evolving metabolic requirements of tumors and suggests promising targets for stage-specific therapy. Changes in choline metabolism and the observed reduction in lactate levels in CRPC point toward a deviation from the classical Warburg effect, indicating a potentially unique metabolic phenotype in advanced disease. Furthermore, the decreased citrate levels and increased creatine levels reflect significant metabolic reprogramming during PCa progression. These metabolic markers offer valuable insights into tumor biology and represent potential diagnostic and therapeutic targets for managing aggressive prostate cancer.

5.1.4 Epigenetic and Epitranscriptomic Studies

Non-mutational events, particularly the dysregulation of DNA and RNA epigenetics, are increasingly recognized as significant contributors to tumor formation. A series of recent studies provides an extensive review of how epigenetic and epitranscriptomic processes influence the development and progression of prostate cancer (PCa) (López et al., 2022). Alterations in epigenetic mechanisms, including DNA methylation and histone modifications, can contribute to the onset and advancement of PCa. According to the study, hypermethylation of promoter regions in tumor suppressor genes (such as GSTP1, PTEN, and CDKN2A) leads to their inactivation, thereby facilitating cancer progression. In PCa, enzymes such as KMT1A, KMT1B, and KMT1E are upregulated, resulting in increased histone methylation and altered gene expression.

Additionally, research on RNA modifications through epitranscriptomics has demonstrated that alterations in m^6A (N6-methyladenosine) RNA methylation—regulated by proteins such as METTL3, FTO, and YTHDF—affect mRNA stability and translation, thus influencing cancer cell behavior (López et al., 2022). Similarly, various other epigenetic and epitranscriptomic modifications have been studied, further enhancing our understanding of PCa progression and aiding in the discovery of potential biomarkers.To summarize, non-mutational processes such as epigenetic and epitranscriptomic changes are essential in the progression of prostate cancer. The hypermethylation of promoters for tumor suppressor genes like GSTP1, PTEN, and CDKN2A leads to their inactivation, while an increase in histone methylation through enzymes such as KMT1A, KMT1B, and KMT1E further disturbs gene regulation. Moreover, alterations in m^6A RNA methylation, driven by METTL3, FTO, and YTHDF proteins, impact mRNA stability and translation, thereby influencing cancer cell behavior. These discoveries underscore the importance of dysregulation in epigenetic and epitranscriptomic processes as both contributors to the disease and potential biomarkers for diagnosing and treating prostate cancer.

5.2 Single-cell RNA sequencing (scRNA-seq) for exposome-related PCa studies

A team of researchers has identified long non-coding RNAs (lncRNAs) that are abundant in cancer cells and the tumor microenvironment (TME) of metastatic castration-resistant prostate cancer (mCRPC) by examining gene expression. They conducted their analysis using single-cell RNA sequencing data obtained from

2,170 cells across 15 different metastatic biopsies from bone, lymph nodes, and liver, collected from 14 patients with mCRPC (Saha et al., 2024).

They identified PCa-related lncRNAs such as PART1, which has been associated with oncogenesis due to its role in promoting cell growth and invasion. The study also uncovered TME-associated lncRNAs in mCRPC, including SMIM25 in monocytes, which has been identified as a specific marker for these cells. Additionally, they identified B-cell-specific and T-cell-specific lncRNAs, namely LINC00926 and PVT1, respectively. They also discovered FAM157C in neutrophils, which has been shown to promote granulocyte proliferation. Furthermore, the study reported that when both copies of the RB1 gene are deleted, the tumor begins to express specific lncRNAs that are active within the TME. This suggests that these lncRNAs are linked to the molecular consequences of RB1 deletion and are associated with a poorer prognosis, including increased treatment resistance (Saha et al., 2024). In summary, single-cell RNA sequencing has illuminated the molecular landscape of the exposome in mCRPC, particularly by identifying lncRNAs present in both cancer cells and the tumor microenvironment. The discovery of oncogenic PCa-lncRNAs such as PART1 and immune cell-specific lncRNAs including SMIM25, LINC00926, PVT1, and FAM157C underscores the complex interplay between tumor and immune components in mCRPC. Notably, the expression of TME-associated lncRNAs following RB1 gene deletion highlights their potential involvement in disease progression, treatment resistance, and poor prognosis. These findings suggest that lncRNAs not only serve as biomarkers of cellular origin and disease state but also represent promising therapeutic targets in advanced prostate cancer.

5.3 Predictive Models For Environmental Contributions To Metastatic Potential

Prostate cancer risk assessment models are crucial tools in clinical settings, helping to identify individuals at increased risk and guiding decisions about screening and treatment. These models combine multiple factors, including clinical data, genetic information, and imaging results, to improve the accuracy of predictions. Conventional models typically rely on clinical indicators such as prostate-specific antigen (PSA) levels, findings from digital rectal examinations (DRE), and biopsy Gleason scores.

To identify disease-associated single nucleotide polymorphisms (SNPs), genome-wide association studies (GWAS) have been conducted. Since 2006, over 76 SNPs linked to prostate cancer (PCa) risk have been identified, accounting for approximately 30% of the heritability of the disease. Assessing risk alleles in individuals alongside PSA levels, family history, and environmental factors may enhance the specificity and sensitivity of PCa diagnostic tests (Gómez-Acebo et al., 2017). Supporting this, a study found that the genetic risk score is significantly more predictive than the environmental score (AUROC for the genetic score: 0.66 compared to 0.57 for the environmental score). This reinforces the notion that prostate cancer has a substantial hereditary component, accounting for roughly 42% of the overall risk, which is the highest among all cancers (Gómez-Acebo et al., 2017).

The study also reported that the only significant independent environmental risk factor linked to prostate cancer was a high consumption of red meat. On average, greater intake of red meat increases the risk of prostate cancer by 31% (Gómez-Acebo et al., 2017). In support of this, another study indicated that consumption of animal fat raises the risk of mortality from prostate cancer, suggesting that animal fat may increase adult sex hormone levels, whereas vegetable fat does not have the same effect (Hebert et al., 1998). In contrast to meat and poultry, fish appears to offer protection against prostate cancer, which might be attributed to omega-3 fatty acids that can slow down the growth of prostate tumors (Hebert et al., 1998).

A meta-analysis cohort also found that the intake of sweetened beverages, vitamin D, folate, dairy products, processed meats, and eggs is associated with an elevated risk of prostate cancer, while consumption of selenium and soy appears to reduce that risk (Cui et al., 2024). In conclusion, nutritional quality can significantly influence the prognosis and progression of prostate cancer.

In summary, GWAS studies have revealed a strong hereditary component to prostate cancer, with over 76 identified SNPs contributing significantly to disease risk. Genetic risk scores have proven more predictive than environmental factors, highlighting the importance of inherited predisposition. Nevertheless, lifestyle and dietary choices remain crucial, as high consumption of red meat and animal fats is linked to increased risk, while fish, selenium, and soy show protective effects. These findings underscore the combined influence of genetics and diet on prostate cancer development and progression, offering opportunities for improved risk assessment and preventive strategies.

6. ENVIRONMENTAL DNA (EDNA), EPIGENETICS, AND CARCINOGENESIS RISK MODELS

6.1 eDNA as a Biomarker For Environmental Exposures In Prostate Cancer Patients

Environmental DNA (eDNA) is defined as the genetic material found in the constructed environment, such as homes, workplaces, hazardous waste sites, lake and river water, air, and other surroundings. Every living organism, including bacteria, humans, and animals, leaves behind genetic material in the environment as they move through different habitats or come into contact with other living beings. Sources of eDNA include human or animal blood, hair, urine, feces, mucus, saliva, secretions, and more (Thakur & Roy, 2020). These genetic "breadcrumbs," left behind or excreted by organisms, can serve as important biological materials for analyzing the relationship between the human exposome and health responses (Thakur & Roy, 2020).

It has also been observed that next-generation sequencing (NGS) of eDNA can be used to evaluate air quality, chemical exposure, and their impacts on human health (Brown et al., 2016). DNA methylation, an epigenetic process, has been exploited to monitor environmental exposure to chemical agents. By identifying altered epigenomes and the epigenetic changes caused by hazardous chemicals stored in eDNA, exposure can be tracked even after extensive prior contact. Exposome and epigenomic markers that change in response to environmental stressors and diseases can be monitored using this technology (Thakur & Roy, 2020).

Therefore, by using eDNA as a non-invasive biomarker, one can analyze and determine the environmental factors that lead to epigenetic changes in the human genome, which may contribute to the progression of prostate cancer.

6.2 Germline Transmission Of Exposure-Induced Epigenetic Changes

Epigenetics is defined as "molecular factors and processes around the DNA that regulate genome activity independent of DNA sequence, and that are mitotically stable" (Klukovich et al., 2019). Epigenetic transgenerational inheritance refers to the process by which epigenetic information and phenotypic changes are passed down through the germline across generations without any ongoing direct exposure to environmental factors or genetic alterations. These epigenetic changes can be induced by environmental factors, including diet or exposure to toxins (Klukovich et al., 2019).

Overweight and obesity significantly contribute to tumor development via various molecular pathways. It has been noted that obese males are more likely to develop prostate cancer (Santos-Pereira et al., 2023). Moreover, the development of androgen-independent prostate cancer (PCa), which significantly decreases the efficacy of androgen deprivation therapy, tends to be directly correlated with hypoandrogenism. Interestingly, leptin has been suggested to regulate androgen-independent PCa proliferation in obese individuals (Santos-Pereira et al., 2023). One study provided experimental evidence that obesity can be transmitted from one generation to another through the paternal line (Fullston et al., 2013). Additionally, family studies reveal that hereditary PCa has a higher inheritance rate in men than any other cancer and tends to develop at a younger age than sporadic PCa (Verhage & Kiemeney, n.d.).

Numerous environmental pollutants have been directly linked to prostate disease and even prostate carcinoma. One study observed that epigenetic transgenerational transmission of alterations in the transcriptome and epigenome of prostate stromal and epithelial cells, which eventually result in prostate disease or even PCa, is caused by ancestral exposure to vinclozolin during a crucial stage of pregnancy (Klukovich et al., 2019). Vinclozolin is an endocrine disruptor and an antiandrogenic substance that binds to the androgen receptor with high affinity. It is a fungicide applied to agricultural crops, including grapes grown for wine production (Anway et al., 2006). Other examples of environmental toxicants that show transgenerational inheritance include permethrin/DEET, dioxin, BPA, and phthalates, all of which have been associated with prostate diseases and carcinoma (Nilsson et al., 2018).

6.3 Epigenetic Biomarkers for Early PCa Detection And Risk Stratification

Epigenetics plays a key role in regulating genes throughout an organism's life by modifying chromatin structure and/or influencing the accessibility of transcription factors (Ferro et al., 2017). This process involves mechanisms such as DNA methylation, histone modifications, and regulation of gene expression after transcription by non-coding RNAs; therefore, it governs gene expression by altering the chromatin structure of DNA (Ferro et al., 2017).

DNA methylation is a process facilitated by enzymes known as DNA methyltransferases. In tumor development, both DNA methylation and demethylation contribute to turning off tumor suppressor genes and turning on oncogenes, respectively (Waddington, 2012). The progression of prostate cancer (PCa) is often linked to widespread DNA hypomethylation observed in metastatic tissues (Yegnasubramanian et al., 2008). In PCa, abnormal DNA methylation—more precisely, promoter hypermethylation—occurs early in cancer development and continues to spread as the disease progresses. This change affects several crucial genes, including tumor suppressor genes, and can be observed in early cancerous conditions such as prostatic intraepithelial neoplasia (PIN) (Perry et al., 2010). For instance, methylation frequency at the promoter of Ras association domain family protein 1 isoform A (RASSF1A) was significantly higher in aggressive tumors compared to less malignant ones (Liu et al., n.d.).

One of the most studied epigenetic enzymes in PCa is the histone methyltransferase EZH2, which is responsible for the trimethylation of H3K27. Its increased expression is particularly observed in metastatic castration-resistant prostate cancer (CRPC) (Cebrià et al., 2002). Another study examined miRNAs and found that the expression of miR-18a was elevated in the peripheral blood of individuals with prostate cancer, suggesting its potential use as a non-invasive biomarker for PCa (Al-Kafaji et al., 2016). In contrast, miRNA-129 was found to be downregulated in prostate cancer and thus may serve as a potential therapeutic target to prevent PCa (Ferro et al., 2017). Collectively, several studies have identified potent epigenetic biomarkers for the early non-invasive detection of PCa.

7. IMPLICATIONS FOR PUBLIC HEALTH AND POLICY RECOMMENDATIONS

7.1 Policy Interventions To Regulate Exposure To Endocrine Disruptors and POPs

A primary global health concern that affects millions of men worldwide is prostate cancer. Therefore, for efficient public health planning, it is crucial to understand its prevalence, risk factors, and outcomes. Exposure to persistent organic pollutants (POPs) and endocrine disruptors has long been known to be linked to an elevated risk of aggressive prostate cancer. Therefore, reducing exposure to hazardous chemicals associated with prostate cancer is essential.

It was found that most of the participants in a qualitative study on public awareness of EDCs were not familiar with the hazardous chemicals (Kelly et al., 2020) Previous research showed that the general public, especially nursing mothers, does not receive enough education about EDCs. Given the effects of EDCs on human health and the level of risk associated with exposure, preventive action is required to increase awareness and interest in EDCs and actually lower exposure.(Park et al., 2022).

7.2 Policies to Reduce Exposure To Endocrine Disruptors

7.2.1 Plant Protection Products And Biocides Regulation:

Pesticides have been prohibited from containing EDCs under EU regulations established in 2009 (Plant Protection Products Regulation) and 2012 (Biocidal Products Regulation), which utilize hazard-based criteria similar to those for CMRs (carcinogens, mutagens, and reproductive toxicants). In 2018, the European Food Safety Authority (EFSA) and the European Chemicals Agency (ECHA) released guidelines to help identify EDCs based on scientific evidence. A chemical qualifies as an EDC if it interferes with the endocrine system and leads to a biologically plausible harmful effect (Kassotis et al., 2020). However, if there is proof that the harmful effect is insignificant to humans (and other non-target organisms) or if exposure is minimal, permission to use the pesticide can still be given even when the requirements are satisfied.

7.2.2 Registration, Evaluation, Authorization, And Restriction Of Chemicals (REACH):

The REACH program, established in 2006, governs chemical use within the European Union across various industries, while excluding specific categories such as pesticides, cosmetics, and pharmaceuticals. It identifies chemicals that are classified as carcinogenic, mutagenic, or toxic to reproduction (CMRs), as well as substances that are persistent, bioaccumulative, toxic, or EDCs that must receive approval from the ECHA for any level of human exposure. REACH employs a risk-based strategy, evaluating both hazards and exposure prior to implementing any restrictions (Kassotis et al., 2020). The chemicals of very high concern (SVHC) list had 205 compounds as of February 2020 (16 due to their endocrine-disrupting qualities).Two of the 43 compounds listed in REACH's annex XIV are recognized as EDCs, indicating the intention to outlaw their usage as soon as technically and financially viable substitutes are found (Kassotis et al., 2020).

However, regulatory efforts and policies have been made but are insufficient to decrease human exposure to EDCs. More substantial restrictions are required in light of the overwhelming scientific evidence that EDCs pose a health risk to humans.

7.3 Integration of Exposome Biomarkers Into Cancer Screening Programs

Exposome is referred to as "the measure of all the exposures of an individual in a lifetime and how those exposures relate to health". Exposomics is an emerging field in science and healthcare that combines information from numerous approaches and calculate the burden of environmental disease, evaluates risk, and fully and cumulatively ascertains the effect of exposure on health. It also seeks to shed light on the alterations in cells and molecules that the exposome mediates (Wan et al., 2025). Exposomics seeks to find significant exposure biomarkers that enable the exploration of theories on the root causes of exposure, dose-response relationships, mechanisms of action, the etiology of illness, and public health measures (Wan et al., 2025). Using exposomics, we can discover new non-invasive biomarkers for the diagnosis of prostate carcinoma.

7.4 Development of Personalized Medicine Approaches Based On Environmental Risk Factors

With the emergence and progressive nature of prostate cancer (PCa), relying solely on standard rectal digital examination and prostate-specific antigen testing often fails to address clinical requirements adequately. For some patients with low-risk cancer, treatment may not be necessary because the tumor is typically small and grows slowly. Here comes the need of active surveillance as a best option to prevent the side effects that come with all these treatments. In cases of high-risk cancer, individual patients often show different responses to the same medication, and the current standard therapy is not always the most effective for every patient. These varying responses to medications could be linked to the genetic variations among individual patients and their tumors. Thus, it becomes a requirement for biomarkers that can target specific cancer genetic abnormalities, which may be utilized to understand oncogenic diversity, enhance the diagnosis of cancer risk and progression, aiding in the prediction of effective therapies through a personalized method (Li et al., 2024). Various types of biomarkers are in current research including molecular biomarkers (genes, noncoding RNAs, and proteins), cellular biomarkers [circulating tumor cells (CTCs), cancer stem cells (CSCs), and circulating endothelial cells (tCECs)], and exosomal biomarkers (RNAs, proteins, DNAs, and lipids) (Li et al., 2024).

7.4.1 Nucleic Acid Biomarkers:

Whenever it comes to identifying, tracking, and treating diseases, nucleic acids are crucial biomarkers. The primary tumor, tumor cells that travel through the bloodstream, micrometastatic deposits that are found at distant locations (like the liver and bone marrow), and normal cell types like hematopoietic and stromal cells are some of the various sources that release cell-free nucleic acids (cfNAs) into the bloodstream (Schwarzenbach et al., 2009). Increased apoptotic and necrotic cell deaths, along with active secretion into the bloodstream, are the physiological processes that cause the blood levels of cfNAs to rise throughout the development and spread of cancer. Therefore, the blood of tumor patients contains both tumor and normal cfNAs (Schwarzenbach et al., 2009). **Table 2**

Table 2. Enlisted are the recent nucleic acid biomarkers which are being used for the diagnosis of prostate cancer.

Sr. no.	Nucleic Acid Biomarkers	Gene name	Function	Diagnostic marker	Reference
1.	UBASH3B	Ubiquitin-Associated and SH3 Domain-Containing B	A gene involved in regulating biological processes which includes cellular signaling and immune regulation. This gene's mRNA and protein expression is elevated during PCa.	Higher expression in PCa than in benign prostatic hyperplasia (BPH). Thus, proving as a potential biomarker.	(Li et al., 2024)
2.	TMPRSS2-ERG gene rearrangement	TMPRSS2 (Transmembrane Protease, Serine 2) and ERG (ETS Related Gene)	TMPRSS2-ERG fusion and rearrangement leads to ERG overexpression leading to PCa development and metastasis.	TMPRSS2-ERG fusion act as a primary molecular factor for prostate cancer and can act as a potential biomarker.	
3.	BRCA1, BRCA 2	Breast Cancer 1 and 2	An important DNA damage repair gene. Mutation in this gene leads to increased risk of prostate cancer (PCa).	This mutation can be used for the early detection of PCa.	
4.	ESRP1	ESR- Related Protein 1	They are involved in alternative DNA splicing and tumor progression.	Potential biomarker for early detection of PCa.	
5.	KIAA1324	Long non-coding RNA	Encodes a transmembrane protein, there role is unclear but are connected with PCa prognosis.	Further studies and researches can make it a promising biomarker.	
6.	SNHG12	Small Nuclear Host Gene 12	It is a long non-coding RNA which act as an oncogene and promotes prostate cancer progression.	It can be a potential biomarker as it is associated with tumor viability and PCa progression.	

7.4.2 Protein Biomarkers

In prostate cancer various proteins are produced and secreted in the blood which can be used as a non-invasive biomarker for the early diagnosis of PCa **Table 3**

Table 3. Enlisted are the protein biomarkers which can help in the non-invasive diagnosis of prostate cancer

Sr. no.	Protein	Protein name	Function	Diagnostic markers	Reference
1.	PSA	Prostate specific antigen	It is a specific glycoprotein which is produced during prostate cancer in prostate alveolar and ductal epithelial cells.	PSA levels are usually elevated in PCa which is used for the detection of prostate cancer.	(Li et al., 2024)
2.	PSMA	Prostate specific membrane antigen	It is a transmembrane glycoprotein with enzymatic activity, primarily produced in the prostate tissue.	It is expressed at low levels in normal condition but its expression increases in PCa which can be used as diagnostic marker.	
3.	EPCA	Early prostate cancer antigen	A cytosolic protein encoded by a gene consisting of eight different exons.	The isoform of EPCA, EPCA1 is highly expressed in PCA which can act as potential biomarker.	
4.	ZIC2	Zinc finger of the cerebellum 2	It is a protein coding gene for early embryonic development particularly in neural tube formation and brain development.	Deletion of ZIC2 protein expression was related with poor prognosis in PCa.	
5.	B7-H4	B7 Homolog 4	A protein involved in immune regulation belonging to B7 family of immune checkpoint.	It has been reported as a potential prognostic biomarker in Prostate cancer by a bioassay.	
6.	CK	Cytokines	A class of molecular proteins that regulate cell-cell communication and involved in immune response and inflammatory responses.	A previous research has reported 21 up-regulated and 17 down-regulated CKs in PCa which can be used as diagnostic biomarker in PCa.	

continued on following page

Table 3. Continued

Sr. no.	Protein	Protein name	Function	Diagnostic markers	Reference
7.	RAMP1	Receptor activity modifying protein 1	A membrane protein involved in regulating receptor activity and signalling.	RAMP1 is expressed at high levels in PCa tissues. Detecting its level in prostate tissue or serum serves as a diagnostic biomarker of PCa.	
8.	SGP	Sialylated glycoprotein	A class of glycoprotein molecules with salivary acid modifications, widely found on cell surfaces and in body fluids.	It has been reported that the expression levels of sialylated glycoproteins are higher in PCa tissues, therefore can be used as PCa diagnostic using blood and urine sample.	

7.4.3 Cell Biomarkers:

It encompass a range of cell types and populations that display unique characteristics with respect to prostate cancer (PCa). These biomarkers consist of circulating tumor cells (CTCs), cancer stem cells (CSCs), and tumor-derived circulating endothelial cells (tCECs), each providing distinct avenues for non-invasive detection, tracking disease progression, and pinpointing therapeutic targets (Li et al., 2024) **Table 4**.

Table 4. Enlisted are the non-invasive cell biomarkers for prostate cancer detection

Sr. no.	Cell biomarkers	Function	Diagnostic markers	Reference
1.	Circulating tumor cells (CTCs)	When a cancerous cell separates from the main tumor and enters the bloodstream. They are present in PCa patients' bone marrow and blood.	CellSearch, an FDA-approved system, relies on the identification and counting of circulating tumor cells (CTCs) through immunomagnetic capture and fluorescence imaging, showcased the efficacy of CTCs as a predictive biomarker for prostate cancer.	(Li et al., 2024)
2.	Cancer stem cells (CSCs)	CSCs are characterized as cells that possess the ability to self-renew within cancerous tissue.	In PCa, CD144 and CD133 (a glycoprotein expressed in various stem cells and endothelial progenitor cells.) are highly expressed. Thus can be used as a prostate biomarker.	
3.	Circulating endothelial cells (tCECs)	They are biomarkers of vascular health, angiogenesis and inflammation.	It has been recognized as a new blood biomarker for cancer that holds clinical importance, exhibiting a negative detection rate exceeding 90% in prostate cancer testing.	

7.4.4 Exosomes biomarkers:

Extracellular vesicles (EVs) are cellular particles that are secreted and expelled from the cell, surrounded by a lipid bilayer. EVs are generated through endocytosis and are released via exocytosis. These vesicles primarily consist of DNA, RNA, proteins, and lipids. EVs are crucial for conveying information among prostate cells and in relation to lesions associated with the prostate gland. They may act as biomarkers for prostate cancer (PCa) in the detection of cancer (Li et al., 2024) **Table 5.**

Table 5. Enlisted are the Exosome Biomarkers for Prostate Cancer

Sr. no.	Exosomes	Diagnostic markers	Reference
1.	miR-21 and miR-375	They are the urinary EVs, through liquid biospies one can better differentiate between prostate patients and healthy individuals.	(Li et al., 2024)
2.	miR-26b-5p and miR-98-5p	They are the exocrine RNAs which have higher accuracy for early detection of PCa in patients	
3.	miR-4732-3p	One study reported its high accuracy in PCa detection compared to PSA technique.	
4.	FABP5	A fatty acid binding protein which enters the urine. Several studies have reported that proteins in urine EV can be used as PCa-specific biomarkers.	
5.	ERG proteins	Its abnormal elevation found in the serum EV are associated with high risk of PCa and also its recurrence.	
6.	Cholesteryl ester (CE)	It is a lipid like substance formed by cholesterol and fat. Level of CE directly correlate with progression of PCa.	

7.5 Development of 3D Organoids for Precision Medicine

Innovative methods have emerged for cultivating both healthy and diseased tissues, leading to the formation of organ-specific miniature 3D structures called "organoids" in laboratory environments. Organoids have been created from both pluripotent stem cells (PSCs) and adult stem cells (SCs) by replicating the processes of cellular and tissue development (Bartucci et al., 2016). These organoids are thought to originate from individual multipotent stem cells or organ progenitors that have the ability to differentiate and can organize themselves on their own, resulting in structures that phenotype and function similarly to the respective organs found in vivo (Bartucci et al., 2016).

There are various limitations; for example, cell lines that are exclusively cultivated in monolayers do not accurately represent the heterogeneity that is seen in patient prostate cancer (PCa). However, while multi-allelic genetically engineered mouse models (GEMMs) enhance our understanding of various stages of tumor formation, they do not accurately replicate PCa progression or the diverse mechanisms behind therapy resistance. Conversely, patient-derived xenografts (PDXs) are good and efficient models for PCa, but they are challenging to establish, costly, and time-consuming; furthermore, tumor clones experience selective engraftment and lack immune regulation. Therefore, this 3D culture system would better mimic the natural in vivo behaviour of PCa tissue, making its in vitro propagation simpler and its use for predicting therapeutic response significantly more dependable (Bartucci et al., 2016).

Three-dimensional organoids are excellent model systems for studying mechanisms and conducting drug screening assays. Various 3D models have been developed, as outlined below. Table 6 A, B, C, D.

Table 6. A: Spheroids

Spheroids		**References**
Production	**These are 3D cell models obtained from cancer cell lines or samples taken from cancer patients, and they are grown in suspension culture using scaffold-based or hydrogel approaches.**	**(Waseem & Wang, 2024)**
Prostaspheres	Prostate-derived spheroids are utilized to investigate genetic and molecular features in in-vitro settings.	(Ellem et al., 2014)
Expressed proteins	They demonstrate elevated levels of AR, CK8, and AMACR proteins akin to those found in the original prostate cancer cells.	(Waseem & Wang, 2024)
Advantages	They are cost-effective 3D models. They are capable of replicating various in vivo tumor characteristics, such as interactions between cells and between cells and the extracellular matrix, which assist in the examination of cell growth, metabolism, oxygen deficiency, and the diversity of tumors in prostate cancer.	(Waseem & Wang, 2024)
Disadvantages	Lack of structured form and consistency in cultural practices.	(Waseem & Wang, 2024)

Table 7. B: Patient-Derived Organoids (PODS)

Institution	Model name	source	Success rate	Key features	References
Memorial Sloan Kettering Cancer Center (MSKCC)	MSK-PCa patient-derived organoid Models	Biopsy of Prostate cancer metastases and circulating tumor cells (CTCs)	15-20%	Formed tumors in SCID (severe combined immunodeficiency) mice, mimicked molecular diversity of PCa subtypes.	(Gao et al., 2014)
Weil Cornell Medicine (WCM)	ORG WCM Organoids	Metastatic PCa biopsies from NEPC patients	16% (4/25 patients)	Used to create PDOXs (patient-derived organoid xenografts) in NOD/SCID mice, expressed NEPC marker genes (MYCN, PEG10, SRRM4, EZH2, SOX2, BRN2, and FOXA2 and low levels of AR signalling), used for drug efficiency testing.	(Puca et al., 2018)

Table 8. C: Induced-Pluripotent Stem Cell (iPSC)-Derived Organoids

Induced-Pluripotent Stem Cell (iPSC)-Derived Organoids		**Reference**
PSC	Organoids derived from pluripotent stem cells which are developed from either induced pluripotent stem cells (iPSCs,) or embryonic stem cells (ESCs)	(Waseem & Wang, 2024)
ASC	Organoids derived from adult stem cell which are utilized to model adult tissue rearrangement.	
Development of iPSCs	They were developed using co-culture methods with urogenital mesenchyme.	
Advantage	iPSC-derived prostate organoids, have been suggested as valuable 3D models for investigating the molecular mechanisms that drive PCa and assessing the effectiveness of drugs for personalized medicine.	
Disadvantage	They lack the formation of tumor microenvironment.	

Table 9. D: Patient-Derived Xenograft (PDX)-Derived Organoids

Patient-Derived Xenograft (PDX)-Derived Organoids		**References**
PDX- derived organoids	**3D organoid cultures, developed from PDXs in animal models.**	**(Waseem & Wang, 2024)**
First PDX model mouse	Lu-CAP PDX model has been notably considered as an advanced prostate cancer PDX.	(Beshiri et al., 2023)
Advantages	Organoids derived from PDX serve as three-dimensional model systems that retain the genetic and genomic characteristics of various prostate cancer patients, making them excellent platforms for researching prostate cancer.	(Waseem & Wang, 2024)
Disadvantages	Developing a reliable PDX-derived organoid for in vitro use continues to be a challenge (low success rate models of CRPC organoids with long term and stable phenotypes).	

7.6 Microfluidic-Based Technology: Human Prostate Cancer-On-Chip

Prostate cancer organoids appear to be encouraging models due to their representation of multicellular complexity at the tissue level, which is relevant to physiological conditions. Nevertheless, this significant complexity presents substantial challenges in exploring and evaluating the roles of individual cell types and the interactions between different cell types to gain a deeper understanding of molecular mechanisms. Additional obstacles faced in organoid experiments include issues related to maturation, the need for nutrient replenishment, waste elimination, and hypoxia (Jiang et al., 2024).

Another innovative technology is microfabrication, commonly known as organ-on-a-chip, which consists of miniaturized organs integrated into a processor or chip-like structure that can be manipulated for drug testing. These compact organ-on-a-chip models are appealing due to their modular design, three-dimensional capabilities, variability in constructing various complex organ systems, and their ability to expedite the production of testable organ environments (Mittal et al., 2019).

In a research study, a cohort demonstrated the creation of an in vitro model for human Prostate Cancer-on-Chip (PCoC), along with findings related to the interaction between the tumor and stroma within the co-culture microenvironment. They made a model illustrating the significance of the prostate stroma in promoting and sustaining normal differentiation of prostate epithelium (Jiang et al., 2024). However, microfluidics is not limited to co-culture devices; it has been utilized in several studies to identify circulating tumor cells and investigate the physical characteristics of cancer cells (Sassi & You, 2024). Table 10.

7.7 PCa Cell Lines Used in Current Microfluidics Systems

The capacity of cell lines to spread to organs like the brain, spine, and lymph nodes makes them a practical and reliable platform for studying PCa (Sassi & You, 2024).

Table 10. Different cell lines used in microfluidics system of prostate cancer

	LNCaP	DU-145	PC3	References
Full name	**Lymph Node Carcinoma of the Prostate**	**DU stands for Duke University, where the cell line was established.**	**Prostate cancer-3**	**(Sassi & You, 2024)**
Isolation	**Derived from a metastatic adenocarcinoma in the lymph node of a 50-year-old Caucasian male.**	**Isolated from a brain adenocarcinoma in a 69-year-old Caucasian male with central nervous system metastasis.**	**Isolated from the vertebrae of a 62-year-old Caucasian male.**	
Features	One of the most widely used androgen-dependent PCa cell line. It exhibits robust growth in culture.	DU-145 cell line has an epithelial morphology and forms adherent layers in cell culture.	PC3 cells are like DU-145 cells, as they lack expression of AR, PSA and hK2 mRNA and proteins.	(Sassi & You, 2024)
Application	Aids in the expression of crucial biomarkers for PCa, including AR, PSA and human kallikrein 2 (hK2) mRNA and protein.	DU-145 cells have been widely used as a standard PCa cell line.	This cell line is androgen-independent and has been widely used to examine castration resistance in PCa.	

Advances in materials science, nanotechnology, and biomedical engineering are driving the rapid evolution of microfluidic technology. Researchers can use microfluidic chips to analyze the mechanical characteristics of castration-resistant prostate cancer cells in order to investigate label-free indicators with diagnostic potential for determining androgen sensitivity and assessing the impact of treatment drugs utilizing in vitro technologies (Sassi & You, 2024).

These microfluidic systems provide flexible platforms for examining tumor biology, drug responses, and the prostate stroma's role in preserving epithelial differentiation. In addition to co-culture models, microfluidics has demonstrated its utility in identifying circulating tumor cells and investigating the mechanics of cancer cells, establishing it as a potent tool for both basic research and translational applications in prostate cancer.

REFERENCES

Abate-Shen, C., & de Almeida, F. N. (2022). Establishment of the LNCaP cell line – the dawn of an era for prostate cancer research. *Cancer Research, 82*(9), 1689–1691. DOI: 10.1158/0008-5472.CAN-22-1065 PMID: 35502546

Ahn, C., & Jeung, E. B. (2023). Endocrine-Disrupting Chemicals and Disease Endpoints. *International Journal of Molecular Sciences, 24*(6), 5342. DOI: 10.3390/ijms24065342 PMID: 36982431

Ai, J., Wang, Y., Dar, J. A., Liu, J., Liu, L., Nelson, J. B., & Wang, Z. (2009). HDAC6 regulates androgen receptor hypersensitivity and nuclear localization via modulating Hsp90 acetylation in castration-resistant prostate cancer. *Molecular Endocrinology (Baltimore, Md.), 23*(12), 1963–1972. DOI: 10.1210/me.2009-0188 PMID: 19855091

Aimola, P., Carmignani, M., Volpe, A. R., Di Benedetto, A., Claudio, L., Waalkes, M. P., van Bokhoven, A., Tokar, E. J., & Claudio, P. P. (2012). Cadmium Induces p53-Dependent Apoptosis in Human Prostate Epithelial Cells. *PLoS One, 7*(3), e33647. DOI: 10.1371/journal.pone.0033647 PMID: 22448262

Al-Kafaji, G., Al-Naieb, Z. T., & Bakhiet, M. (2016). Increased oncogenic microRNA-18a expression in the peripheral blood of patients with prostate cancer: A potential novel non-invasive biomarker. *Oncology Letters, 11*(2), 1201–1206. DOI: 10.3892/ol.2015.4014 PMID: 26893719

. Alemu, R., Sharew, N. T., Arsano, Y. Y., Ahmed, M., Tekola-Ayele, F., Mersha, T. B., & Amare, A. T. (2025). Multi-omics approaches for understanding gene-environment interactions in noncommunicable diseases: techniques, translation, and equity issues. *Human Genomics 2025 19:1, 19*(1), 1–27. DOI: 10.1186/s40246-025-00718-9

Alwadi, D., Felty, Q., Yoo, C., Roy, D., & Deoraj, A. (2023a). Endocrine Disrupting Chemicals Influence Hub Genes Associated with Aggressive Prostate Cancer. *International Journal of Molecular Sciences, 24*(4), 3191. Advance online publication. DOI: 10.3390/ijms24043191 PMID: 36834602

Alwadi, D., Felty, Q., Yoo, C., Roy, D., & Deoraj, A. (2023b). Endocrine Disrupting Chemicals Influence Hub Genes Associated with Aggressive Prostate Cancer. *International Journal of Molecular Sciences, 24*(4), 3191. Advance online publication. DOI: 10.3390/ijms24043191 PMID: 36834602

Anway, M. D., Leathers, C., & Skinner, M. K. (2006). Endocrine disruptor vinclozolin induced epigenetic transgenerational adult-onset disease. *Endocrinology, 147*(12), 5515–5523. DOI: 10.1210/en.2006-0640 PMID: 16973726

Arzuaga, X., Reiterer, G., Majkova, Z., Kilgore, M. W., Toborek, M., & Hennig, B. (2007). PPARα ligands reduce PCB-induced endothelial activation: Possible interactions in inflammation and atherosclerosis. *Cardiovascular Toxicology, 7*(4), 264–272. DOI: 10.1007/s12012-007-9005-8 PMID: 17955387

Audouze, K., & Grandjean, P. (2011). Application of computational systems biology to explore environmental toxicity hazards. *Environmental Health Perspectives, 119*(12), 1754–1759. DOI: 10.1289/ehp.1103533 PMID: 21846611

Baev, A. Y., Vinokurov, A. Y., Potapova, E. V., Dunaev, A. V., Angelova, P. R., & Abramov, A. Y. (2024). Mitochondrial Permeability Transition, Cell Death and Neurodegeneration. *Cells, 13*(7), 648. DOI: 10.3390/cells13070648 PMID: 38607087

. Bahar, M. E., Kim, H. J., & Kim, D. R. (2023). Targeting the RAS/RAF/MAPK pathway for cancer therapy: from mechanism to clinical studies. *Signal Transduction and Targeted Therapy 2023 8:1, 8*(1), 1–38. DOI: 10.1038/s41392-023-01705-z

Bartucci, M., Ferrari, A. C., Kim, I. Y., Ploss, A., Yarmush, M., & Sabaawy, H. E. (2016). Personalized medicine approaches in prostate cancer employing patient derived 3D organoids and humanized mice. *Frontiers in Cell and Developmental Biology, 4*(JUN). Advance online publication. DOI: 10.3389/fcell.2016.00064 PMID: 27446916

Basanta, D., Strand, D. W., Lukner, R. B., Franco, O. E., Cliffel, D. E., Ayala, G. E., Hayward, S. W., & Anderson, A. R. A. (2009). The role of TGF-β mediated tumor-stroma interactions in prostate cancer progression: An integrative approach. *Cancer Research, 69*(17), 7111. DOI: 10.1158/0008-5472.CAN-08-3957 PMID: 19706777

. Basyuni, S., Heskin, L., Degasperi, A., Black, D., Koh, G. C. C., Chmelova, L., Rinaldi, G., Bell, S., Grybowicz, L., Elgar, G., Memari, Y., Robbe, P., Kingsbury, Z., Caldas, C., Abraham, J., Schuh, A., Jones, L., Tischkowitz, M., Brown, M. A., … Nik-Zainal, S. (2024). Large-scale analysis of whole genome sequencing data from formalin-fixed paraffin-embedded cancer specimens demonstrates preservation of clinical utility. *Nature Communications 2024 15:1, 15*(1), 1–12. DOI: 10.1038/s41467-024-51577-2

Ben-Levy, R., Hooper, S., Wilson, R., Paterson, H. F., & Marshall, C. J. (1998). Nuclear export of the stress-activated protein kinase p38 mediated by its substrate MAPKAP kinase-2. *Current Biology, 8*(19), 1049–1057. DOI: 10.1016/S0960-9822(98)70442-7 PMID: 9768359

Beshiri, M., Agarwal, S., Yin, J. J., & Kelly, K. (2023). Prostate organoids: emerging experimental tools for translational research. In *Journal of Clinical Investigation* (Vol. 133, Issue 10). American Society for Clinical Investigation. https://doi.org/ DOI: 10.1172/JCI169616

Bian, X., Wang, W., Abudurexiti, M., Zhang, X., Ma, W., Shi, G., Du, L., Xu, M., Wang, X., Tan, C., Sun, H., He, X., Zhang, C., Zhu, Y., Zhang, M., Ye, D., & Wang, J. (2024a). Integration Analysis of Single-Cell Multi-Omics Reveals Prostate Cancer Heterogeneity. *Advancement of Science*, *11*(18), 2305724. DOI: 10.1002/ advs.202305724 PMID: 38483933

Bian, X., Wang, W., Abudurexiti, M., Zhang, X., Ma, W., Shi, G., Du, L., Xu, M., Wang, X., Tan, C., Sun, H., He, X., Zhang, C., Zhu, Y., Zhang, M., Ye, D., & Wang, J. (2024b). Integration Analysis of Single-Cell Multi-Omics Reveals Prostate Cancer Heterogeneity. *Advancement of Science*, *11*(18), 2305724. DOI: 10.1002/ advs.202305724 PMID: 38483933

Bilancio, A., Bontempo, P., Di Donato, M., Conte, M., Giovannelli, P., Altucci, L., Migliaccio, A., & Castoria, G. (2017). Bisphenol A induces cell cycle arrest in primary and prostate cancer cells through EGFR/ERK/p53 signaling pathway activation. *Oncotarget*, *8*(70), 115620–115631. DOI: 10.18632/oncotarget.23360 PMID: 29383186

Blum, B. C., Lin, W., Lawton, M. L., Liu, Q., Kwan, J., Turcinovic, I., Hekman, R., Hu, P., & Emili, A. (2022). Multiomic Metabolic Enrichment Network Analysis Reveals Metabolite–Protein Physical Interaction Subnetworks Altered in Cancer. *Molecular & Cellular Proteomics*, *21*(1), 100189. DOI: 10.1016/j.mcpro.2021.100189 PMID: 34933084

Brown, E. A., Chain, F. J. J., Zhan, A., MacIsaac, H. J., & Cristescu, M. E. (2016). Early detection of aquatic invaders using metabarcoding reveals a high number of non-indigenous species in Canadian ports. *Diversity & Distributions*, *22*(10), 1045–1059. DOI: 10.1111/ddi.12465

Buchanan, D. L., Ohsako, S., Tohyama, C., Cooke, P. S., & Iguchi, T. (2002). Dioxin Inhibition of Estrogen-Induced Mouse Uterine Epithelial Mitogenesis Involves Changes in Cyclin and Transforming Growth Factor-β Expression. *Toxicological Sciences*, *66*(1), 62–68. DOI: 10.1093/toxsci/66.1.62 PMID: 11861973

. Buñay, J., Kossai, M., Damon-Soubeyrant, C., De Haze, A., Saru, J. P., Trousson, A., de Joussineau, C., Bouchareb, E., Kocer, A., Vialat, M., Dallel, S., Degoul, F., Bost, F., Clavel, S., Penault-Llorca, F., Valli, M. P., Guy, L., Matthews, J., Renaud, Y., … Baron, S. (2023a). Persistent organic pollutants promote aggressiveness in prostate cancer. *Oncogene 2023 42:38, 42*(38), 2854–2867. DOI: 10.1038/s41388-023-02788-2

Buñay, J., Kossai, M., Damon-Soubeyrant, C., De Haze, A., Saru, J. P., Trousson, A., de Joussineau, C., Bouchareb, E., Kocer, A., Vialat, M., Dallel, S., Degoul, F., Bost, F., Clavel, S., Penault-Llorca, F., Valli, M. P., Guy, L., Matthews, J., Renaud, Y., & Baron, S. (2023b). Persistent organic pollutants promote aggressiveness in prostate cancer. *Oncogene*, *42*(38), 2854–2867. DOI: 10.1038/s41388-023-02788-2 PMID: 37587334

Buoso, E., Masi, M., Racchi, M., & Corsini, E. (2020). Endocrine-Disrupting Chemicals' (EDCs) Effects on Tumour Microenvironment and Cancer Progression: Emerging Contribution of RACK1. *International Journal of Molecular Sciences*, *21*(23), 9229. DOI: 10.3390/ijms21239229 PMID: 33287384

Burris-Hiday, S. D., & Scott, E. E. (2021). Steroidogenic Cytochrome P450 17A1 Structure and Function. *Molecular and Cellular Endocrinology*, *528*, 111261. DOI: 10.1016/j.mce.2021.111261 PMID: 33781841

Cai, H., Zhang, B., Ahrenfeldt, J., Joseph, J. V., Riedel, M., Gao, Z., Thomsen, S. K., Christensen, D. S., Bak, R. O., Hager, H., Vendelbo, M. H., Gao, X., Birkbak, N., & Thomsen, M. K. (2024). CRISPR/Cas9 model of prostate cancer identifies Kmt2c deficiency as a metastatic driver by Odam/Cabs1 gene cluster expression. *Nature Communications*, *15*(1), 2088. Advance online publication. DOI: 10.1038/s41467-024-46370-0 PMID: 38453924

Calderon-Gierszal, E. L., & Prins, G. S. (2015). Directed Differentiation of Human Embryonic Stem Cells into Prostate Organoids In Vitro and its Perturbation by Low-Dose Bisphenol A Exposure. *PLoS One*, *10*(7), e0133238. DOI: 10.1371/journal.pone.0133238 PMID: 26222054

. Caneparo, C., Carignan, L., Lonina, E., Goulet, S. M., Pellerin, F. A., Chabaud, S., Bordeleau, F., Bolduc, S., & Pelletier, M. (2024). Impact of Endocrine Disruptors on the Genitourinary Tract. *Journal of Xenobiotics 2024, Vol. 14, Pages 1849-1888, 14*(4), 1849–1888. DOI: 10.3390/jox14040099

Casals-Casas, C., & Desvergne, B. (2011). Endocrine disruptors: From endocrine to metabolic disruption. *Annual Review of Physiology*, *73*(1), 135–162. DOI: 10.1146/annurev-physiol-012110-142200 PMID: 21054169

Casati, L. (2013). Epigenetics and PCBs. *Endocrine Disruptors (Austin, Tex.), 1*(1), e27347. DOI: 10.4161/endo.27347

. Castillo-Rodríguez, C. ;, Serrano-García, R. A. ;, Silva-Adaya, N. ;, Vargas-Cruz, D. ;, Chávez-Cortéz, S. ;, Gallardo-Pérez, E. G. ;, Zavala-Vega, J. C. ;, Cruz-Salgado, S. ;, Magaña-Maldonado, A. ;, Trejo-Solís, C., Angélica Castillo-Rodríguez, R., Serrano-García, N., Silva-Adaya, D., Vargas-Cruz, S., Georgina Chávez-Cortéz, E., Carlos Gallardo-Pérez, J., Zavala-Vega, S., Cruz-Salgado, A., & Magaña-Maldonado, R. (2024). Metabolic Roles of HIF1, c-Myc, and p53 in Glioma Cells. *Metabolites 2024, Vol. 14, Page 249, 14*(5), 249. DOI: 10.3390/metabo14050249

Cebrià, F., Kobayashi, C., Umesono, Y., Nakazawa, M., Mineta, K., Ikeo, K., Gojobori, T., Itoh, M., Taira, M., Sánchez Alvarado, A., & Agata, K. (2002). FGFR-related gene nou-darake restricts brain tissues to the head region of planarians. *Nature, 419*(6907), 620–624. DOI: 10.1038/nature01042 PMID: 12374980

. Chen, Z., Han, F., Du, Y., Shi, H., & Zhou, W. (2023a). Hypoxic microenvironment in cancer: molecular mechanisms and therapeutic interventions. *Signal Transduction and Targeted Therapy 2023 8:1, 8*(1), 1–23. DOI: 10.1038/s41392-023-01332-8

. Chen, Z., Han, F., Du, Y., Shi, H., & Zhou, W. (2023b). Hypoxic microenvironment in cancer: molecular mechanisms and therapeutic interventions. *Signal Transduction and Targeted Therapy 2023 8:1, 8*(1), 1–23. DOI: 10.1038/s41392-023-01332-8

. Chen, Z., Han, F., Du, Y., Shi, H., & Zhou, W. (2023c). Hypoxic microenvironment in cancer: molecular mechanisms and therapeutic interventions. *Signal Transduction and Targeted Therapy 2023 8:1, 8*(1), 1–23. DOI: 10.1038/s41392-023-01332-8

Chen, Z., & Lu, W. (2015). Roles of ubiquitination and SUMOylation on prostate cancer: Mechanisms and clinical implications. *International Journal of Molecular Sciences, 16*(3), 4560–4580. DOI: 10.3390/ijms16034560 PMID: 25734985

Cheong, A., Zhang, X., Cheung, Y. Y., Tang, W. Y., Chen, J., Ye, S. H., Medvedovic, M., Leung, Y. K., Prins, G. S., & Ho, S. M. (2016). DNA methylome changes by estradiol benzoate and bisphenol A links early-life environmental exposures to prostate cancer risk. *Epigenetics, 11*(9), 674–689. DOI: 10.1080/15592294.2016.1208891 PMID: 27415467

Cho, E., Allemang, A., Audebert, M., Chauhan, V., Dertinger, S., Hendriks, G., Marchetti, F., Minocherhomji, S., Pfuhler, S., Roberts, D. J., Trenz, K., & Yauk, C. L. (2023). Oxidative DNA damage leading to chromosomal aberrations and mutations. *OECD Series on Adverse Outcome Pathways, 29*. Advance online publication. DOI: 10.1787/2415170X

Choi, K. Y. G., Wu, B. C., Lee, A. H. Y., Baquir, B., & Hancock, R. E. W. (2020). Utilizing Organoid and Air-Liquid Interface Models as a Screening Method in the Development of New Host Defense Peptides. *Frontiers in Cellular and Infection Microbiology*, *10*, 534019. DOI: 10.3389/fcimb.2020.00228 PMID: 32509598

Chopra, M., & Schrenk, D. (2011). Dioxin toxicity, aryl hydrocarbon receptor signaling, and apoptosis—Persistent pollutants affect programmed cell death. *Critical Reviews in Toxicology*, *41*(4), 292–320. DOI: 10.3109/10408444.2010.524635 PMID: 21323611

Choudhary, V., Kaddour-Djebbar, I., Lakshmikanthan, V., Ghazaly, T., Thangjam, G. S., Sreekumar, A., Lewis, R. W., Mills, I. G., Bollag, W. B., & Kumar, M. V. (2011). Novel Role of Androgens in Mitochondrial Fission and Apoptosis. *Molecular Cancer Research*, *9*(8), 1067–1077. DOI: 10.1158/1541-7786.MCR-10-0445 PMID: 21724752

Chung, H. Y., Kim, J. H., Han, I. H., & Ryu, J. S. (2020). Polarization of M2 Macrophages by Interaction between Prostate Cancer Cells Treated with Trichomonas vaginalis and Adipocytes. *Korean Journal of Parasitology*, *58*(3), 217–227. DOI: 10.3347/kjp.2020.58.3.217 PMID: 32615735

Coffey, K., & Robson, C. N. (2012). Regulation of the androgen receptor by post-translational modifications. *The Journal of Endocrinology*, *215*(2), 221–237. DOI: 10.1530/JOE-12-0238 PMID: 22872761

Coffey, K., Rogerson, L., Ryan-Munden, C., Alkharaif, D., Stockley, J., Heer, R., Sahadevan, K., O'Neill, D., Jones, D., Darby, S., Staller, P., Mantilla, A., Gaughan, L., & Robson, C. N. (2013). The lysine demethylase, KDM4B, is a key molecule in androgen receptor signalling and turnover. *Nucleic Acids Research*, *41*(8), 4433–4446. DOI: 10.1093/nar/gkt106 PMID: 23435229

Conteduca, V., Hess, J., Yamada, Y., Ku, S. Y., & Beltran, H. (2021). Epigenetics in prostate cancer: Clinical implications. *Translational Andrology and Urology*, *10*(7), 3104–3116. DOI: 10.21037/tau-20-1339 PMID: 34430414

Corn, P. G. (2012). The tumor microenvironment in prostate cancer: Elucidating molecular pathways for therapy development. *Cancer Management and Research*, *4*(1), 183. DOI: 10.2147/CMAR.S32839 PMID: 22904640

Corti, M., Lorenzetti, S., Ubaldi, A., Zilli, R., & Marcoccia, D. (2022). Endocrine Disruptors and Prostate Cancer. *International Journal of Molecular Sciences*, *23*(3), 1216. DOI: 10.3390/ijms23031216 PMID: 35163140

Corton, J. C., & Lapinskas, P. J. (2005). Peroxisome Proliferator-Activated Receptors: Mediators of Phthalate Ester-Induced Effects in the Male Reproductive Tract? *Toxicological Sciences*, *83*(1), 4–17. DOI: 10.1093/toxsci/kfi011 PMID: 15496498

Crea, F., Sun, L., Mai, A., Chiang, Y. T., Farrar, W. L., Danesi, R., & Helgason, C. D. (2012). The emerging role of histone lysine demethylases in prostate cancer. *Molecular Cancer*, *11*(1), 52. DOI: 10.1186/1476-4598-11-52 PMID: 22867098

Cross, A. J., Leitzmann, M. F., Gail, M. H., Hollenbeck, A. R., Schatzkin, A., & Sinha, R. (2007). A Prospective Study of Red and Processed Meat Intake in Relation to Cancer Risk. *PLoS Medicine*, *4*(12), e325. DOI: 10.1371/journal.pmed.0040325 PMID: 18076279

Crumbaker, M., Khoja, L., & Joshua, A. M. (2017). AR Signaling and the PI3K Pathway in Prostate Cancer. *Cancers (Basel)*, *9*(4), 34. DOI: 10.3390/cancers9040034 PMID: 28420128

Cui, H., Zhang, W., Zhang, L., Qu, Y., Xu, Z., Tan, Z., Yan, P., Tang, M., Yang, C., Wang, Y., Chen, L., Xiao, C., Zou, Y., Liu, Y., Zhang, L., Yang, Y., Yao, Y., Li, J., Liu, Z., & Zhang, B. (2024). Risk factors for prostate cancer: An umbrella review of prospective observational studies and mendelian randomization analyses. *PLoS Medicine*, *21*(3), e1004362. Advance online publication. DOI: 10.1371/journal.pmed.1004362 PMID: 38489391

. Dahmani, A., & Delisle, J. S. (2018). TGF-? in T Cell Biology: Implications for Cancer Immunotherapy. *Cancers 2018, Vol. 10, Page 194*, *10*(6), 194. DOI: 10.3390/cancers10060194

Damaschke, N. A., Yang, B., Bhusari, S., Svaren, J. P., & Jarrard, D. F. (2013). Epigenetic susceptibility factors for prostate cancer with aging. *The Prostate*, *73*(16), 1721–1730. DOI: 10.1002/pros.22716 PMID: 23999928

Das, R., Sjöström, M., Shrestha, R., Yogodzinski, C., Egusa, E. A., Chesner, L. N., Chen, W. S., Chou, J., Dang, D. K., Swinderman, J. T., Ge, A., Hua, J. T., Kabir, S., Quigley, D. A., Small, E. J., Ashworth, A., Feng, F. Y., & Gilbert, L. A. (2021). An integrated functional and clinical genomics approach reveals genes driving aggressive metastatic prostate cancer. *Nature Communications*, *12*(1), 4601. Advance online publication. DOI: 10.1038/s41467-021-24919-7 PMID: 34326322

De Coster, S., & Van Larebeke, N. (2012). Endocrine-Disrupting Chemicals: Associated Disorders and Mechanisms of Action. *Journal of Environmental and Public Health*, *713696*, 1–52. Advance online publication. DOI: 10.1155/2012/713696 PMID: 22991565

. De Falco, M., Laforgia, V., La Rocca, C., Di Nardo, G., & Cristina Varese, G. (2021). Combined Effects of Different Endocrine-Disrupting Chemicals (EDCs) on Prostate Gland. *International Journal of Environmental Research and Public Health 2021, Vol. 18, Page 9772, 18*(18), 9772. DOI: 10.3390/ijerph18189772

De Marzo, A. M., Platz, E. A., Sutcliffe, S., Xu, J., Grönberg, H., Drake, C. G., Nakai, Y., Isaacs, W. B., & Nelson, W. G. (2007). Inflammation in prostate carcinogenesis. *Nature Reviews. Cancer, 7*(4), 256–269. DOI: 10.1038/nrc2090 PMID: 17384581

Dehm, S. M., & Tindall, D. J. (2011). Alternatively Spliced Androgen Receptor Variants. *Endocrine-Related Cancer, 18*(5), R183–R196. DOI: 10.1530/ERC-11-0141 PMID: 21778211

Di Donato, M., Cernera, G., Giovannelli, P., Galasso, G., Bilancio, A., Migliaccio, A., & Castoria, G. (2017). Recent advances on bisphenol-A and endocrine disruptor effects on human prostate cancer. *Molecular and Cellular Endocrinology, 457*, 35–42. DOI: 10.1016/j.mce.2017.02.045 PMID: 28257827

. Drost, J., Karthaus, W. R., Gao, D., Driehuis, E., Sawyers, C. L., Chen, Y., & Clevers, H. (2016). Organoid culture systems for prostate epithelial and cancer tissue. *Nature Protocols 2016 11:2, 11*(2), 347–358. DOI: 10.1038/nprot.2016.006

. Ebnet, K. (2008). Organization of multiprotein complexes at cell–cell junctions. *Histochemistry and Cell Biology 2008 130:1, 130*(1), 1–20. DOI: 10.1007/s00418-008-0418-7

Ellem, S. J., De-Juan-Pardo, E. M., & Risbridger, G. P. (2014). In vitro modeling of the prostate cancer microenvironment. In *Advanced Drug Delivery Reviews* (Vol. 79, pp. 214–221). Elsevier B.V., DOI: 10.1016/j.addr.2014.04.008

Erlandsson, A., Carlsson, J., Lundholm, M., Fält, A., Andersson, S. O., Andrén, O., & Davidsson, S. (2018). M2 macrophages and regulatory T cells in lethal prostate cancer. *The Prostate, 79*(4), 363–369. DOI: 10.1002/pros.23742 PMID: 30500076

Fatma Karaman, E., Caglayan, M., Sancar-Bas, S., Ozal-Coskun, C., Arda-Pirincci, P., & Ozden, S. (2019). Global and region-specific post-transcriptional and post-translational modifications of bisphenol A in human prostate cancer cells. *Environmental Pollution, 255*, 113318. DOI: 10.1016/j.envpol.2019.113318 PMID: 31610501

. Faustino, A., Oliveira, P. A., Santos, L. L., Zhang, Y., Campbell, B. K., Stylli, S. S., Corcoran, N. M., & Hovens, C. M. (2022). The Prostate Cancer Immune Microenvironment, Biomarkers and Therapeutic Intervention. *Uro 2022, Vol. 2, Pages 74-92, 2*(2), 74–92. DOI: 10.3390/uro2020010

. Fernández-Cancio, M., Camats, N., Flück, C. E., Zalewski, A., Dick, B., Frey, B. M., Monné, R., Torán, N., Audí, L., & Pandey, A. V. (2018). Mechanism of the Dual Activities of Human CYP17A1 and Binding to Anti-Prostate Cancer Drug Abiraterone Revealed by a Novel V366M Mutation Causing 17,20 Lyase Deficiency. *Pharmaceuticals 2018, Vol. 11, Page 37, 11*(2), 37. DOI: 10.3390/ph11020037

Ferro, M., Ungaro, P., Cimmino, A., Lucarelli, G., Busetto, G. M., Cantiello, F., Damiano, R., & Terracciano, D. (2017). Epigenetic signature: A new player as predictor of clinically significant prostate cancer (PCa) in patients on active surveillance (AS). In International Journal of Molecular Sciences (Vol. 18, Issue 6). MDPI AG. https://doi.org/DOI: 10.3390/ijms18061146

Foley, R., Marignol, L., Keane, J. P., Lynch, T. H., & Hollywood, D. (2011). Androgen hypersensitivity in prostate cancer: Molecular perspectives on androgen deprivation therapy strategies. *The Prostate, 71*(5), 550–557. DOI: 10.1002/pros.21266 PMID: 20945429

. Fontana, F., Anselmi, M., & Limonta, P. (2023). Unraveling the Peculiar Features of Mitochondrial Metabolism and Dynamics in Prostate Cancer. *Cancers 2023, Vol. 15, Page 1192, 15*(4), 1192. https://doi.org/DOI: 10.3390/cancers15041192

Fullston, T., Teague, E. M. C. O., Palmer, N. O., Deblasio, M. J., Mitchell, M., Corbett, M., Print, C. G., Owens, J. A., & Lane, M. (2013). Paternal obesity initiates metabolic disturbances in two generations of mice with incomplete penetrance to the F2 generation and alters the transcriptional profile of testis and sperm microRNA content. *The FASEB Journal, 27*(10), 4226–4243. DOI: 10.1096/fj.12-224048 PMID: 23845863

Gao, D., Vela, I., Sboner, A., Iaquinta, P. J., Karthaus, W. R., Gopalan, A., Dowling, C., Wanjala, J. N., Undvall, E. A., Arora, V. K., Wongvipat, J., Kossai, M., Ramazanoglu, S., Barboza, L. P., Di, W., Cao, Z., Zhang, Q. F., Sirota, I., Ran, L., & Chen, Y. (2014). Organoid cultures derived from patients with advanced prostate cancer. *Cell, 159*(1), 176–187. DOI: 10.1016/j.cell.2014.08.016 PMID: 25201530

Gao, H., Chen, X., Cai, Q., Shang, Z., & Niu, Y. (2018). Increased KIF4a expression is a potential prognostic factor in prostate cancer. *Oncology Letters, 15*(5), 7941–7947. DOI: 10.3892/ol.2018.8322 PMID: 29725481

Gao, M., Li, H., Dang, F., Chen, L., Liu, X., & Gao, J. (2020). Induction of proliferative and mutagenic activity by benzo(a)pyrene in PC-3 cells via JAK2/STAT3 pathway. *Mutation Research. Fundamental and Molecular Mechanisms of Mutagenesis, 821*, 111720. DOI: 10.1016/j.mrfmmm.2020.111720 PMID: 32841893

Gao, S., Chen, S., Han, D., Wang, Z., Li, M., Han, W., Besschetnova, A., Liu, M., Zhou, F., Barrett, D., Luong, M. P., Owiredu, J., Liang, Y., Ahmed, M., Petricca, J., Patalano, S., Macoska, J. A., Corey, E., Chen, S., & Cai, C. (2020). Chromatin binding of FOXA1 is promoted by LSD1-mediated demethylation in prostate cancer. *Nature Genetics*, *52*(10), 1011–1017. DOI: 10.1038/s41588-020-0681-7 PMID: 32868907

Gao, W., Wang, Y., Yu, S., Wang, Z., Ma, T., Chan, A. M. L., Chiu, P. K. F., Ng, C. F., Wu, D., & Chan, F. L. (2022). Endothelial nitric oxide synthase (eNOS)-NO signaling axis functions to promote the growth of prostate cancer stem-like cells. *Stem Cell Research & Therapy*, *13*(1), 188. Advance online publication. DOI: 10.1186/s13287-022-02864-6 PMID: 35526071

Garcia-Bermudez, J., & Birsoy, K. (2016). Drugging ACAT1 for Cancer Therapy. *Molecular Cell*, *64*(5), 856–857. DOI: 10.1016/j.molcel.2016.11.023 PMID: 27912096

Garofoli, M., Maiorano, B. A., Bruno, G., Giordano, G., Di Tullio, P., Maselli, F. M., Landriscina, M., & Conteduca, V. (2024). Androgen receptor, PARP signaling, and tumor microenvironment: The 'perfect triad' in prostate cancer? *Therapeutic Advances in Medical Oncology*, *16*, 17588359241258444. DOI: 10.1177/17588359241258443 PMID: 38887656

Ghalehbandi, S., Yuzugulen, J., Pranjol, M. Z. I., & Pourgholami, M. H. (2023). The role of VEGF in cancer-induced angiogenesis and research progress of drugs targeting VEGF. *European Journal of Pharmacology*, *949*, 175586. DOI: 10.1016/j.ejphar.2023.175586 PMID: 36906141

. Gholami, N., Haghparast, A., Alipourfard, I., & Nazari, M. (2022). Prostate cancer in omics era. *Cancer Cell International 2022 22:1, 22*(1), 1–15. DOI: 10.1186/s12935-022-02691-y

Gómez-Acebo, I., Dierssen-Sotos, T., Fernandez-Navarro, P., Palazuelos, C., Moreno, V., Aragonés, N., Castaño-Vinyals, G., Jiménez-Monleón, J. J., Ruiz-Cerdá, J. L., Pérez-Gómez, B., Ruiz-Dominguez, J. M., Molero, J. A., Pollán, M., Kogevinas, M., & Llorca, J. (2017). Risk Model for Prostate Cancer Using Environmental and Genetic Factors in the Spanish Multi-Case-Control (MCC). *Scientific Reports*, *7*(1), 8994. Advance online publication. DOI: 10.1038/s41598-017-09386-9 PMID: 28827750

Gómez-Olarte, S., Mailänder, V., Castro-Neves, J., Stojanovska, V., Schumacher, A., Meyer, N., & Zenclussen, A. C. (2024). The ENDOMIX perspective: How everyday chemical mixtures impact human health and reproduction by targeting the immune system. *Biology of Reproduction*, *111*(6), 1170–1187. DOI: 10.1093/biolre/ioae142 PMID: 39446589

Gou, Z., Li, J., Liu, J., & Yang, N. (2024). The hidden messengers: Cancer associated fibroblasts—derived exosomal miRNAs as key regulators of cancer malignancy. *Frontiers in Cell and Developmental Biology, 12*, 1378302. DOI: 10.3389/fcell.2024.1378302 PMID: 38694824

Granata, I., & Barboro, P. (2024). Identification of Molecular Markers Associated with Prostate Cancer Subtypes: An Integrative Bioinformatics Approach. *Biomolecules, 14*(1), 87. DOI: 10.3390/biom14010087 PMID: 38254687

Greco, T., Poole, E. M., Young, A. C., & Alexander, J. K. (2024). Application of the Bayesian network theory in clinical trial data: Severity shift in spasticity numeric rating scale in patients with multiple sclerosis. *Multiple Sclerosis and Related Disorders, 83*, 105466. DOI: 10.1016/j.msard.2024.105466 PMID: 38310831

Grypari, I. M., Tzelepi, V., & Gyftopoulos, K. (2023). DNA Damage Repair Pathways in Prostate Cancer: A Narrative Review of Molecular Mechanisms, Emerging Biomarkers and Therapeutic Targets in Precision Oncology. *International Journal of Molecular Sciences, 24*(14), 11418. DOI: 10.3390/ijms241411418 PMID: 37511177

. Gu, X., Wei, S., & Lv, X. (2024). Circulating tumor cells: from new biological insights to clinical practice. *Signal Transduction and Targeted Therapy 2024 9:1, 9*(1), 1–35. DOI: 10.1038/s41392-024-01938-6

Guo, T., Meng, X., Liu, X., Wang, J., Yan, S., Zhang, X., Wang, M., Ren, S., & Huang, Y. (2023). Associations of phthalates with prostate cancer among the US population. *Reproductive Toxicology (Elmsford, N.Y.), 116*, 108337. Advance online publication. DOI: 10.1016/j.reprotox.2023.108337 PMID: 36646329

. Hahm, J. Y., Park, J., Jang, E. S., & Chi, S. W. (2022). 8-Oxoguanine: from oxidative damage to epigenetic and epitranscriptional modification. *Experimental & Molecular Medicine 2022 54:10, 54*(10), 1626–1642. DOI: 10.1038/s12276-022-00822-z

Harris, A. E., Metzler, V. M., Lothion-Roy, J., Varun, D., Woodcock, C. L., Haigh, D. B., Endeley, C., Haque, M., Toss, M. S., Alsaleem, M., Persson, J. L., Gudas, L. J., Rakha, E., Robinson, B. D., Khani, F., Martin, L. M., Moyer, J. E., Brownlie, J., Madhusudan, S., & Jeyapalan, J. N. (2022). Exploring anti-androgen therapies in hormone dependent prostate cancer and new therapeutic routes for castration resistant prostate cancer. *Frontiers in Endocrinology, 13*, 1006101. DOI: 10.3389/fendo.2022.1006101 PMID: 36263323

Hartley, A., & Ahmad, I. (2022). The role of PPARγ in prostate cancer development and progression. *British Journal of Cancer, 128*(6), 940–945. DOI: 10.1038/s41416-022-02096-8 PMID: 36510001

. He, Y., Sun, M. M., Zhang, G. G., Yang, J., Chen, K. S., Xu, W. W., & Li, B. (2021). Targeting PI3K/Akt signal transduction for cancer therapy. *Signal Transduction and Targeted Therapy 2021 6:1, 6*(1), 1–17. DOI: 10.1038/s41392-021-00828-5

Hebert, J. R., Hurley, T. G., Olendzki, B. C., Teas, J., Ma, Y., & Hampl, J. S. (1998). *Nutritional and Socioeconomic Factors in Relation to Prostate Cancer Mortality: a Cross-National Study*. https://academic.oup.com/jnci/article/90/21/1637/2520516

Heery, D. M., Kalkhoven, E., Hoare, S., & Parker, M. G. (1997). A signature motif in transcriptional co-activators mediates binding to nuclear receptors. *Nature, 387*(6634), 733–736. DOI: 10.1038/42750 PMID: 9192902

Hess-Wilson, J. K., Webb, S. L., Daly, H. K., Leung, Y. K., Boldison, J., Comstock, C. E. S., Sartor, M. A., Ho, S. M., & Knudsen, K. E. (2007). Unique Bisphenol A Transcriptome in Prostate Cancer: Novel Effects on ERβ Expression That Correspond to Androgen Receptor Mutation Status. *Environmental Health Perspectives, 115*(11), 1646–1653. DOI: 10.1289/ehp.10283 PMID: 18007998

. Hirz, T., Mei, S., Sarkar, H., Kfoury, Y., Wu, S., Verhoeven, B. M., Subtelny, A. O., Zlatev, D. V., Wszolek, M. W., Salari, K., Murray, E., Chen, F., Macosko, E. Z., Wu, C. L., Scadden, D. T., Dahl, D. M., Baryawno, N., Saylor, P. J., Kharchenko, P. V., & Sykes, D. B. (2023). Dissecting the immune suppressive human prostate tumor microenvironment via integrated single-cell and spatial transcriptomic analyses. *Nature Communications 2023 14:1, 14*(1), 1–20. DOI: 10.1038/s41467-023-36325-2

Ho, S. M., Johnson, A., Tarapore, P., Janakiram, V., Zhang, X., & Leung, Y. K. (2012). Environmental Epigenetics and Its Implication on Disease Risk and Health Outcomes. *ILAR Journal, 53*(3–4), 289–305. DOI: 10.1093/ilar.53.3-4.289 PMID: 23744968

Hockley, S. L., Arlt, V. M., Brewer, D., Te Poele, R., Workman, P., Giddings, I., & Phillips, D. H. (2007). AHR- and DNA-damage-mediated gene expression responses induced by benzo(a)pyrene in human cell lines. *Chemical Research in Toxicology, 20*(12), 1797–1810. DOI: 10.1021/tx700252n PMID: 17944540

Hodgson, M. C., Shen, H. C., Hollenberg, A. N., & Balk, S. P. (2008). Structural basis for nuclear receptor corepressor recruitment by antagonist-liganded androgen receptor. *Molecular Cancer Therapeutics, 7*(10), 3187–3194. DOI: 10.1158/1535-7163.MCT-08-0461 PMID: 18852122

Home - HEAP. (n.d.). Retrieved 14 April 2025, from https://heap-exposome.eu/?utm_source=chatgpt.com

Hu, W. Y., Shi, G., Hu, D.-P., Nelles, J. L., & Prins, G. S. (2011). Actions of Estrogens and Endocrine Disrupting Chemicals on Human Prostate Stem/Progenitor Cells and Prostate Cancer Risk. *Molecular and Cellular Endocrinology*, *354*(1–2), 63–73. DOI: 10.1016/j.mce.2011.08.032 PMID: 21914459

Humphrey, K. M., Pandey, S., Martin, J., Hagoel, T., Grand'Maison, A., & Ohm, J. E. (2018). Establishing a role for environmental toxicant exposure induced epigenetic remodeling in malignant transformation. *Seminars in Cancer Biology*, *57*, 86–94. DOI: 10.1016/j.semcancer.2018.11.002 PMID: 30453042

Humphrey, K. M., Pandey, S., Martin, J., Hagoel, T., Grand'Maison, A., & Ohm, J. E. (2018). Establishing a role for environmental toxicant exposure induced epigenetic remodeling in malignant transformation. *Seminars in Cancer Biology*, *57*, 86–94. DOI: 10.1016/j.semcancer.2018.11.002 PMID: 30453042

Huttunen, J., Aaltonen, N., Helminen, L., Rilla, K., & Paakinaho, V. (2024). EP300/CREBBP acetyltransferase inhibition limits steroid receptor and FOXA1 signaling in prostate cancer cells. *Cellular and Molecular Life Sciences : CMLS*, *81*(1), 1–21. DOI: 10.1007/s00018-024-05209-z PMID: 38564048

Hwang, G. C., Wankowicz, J., Zhang, S. A. M., Liu, Z., Cibulskis, D., Gaviola, C., Ghazikhanian, G. C., Mc, V., Kay, R. R., Bubley, G. J., Carter, S. L., Balk, S. P., Hahn, W. C., Taplin, M.-E., & Van Allen, E. M. (2017). Genomic resistance patterns to second-generation androgen blockade in paired tumor biopsies of metastatic castration-resistant prostate cancer. *JCO Precision Oncology*, (1), 1–11. DOI: 10.1200/PO.17.00140 PMID: 32913968

Imamura, Y., & Sadar, M. D. (2016). Androgen receptor targeted therapies in castration-resistant prostate cancer: Bench to clinic. *International Journal of Urology*, *23*(8), 654–665. DOI: 10.1111/iju.13137 PMID: 27302572

Imir, O. B., Kaminsky, A. Z., Zuo, Q. Y., Liu, Y. J., Singh, R., Spinella, M. J., Irudayaraj, J., Hu, W. Y., Prins, G. S., & Erdogan, Z. M. (2021). Per- and Polyfluoroalkyl Substance Exposure Combined with High-Fat Diet Supports Prostate Cancer Progression. *Nutrients*, *13*(11), 3902. Advance online publication. DOI: 10.3390/nu13113902 PMID: 34836157

. Jarnicki, A. G., Lysaght, J., Todryk, S., & Mills, K. H. G. (2006). Suppression of antitumor immunity by IL-10 and TGF-beta-producing T cells infiltrating the growing tumor: influence of tumor environment on the induction of CD4+ and CD8+ regulatory T cells. *Journal of Immunology (Baltimore, Md. : 1950)*, *177*(2), 896–904. DOI: 10.4049/jimmunol.177.2.896

Jiang, L., Khawaja, H., Tahsin, S., Clarkson, T. A., Miranti, C. K., & Zohar, Y. (2024). Microfluidic-based human prostate-cancer-on-chip. *Frontiers in Bioengineering and Biotechnology, 12*, 1302223. Advance online publication. DOI: 10.3389/fbioe.2024.1302223 PMID: 38322789

. Jin, M. Z., & Jin, W. L. (2020). The updated landscape of tumor microenvironment and drug repurposing. *Signal Transduction and Targeted Therapy 2020 5:1, 5*(1), 1–16. DOI: 10.1038/s41392-020-00280-x

Kahn, L. G., Philippat, C., Nakayama, S. F., Slama, R., & Trasande, L. (2020). Endocrine-disrupting chemicals: implications for human health. In *The Lancet Diabetes and Endocrinology* (Vol. 8, Issue 8, pp. 703–718). Lancet Publishing Group. DOI: 10.1016/S2213-8587(20)30129-7

Kamada, S., Takeiwa, T., Ikeda, K., Horie-Inoue, K., & Inoue, S. (2020). Long Non-coding RNAs Involved in Metabolic Alterations in Breast and Prostate Cancers. *Frontiers in Oncology, 10*, 593200. DOI: 10.3389/fonc.2020.593200 PMID: 33123488

Karthaus, W. R., Chan, J., Setty, M., Love, J. R., Zaidi, S., Choo, Z., Persad, S., LaClair, J., Lawrence, K. E., Chaudhary, O., Xu, T., Masilionis, I., Mazutis, L., Chaligne, R., Pe'er, D., & Sawyers, C. L. (2021). Reversal of lineage plasticity in RB1/TP53-deleted prostate cancer through FGFR and Janus kinase inhibition. *BioRxiv*, 2021.11.01.466615. DOI: 10.1101/2021.11.01.466615

Kassotis, C. D., Vandenberg, L. N., Demeneix, B. A., Porta, M., Slama, R., & Trasande, L. (2020). Endocrine-disrupting chemicals: economic, regulatory, and policy implications. In *The Lancet Diabetes and Endocrinology* (Vol. 8, Issue 8, pp. 719–730). Lancet Publishing Group. https://doi.org/DOI: 10.1016/S2213-8587(20)30128-5

. Kaufhold, S., & Bonavida, B. (2014). Central role of Snail1 in the regulation of EMT and resistance in cancer: a target for therapeutic intervention. *Journal of Experimental & Clinical Cancer Research 2014 33:1, 33*(1), 1–19. DOI: 10.1186/s13046-014-0062-0

Kaupang, Å., Paulsen, S. M., Steindal, C. C., Ravna, A. W., Sylte, I., Halvorsen, T. G., Thoresen, G. H., & Hansen, T. V. (2002). Structural basis for antagonist-mediated recruitment of nuclear co-repressors by PPARalpha. *Nature, 415*(6873), 229–236. DOI: 10.1038/415813a PMID: 11845213

Kelly, M., Connolly, L., & Dean, M. (2020). Public awareness and risk perceptions of endocrine disrupting chemicals: A qualitative study. *International Journal of Environmental Research and Public Health, 17*(21), 1–16. DOI: 10.3390/ijerph17217778 PMID: 33114266

Khan, M. M., Mohsen, M. T., Malik, M. Z., Bagabir, S. A., Alkhanani, M. F., Haque, S., Serajuddin, M., & Bharadwaj, M. (2022). Identification of Potential Key Genes in Prostate Cancer with Gene Expression, Pivotal Pathways and Regulatory Networks Analysis Using Integrated Bioinformatics Methods. *Genes*, *13*(4), 655. DOI: 10.3390/genes13040655 PMID: 35456461

Khatiwada, P., Rimal, U., Han, Z., & Shemshedini, L. (2024). MDM2 regulates the stability of AR, AR-V7, and TM4SF3 proteins in prostate cancer. *Endocrine Oncology*, *4*(1). Advance online publication. DOI: 10.1530/EO-23-0017 PMID: 38410785

Khurana, N., & Sikka, S. C. (2018). Targeting Crosstalk between Nrf-2, NF-κB and Androgen Receptor Signaling in Prostate Cancer. *Cancers (Basel)*, *10*(10), 352. DOI: 10.3390/cancers10100352 PMID: 30257470

Kim, H. M., & Kang, J. S. (2021). Metabolomic Studies for the Evaluation of Toxicity Induced by Environmental Toxicants on Model Organisms. *Metabolites*, *11*(8), 485. DOI: 10.3390/metabo11080485 PMID: 34436425

Kiyama, R. (2016). Endocrine disruptor actions through receptor crosstalk. *Environmental Biotechnology*, *12*(1), 1–16. DOI: 10.14799/ebms262

Klukovich, R., Nilsson, E., Sadler-Riggleman, I., Beck, D., Xie, Y., Yan, W., & Skinner, M. K. (2019). Environmental Toxicant Induced Epigenetic Transgenerational Inheritance of Prostate Pathology and Stromal-Epithelial Cell Epigenome and Transcriptome Alterations: Ancestral Origins of Prostate Disease. *Scientific Reports*, *9*(1), 2209. Advance online publication. DOI: 10.1038/s41598-019-38741-1 PMID: 30778168

Klukovich, R., Nilsson, E., Sadler-Riggleman, I., Beck, D., Xie, Y., Yan, W., & Skinner, M. K. (2019). Environmental Toxicant Induced Epigenetic Transgenerational Inheritance of Prostate Pathology and Stromal-Epithelial Cell Epigenome and Transcriptome Alterations: Ancestral Origins of Prostate Disease. *Scientific Reports*, *9*(1), 2209. Advance online publication. DOI: 10.1038/s41598-019-38741-1 PMID: 30778168

Kodanch, S. M., Mukherjee, S., Prabhu, N. B., Kabekkodu, S. P., Bhat, S. K., & Rai, P. S. (2024). Altered mitochondrial homeostasis on bisphenol-A exposure and its association in developing polycystic ovary syndrome: A comprehensive review. *Reproductive Toxicology (Elmsford, N.Y.)*, *130*, 108700. DOI: 10.1016/j.reprotox.2024.108700 PMID: 39181417

Koistinen, H., Künnapuu, J., & Jeltsch, M. (2021). KLK3 in the Regulation of Angiogenesis—Tumorigenic or Not? *International Journal of Molecular Sciences*, *22*(24), 13545. DOI: 10.3390/ijms222413545 PMID: 34948344

Kokai, D., Stanic, B., Tesic, B., Samardzija Nenadov, D., Pogrmic-Majkic, K., Fa Nedeljkovic, S., & Andric, N. (2022). Dibutyl phthalate promotes angiogenesis in EA.hy926 cells through estrogen receptor-dependent activation of ERK1/2, PI3K-Akt, and NO signaling pathways. *Chemico-Biological Interactions*, *366*, 110174. DOI: 10.1016/j.cbi.2022.110174 PMID: 36089060

Kulkarni, P., Dasgupta, P., Bhat, N. S., Hashimoto, Y., Saini, S., Shahryari, V., Yamamura, S., Shiina, M., Tanaka, Y., Dahiya, R., & Majid, S. (2020). Role of the PI3K/Akt pathway in cadmium induced malignant transformation of normal prostate epithelial cells. *Toxicology and Applied Pharmacology*, *409*, 115308. DOI: 10.1016/j.taap.2020.115308 PMID: 33129824

Kuo, C. H., Yang, S. N., Kuo, P. L., & Hung, C. H. (2012). Immunomodulatory effects of environmental endocrine disrupting chemicals. *The Kaohsiung Journal of Medical Sciences*, *28*(7, SUPPL.), S37–S42. DOI: 10.1016/j.kjms.2012.05.008 PMID: 22871600

. Lacouture, A., Lafront, C., Peillex, C., Pelletier, M., & Audet-Walsh, É. (2022). Impacts of endocrine-disrupting chemicals on prostate function and cancer. *Environmental Research, 204*(Pt B). DOI: 10.1016/j.envres.2021.112085

Latonen, L., Afyounian, E., Jylhä, A., Nättinen, J., Aapola, U., Annala, M., Kivinummi, K. K., Tammela, T. T. L., Beuerman, R. W., Uusitalo, H., Nykter, M., & Visakorpi, T. (2018). Integrative proteomics in prostate cancer uncovers robustness against genomic and transcriptomic aberrations during disease progression. *Nature Communications*, *9*(1), 1176. Advance online publication. DOI: 10.1038/s41467-018-03573-6 PMID: 29563510

Launonen, K. M., Varis, V., Aaltonen, N., Niskanen, E. A., Varjosalo, M., Paakinaho, V., & Palvimo, J. J. (2024). Central role of SUMOylation in the regulation of chromatin interactions and transcriptional outputs of the androgen receptor in prostate cancer cells. *Nucleic Acids Research*, *52*(16), 9519–9535. DOI: 10.1093/nar/gkae653 PMID: 39106160

Laury, A. R., Zheng, S., Aho, N., Fallegger, R., Hänninen, S., Saez-Rodriguez, J., Tanevski, J., Youssef, O., Tang, J., & Carpén, O. M. (2024). Opening the Black Box: Spatial Transcriptomics and the Relevance of Artificial Intelligence–Detected Prognostic Regions in High-Grade Serous Carcinoma. *Modern Pathology*, *37*(7), 100508. DOI: 10.1016/j.modpat.2024.100508 PMID: 38704029

. Lawrence, O., Woldegiorgis, S., Ahmed, R. C., Zhen, Y., Erdmann, C. A., Russell, M. L., & Goth-Goldstein, R. (2002). *LBNL-50365 Genetic Polymorphism in Three Glutathione S-Transferase Genes and Breast Cancer Risk.*

. Lee, S., Kim, G., Lee, J. Y., Lee, A. C., & Kwon, S. (2024). Mapping cancer biology in space: applications and perspectives on spatial omics for oncology. *Molecular Cancer 2024 23:1, 23*(1), 1–27. DOI: 10.1186/s12943-024-01941-z

Leng, L., Chen, X., Li, C. P., Luo, X. Y., & Tang, N. J. (2014). 2,3,7,8-Tetrachlorodibezo-p-dioxin exposure and prostate cancer: A meta-analysis of cohort studies. *Public Health, 128*(3), 207–213. DOI: 10.1016/j.puhe.2013.10.006 PMID: 24461260

Li, D., Chang, B., & Huang, Q. (2025). Using XBGoost, an interpretable machine learning model, for diagnosing prostate cancer in patients with PSA <20 ng/ml based on the PSAMR indicator. *Scientific Reports, 15*(1), 1532. DOI: 10.1038/s41598-025-85963-7 PMID: 39789130

Li, J., & Bluth, M. H. (2011). Pharmacogenomics of drug metabolizing enzymes and transporters: Implications for cancer therapy. *Pharmacogenomics and Personalized Medicine, 4*(1), 11. DOI: 10.2147/PGPM.S18861 PMID: 23226051

. Li, K., Wang, H., Jiang, B., & Jin, X. (2025). The impact of dysregulation SUMOylation on prostate cancer. *Journal of Translational Medicine 2025 23:1, 23*(1), 1–16. DOI: 10.1186/s12967-025-06271-2

Li, K., Wang, Q., Tang, X., Akakuru, O. U., Li, R., Wang, Y., Zhang, R., Jiang, Z., & Yang, Z. (2024). Advances in Prostate Cancer Biomarkers and Probes. In *Cyborg and Bionic Systems* (Vol. 5). American Association for the Advancement of Science., DOI: 10.34133/cbsystems.0129

Li, Q., Wang, Y., Chen, J., Zeng, K., Wang, C., Guo, X., Hu, Z., Hu, J., Liu, B., Xiao, J., & Zhou, P. (2024). Machine learning based androgen receptor regulatory gene-related random forest survival model for precise treatment decision in prostate cancer. *Heliyon, 10*(17), e37256. DOI: 10.1016/j.heliyon.2024.e37256 PMID: 39296076

Li, S., Kang, Y., & Zeng, Y. (2024). Targeting tumor and bone microenvironment: Novel therapeutic opportunities for castration-resistant prostate cancer patients with bone metastasis. *Biochimica et Biophysica Acta. Reviews on Cancer, 1879*(1), 189033. Advance online publication. DOI: 10.1016/j.bbcan.2023.189033 PMID: 38040267

. Li, S., Sampson, C., Liu, C., Piao, H. long, & Liu, H. X. (2023). Integrin signaling in cancer: bidirectional mechanisms and therapeutic opportunities. *Cell Communication and Signaling 2023 21:1, 21*(1), 1–19. DOI: 10.1186/s12964-023-01264-4

Li, Y., Zhou, T., Liu, Z., Zhu, X., Wu, Q., Meng, C., & Deng, Q. (2025). Air pollution and prostate cancer: Unraveling the connection through network toxicology and machine learning. *Ecotoxicology and Environmental Safety, 292*, 117966. Advance online publication. DOI: 10.1016/j.ecoenv.2025.117966 PMID: 40022828

Liang, Y., Chu, P. H., Tian, L., Ho, K. F., Ip, M. S. M., & Mak, J. C. W. (2022). Targeting mitochondrial permeability transition pore ameliorates PM2.5-induced mitochondrial dysfunction in airway epithelial cells. *Environmental Pollution, 295*, 118720. Advance online publication. DOI: 10.1016/j.envpol.2021.118720 PMID: 34953947

. Lin, K. X., Wu, Z. Y., Qin, M. L., & Zeng, H. C. (2025). Bisphenol S Induces Lipid Metabolism Disorders in HepG2 and SK-Hep-1 Cells via Oxidative Stress. *Toxics 2025, Vol. 13, Page 44, 13*(1), 44. DOI: 10.3390/toxics13010044

Lin, S., Chai, Y., Zheng, X., & Xu, X. (2024). The role of HIF in angiogenesis, lymphangiogenesis, and tumor microenvironment in urological cancers. *Molecular Biology Reports, 51*(1), 1–13. DOI: 10.1007/s11033-023-08931-2 PMID: 38085375

Lin, Z., & Chou, W. C. (2022). Machine Learning and Artificial Intelligence in Toxicological Sciences. *Toxicological Sciences, 189*(1), 7–19. DOI: 10.1093/toxsci/kfac075 PMID: 35861448

Liu, C., Yang, J., Fu, W., Qi, S., Wang, C., Quan, C., & Yang, K. (2014). Coactivation of the PI3K/Akt and ERK signaling pathways in PCB153-induced NF-κB activation and caspase inhibition. *Toxicology and Applied Pharmacology, 277*(3), 270–278. DOI: 10.1016/j.taap.2014.03.027 PMID: 24726520

. Liu, L., Yoon, J.-H., Dammann, R., & Pfeifer, G. P. (n.d.). Frequent hypermethylation of the RASSF1A gene in prostate cancer. https://doi.org/DOI: 10.1038/sj.onc

. Liu, N., Wang, A., Xue, M., Zhu, X., Liu, Y., & Chen, M. (2024). FOXA1 and FOXA2: the regulatory mechanisms and therapeutic implications in cancer. *Cell Death Discovery 2024 10:1, 10*(1), 1–15. DOI: 10.1038/s41420-024-01936-1

Liu, Q., Harvey, C. T., Geng, H., Xue, C., Chen, V., Beer, T. M., & Qian, D. Z. (2013). Malate dehydrogenase 2 confers docetaxel resistance via regulations of JNK signaling and oxidative metabolism. *The Prostate, 73*(10), 1028–1037. DOI: 10.1002/pros.22650 PMID: 23389923

Liu, Y., Asnani, A., Zou, L., Bentley, V. L., Yu, M., Wang, Y., Dellaire, G., Sarkar, K. S., Dai, M., Chen, H. H., Sosnovik, D. E., Shin, J. T., Haber, D. A., Berman, J. N., Chao, W., & Peterson, R. T. (2014). Visnagin protects against doxorubicin-induced cardiomyopathy through modulation of mitochondrial malate dehydrogenase. *Science Translational Medicine, 6*(266). Advance online publication. DOI: 10.1126/scitranslmed.3010189 PMID: 25504881

Liu, Y., Horn, J. L., Banda, K., Goodman, A. Z., Lim, Y., Jana, S., Arora, S., Germanos, A. A., Wen, L., Hardin, W. R., Yang, Y. C., Coleman, I. M., Tharakan, R. G., Cai, E. Y., Uo, T., Pillai, S. P. S., Corey, E., Morrissey, C., Chen, Y., & Hsieh, A. C. (2019). The androgen receptor regulates a druggable translational regulon in advanced prostate cancer. *Science Translational Medicine*, *11*(503), eaaw4993. Advance online publication. DOI: 10.1126/scitranslmed.aaw4993 PMID: 31366581

Liu, Z., Hu, M., Yang, Y., Du, C., Zhou, H., Liu, C., Chen, Y., Fan, L., Ma, H., Gong, Y., & Xie, Y. (2022). An overview of PROTACs: A promising drug discovery paradigm. *Molecular Biomedicine*, *3*(1), 46. DOI: 10.1186/s43556-022-00112-0 PMID: 36536188

Loehr, A., Hussain, A., Patnaik, A., Bryce, A. H., Castellano, D., Font, A., Shapiro, J., Zhang, J., Sautois, B., Vogelzang, N. J., Chatta, G., Courtney, K., Harzstark, A., Ricci, F., Despain, D., Watkins, S., King, C., Nguyen, M., Simmons, A. D., & Abida, W. (2023). Emergence of BRCA Reversion Mutations in Patients with Metastatic Castration-resistant Prostate Cancer After Treatment with Rucaparib. *European Urology*, *83*(3), 200–209. DOI: 10.1016/j.eururo.2022.09.010 PMID: 36243543

López, J., Añazco-Guenkova, A. M., Monteagudo-García, Ó., & Blanco, S. (2022). Epigenetic and Epitranscriptomic Control in Prostate Cancer. *Genes*, *13*(2), 378. DOI: 10.3390/genes13020378 PMID: 35205419

Luccio-Camelo, D. C., & Prins, G. S. (2011). Disruption of androgen receptor signaling in males by environmental chemicals. *The Journal of Steroid Biochemistry and Molecular Biology*, *127*(1–2), 74–82. DOI: 10.1016/j.jsbmb.2011.04.004 PMID: 21515368

. Luis-García, E. R., Becerril, C., Salgado-Aguayo, A., Aparicio-Trejo, O. E., Romero, Y., Flores-Soto, E., Mendoza-Milla, C., Montaño, M., Chagoya, V., Pedraza-Chaverri, J., El Hafidi, M., Orozco-Ibarra, M., Pardo, A., & Selman, M. (2021). Mitochondrial Dysfunction and Alterations in Mitochondrial Permeability Transition Pore (mPTP) Contribute to Apoptosis Resistance in Idiopathic Pulmonary Fibrosis Fibroblasts. *International Journal of Molecular Sciences 2021, Vol. 22, Page 7870*, *22*(15), 7870. DOI: 10.3390/ijms22157870

Luo, J., Chen, Z., Qiao, Y., Tien, J. C.-Y., Young, E., Mannan, R., Mahapatra, S., He, T., Eyunni, S., Zhang, Y., Zheng, Y., Su, F., Cao, X., Wang, R., Cheng, Y., Seri, R., George, J., Shahine, M., Miner, S. J., . . . Chinnaiyan, A. M. (2024). p300/CBP degradation is required to disable the active AR enhanceosome in prostate cancer. BioRxiv, 2024.03.29.587346. https://doi.org/DOI: 10.1101/2024.03.29.587346

Maeda, K., Habara, M., Kawaguchi, M., Matsumoto, H., Hanaki, S., Masaki, T., Sato, Y., Matsuyama, H., Kunieda, K., Nakagawa, H., & Shimada, M. (2022). FKBP51 and FKBP52 regulate androgen receptor dimerization and proliferation in prostate cancer cells. *Molecular Oncology*, *16*(4), 940–956. DOI: 10.1002/1878-0261.13030 PMID: 34057812

Manzar, N., Khan, U. K., Goel, A., Carskadon, S., Gupta, N., Palanisamy, N., & Ateeq, B. (2024). An integrative proteomics approach identifies tyrosine kinase KIT as a therapeutic target for SPINK1-positive prostate cancer. *iScience*, *27*(3), 108794. Advance online publication. DOI: 10.1016/j.isci.2024.108794 PMID: 38384854

Marquez, J., Ángel, J., Sandoval, C., Erb, H. H. H., Polishchuk, N., Stasyk, O., Gur Kahya, U. ˘., Weigel, M. M., Dubrovska, A., & Dresden-Rossendorf, H.-Z. (2024). Glutamine Metabolism and Prostate Cancer. *Cancers (Basel)*, *16*(16), 2871. DOI: 10.3390/cancers16162871 PMID: 39199642

McGirt, L. Y., Jia, P., Baerenwald, D. A., Duszynski, R. J., Dahlman, K. B., Zic, J. A., Zwerner, J. P., Hucks, D., Dave, U., Zhao, Z., & Eischen, C. M. (2015). Whole-genome sequencing reveals oncogenic mutations in mycosis fungoides. *Blood*, *126*(4), 508–519. DOI: 10.1182/blood-2014-11-611194 PMID: 26082451

Mediwala, S. N., Sun, H., Szafran, A. T., Hartig, S. M., Sonpavde, G., Hayes, T. G., Thiagarajan, P., Mancini, M. A., & Marcelli, M. (2013). The activity of the androgen receptor variant AR-V7 is regulated by FOXO1 in a PTEN-PI3K-AKT-dependent way. *The Prostate*, *73*(3), 267–277. DOI: 10.1002/pros.22566 PMID: 22821817

Meng, L., Zheng, Y., Liu, H., & Fan, D. (2024). The tumor microenvironment: A key player in multidrug resistance in cancer. *Oncologie*, *26*(1), 41–58. DOI: 10.1515/oncologie-2023-0459

Mishra, R., Haldar, S., Suchanti, S., & Bhowmick, N. A. (2019). Epigenetic changes in fibroblasts drive cancer metabolism and differentiation. *Endocrine-Related Cancer*, *26*(12), R673–R688. DOI: 10.1530/ERC-19-0347 PMID: 31627186

Mittal, R., Woo, F. W., Castro, C. S., Cohen, M. A., Karanxha, J., Mittal, J., Chhibber, T., & Jhaveri, V. M. (2019). Organ-on-chip models: Implications in drug discovery and clinical applications. In *Journal of Cellular Physiology* (Vol. 234, Issue 6, pp. 8352–8380). Wiley-Liss Inc. https://doi.org/DOI: 10.1002/jcp.27729

Miura, R., Ikeda-Araki, A., Ishihara, T., Miyake, K., Miyashita, C., Nakajima, T., Kobayashi, S., Ishizuka, M., Kubota, T., & Kishi, R. (2021). Effect of prenatal exposure to phthalates on epigenome-wide DNA methylations in cord blood and implications for fetal growth: The Hokkaido Study on Environment and Children's Health. *The Science of the Total Environment, 783*, 147035. DOI: 10.1016/j.scitotenv.2021.147035 PMID: 33872906

Modica, R., Benevento, E., & Colao, A. (2023). Endocrine-disrupting chemicals (EDCs) and cancer: New perspectives on an old relationship. *Journal of Endocrinological Investigation, 46*(4), 667–677. DOI: 10.1007/s40618-022-01983-4 PMID: 36526827

Moldogazieva, N. T., Mokhosoev, I. M., & Terentiev, A. A. (2020). Metabolic Heterogeneity of Cancer Cells: An Interplay between HIF-1, GLUTs, and AMPK. *Cancers (Basel), 12*(4), 862. DOI: 10.3390/cancers12040862 PMID: 32252351

Montoya-Novoa, I., Gardeazábal-Torbado, J. L., Alegre-Martí, A., Fuentes-Prior, P., & Estébanez-Perpiñá, E. (2024). Androgen receptor post-translational modifications and their implications for pathology. *Biochemical Society Transactions, 52*(4), 1673–1694. DOI: 10.1042/BST20231082 PMID: 38958586

Mukhopadhyay, S., Huang, H. Y., Lin, Z., Ranieri, M., Li, S., Sahu, S., Liu, Y., Ban, Y., Guidry, K., Hu, H., Lopez, A., Sherman, F., Tan, Y. J., Lee, Y. T., Armstrong, A. P., Dolgalev, I., Sahu, P., Zhang, T., Lu, W., & Neel, B. G. (2023). Genome-Wide CRISPR Screens Identify Multiple Synthetic Lethal Targets That Enhance KRASG12C Inhibitor Efficacy. *Cancer Research, 83*(24), 4095–4111. DOI: 10.1158/0008-5472.CAN-23-2729 PMID: 37729426

Na, A. Y., Choi, S., Yang, E., Liu, K. H., Kim, S., Jung, H. J., Choe, Y., Ha, Y. S., Kwon, T. G., Lee, J. N., & Lee, S. (2021). Characterization of novel progression factors in castration-resistant prostate cancer based on global comparative proteome analysis. *Cancers (Basel), 13*(14), 3432. Advance online publication. DOI: 10.3390/cancers13143432 PMID: 34298646

. Nayak, D., Adiga, D., Khan, N. G., Rai, P. S., Dsouza, H. S., Chakrabarty, S., Gassman, N. R., & Kabekkodu, S. P. (2022). Impact of Bisphenol A on Structure and Function of Mitochondria: A Critical Review. *Reviews of Environmental Contamination and Toxicology 2022 260:1, 260*(1), 1–23. DOI: 10.1007/s44169-022-00011-z

Nemmiche, S., & Guiraud, P. (2016). Cadmium-induced oxidative damages in the human BJAB cells correlate with changes in intracellular trace elements levels and zinc transporters expression. *In Vitro, 37*, 169–177. DOI: 10.1016/j.tiv.2016.09.014 PMID: 27647474

Nevedomskaya, E., & Haendler, B. (2022). From Omics to Multi-Omics Approaches for In-Depth Analysis of the Molecular Mechanisms of Prostate Cancer. In *International Journal of Molecular Sciences* (Vol. 23, Issue 11). MDPI. https://doi.org/ DOI: 10.3390/ijms23116281

Nientiedt, C., Budczies, J., Endris, V., Kirchner, M., Schwab, C., Jurcic, C., Behnisch, R., Hoveida, S., Lantwin, P., Kaczorowski, A., Geisler, C., Dieffenbacher, S., Falkenbach, F., Franke, D., Görtz, M., Heller, M., Himmelsbach, R., Pecqueux, C., Rath, M., & Duensing, S. (2022). Mutations in TP53 or DNA damage repair genes define poor prognostic subgroups in primary prostate cancer. *Urologic Oncology, 40*(1), 8.e11–8.e18. DOI: 10.1016/j.urolonc.2021.06.024 PMID: 34325986

Nilsson, E. E., Sadler-Riggleman, I., & Skinner, M. K. (2018). Environmentally induced epigenetic transgenerational inheritance of disease. In Environmental Epigenetics (Vol. 4, Issue 2, pp. 1–13). Oxford University Press. https://doi.org/DOI: 10.1093/eep/dvy016

Nock, N. L., Liu, X., Cicek, M. S., Li, L., Macarie, F., Rybicki, B. A., Plummer, S. J., MacLennan, G. T., Casey, G., & Witte, J. S. (2006). Polymorphisms in polycyclic aromatic hydrocarbon metabolism and conjugation genes, interactions with smoking and prostate cancer risk. *Cancer Epidemiology, Biomarkers & Prevention, 15*(4), 756–761. DOI: 10.1158/1055-9965.EPI-05-0826 PMID: 16614120

. Ofner, H., Kramer, G., Shariat, S. F., & Hassler, M. R. (2025). TP53 Deficiency in the Natural History of Prostate Cancer. *Cancers 2025, Vol. 17, Page 645, 17*(4), 645. DOI: 10.3390/cancers17040645

Pandiri, A. R., Auerbach, S. S., Stevens, J. L., & Blomme, E. A. G. (2024). Toxicogenomics approaches to address toxicity and carcinogenicity in the liver. *Toxicologic Pathology, 51*(7–8), 470–481. DOI: 10.1177/01926233241227942 PMID: 38288963

. Parfenyev, S. E., Daks, A. A., Shuvalov, O. Y., Fedorova, O. A., Pestov, N. B., Korneenko, T. V., & Barlev, N. A. (2025). Dualistic role of ZEB1 and ZEB2 in tumor progression. *Biology Direct 2025 20:1, 20*(1), 1–16. DOI: 10.1186/s13062-025-00604-3

Park, J., Lee, H., Lee, S., & Lee, H. (2022). Interventions on Reducing Exposure to Endocrine Disrupting Chemicals in Human Health Care Context: A Scoping Review. In *Risk Management and Healthcare Policy* (Vol. 15, pp. 779–791). Dove Medical Press Ltd. https://doi.org/DOI: 10.2147/RMHP.S358561

Pereira, S. A., & Antunes, A. M. M. (2019). Special issue 'Adductomics: Elucidating the environmental causes of disease'. *High-Throughput, 8*(3), 17. Advance online publication. DOI: 10.3390/ht8030017 PMID: 31370290

Perry, A. S., Watson, R. W. G., Lawler, M., & Hollywood, D. (2010). The epigenome as a therapeutic target in prostate cancer. In Nature Reviews Urology (Vol. 7, Issue 12, pp. 668–680). https://doi.org/DOI: 10.1038/nrurol.2010.185

Portugal, J., Mansilla, S., & Piña, B. (2022). Perspectives on the Use of Toxicogenomics to Assess Environmental Risk. *Frontiers in Bioscience (Landmark Edition)*, *27*(10), 294. Advance online publication. DOI: 10.31083/j.fbl2710294 PMID: 36336867

Prakash, P., Verma, S., & Gupta, S. (2024). Risk factors influencing chronic inflammation in neoplastic transition to prostate cancer. *Journal of Translational Genetics and Genomics*, *8*(4), 312–327. DOI: 10.20517/jtgg.2024.52

Prins, G. S. (2008). Endocrine disruptors and prostate cancer risk. *Endocrine-Related Cancer*, *15*(3), 649–656. DOI: 10.1677/ERC-08-0043 PMID: 18524946

Prins, G. S. (2008). Endocrine disruptors and prostate cancer risk. *Endocrine-Related Cancer*, *15*(3), 649–656. DOI: 10.1677/ERC-08-0043 PMID: 18524946

Prins, G. S., Ye, S. H., Birch, L., Zhang, X., Cheong, A., Lin, H., Calderon-Gierszal, E., Groen, J., Hu, W. Y., Ho, S. M., & Van Breemen, R. B. (2017). Prostate Cancer Risk and DNA Methylation Signatures in Aging Rats following Developmental BPA Exposure: A Dose-Response Analysis. *Environmental Health Perspectives*, *125*(7), 077007. Advance online publication. DOI: 10.1289/EHP1050 PMID: 28728135

Puca, L., Bareja, R., Prandi, D., Shaw, R., Benelli, M., Karthaus, W. R., Hess, J., Sigouros, M., Donoghue, A., Kossai, M., Gao, D., Cyrta, J., Sailer, V., Vosoughi, A., Pauli, C., Churakova, Y., Cheung, C., Deonarine, L. D., McNary, T. J., & Beltran, H. (2018). Patient derived organoids to model rare prostate cancer phenotypes. *Nature Communications*, *9*(1), 2404. Advance online publication. DOI: 10.1038/s41467-018-04495-z PMID: 29921838

Quagliariello, V., Rossetti, S., Cavaliere, C., Di Palo, R., Lamantia, E., Castaldo, L., Nocerino, F., Ametrano, G., Cappuccio, F., Malzone, G., Montanari, M., Vanacore, D., Romano, F. J., Piscitelli, R., Iovane, G., Pepe, M. F., Berretta, M., D'Aniello, C., Perdonà, S., & Facchini, G. (2017). Metabolic syndrome, endocrine disruptors and prostate cancer associations: Biochemical and pathophysiological evidences. *Oncotarget*, *8*(18), 30606–30616. DOI: 10.18632/oncotarget.16725 PMID: 28389628

Querol Cano, L., Lavery, D. N., & Bevan, C. L. (2013). Mini-review: Foldosome regulation of androgen receptor action in prostate cancer. *Molecular and Cellular Endocrinology*, *369*(1–2), 52–62. DOI: 10.1016/j.mce.2013.01.023 PMID: 23395916

Rajdeo, P., Aronow, B., & Surya Prasath, V. B. (2024). Deep learning-based multimodal spatial transcriptomics analysis for cancer. *Advances in Cancer Research, 163*, 1–38. DOI: 10.1016/bs.acr.2024.08.001 PMID: 39271260

Ralph, J. L., Orgebin-Crist, M. C., Lareyre, J. J., & Nelson, C. C. (2003a). Disruption of androgen regulation in the prostate by the environmental contaminant hexachlorobenzene. In *Environmental Health Perspectives* (Vol. 111, Issue 4, pp. 461–466). Public Health Services, US Dept of Health and Human Services. DOI: 10.1289/ehp.5919

Ralph, J. L., Orgebin-Crist, M. C., Lareyre, J. J., & Nelson, C. C. (2003b). Disruption of androgen regulation in the prostate by the environmental contaminant hexachlorobenzene. *Environmental Health Perspectives, 111*(4), 461–466. DOI: 10.1289/ehp.5919 PMID: 12676599

Rappaport, S. M. (2011). Implications of the exposome for exposure science. *Journal of Exposure Science & Environmental Epidemiology, 21*(1), 5–9. DOI: 10.1038/jes.2010.50 PMID: 21081972

Rathkopf, D. E., Smith, M. R., Ryan, C. J., Berry, W. R., Shore, N. D., Liu, G., Higano, C. S., Alumkal, J. J., Hauke, R., Tutrone, R. F., Saleh, M., Maneval, E. C., Thomas, S., Ricci, D. S., Yu, M. K., de Boer, C. J., Trinh, A., Kheoh, T., Bandekar, R., & Antonarakis, E. S. (2017). Androgen receptor mutations in patients with castration-resistant prostate cancer treated with apalutamide. *Annals of Oncology : Official Journal of the European Society for Medical Oncology, 28*(9), 2264–2271. DOI: 10.1093/annonc/mdx283 PMID: 28633425

Risdon, E. N., Chau, C. H., Price, D. K., Sartor, O., & Figg, W. D. (2020). PARP Inhibitors and Prostate Cancer: To Infinity and Beyond BRCA. *The Oncologist, 26*(1), e115–e129. DOI: 10.1634/theoncologist.2020-0697 PMID: 32790034

Ronsmans, S., Sørig Hougaard, K., Nawrot, T. S., Plusquin, M., Huaux, F., Jesús Cruz, M., Moldovan, H., Verpaele, S., Jayapala, M., Tunney, M., Humblet-Baron, S., Dirven, H., Cecilie Nygaard, U., Lindeman, B., Duale, N., Liston, A., Flachs, E. M., Kastaniegaard, K., Ketzel, M., & Yserbyt, J. (2022). The EXIMIOUS project—Mapping exposure-induced immune effects: Connecting the exposome and the immunome. *Environmental Epidemiology (Philadelphia, Pa.), 6*(1), e193. DOI: 10.1097/EE9.0000000000000193 PMID: 35169671

Roux, P. P., & Blenis, J. (2004). ERK and p38 MAPK-Activated Protein Kinases: A Family of Protein Kinases with Diverse Biological Functions. *Microbiology and Molecular Biology Reviews : MMBR, 68*(2), 320–344. DOI: 10.1128/MMBR.68.2.320-344.2004 PMID: 15187187

. Rozelle, A. L., Cheun, Y., Vilas, C. K., Koag, M. C., & Lee, S. (2021). DNA interstrand cross-links induced by the major oxidative adenine lesion 7,8-dihydro-8-oxoadenine. *Nature Communications 2021 12:1, 12*(1), 1–16. DOI: 10.1038/s41467-021-22273-2

Ruan, Y., Fang, X., Guo, T., Liu, Y., Hu, Y., Wang, X., Hu, Y., Gao, L., Li, Y., Pi, J., & Xu, Y. (2022). Metabolic reprogramming in the arsenic carcinogenesis. *Ecotoxicology and Environmental Safety, 229*, 113098. DOI: 10.1016/j.ecoenv.2021.113098 PMID: 34952379

Ruggeri, R. M., Minuti, A., Gianì, F., Masto, R., Romano, D., Aliquò, F., Campennì, A., Campo, S., Cannavò, S., & D'Ascola, A. (2025). Polychlorinated Biphenyls (PCBS)-induced oxidative stress and inflammation in human thyrocytes: Involvement of AhR and NRF-2/HO-1 pathway. *Endocrine, 87*(1), 252–261. Advance online publication. DOI: 10.1007/s12020-024-04005-w PMID: 39174753

Rusiecki, J. A., Beane Freeman, L. E., Bonner, M. R., Alexander, M., Chen, L., Andreotti, G., Barry, K. H., Moore, L. E., Byun, H. M., Kamel, F., Alavanja, M., Hoppin, J. A., & Baccarelli, A. (2017). High pesticide exposure events and DNA methylation among pesticide applicators in the agricultural health study. *Environmental and Molecular Mutagenesis, 58*(1), 19–29. DOI: 10.1002/em.22067 PMID: 27996157

Ryeom, S. W., Paul, D., & Goodenough, D. A. (2000). Truncation mutants of the tight junction protein ZO-1 disrupt corneal epithelial cell morphology. *Molecular Biology of the Cell, 11*(5), 1687–1696. DOI: 10.1091/mbc.11.5.1687 PMID: 10793144

. Saber, S. H., Ali, H. E. A., Gaballa, R., Gaballah, M., Ali, H. I., Zerfaoui, M., & Elmageed, Z. Y. A. (2020). Exosomes are the Driving Force in Preparing the Soil for the Metastatic Seeds: Lessons from the Prostate Cancer. *Cells 2020, Vol. 9, Page 564, 9*(3), 564. DOI: 10.3390/cells9030564

Sadar, M. D., & Gleave, M. E. (2000). Ligand-independent Activation of the Androgen Receptor by the Differentiation Agent Butyrate in Human Prostate Cancer Cells 1. In *CANCER RESEARCH* (Vol. 60).

Saha, D., Dang, H. X., Zhang, M., Quigley, D. A., Feng, F. Y., & Maher, C. A. (2024). Single cell-transcriptomic analysis informs the lncRNA landscape in metastatic castration resistant prostate cancer. *NPJ Genomic Medicine, 9*(1), 14. Advance online publication. DOI: 10.1038/s41525-024-00401-3 PMID: 38396008

Salian, S., Doshi, T., & Vanage, G. (2009). Impairment in protein expression profile of testicular steroid receptor coregulators in male rat offspring perinatally exposed to Bisphenol A. *Life Sciences*, *85*(1–2), 11–18. DOI: 10.1016/j.lfs.2009.04.005 PMID: 19379760

Santos-Pereira, M., Pereira, S. C., Rebelo, I., Spadella, M. A., Oliveira, P. F., & Alves, M. G. (2023). Decoding the Influence of Obesity on Prostate Cancer and Its Transgenerational Impact. In Nutrients (Vol. 15, Issue 23). Multidisciplinary Digital Publishing Institute (MDPI). https://doi.org/DOI: 10.3390/nu15234858

Sardar, S., McNair, C. M., Ravindranath, L., Chand, S. N., Yuan, W., Bogdan, D., Welti, J., Sharp, A., Ryan, N. K., Schiewer, M. J., DeArment, E. G., Janas, T., Su, X. A., Butler, L. M., de Bono, J. S., Frese, K., Brooks, N., Pegg, N., Knudsen, K. E., & Shafi, A. A. (2024). AR coactivators, CBP/p300, are critical mediators of DNA repair in prostate cancer. BioRxiv, 2024.05.07.592966. DOI: 10.1101/2024.05.07.592966

Sarkar, A., Paul, A., Banerjee, T., Maji, A., Saha, S., Bishayee, A., & Maity, T. K. (2023). Therapeutic advancements in targeting BCL-2 family proteins by epigenetic regulators, natural, and synthetic agents in cancer. *European Journal of Pharmacology*, *944*, 175588. DOI: 10.1016/j.ejphar.2023.175588 PMID: 36791843

Sassi, A., & You, L. (2024). Microfluidics-Based Technologies for the Assessment of Castration-Resistant Prostate Cancer. In *Cells* (Vol. 13, Issue 7). Multidisciplinary Digital Publishing Institute (MDPI). https://doi.org/DOI: 10.3390/cells13070575

Schuler, M. S., & Rose, S. (2017). Targeted Maximum Likelihood Estimation for Causal Inference in Observational Studies. *American Journal of Epidemiology*, *185*(1), 65–73. DOI: 10.1093/aje/kww165 PMID: 27941068

Schulz, H., Abdelfattah, F., Heinrich, A., Melnik, D., Sandt, V., Krüger, M., Wehland, M., Hoffmann, P., Cortés-Sánchez, J. L., Evert, M., Evert, K., & Grimm, D. (2025). Omics Investigations of Prostate Cancer Cells Exposed to Simulated Microgravity Conditions. *Biomolecules*, *15*(2), 303. DOI: 10.3390/biom15020303 PMID: 40001606

Schwarzenbach, H., Alix-Panabières, C., Müller, I., Letang, N., Vendrell, J. P., Rebillard, X., & Pantel, K. (2009). Cell-free tumor DNA in blood plasma as a marker for circulating tumor cells in prostate cancer. *Clinical Cancer Research*, *15*(3), 1032–1038. DOI: 10.1158/1078-0432.CCR-08-1910 PMID: 19188176

Segovia-Mendoza, M., Nava-Castro, K. E., Palacios-Arreola, M. I., Garay-Canales, C., & Morales-Montor, J. (2020). How microplastic components influence the immune system and impact on children health: Focus on cancer. *Birth Defects Research*, *112*(17), 1341–1361. DOI: 10.1002/bdr2.1779 PMID: 32767490

Shafi, A. A., Yen, A. E., & Weigel, N. L. (2013). Androgen receptors in hormone-dependent and castration-resistant prostate cancer. *Pharmacology & Therapeutics, 140*(3), 223–238. DOI: 10.1016/j.pharmthera.2013.07.003 PMID: 23859952

Shin, H. J., Hua, J. T., & Li, H. (2023). Recent advances in understanding DNA methylation of prostate cancer. *Frontiers in Oncology, 13*, 1182727. DOI: 10.3389/fonc.2023.1182727 PMID: 37234978

Shorning, B. Y., Dass, M. S., Smalley, M. J., & Pearson, H. B. (2020). The PI3K-AKT-mTOR Pathway and Prostate Cancer: At the Crossroads of AR, MAPK, and WNT Signaling. *International Journal of Molecular Sciences, 21*(12), 4507. DOI: 10.3390/ijms21124507 PMID: 32630372

. Shukla, S., Srivastava, J. K., Shankar, E., Kanwal, R., Nawab, A., Sharma, H., Bhaskaran, N., Ponsky, L. E., Fu, P., MacLennan, G. T., & Gupta, S. (2020). Oxidative Stress and Antioxidant Status in High-Risk Prostate Cancer Subjects. *Diagnostics 2020, Vol. 10, Page 126, 10*(3), 126. DOI: 10.3390/diagnostics10030126

Silkina, M. O., Razumovskaya, A. V., Nikulin, S. V., Tonevitsky, A. G., & Alekseev, B. Y. (2023). Assessing the Efficacy of Anti-Cancer Drugs on Organoid Models Derived from Prostate Cancer. *Doklady. Biochemistry and Biophysics, 513*(S1, Suppl 1), S96–S99. Advance online publication. DOI: 10.1134/S1607672923700692 PMID: 38337100

Singh, A. V., Bhardwaj, P., Laux, P., Pradeep, P., Busse, M., Luch, A., Hirose, A., Osgood, C. J., & Stacey, M. W. (2024). AI and ML-based risk assessment of chemicals: Predicting carcinogenic risk from chemical-induced genomic instability. *Frontiers in Toxicology, 6*, 1461587. DOI: 10.3389/ftox.2024.1461587 PMID: 39659701

Singh, D. D. (2024). Epigenetic Mechanisms of Endocrine-Disrupting Chemicals in Breast Cancer and Their Impact on Dietary Intake. *Journal of Xenobiotics, 15*(1), 1. DOI: 10.3390/jox15010001 PMID: 39846533

Singh, G., Trehan, S., Singh, A., Goswami, K., Farooq, A., Antil, P., Puri, P., Bector, G., Jain, A., Azhar, W., Singh, G., Trehan, S., Singh, A., Goswami, K., Farooq, A., Antil, P., Puri, P., Bector, G., Jain, A., & Azhar, W. (2024). Aryl Hydrocarbon Receptor Signaling in Prostate Cancer Therapy: A Review of Implications for Anti-androgen Treatment Strategies and Resistance. *Cureus, 16*(7). Advance online publication. DOI: 10.7759/cureus.65247 PMID: 39184676

Singh, P., Lanman, N. A., Kendall, H. L. R., Wilson, L., Long, R., Franco, O. E., Buskin, A., Miles, C. G., Hayward, S. W., Heer, R., & Robson, C. N. (2023). Human prostate organoid generation and the identification of prostate development drivers using inductive rodent tissues. *Development (Cambridge, England), 150*(13), dev201328. Advance online publication. DOI: 10.1242/dev.201328 PMID: 37376888

Singh, V. K., Pal, R., Srivastava, P., Misra, G., Shukla, Y., & Sharma, P. K. (2021). Exposure of androgen mimicking environmental chemicals enhances proliferation of prostate cancer (LNCaP) cells by inducing AR expression and epigenetic modifications. *Environmental Pollution, 272*, 116397. Advance online publication. DOI: 10.1016/j.envpol.2020.116397 PMID: 33433340

Skakkebaek, N. E., Rajpert-De Meyts, E., Buck Louis, G. M., Toppari, J., Andersson, A. M., Eisenberg, M. L., Jensen, T. K., Jørgensen, N., Swan, S. H., Sapra, K. J., Ziebe, S., Priskorn, L., & Juul, A. (2016). Male Reproductive Disorders and Fertility Trends: Influences of Environment and Genetic Susceptibility. *Physiological Reviews, 96*(1), 55–97. DOI: 10.1152/physrev.00017.2015 PMID: 26582516

Snyder, L. B., Neklesa, T. K., Willard, R. R., Gordon, D. A., Pizzano, J., Vitale, N., Robling, K., Dorso, M. A., Moghrabi, W., Landrette, S., Gedrich, R., Lee, S. H., Taylor, I. C. A., & Houston, J. G. (2025). Preclinical Evaluation of Bavdegalutamide (ARV-110), a Novel PROteolysis TArgeting Chimera Androgen Receptor Degrader. *Molecular Cancer Therapeutics, 24*(4), 511–522. DOI: 10.1158/1535-7163.MCT-23-0655 PMID: 39670468

Soto, A. M., & Sonnenschein, C. (2010). Environmental causes of cancer: Endocrine disruptors as carcinogens. In *Nature Reviews Endocrinology* (Vol. 6, Issue 7, pp. 363–370). DOI: 10.1038/nrendo.2010.87

Sreekumar, A., & Saini, S. (2022). Role of MicroRNAs in Neuroendocrine Prostate Cancer. *Non-Coding RNA, 8*(2), 25. DOI: 10.3390/ncrna8020025 PMID: 35447888

St. John, J., Powell, K., Katie Conley-LaComb, M., & Chinni, S. R. (2012). TMPRSS2-ERG Fusion Gene Expression in Prostate Tumor Cells and Its Clinical and Biological Significance in Prostate Cancer Progression. *Journal of Cancer Science & Therapy, 4*(4), 94. DOI: 10.4172/1948-5956.1000119 PMID: 23264855

Steroid 5 alpha-reductase 2 enzyme variants, biomass exposure and tobacco use in Mexican patients with prostate cancer. (n.d.). Retrieved 14 April 2025, from https://www.spandidos-publications.com/10.3892/ol.2020.12124?utm_source=chatgpt.com

Tan, K., & Naylor, M. J. (2022). The Influence of Modifiable Factors on Breast and Prostate Cancer Risk and Disease Progression. *Frontiers in Physiology*, *13*, 840826. DOI: 10.3389/fphys.2022.840826 PMID: 35330933

. Tan, M. E., Li, J., Xu, H. E., Melcher, K., & Yong, E. L. (2014a). Androgen receptor: structure, role in prostate cancer and drug discovery. *Acta Pharmacologica Sinica 2015 36:1, 36*(1), 3–23. DOI: 10.1038/aps.2014.18

. Tan, M. E., Li, J., Xu, H. E., Melcher, K., & Yong, E. L. (2014b). Androgen receptor: structure, role in prostate cancer and drug discovery. *Acta Pharmacologica Sinica 2015 36:1, 36*(1), 3–23. DOI: 10.1038/aps.2014.18

. Tătaru, O. S., Vartolomei, M. D., Rassweiler, J. J., Virgil, O., Lucarelli, G., Porpiglia, F., Amparore, D., Manfredi, M., Carrieri, G., Falagario, U., Terracciano, D., de Cobelli, O., Busetto, G. M., Del Giudice, F., & Ferro, M. (2021). Artificial Intelligence and Machine Learning in Prostate Cancer Patient Management—Current Trends and Future Perspectives. *Diagnostics 2021, Vol. 11, Page 354, 11*(2), 354. DOI: 10.3390/diagnostics11020354

Thakur, I. S., & Roy, D. (2020). Environmental DNA and RNA as records of human exposome, including biotic/abiotic exposures and its implications in the assessment of the role of environment in chronic diseases. In International Journal of Molecular Sciences (Vol. 21, Issue 14, pp. 1–15). MDPI AG. https://doi.org/DOI: 10.3390/ijms21144879

. Thomas, R., Jerome, J. M., Krieger, K. L., Ashraf, N., & Rowley, D. R. (2024). The reactive stroma response regulates the immune landscape in prostate cancer. *J Transl Genet Genom 2024;8:249-77., 8*(3), 249–277. DOI: 10.20517/jtgg.2024.15

Thompson, P. A., Khatami, M., Baglole, C. J., Sun, J., Harris, S. A., Moon, E. Y., Al-Mulla, F., Al-Temaimi, R., Brown, D. G., Colacci, A. M., Mondello, C., Raju, J., Ryan, E. P., Woodrick, J., Ivana Scovassi, A., Singh, N., Vaccari, M., Roy, R., Forte, S., & Bisson, W. H. (2015). Environmental immune disruptors, inflammation and cancer risk. *Carcinogenesis*, *36*(Suppl 1), S232–S253. DOI: 10.1093/carcin/bgv038 PMID: 26106141

Trudeau, V. L., Iguchi, T., Di Donato, M., Maradonna, F., & Carnevali, O. (2018). Lipid Metabolism Alteration by Endocrine Disruptors in Animal Models: An Overview. *Frontiers in Endocrinology*, *9*, 654. DOI: 10.3389/fendo.2018.00654 PMID: 30467492

Trummer, O., Langsenlehner, U., Krenn-Pilko, S., Pieber, T. R., Obermayer-Pietsch, B., Gerger, A., Renner, W., & Langsenlehner, T. (2016). Vitamin D and prostate cancer prognosis: A Mendelian randomization study. *World Journal of Urology, 34*(4), 607–611. DOI: 10.1007/s00345-015-1646-9 PMID: 26209090

Ueda, T., Mawji, N. R., Bruchovsky, N., & Sadar, M. D. (2002). Ligand-independent activation of the androgen receptor by interleukin-6 and the role of steroid receptor coactivator-1 in prostate cancer cells. *The Journal of Biological Chemistry, 277*(41), 38087–38094. DOI: 10.1074/jbc.M203313200 PMID: 12163482

Unno, K., Roh, M., Yoo, Y. A., Al-Shraideh, Y., Wang, L., Nonn, L., Abdulkadir, S. A., Unno, K., Roh, M., Yoo, Y. A., Al-Shraideh, Y., Wang, L., Nonn, L., & Abdulkadir, S. A. (2017). Modeling African American prostate adenocarcinoma by inducing defined genetic alterations in organoids. *Oncotarget, 8*(31), 51264–51276. DOI: 10.18632/oncotarget.17230 PMID: 28881646

Urade, R., Chou, C. K., Chou, H. L., Chen, B. H., Wang, T. N., Tsai, E. M., Hung, C. T., Wu, S. J., & Chiu, C. C. (2023). Phthalate derivative DEHP disturbs the anti-proliferative effect of camptothecin in human lung cancer cells by attenuating DNA damage and activating Akt/NF-κB signaling pathway. *Environmental Toxicology, 38*(2), 332–342. DOI: 10.1002/tox.23686 PMID: 36394428

Vaiserman, A. (2014). Early-life Exposure to Endocrine Disrupting Chemicals and Later-life Health Outcomes: An Epigenetic Bridge? *Aging and Disease, 5*(6), 419. DOI: 10.14336/ad.2014.0500419 PMID: 25489493

van Dessel, L. F., van Riet, J., Smits, M., Zhu, Y., Hamberg, P., van der Heijden, M. S., Bergman, A. M., van Oort, I. M., de Wit, R., Voest, E. E., Steeghs, N., Yamaguchi, T. N., Livingstone, J., Boutros, P. C., Martens, J. W. M., Sleijfer, S., Cuppen, E., Zwart, W., van de Werken, H. J. G., & Lolkema, M. P. (2019). The genomic landscape of metastatic castration-resistant prostate cancers reveals multiple distinct genotypes with potential clinical impact. *Nature Communications, 10*(1), 5251. Advance online publication. DOI: 10.1038/s41467-019-13084-7 PMID: 31748536

Van Hée, V. F., Labar, D., Dehon, G., Grasso, D., Grégoire, V., Muccioli, G. G., Frédérick, R., & Sonveaux, P. (2017). *Radiosynthesis and validation of (±)-[18 F]-3-fluoro-2-hydroxypropionate ([18 F]-FLac) as a PET tracer of lactate to monitor MCT1-dependent lactate uptake in tumors*. www.impactjournals.com/oncotarget

Van Hemelryk, A., Mout, L., Erkens-Schulze, S., French, P. J., van Weerden, W. M., & van Royen, M. E. (2021). Modeling prostate cancer treatment responses in the organoid era: 3D environment impacts drug testing. *Biomolecules, 11*(11), 1572. DOI: 10.3390/biom11111572 PMID: 34827570

Van Hemelryk, A., Tomljanovic, I., de Ridder, C. M. A., Stuurman, D. C., Teubel, W. J., Erkens-Schulze, S., Verhoef, E. I., Remmers, S., Mahes, A. J., van Leenders, G. J. L. H., van Royen, M. E., van de Werken, H. J. G., Grudniewska, M., Jenster, G. W., & van Weerden, W. M. (2022). Patient-Derived Xenografts and Organoids Recapitulate Castration-Resistant Prostate Cancer with Sustained Androgen Receptor Signaling. *Cells*, *11*(22), 3632. DOI: 10.3390/cells11223632 PMID: 36429059

Varnai, R., Koskinen, L. M., Mäntylä, L. E., Szabo, I., Fitzgerald, L. M., & Sipeky, C. (2019). Pharmacogenomic Biomarkers in Docetaxel Treatment of Prostate Cancer: From Discovery to Implementation. *Genes*, *10*(8), 599. DOI: 10.3390/genes10080599 PMID: 31398933

Vazquez, J. P., Pulido, E. G., & Aparicio, L. M. A. (2012). Cytokine and endocrine signaling in prostate cancer. *Medical Oncology (Northwood, London, England)*, *29*(3), 1956–1963. DOI: 10.1007/s12032-011-0036-4 PMID: 21858553

. Verhage, B. A. J., & Kiemeney, L. A. L. M. (n.d.). Inherited predisposition to prostate cancer.

Waddell, A. R., Huang, H., & Liao, D. (2021a). CBP/p300: Critical Co-Activators for Nuclear Steroid Hormone Receptors and Emerging Therapeutic Targets in Prostate and Breast Cancers. *Cancers (Basel)*, *13*(12), 2872. DOI: 10.3390/cancers13122872 PMID: 34201346

. Waddell, A. R., Huang, H., & Liao, D. (2021b). CBP/p300: Critical Co-Activators for Nuclear Steroid Hormone Receptors and Emerging Therapeutic Targets in Prostate and Breast Cancers. *Cancers 2021, Vol. 13, Page 2872*, *13*(12), 2872. DOI: 10.3390/cancers13122872

Waddington, C. H. (2012). The epigenotype. 1942. *International Journal of Epidemiology*, *41*(1), 10–13. DOI: 10.1093/ije/dyr184 PMID: 22186258

Waltering, K. K., Helenius, M. A., Sahu, B., Manni, V., Linja, M. J., Jänne, O. A., & Visakorpi, T. (2009). Increased expression of androgen receptor sensitizes prostate cancer cells to low levels of androgens. *Cancer Research*, *69*(20), 8141–8149. DOI: 10.1158/0008-5472.CAN-09-0919 PMID: 19808968

Wan, M., Simonin, E. M., Johnson, M. M., Zhang, X., Lin, X., Gao, P., Patel, C. J., Yousuf, A., Snyder, M. P., Hong, X., Wang, X., Sampath, V., & Nadeau, K. C. (2025). Exposomics: a review of methodologies, applications, and future directions in molecular medicine. In *EMBO Molecular Medicine*. Springer Science and Business Media Deutschland GmbH. https://doi.org/DOI: 10.1038/s44321-025-00191-w

Wang, H., Liu, B., Chen, H., Xu, P., Xue, H., & Yuan, J. (2023). Dynamic changes of DNA methylation induced by benzo(a)pyrene in cancer. *Genes and Environment : the Official Journal of the Japanese Environmental Mutagen Society*, *45*(1), 21. DOI: 10.1186/s41021-023-00278-1 PMID: 37391844

Wang, K., & Zhao, Z. pharmacotherapy, W. J.-B. &, & 2019, undefined. (n.d.). Bisphenol A induces apoptosis, oxidative stress and inflammatory response in colon and liver of mice in a mitochondria-dependent manner. *ElsevierK Wang, Z Zhao, W JiBiomedicine & Pharmacotherapy, 2019•Elsevier*. Retrieved 3 April 2025, from https://www.sciencedirect.com/science/article/pii/S0753332219323017

. Wang, M. ;, Erb, H., Waseem, M., & Wang, B.-D. (2024). Organoids: An Emerging Precision Medicine Model for Prostate Cancer Research. *International Journal of Molecular Sciences 2024, Vol. 25, Page 1093*, *25*(2), 1093. DOI: 10.3390/ijms25021093

Wang, X., Hu, Z., Jin, Y., Yang, M., Zhang, Z., Zhou, X., Qiu, S., & Zou, X. (2024). Exploring the relationships between exposure levels of bisphenols and phthalates and prostate cancer occurrence. *Journal of Hazardous Materials*, *474*, 134736. Advance online publication. DOI: 10.1016/j.jhazmat.2024.134736 PMID: 38815394

Waseem, M., & Wang, B. D. (2024). Organoids: An Emerging Precision Medicine Model for Prostate Cancer Research. In *International Journal of Molecular Sciences* (Vol. 25, Issue 2). Multidisciplinary Digital Publishing Institute (MDPI). https://doi.org/DOI: 10.3390/ijms25021093

Westaby, D., Jiménez-Vacas, J. M., Figueiredo, I., Rekowski, J., Pettinger, C., Gurel, B., Lundberg, A., Bogdan, D., Buroni, L., Neeb, A., Padilha, A., Taylor, J., Zeng, W., Das, S., Hobern, E., Riisnaes, R., Crespo, M., Miranda, S., Ferreira, A., & Sharp, A. (2024). BCL2 expression is enriched in advanced prostate cancer with features of lineage plasticity. *The Journal of Clinical Investigation*, *134*(18), e179998. Advance online publication. DOI: 10.1172/JCI179998 PMID: 39286979

Wild, C. P. (2005). Complementing the genome with an 'exposome': The outstanding challenge of environmental exposure measurement in molecular epidemiology. *Cancer Epidemiology, Biomarkers & Prevention*, *14*(8), 1847–1850. DOI: 10.1158/1055-9965.EPI-05-0456 PMID: 16103423

. Wu, L., Yang, Y., Guo, X., Shu, X. O., Cai, Q., Shu, X., Li, B., Tao, R., Wu, C., Nikas, J. B., Sun, Y., Zhu, J., Roobol, M. J., Giles, G. G., Brenner, H., John, E. M., Clements, J., Grindedal, E. M., Park, J. Y., … Riboli, E. (2020). An integrative multi-omics analysis to identify candidate DNA methylation biomarkers related to prostate cancer risk. *Nature Communications 2020 11:1, 11*(1), 1–11. https://doi .org/DOI: 10.1038/s41467-020-17673-9

Xiao, W., & Goswami, P. C. (2015). Down-regulation of peroxisome proliferator activated receptor γ coactivator 1α induces oxidative stress and toxicity of 1-(4-Chlorophenyl)-benzo-2,5-quinone in HaCaT human keratinocytes. *Toxicology In Vitro, 29*(7), 1332–1338. DOI: 10.1016/j.tiv.2015.05.009 PMID: 26004620

. Xu, J., Ye, Y., Huang, F., Chen, H., Wu, H., Huang, J., Hu, J., Xia, D., & Wu, Y. (2016). Association between dioxin and cancer incidence and mortality: a meta-analysis. *Scientific Reports 2016 6:1, 6*(1), 1–17. DOI: 10.1038/srep38012

Xu, K., Shimelis, H., Linn, D. E., Jiang, R., Yang, X., Sun, F., Guo, Z., Chen, H., Li, W., Chen, H., Kong, X., Melamed, J., Fang, S., Xiao, Z., Veenstra, T. D., & Qiu, Y. (2009). Regulation of androgen receptor transcriptional activity and specificity by RNF6-induced ubiquitination. *Cancer Cell, 15*(4), 270–282. DOI: 10.1016/j.ccr.2009.02.021 PMID: 19345326

Xu, K., Wu, Z. J., Groner, A. C., He, H. H., Cai, C., Lis, R. T., Wu, X., Stack, E. C., Loda, M., Liu, T., Xu, H., Cato, L., Thornton, J. E., Gregory, R. I., Morrissey, C., Vessella, R. L., Montironi, R., Magi-Galluzzi, C., Kantoff, P. W., & Brown, M. (2012). EZH2 Oncogenic Activity in Castration Resistant Prostate Cancer Cells is Polycomb-Independent. *Science, 338*(6113), 1465–1469. DOI: 10.1126/science.1227604 PMID: 23239736

Yadav, R., Petrunak, E. M., Estrada, D. F., & Scott, E. E. (2016). Structural Insights into the Function of Steroidogenic Cytochrome P450 17A1. *Molecular and Cellular Endocrinology, 441*, 68–75. DOI: 10.1016/j.mce.2016.08.035 PMID: 27566228

Yao, T. P., Ku, G., Zhou, N., Scully, R., & Livingston, D. M. (1996). The nuclear hormone receptor coactivator SRC-1 is a specific target of p300. *Proceedings of the National Academy of Sciences of the United States of America, 93*(20), 10626–10631. DOI: 10.1073/pnas.93.20.10626 PMID: 8855229

Yaqinuddin, A., Qureshi, S. A., Pervez, S., Bashir, M. U., Nazir, R., & Abbas, F. (2013). Frequent DNA Hypermethylation at the RASSF1A and APC Gene Loci in Prostate Cancer Patients of Pakistani Origin. *ISRN Urology, 627249*, 1–4. Advance online publication. DOI: 10.1155/2013/627249 PMID: 23431474

Yegnasubramanian, S., Haffner, M. C., Zhang, Y., Gurel, B., Cornish, T. C., Wu, Z., Irizarry, R. A., Morgan, J., Hicks, J., DeWeese, T. L., Isaacs, W. B., Bova, G. S., De Marzo, A. M., & Nelson, W. G. (2008). DNA hypomethylation arises later in prostate cancer progression than CpG island hypermethylation and contributes to metastatic tumor heterogeneity. *Cancer Research*, *68*(21), 8954–8967. DOI: 10.1158/0008-5472.CAN-07-6088 PMID: 18974140

Ylitalo, E. B., Thysell, E., Landfors, M., Brattsand, M., Jernberg, E., Crnalic, S., Widmark, A., Hultdin, M., Bergh, A., Degerman, S., & Wikström, P. (2021). A novel DNA methylation signature is associated with androgen receptor activity and patient prognosis in bone metastatic prostate cancer. *Clinical Epigenetics*, *13*(1), 1–15. DOI: 10.1186/s13148-021-01119-0 PMID: 34193246

Yu, S. Y., Koh, E. J., Kim, S. H., Lee, S. Y., Lee, J. S., Son, S. W., & Hwang, S. Y. (2021). Integrated analysis of multi-omics data on epigenetic changes caused by combined exposure to environmental hazards. *Environmental Toxicology*, *36*(6), 1001–1010. DOI: 10.1002/tox.23099 PMID: 33438815

Yusufi, A. (n.d.). *Studies on Hexachlorobenzene (HCB) Induced Toxicity and Oxidative Damage in the Kidney and Other Rat Tissues*. Retrieved 3 April 2025, from https://www.academia.edu/127701788/Studies_on_Hexachlorobenzene_HCB_Induced_Toxicity_and_Oxidative_Damage_in_the_Kidney_and_Other_Rat_Tissues

Zaman, N., Giannopoulos, P. N., Chowdhury, S., Bonneil, E., Thibault, P., Wang, E., Trifiro, M., & Paliouras, M. (2014). Proteomic-Coupled-Network Analysis of T877A-Androgen Receptor Interactomes Can Predict Clinical Prostate Cancer Outcomes between White (Non-Hispanic) and African-American Groups. *PLoS One*, *9*(11), e113190. DOI: 10.1371/journal.pone.0113190 PMID: 25409505

Zhang, F., Ma, Y., Li, D., Wei, J., Chen, K., Zhang, E., Liu, G., Chu, X., Liu, X., Liu, W., Tian, X., & Yang, Y. (2024a). Cancer associated fibroblasts and metabolic reprogramming: Unraveling the intricate crosstalk in tumor evolution. *Journal of Hematology & Oncology*, *17*(1), 80. DOI: 10.1186/s13045-024-01600-2 PMID: 39223656

Zhang, F., Ma, Y., Li, D., Wei, J., Chen, K., Zhang, E., Liu, G., Chu, X., Liu, X., Liu, W., Tian, X., & Yang, Y. (2024b). Cancer associated fibroblasts and metabolic reprogramming: Unraveling the intricate crosstalk in tumor evolution. *Journal of Hematology & Oncology*, *17*(1), 80. DOI: 10.1186/s13045-024-01600-2 PMID: 39223656

Zhang, H., Gao, H., Gu, Y., John, A., Wei, L., Huang, M., Yu, J., Adeosun, A. A., Weinshilboum, R. M., & Wang, L. (2022). 3D CRISPR screen in prostate cancer cells reveals PARP inhibitor sensitization through TBL1XR1-SMC3 interaction. *Frontiers in Oncology, 12*, 999302. DOI: 10.3389/fonc.2022.999302 PMID: 36523978

Zhang, L., & Shiverick, K. T. (1997). Benzo(a)pyrene, but not 2,3,7,8-tetrachlorodibenzo-p-dioxin, alters cell proliferation and c-myc and growth factor expression in human placental choriocarcinoma JEG-3 cells. *Biochemical and Biophysical Research Communications, 231*(1), 117–120. DOI: 10.1006/bbrc.1997.6053 PMID: 9070231

Zhang, Y., Huang, Z., Li, K., Xie, G., Feng, Y., Wang, Z., Li, N., Liu, R., Ding, Y., Wang, J., Yang, J., & Jia, Z. (2024). TrkA promotes MDM2-mediated AGPS ubiquitination and degradation to trigger prostate cancer progression. *Journal of Experimental & Clinical Cancer Research : CR, 43*(1), 16. Advance online publication. DOI: 10.1186/s13046-023-02920-w PMID: 38200609

. Zhang, Y., Wang, D., Peng, M., Tang, L., Ouyang, J., Xiong, F., Guo, C., Tang, Y., Zhou, Y., Liao, Q., Wu, X., Wang, H., Yu, J., Li, Y., Li, X., Li, G., Zeng, Z., Tan, Y., & Xiong, W. (2021). Single-cell RNA sequencing in cancer research. *Journal of Experimental & Clinical Cancer Research 2021 40:1, 40*(1), 1–17. DOI: 10.1186/s13046-021-01874-1

Zhang, Z., Cheng, L., Li, J., Farah, E., Atallah, N. M., Pascuzzi, P. E., Gupta, S., & Liu, X. (2018). Inhibition of the Wnt/b-catenin pathway overcomes resistance to enzalutamide in castration-resistant prostate cancer. *Cancer Research, 78*(12), 3147–3162. DOI: 10.1158/0008-5472.CAN-17-3006 PMID: 29700003

Zhao, F., Zhang, T., Wei, J., Chen, L., Liu, Z., Jin, Y., Liu, M., Zhou, H., Hu, Y., & Sheng, X. (2024). Integrated single-cell transcriptomic analyses identify a novel lineage plasticity-related cancer cell type involved in prostate cancer progression. *EBioMedicine, 109*, 105398. DOI: 10.1016/j.ebiom.2024.105398 PMID: 39418984

Zhao, J., Shi, Y., & Cao, G. (2023). The Application of Single-Cell RNA Sequencing in the Inflammatory Tumor Microenvironment. *Biomolecules, 13*(2), 344. DOI: 10.3390/biom13020344 PMID: 36830713

Zheng, H., Zhu, Y., Shao, X., Cai, A., Dong, B., Xue, W., & Gao, H. (2020). Distinct Metabolic Signatures of Hormone-Sensitive and Castration-Resistant Prostate Cancer Revealed by a 1H NMR-Based Metabolomics of Biopsy Tissue. *Journal of Proteome Research, 19*(9), 3741–3749. DOI: 10.1021/acs.jproteome.0c00282 PMID: 32702989

Zheng, L., Zhang, X., Gao, Z., Zhong, C., Qiu, D., & Yan, Q. (2024). The association between polychlorinated dibenzo-p-dioxin exposure and cancer mortality in the general population: A cohort study. *Frontiers in Public Health*, *12*, 1354149. Advance online publication. DOI: 10.3389/fpubh.2024.1354149 PMID: 38410662

Zhou, L., Zhang, C., Zhang, Y., & Shi, C. (2021a). Application of Organoid Models in Prostate Cancer Research. *Frontiers in Oncology*, *11*, 736431. DOI: 10.3389/fonc.2021.736431 PMID: 34646778

Zhou, L., Zhang, C., Zhang, Y., & Shi, C. (2021b). Application of Organoid Models in Prostate Cancer Research. *Frontiers in Oncology*, *11*, 736431. DOI: 10.3389/fonc.2021.736431 PMID: 34646778

Zhou, W., Liotta, L. A., & Petricoin, E. F. (2012). Cancer Metabolism: What we Can Learn from Proteomic Analysis by Mass Spectrometry. *Cancer Genomics & Proteomics*, *9*(6), 373. https://pmc.ncbi.nlm.nih.gov/articles/PMC5547437/ PMID: 23162076

Zhu, M., Huang, C., Ma, X., Wu, R., Zhu, W., Li, X., Liang, Z., Deng, F., Wu, J., Geng, S., Xie, C., & Zhong, C. (2018). Phthalates promote prostate cancer cell proliferation through activation of ERK5 and p38. *Environmental Toxicology and Pharmacology*, *63*, 29–33. DOI: 10.1016/j.etap.2018.08.007 PMID: 30125794

Zhu, W., Liu, H., Wang, X., Lu, J., Zhang, H., Wang, S., & Yang, W. (2019). Associations of CYP1 polymorphisms with risk of prostate cancer: An updated meta-analysis. *Bioscience Reports*, *39*(3), BSR20181876. Advance online publication. DOI: 10.1042/BSR20181876 PMID: 30765615

Zou, Z., Yoshimura, Y., Yamanishi, Y., & Oki, S. (2023). Elucidating disease-associated mechanisms triggered by pollutants via the epigenetic landscape using large-scale ChIP-Seq data. *Epigenetics & Chromatin*, *16*(1), 1–15. DOI: 10.1186/s13072-023-00510-w PMID: 37743474

Chapter 5
The Interplay Between CES1 Gene Polymorphisms and Environmental Exposures in Chemotherapy Toxicity in Breast Cancer:
CES1 Variants and Environment in Chemo Toxicity

Duygu Aygunes Jafari
https://orcid.org/0000-0003-4756-7365
Ege University Faculty of Medicine, Turkey

Canfeza Sezgin
Biruni University Faculty of Medicine, Turkey

Buket Kosova
Ege University Faculty of Medicine, Turkey

ABSTRACT

Breast cancer remains one of the most prevalent malignancies worldwide, with chemotherapy serving as a cornerstone of treatment despite its substantial toxicity risks. Carboxylesterase 1 (CES1), a critical drug-metabolizing enzyme, plays a central role in the activation and clearance of various chemotherapeutic agents, including capecitabine. Genetic polymorphisms in CES1, together with environmental expo-

DOI: 10.4018/979-8-3373-5796-6.ch005

Copyright © 2026, IGI Global Scientific Publishing. Copying or distributing in print or electronic forms without written permission of IGI Global Scientific Publishing is prohibited.

sures such as pollutants, diet, and lifestyle factors, contribute to the interindividual variability in chemotherapy metabolism and toxicity profiles. This chapter examines the complex gene–environment interplay influencing treatment outcomes in breast cancer and highlights emerging strategies for integrating genetic and environmental assessments. A deeper understanding of these interactions paves the way for precision oncology approaches that personalize therapy, improve tolerability, and ultimately enhance patient outcomes in breast cancer care.

INTRODUCTION

As one of the most frequently occurring cancers worldwide, breast cancer continues to account for a substantial proportion of cancer mortality in the female population (Yüksel et al., 2019). Standard treatment often includes chemotherapy, which has significantly improved survival rates and reduced recurrence for patients with breast cancer . However, chemotherapy is a double-edged sword: while it targets rapidly dividing tumor cells, it also causes systemic toxicity that can vary widely among individuals. This variability in chemotherapy-induced toxicity is a major clinical challenge, as some patients experience severe adverse effects that necessitate dose reductions or even treatment discontinuation. Understanding the factors that underlie differences in toxicity profiles is therefore critical for optimizing breast cancer care and improving patient outcomes.

Chemotherapy toxicity is influenced by a combination of genetic factors (such as inherited polymorphisms in drug metabolism genes) and environmental factors (such as exposure to pollutants, lifestyle, and concurrent medications). The field of pharmacogenetics has demonstrated that patients' genetic makeup can substantially affect how they metabolize and respond to chemotherapeutic drugs (Wu & Xiong, 2024). In parallel, environmental exposures throughout a patient's life can modulate biological pathways through epigenetic changes or enzyme induction/inhibition, thereby altering drug efficacy and toxicity (Panahi et al., 2016; Kim et al., 2012; Alam et al., 2021; Swagatika & Tomar, 2016; Hu & Yu, 2019). Among the genetic factors, increasing attention has been given to polymorphisms in genes encoding drug-metabolizing enzymes. One such enzyme is Carboxylesterase 1 (*CES1*), a liver enzyme involved in the metabolism of various chemotherapeutic agents and prodrugs (Qian & Markowitz, 2020). Variations in the *CES1* gene may lead to altered enzyme activity, influencing the breakdown of chemotherapy drugs and consequently the intensity of side effects (Yüksel et al., 2019).

The interplay between *CES1* gene polymorphisms and environmental exposures represents a rapidly expanding area of research with significant implications for breast cancer therapy. *CES1* exhibits considerable genetic variability and is also subject to modulation by non-genetic factors, positioning it as a representative model of gene and environment interaction. This chapter presents a comprehensive analysis of how *CES1* polymorphisms and environmental exposures together influence chemotherapy-induced toxicity in breast cancer. It begins with an overview of pharmacogenetics in breast cancer treatment, followed by a detailed examination of the structure and function of the *CES1* enzyme and its common genetic variants. The chapter then addresses the range of chemotherapy-related toxicities and explores how both genetic predisposition, particularly involving *CES1* variants, and environmental exposures such as pollutants, dietary factors, and lifestyle choices may modulate these adverse effects. Mechanistic insights into gene and environment interactions are discussed alongside clinical data from real-world settings. The final sections consider the clinical applications of this knowledge for personalized therapy, the research methodologies used to investigate gene and environment interactions, and future directions involving emerging technologies, novel therapeutic strategies, and relevant policy frameworks. The overall aim is to clarify the complex contributors to chemotherapy toxicity and to identify practical pathways toward more precise and individualized treatment approaches in breast cancer care.

PHARMACOGENETICS OF BREAST CANCER

Pharmacogenetics (and pharmacogenomics) refers to the field that explores how inter-individual genetic differences shape responses to medications, with implications for optimizing drug therapy. In the context of breast cancer, pharmacogenetic approaches form the cornerstone of personalized medicine by tailoring treatment based on a patient's genetic profile (Wu & Xiong, 2024). This personalized strategy is especially relevant in chemotherapy, where the same drug regimen can be highly effective for some patients but cause severe toxicity or inadequate response in others. By identifying genetic polymorphisms that affect drug metabolism, transport, or targets, clinicians can adjust chemotherapy choices and dosages to maximize efficacy while minimizing adverse effects (Wu & Xiong, 2024).

One major application of pharmacogenetics in breast cancer is in guiding the use of specific chemotherapeutic drugs known to have pharmacogenetic markers. A classic example is the use of *fluoropyrimidines* such as 5-fluorouracil (5-FU) and its oral prodrug capecitabine. Variations in the gene *DPYD*, that encodes the dihydropyrimidine dehydrogenase enzyme, are known to cause severe toxicity to 5-FU/capecitabine; hence, DPYD genotyping is recommended before starting these drugs to identify patients at high risk of life-threatening toxicity. Beyond DPYD, recent studies highlight that other genes, including *CES1*, may also influence fluoropyrimidine activation and toxicity. Another example is *CYP2D6* polymorphisms affecting the efficacy of tamoxifen (an endocrine therapy often used in breast cancer), although tamoxifen is not a chemotherapy drug per se. For chemotherapeutic agents like the anthracyclines and taxanes, research has identified various polymorphisms that can impact outcomes, for instance, polymorphisms in drug transporters (like *ABCB1*) affecting taxane clearance, or variants in metabolizing enzymes influencing cyclophosphamide activation (Longo et al., 2010). While many of these findings are still emerging, they underscore the broader point that genetic makeup can determine both how well a patient's tumor responds to chemotherapy and how severely the patient is affected by side effects (Wu & Xiong, 2024).

Personalizing breast cancer treatment through pharmacogenetics has demonstrated tangible benefits. Patients who receive genotype-guided therapy often experience improved treatment efficacy and reduced toxicity. For example, in patients with germline genomic variants known to affect drug metabolism, dose adjustments or alternative regimens can preemptively mitigate adverse outcomes (Harnden et al., 2019). Pharmacogenetic stratification can also identify those unlikely to benefit from a given therapy, sparing them unnecessary toxicity and allowing a switch to more promising treatments. In sum, pharmacogenetics adds a critical layer of decision-making in breast cancer care, alongside tumor characteristics and clinical factors, to achieve truly precision oncology where treatment is customized to the genetic and molecular profile of each patient (Wu & Xiong, 2024).

It is important to highlight breast cancer pharmacogenetics extends beyond single gene-drug pairs. Increasingly, a polygenic approach is being recognized, where multiple genetic variants are considered together to predict therapy outcomes. This is especially relevant for drugs like capecitabine and others metabolized via complex pathways involving several enzymes (*CES1*, CES2, CYPs, etc.). The concept of a polygenic risk score for chemotherapy toxicity is emerging, which would integrate information from various genetic loci to estimate a patient's risk of adverse effects. While such tools are still in development, they represent the future direction of personalized medicine: moving from one-size-fits-all to genetically guided dosing algorithms for every patient (García-González et al., 2015).

CES1 GENE AND ITS POLYMORPHISMS

The *CES1* gene encodes carboxylesterase 1 enzyme, which is a serine esterase that plays an important role in drug metabolism and detoxification. *CES1* is highly expressed in the liver, where it is the most abundant drug-metabolizing enzyme, accounting for roughly 1% of the total liver protein content. Functionally, *CES1* is responsible for approximately 80-95% of the hydrolytic activity in human liver tissue (Her & Zhu, 2020). This enzyme excels at hydrolyzing ester and amide bonds, which means it is critically involved in the metabolism of numerous esterified prodrugs and other medications. Examples of *CES1* substrates include the anticoagulant dabigatran etexilate, the antiviral prodrug oseltamivir, the ADHD medication methylphenidate, certain ACE inhibitors like imidapril, and the antiplatelet drug clopidogrel (Merali et al., 2014). In the chemotherapy realm, *CES1* is instrumental in the activation of capecitabine (an oral prodrug of 5-FU) as it hydrolyzes capecitabine into its intermediate metabolites (Yuksel et al., 2019; Matsumoto et al., 2020). Beyond pharmaceuticals, *CES1* also helps metabolize some pesticides and environmental toxicants, reflecting its broad role in clearing xenobiotics from the body (Matsumoto, 2020).

Genetic polymorphisms in the *CES1* gene lead to marked interindividual variability in *CES1* enzyme expression and activity. These polymorphisms can be single-nucleotide polymorphisms (SNPs), deletions/ insertions, or copy number variations. Among the SNPs, the most well-characterized is a missense variant known as G143E (a glycine-to-glutamic acid substitution at position 143, rs71647871). The G143E variant is a loss-of-function mutation; it significantly reduces or abolishes *CES1* enzymatic activity in carriers (Her & Zhu, 2020). Although relatively rare in the general population, its allele frequency shows ethnic variability: it has been reported in around 3-4% of individuals of European or African ancestry, but is virtually absent in East Asian populations (Cha et al., 2014). Clinically, G143E has been linked to altered metabolism of several drugs; for instance, carriers of the G143E variant display reduced activation of clopidogrel (leading to lower anti-platelet effect) and altered pharmacokinetics of methylphenidate (Cura et al., 2023; Her & Zhu, 2020). Within the context of chemotherapy, this variant has also been examined for its potential influence on capecitabine metabolism and associated toxicity, as will be discussed in subsequent sections.

Besides G143E, other common *CES1* polymorphisms have been identified, some of which affect gene regulation rather than enzyme structure. For example, a promoter region variant *-75 T>G* (rs3815583) has been studied for its influence on *CES1* expression levels and was suggested to correlate with appetite loss in chemotherapy patients (National Center for Biotechnology Information [NCBI], 2024). Another SNP, *rs2244613*, located in an intronic region of *CES1*, has been frequently reported in pharmacogenetic studies and may serve as a tag for certain *CES1* haplotypes (Cura et al., 2023). Population-based analyses reveal that *CES1* has multiple haplotypes with distinct frequencies; for instance, in Asian populations a haplotype involving the -816A>C variant is relatively common (~24-30% in Chinese and Japanese), whereas the functional G143E variant is absent (Cha et al., 2014). Some *CES1* polymorphisms are benign in effect, while others can increase or decrease enzymatic activity. For example, certain rare variants have been found that increase *CES1* activity, potentially leading to ultra-rapid metabolism of drugs (though such cases are less documented compared to loss-of-function scenarios).

Functionally, the impact of *CES1* polymorphisms on drug metabolism can be significant. A high-activity variant could cause a chemotherapeutic prodrug to be converted to its active (and possibly toxic) form more quickly, raising the risk of toxicity. Conversely, a low-activity variant like G143E might result in slower drug activation or clearance, possibly leading to drug accumulation or insufficient active drug levels. For breast cancer chemotherapy, consider capecitabine: reduced *CES1* activity might slow its conversion to 5-FU, potentially decreasing efficacy but also altering the profile of side effects if intermediate metabolites build up. Indeed, studies have aimed to correlate *CES1* genotypes with capecitabine outcomes. One study in breast and colorectal cancer patients genotyped a *CES1* variant and measured capecitabine pharmacokinetics and side effects (Yüksel et al., 2019). Although that small study did not find statistically significant differences due to the variant (likely owing to limited sample size of 7 patients), it highlighted a trend toward different adverse effect profiles (with diarrhea, asthenia, anemia, etc. observed variably among genotypes) (Yüksel et al., 2019). More recent and larger studies have strengthened the evidence that *CES1* variants matter: for instance, patients carrying the *CES1* 143E variant allele have been shown to have higher risk of severe hand-foot syndrome when treated with capecitabine (Cura et al., 2023). Such findings underscore that *CES1* polymorphisms, even if not as common as some other pharmacogenes, can be clinically relevant modifiers of chemotherapy toxicity.

Three *CES1* nonsynonymous polymorphisms; namely I49V, N75S, and H199; were previously investigated in a cohort of metastatic breast cancer patients (Aygüneş, 2008). Unlike the extensively studied G143E variant, these polymorphisms are less characterized in the existing literature. In that investigation, the H199R variant was not detected in any of the 80 individuals assessed, including both the capecitabine-treated group and the control group, with all participants carrying the wild-type H/H genotype at this locus. In contrast, the N75S and I49V variants were identified with moderate frequency. The combined cohort exhibited a minor allele frequency of approximately 20.6% for N75S (S allele) and 39.4% for I49V (V allele). Furthermore, the genotype distributions of N75S and I49V were comparable between capecitabine-treated patients (n=20) and control patients (n=60), with no statistically significant differences observed (chi-square tests, $p > 0.05$ for each polymorphism). These findings provided a baseline characterization of *CES1* genetic variability in a metastatic breast cancer population (Aygüneş, 2008).

It is also noteworthy that *CES1* has a closely related pseudogene, *CES1*P1, and several *CES1* gene copies or isoforms exist, which can complicate genotyping analyses (Matsumoto et al., 2020). Copy number variations (duplications or deletions of the *CES1* gene) could potentially alter overall enzyme levels, though research in this area is still emerging. Moreover, non-genetic regulators (discussed later) such as induction or inhibition by co-administered drugs and diet can mimic the effects of polymorphisms. As of now, the G143E SNP is considered the only definitively "actionable" *CES1* variant in clinical settings (Her & Zhu, 2020), but ongoing research is likely to reveal additional polymorphisms with significant effects. In summary, *CES1*'s genetic diversity translates into functional diversity, making it a crucial factor in the metabolism of chemotherapeutic drugs and a focal point for precision medicine efforts in breast cancer.

CHEMOTHERAPY INDUCED TOXICITY

Chemotherapy induced toxicity refers to the spectrum of adverse effects that result from the damage chemotherapy inflicts on normal, healthy tissues. Because chemotherapeutic agents target proliferating cells, they commonly affect the bone marrow, gastrointestinal tract, skin, and other rapidly renewing tissues, as well as certain vital organs like the heart (Nurgalieva et al., 2011). Breast cancer chemotherapy regimens, which often include drugs such as anthracyclines (e.g., doxorubicin or epirubicin), taxanes (e.g., paclitaxel or docetaxel), antimetabolites (e.g., 5-FU or capecitabine), and alkylating agents (e.g., cyclophosphamide), are associated with a range of well-characterized toxicities (Capri et al., 1996; Mayer & Burstein, 2016). These toxicities not only impact a patient's quality of life but can also necessitate dose modifications that potentially compromise the efficacy of cancer treatment (Shimozuma et al., 2012). Below it is outlined that some of the common toxicity profiles of breast cancer chemotherapy, along with their clinical presentation and relevance:

Gastrointestinal (GI) Toxicity

GI side effects are among the most frequent chemotherapeutic toxicities. They include nausea and vomiting (especially prominent with anthracyclines like doxorubicin, although modern antiemetics have greatly improved control of these symptoms), diarrhea (notably with 5-FU and capecitabine), oral mucositis or stomatitis (inflammation and ulceration of the mouth, common with antimetabolites), and abdominal pain. Diarrhea can be dose-limiting, as in the case of fluoropyrimidines where severe diarrhea may indicate DPD enzyme deficiency or overdose. Stomatitis is often a precursor to more severe GI syndrome. These toxicities arise from damage to the rapidly dividing epithelial cells lining the GI tract. For example, capecitabine and 5-FU can cause a syndrome of diarrhea, abdominal cramping, and mucositis that mirrors an extreme form of GI inflammation. Monitoring for signs of dehydration, electrolyte imbalance, and nutritional status is essential in patients with significant GI toxicity. In severe cases, treatment breaks, dose reductions, or supportive care with fluids and medications (like loperamide for diarrhea) are required to manage these effects (Cura et al., 2023).

Hand-Foot Syndrome (HFS)

Also known as palmar-plantar erythrodysesthesia, HFS is a distinctive dermatologic toxicity characterized by redness, swelling, pain, and peeling of the skin on the palms of the hands and soles of the feet. It is most classically associated with capecitabine and continuous-infusion 5-FU. In breast cancer, capecitabine (often used in metastatic or adjuvant settings) frequently causes HFS, which can range from mild tingling and redness to severe pain and blistering that impairs daily activities. HFS pathophysiology is not fully understood, but it is thought that small amounts of drug and its metabolites leak out of capillaries in the extremities, causing local tissue injury. Pharmacogenetic factors can influence HFS; for instance, as mentioned earlier, a *CES1* polymorphism (rs71647871 A-allele) was found to be related with a higher risk of severe HFS in patients on capecitabine.

In a separate cohort of metastatic breast cancer patients treated with capecitabine, 35% of individuals (7 out of 20) were found to develop clinically significant treatment-related toxicity, encompassing severe HFS and gastrointestinal side effects such as diarrhea and stomatitis (Aygüneş, 2008). The potential role of *CES1* polymorphisms, specifically I49V and N75S, in influencing this toxicity was evaluated. Although most patients with toxicity carried the I/V genotype, no statistically significant relation was observed between these variants and toxicity occurrence ($p > 0.05$). Furthermore, none of the individuals with the rare S/S genotype experienced notable adverse effects. These findings suggest that, unlike the G143E variant, the I49V and N75S polymorphisms do not meaningfully alter the risk of capecitabine-induced toxicity (Aygüneş, 2008).

Clinically, HFS is managed by dose interruptions and reductions, supportive measures like cooling and emollients, and sometimes pyridoxine or corticosteroids, although definitive preventative strategies are limited. Early recognition is important, as grade 3 HFS (severe pain and functional impairment) often necessitates stopping the drug until recovery (Cura et al., 2023).

Myelosuppression

Many chemotherapy drugs used in breast cancer cause myelosuppression, the decreased production of blood cells by the bone marrow. Neutropenia (low white blood cell count, especially neutrophils) is a dangerous side effect because it increases the risk of infection and febrile neutropenia can be life-threatening. Anthracyclines, taxanes, and cyclophosphamide all contribute to neutropenia, often most pronounced 7-14 days after dosing (the nadir period). Anemia (low red blood cells) and thrombocytopenia (low platelets) can also occur, though moderate anemia is common and often multifactorial (chemo effect, cancer, etc.). Myelosuppression is typically monitored with regular complete blood counts. Prophylactic use of G-CSF (growth factor support) may be indicated in high-risk regimens to prevent neutropenic complications. Dose adjustments are often based on blood counts; for example, a cycle might be delayed if neutrophils or platelets have not recovered to safe levels (Krol et al., 2006; Staudigl et al., 2012).

Cardiotoxicity

A notorious toxicity of the anthracycline class (doxorubicin, epirubicin) is cumulative dose dependent cardiotoxicity, that can take to cardiomyopathy and congestive heart failure. Doxorubicin's intercalation into DNA and generation of reactive oxygen species in cardiac myocytes are believed to underpin this toxicity. Clinically, patients receiving anthracyclines undergo monitoring of left ventricular ejection fraction (LVEF) via echocardiograms or MUGA scans at baseline and periodically during treatment. Early signs of cardiac dysfunction (e.g., an asymptomatic drop in LVEF or elevated cardiac biomarkers like troponin) may prompt changes in therapy; such as switching to a liposomal formulation of doxorubicin or limiting the cumulative dose. Additionally, anti-HER2 therapy (trastuzumab), often used concurrently or sequentially in HER2-positive breast cancer, can also cause reversible cardiotoxicity, compounding the need for cardiac monitoring. While not a metabolic toxicity per se, genetic susceptibility (for instance, variants in genes related to oxidative stress responses or drug transport) has been investigated in anthracycline cardiotoxicity (Rochette et al., 2015; Shen et al., 2015; Xia et al., 2024). Some studies suggest polymorphisms in the *RARG* gene or others might predispose to this side effect, highlighting again the interplay of genetics with toxicity risk (Rofaiel et al., 2010).

Neurotoxicity

Peripheral neuropathy is primarily associated with the taxane drugs (paclitaxel and docetaxel). Patients may experience numbness, tingling, or pain in hands and feet, which can progress with cumulative dosing. In severe cases, neuropathy can interfere with fine motor skills or balance, necessitating dose reductions. There is variability in who develops neuropathy; pharmacogenomic research has pointed to possible genetic contributors (e.g., variants in *EPHA* genes or *CYP2C8* affecting paclitaxel metabolism) although findings are not yet conclusive enough for clinical use. Other neurotoxic effects can include chemotherapy-related cognitive impairment (sometimes called "chemo brain"), though its mechanisms are multifactorial and not limited to a single drug or pathway.

Other Organ Toxicities

Certain chemotherapies have organ-specific toxicities. Cyclophosphamide can cause hemorrhagic cystitis (blood in urine due to bladder irritation by toxic metabolites; this is more common with higher doses and usually prevented by coadministration of mesna and fluids in those cases). 5-FU can, in rare instances, cause coronary vasospasm leading to chest pain (an acute cardiotoxicity different from anthracycline cardiomyopathy). Taxanes can cause hypersensitivity reactions during infusion (often due to the solvent; premedication with steroids and antihistamines mitigates this). Capecitabine and 5-FU can cause hyperbilirubinemia by liver enzyme elevation. Each drug thus has a unique toxicity "fingerprint" that clinicians must manage through dose scheduling, supportive care, and patient education.

To manage these toxicities, clinicians employ a variety of clinical biomarkers and monitoring strategies. Before and during chemotherapy, patients undergo routine laboratory tests: complete blood counts to track white cells, hemoglobin, and platelets; metabolic panels to check liver and kidney function (as liver enzymes might indicate drug-induced hepatitis and creatinine indicates renal function which can affect drug clearance); and specific tests like cardiac ejection fraction for those on cardiotoxic agents (Bacchiani & Cardinal, 2017). The presence of side effects is also systematically recorded, often using standardized grading systems such as the National Cancer Institute's Common Terminology Criteria for Adverse Events (CTCAE) (Cura et al., 2023). This grading helps determine when to hold or adjust doses. For example, a CTCAE grade 3 neutropenia or any fever with neutropenia will trigger interventions such as growth factor support or antibiotic prophylaxis. A grade 3 or 4 diarrhea will necessitate IV fluids, possible hospitalization, and dose reduction in subsequent cycles.

Emerging *biomarkers* for toxicity risk include germline genetic tests; a form of proactive monitoring. As discussed, testing for DPYD variants prior to 5-FU/capecitabine treatment is becoming standard in some guidelines to predict severe GI toxicity (Zhang et al., 2022). Similarly, testing for *UGT1A1* polymorphisms is standard before using the drug irinotecan (not commonly used in breast cancer, but relevant in other cancers) to predict risk of neutropenia. In the context of *CES1*, while not yet routine, research suggests that genotyping key *CES1* variants like G143E could identify patients who might experience atypical metabolism of capecitabine; either higher toxicity or reduced efficacy. Another area of interest is the use of pharmacokinetic monitoring; for example, measuring drug or metabolite levels in plasma to see if a patient is accumulating a toxic level. This is not common in routine practice for chemotherapy (unlike some other drugs with narrow therapeutic windows), but studies have shown that patients with higher AUC (area-under-curve) of capecitabine metabolites had more severe toxicities (Cura et al., 2023).

In summary, chemotherapy-induced toxicities in breast cancer are diverse and require careful management. Through clinical monitoring and supportive care, many side effects can be mitigated. Importantly, the variability in toxicity between patients has spurred research into predictive factors, including genetic polymorphisms, that could foresee who is at risk. This is where the interplay between genes like *CES1* and the patient's environment and lifestyle becomes crucial, as these factors together shape the body's handling of chemotherapy.

ENVIRONMENTAL INFLUENCES ON CHEMOTHERAPY OUTCOMES

Environmental exposures throughout life can profoundly influence health outcomes, including the efficacy and toxicity of chemotherapy in breast cancer. The term "environment" in this context encompasses a wide range of external factors; from chemical pollutants in air, water, and food to lifestyle choices such as diet, alcohol consumption, and physical activity. These factors can modulate drug metabolism enzymes (like *CES1*), alter DNA and epigenetic regulation, and affect the overall physiological state in which chemotherapy is delivered. Understanding environmental influences is thus key to painting a complete picture of interindividual variability in chemotherapy response.

Environmental Pollutants and Toxins

Certain environmental pollutants have been identified as risk factors for developing breast cancer and may also impact how patients respond to therapy. Notably, many of these pollutants are persistent organic pollutants (POPs) that accumulate in human tissue and exert hormonal or genotoxic effects (He et al., 2016; Joyce & Hou, 2015). Examples include:

Polychlorinated dibenzodioxins (PCDDs)

Commonly referred to as dioxins, these are byproducts of industrial processes and waste incineration. Dioxins are highly lipophilic and can accumulate in fat tissue. They are known to disrupt hormone signaling and have been linked to cancers, including breast cancer (VoPham et al., 2020; Benoit et al., 2022). In the context of chemotherapy, dioxins (and related compounds like polychlorinated biphenyls) can activate the aryl hydrocarbon receptor (AhR) pathway, potentially altering the expression of drug-metabolizing enzymes. For example, exposure to dioxin has been shown to change the expression levels of certain cytochrome P450 enzymes and could conceivably modulate *CES1* expression or activity indirectly. Such changes might influence how quickly chemotherapy drugs are metabolized, thereby impacting toxicity or effectiveness (Lee & Riddick, 2012).

Organochlorine Pesticides (e.g., DDT)

Dichlorodiphenyltrichloroethane (DDT) is a once-widely used pesticide that, despite being banned in many countries decades ago, persists in the environment and human tissues. DDT and its metabolites are known as endocrine disruptors; they can mimic or interfere with estrogen and other hormone pathways (Martyniuk et al., 2020; Bratton et al., 2012). Chronic exposure to DDT has been associated with an increased risk of breast cancer, particularly for exposures during windows of breast development (e.g., puberty). In terms of chemotherapy, organochlorines could potentially induce or inhibit metabolic enzymes. While specific data on DDT's effect on *CES1* are limited, it's plausible that sustained exposure may lead to liver enzyme induction as part of the body's attempt to eliminate the toxin. If *CES1* expression is upregulated or downregulated by such exposure, it could alter the breakdown of chemotherapy drugs that are *CES1* substrates.

Heavy Metals (Cadmium, Lead, Arsenic)

Heavy metals are inorganic pollutants that can enter the body through contaminated food, water, air, or occupational exposure. *Cadmium* in particular has been implicated in breast cancer risk due to its estrogen-mimicking effects (it's considered a metalloestrogen) (Byrne et al., 2013; Aquino et al., 2012; Vu et al., 2019). Cadmium and lead also cause oxidative stress and DNA damage. These metals can interfere with the function of the liver and kidneys; the critical organs for drug metabolism and excretion. Chronic arsenic exposure (through drinking water, for example) is a well-known carcinogen and can impair various metabolic enzymes. Heavy metals may bind to sulfhydryl groups on proteins, potentially inhibiting enzyme function, or they may activate stress-response pathways like Nrf2 which in turn affects expression of detoxification enzymes (Gavito-Covarrubias et al., 2024). If a breast cancer patient has high body burdens of heavy metals, her ability to metabolize chemo drugs could be affected; for instance, metal-induced liver injury might reduce *CES1* activity or availability, leading to higher circulating levels of a given drug and more toxicity.

These environmental carcinogens and pollutants not only increase *breast cancer susceptibility* but can also modulate treatment outcomes. They often accumulate in adipose tissue (which is particularly relevant in breast tissue, a fatty organ) and may cause chronic inflammation or endocrine disruption that affects how cancer cells and normal cells react to chemotherapy (du Plessis et al., 2023; Iyengar et al., 2013; Crespi et al., 2016). Moreover, studies suggest that certain pollutants can cause epigenetic modifications; such as DNA methylation changes; in genes responsible for drug metabolism (Peng et al., 2025; Teti, 2014). For example, early-life or pubertal exposures to mixtures of environmental chemicals have been shown to leave epigenetic marks that persist and may contribute to breast cancer risk and potentially influence genes like *CES1* involved in detoxification (Georgiadis et al., 2013; Zhang et al., 2024).

Lifestyle Factors (Diet, Alcohol, and Physical Activity)

Lifestyle factors are a modifiable subset of environmental influences that significantly shape a patient's overall health and can impact chemotherapy tolerance:

Diet

A diet high in fruits and vegetables provides antioxidants and phytochemicals that can protect cells from damage and may modulate enzyme systems. Conversely, a diet rich in saturated fats and low in nutrients can exacerbate inflammation and possibly affect drug metabolism. For instance, compounds in cruciferous vegetables (like broccoli) can induce phase II detox enzymes, while charred meats contain polycyclic aromatic hydrocarbons (PAHs) that induce certain cytochrome P450s (Inbathamizh, 2020; Sinha et al., 1994). The effect of diet on *CES1* specifically is not well-characterized, but a well-nourished liver is generally more efficient at drug metabolism than one burdened by fatty infiltration or micronutrient deficiencies. Malnutrition or specific vitamin deficiencies could impair the synthesis of metabolic enzymes. Obesity, which is partly dietary, is associated with chronic inflammation and altered pharmacokinetics of drugs; chemotherapy dosages are often calculated on body surface area, but distribution and clearance can differ in obese patients (Zarezadeh et al., 2020). Recent research underscores that a balanced diet might improve chemotherapy outcomes, whereas certain foods or supplements might interact adversely with treatment. For example, high-dose antioxidant supplements during chemo are controversial; they might reduce oxidative damage (and thus side effects) but could also theoretically protect tumor cells from oxidative stress intended by the chemotherapy.

Alcohol Consumption

Alcohol is a known modulator of drug metabolism. Chronic alcohol use can induce some liver enzymes (like CYP2E1) but also cause liver damage that overall reduces metabolic capacity. Intriguingly, as noted in the *CES1* context, ethanol is considered a potent inhibitor of *CES1* activity (Her & Zhu, 2020). This means that patients who consume alcohol heavily might have suppressed *CES1* function, leading to slower metabolism of *CES1* substrate drugs. In a chemotherapy setting, such an effect could increase drug exposure and toxicity (Stoeva et al., 2020). On the other hand, mild to moderate alcohol consumption's impact on chemo efficacy is less clear, but heavy drinkers are certainly at risk of liver dysfunction which complicates chemotherapy dosing (Hussein & Jensen, 2023). Additionally, alcohol can exacerbate certain side effects (e.g., it can be dehydrating and worsen chemotherapy-related liver toxicity or peripheral neuropathy from nutrients deficiencies like B vitamins). From a cancer risk perspective, alcohol is an established risk factor for breast cancer due to its effects on estrogen metabolism and DNA damage; from a treatment perspective, advising patients to limit alcohol is prudent to avoid undue stress on metabolic pathways . Indeed, *CES1* being inhibited by alcohol is a concrete example of gene-environment (where environment = alcohol intake) interaction that could be relevant when a drug like capecitabine is used, as alcohol might raise capecitabine levels or alter its toxicity profile (Stoeva et al., 2020; Liang et al., 2014).

Physical Activity

Exercise has systemic benefits, including improving cardiovascular health, reducing inflammation, and modulating hormone levels. Physically active patients often have better chemotherapy tolerance and fewer complications like blood clots or fatigue (Caetano et al., 2020; Labourey, 2007). There isn't a direct known link between exercise and *CES1* expression, but exercise can improve liver function and possibly epigenetic regulation of genes. Some studies indicate that exercise can influence gene expression patterns in the liver and adipose tissue. Moreover, exercise can help mitigate certain chemo side effects (for example, light exercise can help with fatigue and neuropathy) (May et al., 2014). Sedentary behavior, in contrast, may worsen insulin resistance and fatty liver, potentially impairing drug metabolism. Epidemiologically, higher physical activity is associated with improved cancer outcomes and lower risk of recurrence, likely due to a combination of better physiologic reserve and reduced comorbid conditions.

Smoking

Though not explicitly mentioned in the section prompt, smoking is another lifestyle factor worth noting. Tobacco smoke contains PAHs and nitrosamines that induce various metabolizing enzymes and also cause DNA methylation changes. Smoking can increase clearance of some drugs but also heighten cardiopulmonary stress, which can complicate chemotherapy (e.g., smokers might have worse lung tolerance to certain drugs or radiation). Quitting smoking is always advised, as it can improve oxygenation and healing during treatment.

Air Pollution and Epigenetic Regulation

Air pollution; particularly fine particulate matter (PM2.5 and PM10) and traffic-related pollutants like PAHs, benzene, and others; has gained attention as a factor that can influence cancer outcomes via epigenetic mechanisms. Chronic inhalation of polluted air exposes individuals to oxidative stress and inflammatory stimuli that can lead to changes in DNA methylation, histone modification, and microRNA expression (McCullough et al., 2017; Silveyra & Floros, 2012). These epigenetic changes can silence or activate genes without altering the underlying DNA sequence. For instance, exposure to air pollution has been associated with methylation changes in genes involved in immune responses and xenobiotic metabolism (Mukherjee et al., 2021; Rider & Carlsten, 2019). If a gene like *CES1* were subject to such regulation, one could hypothesize that people in high air pollution environments might have different *CES1* expression levels than those in cleaner environments, although direct evidence for *CES1* specifically is still needed. However, research has documented that xenobiotic metabolism genes broadly can be affected by air quality. A study by Lee et al. (2021) examined interactions between exposure to polycyclic aromatic hydrocarbons (a component of air pollution) and genetic variants in xenobiotic metabolism genes in relation to breast cancer risk. Such studies hint that the combination of genetic susceptibility and pollutant exposure is critical; which is exactly the gene-environment interplay theme (Lee et al., 2021).

Epigenetic regulation is a key way environment interfaces with the genome. For example, Natarajan et al. (2020) demonstrated that environmental exposures during puberty; a critical developmental window; can lead to epigenetic damage that increases breast cancer risk later in life. Some of these epigenetic marks may persist into adulthood and could alter how genes respond when a patient is later exposed to chemotherapy. Additionally, exposure to diesel exhaust or heavy pollution has been shown to alter microRNA profiles; microRNAs could in turn downregulate enzymes like *CES1*. Although research directly linking air pollution to chemotherapy toxicity is nascent, it stands to reason that a lifetime of environmental stressors affects the baseline state of organs that handle chemotherapy (Natarajan et al., 2020).

In summary, environmental influences, from toxic chemicals to everyday lifestyle habits, create a backdrop against which chemotherapy operates. These factors can affect the pharmacokinetics and pharmacodynamics of cancer drugs. For instance, a patient with significant exposure to enzyme-inducing pollutants might metabolize a drug faster, reducing efficacy, whereas another patient with an enzyme-inhibiting exposure (like chronic alcohol use inhibiting *CES1*) might metabolize the same drug more slowly, increasing toxicity. Recognizing these influences offers opportunities to adjust treatment (for example, providing more aggressive detoxification support, antioxidant supplementation, or simply tailoring the drug dose) and highlights the importance of a holistic approach to patient care that includes environmental history. It also underscores public health needs: reducing harmful exposures in the population could improve not just cancer incidence but also outcomes for those undergoing cancer treatment.

Gene-Environment Interactions

The convergence of genetic and environmental factors (gene-environment interactions) is crucial to understanding the full variability in chemotherapy responses among breast cancer patients. Gene-environment interactions occur when the effect of an environmental exposure on an outcome (like chemotherapy toxicity) is conditional on a person's genotype, or conversely, when the effect of a genetic variant depends on environmental context. In other terms, certain genetic predispositions might only manifest as clinical differences in the presence of specific environmental triggers, and vice versa.

Mechanistically, gene-environment interactions can be explained by a variety of biological processes:

- **Regulation of Gene Expression by Environmental Factors:** Environmental exposures can influence the transcription and translation of genes. As discussed, carcinogens or drugs can induce or inhibit enzyme expression via receptor-mediated pathways (e.g., AhR, PXR, Nrf2 pathways). If an individual carries a genetic variant that already affects gene expression or enzyme activity, an environmental factor could amplify or mitigate that effect. For *CES1*, for instance, an individual with a hypomorphic *CES1* allele (one that gives moderately lower activity). If this person is also exposed chronically to an environmental *CES1* inhibitor (like alcohol) or a pollutant that downregulates *CES1*, the combined impact could be a dramatically reduced capacity to metabolize *CES1*-dependent drugs (Her & Zhu, 2020). Conversely, if someone with a risk allele is in a very clean environment with no additional stressors on metabolism, the genetic risk might not translate into noticeable differences clinically.

- **Environmental Activation of Compensatory Pathways:** Sometimes, the body can compensate for a genetic deficiency if the environment provides a stimulus. For example, a person with a slower-metabolizing genotype might, upon exposure to certain dietary inducers, ramp up other enzymes to compensate. However, compensation might fail under heavy pollutant burden or polypharmacy (multiple drugs), revealing the genetic weakness.
- **Synergistic Toxicity:** In some cases, having both a genetic susceptibility and an environmental exposure leads to outcomes worse than the sum of their parts. A classic case outside of chemotherapy is the combination of the BRCA gene mutation and radiation exposure increasing cancer risk more than either alone. In chemotherapy toxicity, one could postulate that, for example, a patient with a *CES1* poor metabolizer genotype who also has high exposure to organochlorine pollutants (which may cause liver stress) could experience particularly severe toxicity from a drug like capecitabine, because their body is both less equipped to detoxify the drug and is under environmental stress that heightens vulnerability.

Real-world evidence of gene-environment interactions in chemotherapy is beginning to accumulate. A study by Cui et al. (2017) in non-small cell lung cancer patients is an illustrative example beyond breast cancer: it showed that gene-gene and gene-environment interactions influenced platinum-based chemotherapy response and toxicity (Cui et al., 2017). This implies that factors such as smoking status combined with certain DNA repair gene polymorphisms jointly determined who had more side effects from platinum chemotherapy. Bringing the focus back to breast cancer, consider an example in the context of *CES1*: A breast cancer patient with the *CES1* G143E variant (which reduces *CES1* function) might normally metabolize capecitabine slower. If this patient also happens to consume a lot of grapefruit juice; a dietary element known to inhibit various drug-metabolizing enzymes (though more famously CYP3A4, but hypothetically if it or some flavonoids inhibited *CES1*); the result could be dangerously high drug levels. Or, if the same patient has high exposure to activating compounds (perhaps some herbal supplement that induces detox enzymes), the effect of the G143E might be lessened because other pathways clear the drug.

Specific data on *CES1 per se* and environment are limited, but there is evidence on fluoropyrimidine toxicity that indicates multiple factors at play. As mentioned earlier, Maslarinou et al. (2023) argue for a *polygenic algorithm* for fluoropyrimidine dosing, which inherently would account for various genetic factors (DPYD, *CES1*, etc.) (Maslarinou et al., 2023). This concept could also be extended to include a 'polyenvironmental' perspective, factoring in things like liver function (could be impacted by alcohol or hepatitis), nutritional status (folate deficiency could worsen 5-FU toxicity since it affects 5-FU's target pathway), and exposure history. In a study of capecitabine-treated patients, overall toxicity was associated with the *CES1* rs71647871 variant, but in analyzing their data, researchers often adjust for things like patient age, which could be a surrogate for accumulated exposures or organ function (Cura et al., 2023). Some evidence suggests smokers on chemotherapy may have different toxicity profiles than non-smokers, possibly due to enzyme induction by smoking or differences in drug distribution.

In line with this, findings from a cohort of capecitabine-treated metastatic breast cancer patients indicated that genetic predispositions to chemotherapy toxicity may only manifest under specific environmental or lifestyle conditions (Aygüneş, 2008). In that analysis, no significant association was observed between *CES1* I49V and N75S polymorphisms and capecitabine-induced toxicity; however, it was proposed that the lack of association could reflect an absence of environmental triggers necessary for these genotypic differences to exert clinical effects. It was suggested that *CES1* polymorphisms might influence capecitabine metabolism predominantly in the presence of enzyme modulators found in diet, concurrent medications, or environmental pollutants (Aygüneş, 2008).

A hypothetical but plausible scenario of gene-environment interaction: dietary folate and DPYD genotype; patients with certain DPYD polymorphisms (genetic) have reduced ability to catabolize 5-FU, and low folate diet (environmental) could exacerbate 5-FU toxicity because 5-FU's mechanism involves folate-dependent pathways. In the case of *CES1*, alcohol intake and *CES1* genotype is a concrete example: as noted, alcohol can inhibit *CES1*, so even a person without a *CES1* genetic variant might exhibit "phenocopied" poor metabolizer status if they drink heavily (Her & Zhu, 2020). If that person also has a *CES1* slow allele, the effect is doubled, potentially leading to unexpectedly high toxicity from a standard dose of a *CES1*-metabolized drug.

Another angle of gene-environment interplay is how environment can cause mutations or polymorphisms (not inherited ones, but somatic changes or rare acquired variations). For instance, long-term toxin exposure might select for certain genetic traits in cells. However, chemotherapy pharmacogenetics deals mostly with germline (inherited) variants.

Clinically, recognizing gene-environment interactions has important implications for dosing and toxicity management. It suggests that oncologists should gather a thorough history of environmental exposures and lifestyle factors when planning treatment, in tandem with genetic testing. For example, two patients might both carry a risk allele for toxicity, but if one has a mitigating environment (healthy lifestyle, no pollutant exposures, robust organ function) and the other has multiple environmental risk factors (e.g., smoker, heavy drinker, occupational chemical exposures), the latter might need more aggressive dose reduction or closer monitoring. Case studies reflect this: there have been reports where patients with unexpected severe toxicity were later found to have both a genetic predisposition and an environmental trigger. In one report, a patient with severe capecitabine-induced toxicity had both a DPYD mutation and was on a medication (environment in broad sense) that inhibited fluoropyrimidine clearance. Similarly, suppose a breast cancer patient experiences severe hand-foot syndrome beyond what their genotype alone would predict; an inquiry might reveal she had been routinely consuming an herbal tea with unknown enzyme-inhibiting properties; illustrating that environment can tip the balance.

Expanding on this, the evaluation of *CES1* polymorphisms such as I49V, N75S, and H199R in a Turkish metastatic breast cancer cohort receiving capecitabine did not reveal significant associations with chemotherapy-induced toxicity (Aygüneş, 2008). This contrasts with the established clinical relevance of other fluoropyrimidine pharmacogenetic markers, such as DPYD, and may indicate that *CES1* I49V and N75S variants are functionally neutral in this therapeutic context. However, the limited sample size remains a constraint, underscoring the need for larger, multicenter studies. Future investigations should incorporate polygenic risk models and systematically explore potential gene-environment interactions that could modulate *CES1*-related drug metabolism and toxicity risk. The integration of both genetic and environmental assessments is essential for advancing precision oncology and tailoring chemotherapy to individual patient profiles.

In research settings, investigators sometimes stratify clinical trial participants by certain environmental factors (like hepatic function or region of residence as a proxy for exposures) when analyzing pharmacogenomic data. This helps isolate true gene effects by minimizing environmental noise, or conversely helps identify when an environmental factor is only relevant in a subset with a particular genotype.

In summary, gene-environment interactions add a layer of complexity to precision medicine. They remind us that genes do not operate in a vacuum: the environment can modulate genetic effects. For breast cancer chemotherapy, this means that optimizing therapy may require both genetic testing and environmental/lifestyle assessments. Personalized medicine thus becomes a multi-dimensional puzzle; not only "which genes does this patient have?" but also "what environmental exposures has this patient had, and how might those interact with their genetic makeup during treatment?" Addressing this interplay can lead to more nuanced and effective chemotherapy management, reducing the trial-and-error approach in dosing and minimizing severe toxicity surprises (Table 1).

Table 1. CES1 Polymorphisms – Drug and Environmental Interactions

Polymorphism	Drug(s)	Effect	Environmental Modulator(s)	Source
G143E (rs71647871)	Methylphenidate, Enalapril, Clopidogrel, Oseltamivir	Significantly reduced CES1 activity	Alcohol (inhibitor)	(Her & Zhu, 2020),
L40T, G142E, G147C, Y170D, R171C	Enalapril, Clopidogrel, Sacubitril	Partial or complete loss of CES1 function	-	(Wang et al, 2017; Hussain et al, 2024)
CES1A2 -816A/C	Imidapril	Increased transcription → increased CES1 activity	Variation in Sp1 binding site	(Yoshimura et al, 2008)
A158V, E220G, R199H	Enalapril, Clopidogrel	Mild reduction in CES1 activity (substrate-specific)	-	(Wang et al, 2017)
(Not a polymorphism)	Methylphenidate, Oseltamivir, Clopidogrel	CES1 inhibition	Quercetin, naringenin, THC, oleanolic acid, etc.	(Qian & Markowitz, 2020)

CLINICAL APPLICATIONS AND PERSONALIZED TREATMENT

Translating the understanding of *CES1* polymorphisms and environmental factors into clinical practice is the next critical step. The ultimate goal is to refine breast cancer treatment so that it is *personalized*, each patient's chemotherapy regimen is optimized for their genetic profile and environmental context. There are several emerging and potential clinical applications of this knowledge:

1. ***CES1* Genotyping in Clinical Decision-Making:** Given the evidence that *CES1* variants (like G143E) can impact drug metabolism and toxicity, one application is to genotype patients for key *CES1* polymorphisms before starting certain chemotherapies. For instance, in a patient scheduled to receive capecitabine, knowing if she carries the *CES1* G143E loss-of-function allele could inform the oncologist to be more cautious. If the patient is a carrier of the high-risk allele, the clinician might opt to start at a lower dose and escalate carefully, or to use an alternative 5-FU delivery method (such as continuous infusion 5-FU, where metabolism doesn't rely on *CES1* to the same extent) if appropriate. While *CES1* testing is not yet standard of care (unlike DPYD testing for fluoropyrimidines), guidelines for incorporating pharmacogenetic testing are evolving. The inclusion of *CES1* in multi-gene pharmacogenetic panels for cancer therapy could soon be justified as data accumulate. If implemented, such testing would enable the

identification of patients who metabolize drugs unusually fast or slow, allowing proactive dose adjustments. This approach exemplifies moving from reactive management of toxicity to *preemptive* personalization of chemotherapy (Yüksel et al., 2019; de With et al., 2023).

2. **Dose Adjustments and Alternative Therapies:** Personalized treatment means not only choosing the right drug but also the right dose. In patients with genetic variants that predict higher risk of toxicity, dose adjustments can be made from the outset. For example, a patient with multiple pharmacogenetic risk factors for 5-FU toxicity (say, a DPYD variant plus a *CES1* variant) might start at 75% of the full dose and then titrate up if tolerated, rather than the standard full dose that could result in hospitalization with severe toxicity. Alternatively, if the risk of a certain drug is deemed too high, an alternative therapy could be chosen. In breast cancer, there are often several regimen options; for example, if capecitabine is contraindicated by genotype, perhaps vinorelbine or another agent could be used for metastatic disease. Or if standard anthracycline dosing might be risky (due to gene variants in drug transport or metabolism), a non-anthracycline regimen could be considered. This decision-making is nuanced and must balance efficacy (to avoid inadequate cancer treatment) with safety, but genetic information can inform clinical decisions in borderline scenarios.
3. **Integrating Environmental Risk Assessments:** A truly personalized approach would consider environment and lifestyle alongside genetics. This could involve taking a detailed exposure history and possibly some form of environmental risk assessment questionnaire when planning treatment (Elespuru & Fischer, 2021). If a patient reports significant exposures (e.g., she works in a chemical factory, or lives in an area with high air pollution, or has a heavy alcohol intake), the oncologist might choose a regimen with a different toxicity profile or ensure more intensive monitoring. For example, a patient with mild liver dysfunction from alcohol use might avoid certain drugs that are hepatically cleared in favor of others, or receive lower doses with more frequent liver function tests (Gripshover et al., 2022). In the future, it could be envisioned that clinical decision support systems that take input such as "*CES1* genotype: poor metabolizer; Alcohol use: yes, daily; Smoking: no; BMI: high" and output a recommended chemo dose adjustment or regimen selection. Lifestyle interventions can also be part of personalized treatment: encouraging modifications such as quitting alcohol or smoking before therapy, improving diet to support liver health, or increasing exercise can potentially improve how a patient handles chemotherapy (Kim et al., 2019). The environment is inherently dynamic and, in many cases, modifiable. Identifying environmental risk factors that can be altered offers an opportunity to incorporate environmental modification into personalized care

strategies. For instance, patients may benefit from targeted interventions aimed at reducing exposure to specific toxins or enhancing nutritional support.

4. **Clinical Monitoring and Support Tailored to Risk:** If it is known that a patient is at high risk of a certain toxicity due to gene-environment factors, the monitoring plan could be tailored. A patient genetically prone to neutropenia might receive prophylactic G-CSF after each cycle to prevent complications (Crea et al., 2009). Someone at risk of cardiotoxicity could get more frequent cardiac imaging or be referred to a cardio-oncologist early. High-risk for hand-foot syndrome might prompt prophylactic use of cooling measures or dose interruptions at the earliest skin changes. These are adjustments not in the drug itself but in the supportive care accompanying it.
5. **Precision Oncology Frameworks:** Many cancer centers are developing precision oncology programs that include molecular tumor boards for genomics of the tumor. A parallel development is pharmacogenomics boards or consultations that focus on the patient's own genome in relation to therapy. Incorporating *CES1* and other relevant pharmacogenes into these discussions would formalize their role. The frameworks involve cross-disciplinary teams: oncologists, pharmacists, geneticists, and sometimes epidemiologists or environmental health experts to interpret how best to tailor treatment. One might envision a future breast cancer case discussion where the team says, "This patient has an ER-positive tumor (which guides choice of chemo/hormone therapy) and also has *CES1* and CYP2C8 variants (which guide adjustments to the chemo dosing), and she has a history of heavy pesticide exposure (perhaps suggest monitoring for certain toxicities or adding protective agents)." This comprehensive view would be the epitome of personalized medicine.

Despite the promise, challenges to implementing personalized treatment plans exist. One practical hurdle is the need for evidence-based guidelines. Current research on *CES1* and related genes remains in progress, and the development of clinical guidelines often lags behind until a sufficient body of evidence and expert consensus is established. Palmirotta et al. (2018) likened the effort of using SNPs to predict chemo outcomes to "walking through quicksand" an indication that it's tricky and fraught with inconsistencies (Palmirotta et al., 2018). Another challenge is the cost and logistics of broad genetic testing and environmental assessment. However, the cost of genetic testing has dropped dramatically, and many hospitals already have infrastructure for some pharmacogenetic tests. Environmental assessments can be done via patient questionnaires, which is economical, albeit with limited precision.

Ethically, clinicians must ensure that personalization doesn't inadvertently cause disparities; for example, genetic tests must be accessible to all patients, and one must be careful not to deny standard treatments solely on genetic results if the evidence for doing so is not solid. If a patient has a high-risk genotype but few alternatives exist, careful dose management is needed rather than withholding effective therapy.

Ultimately, the benefits of personalized interventions are better outcomes and improved safety. Patients experience less severe toxicity, maintain better quality of life, and can stay on effective treatments longer if those treatments are tuned to their tolerance (Jiang & Wang, 2010). There is also a psychological benefit: patients feel more secure knowing their treatment is customized and that their providers have taken into account their unique makeup, this can improve adherence and satisfaction. There's evidence that patients who avoid severe toxicities (through dose tailoring or prophylactic measures) have better overall survival, since they can receive the intended therapy intensity without interruptions or reductions except those deliberately planned.

In summary, clinical application of gene-environment knowledge is advancing. For *CES1* in particular, testing and considering its activity might become part of precision oncology protocols. Personalized medicine in breast cancer is moving from a theoretical concept to a practical approach that integrates multi-omic data (genomics, maybe exposomics) for each patient. The goal is to ensure that each patient gets the right drug at the right dose and at the right time, with supportive measures suited to their personal risk factors. Such approaches have the potential to enhance therapeutic efficacy; the tumor is more likely to be adequately treated; and safety, the patient is less likely to suffer preventable harm.

RESEARCH METHODOLOGIES AND CHALLENGES

Studying the interplay of genetics and environment in chemotherapy toxicity requires sophisticated research methodologies that can capture the complexity of these interactions. Researchers employ a variety of approaches, each with its strengths and limitations. At the same time, the field faces challenges ranging from technical hurdles to ethical considerations.

1. Genetic Analysis Approaches

To investigate how genetic polymorphisms influence chemotherapy outcomes, scientists use several genomic techniques:

- *Candidate Gene Studies:* Early research often focused on known drug metabolism genes. For instance, researchers specifically genotyped single nucleotide polymorphisms (SNPs) in genes like *CES1* in cohorts of chemotherapy patients to see if variants correlated with toxicity or drug levels (Yüksel et al., 2019). An example is genotyping *CES1* G143E in a group of breast cancer patients on capecitabine and comparing toxicity between carriers and non-carriers.

- *Genome-Wide Association Studies (GWAS):* This unbiased approach scans the entire genome for variants associated with a phenotype (e.g., severe neutropenia or neuropathy in chemo patients). GWAS can discover novel genes not previously suspected. However, GWAS for chemotherapy toxicity require large sample sizes to achieve statistical power, and they can be confounded by population stratification.
- *Whole Genome or Exome Sequencing:* Sequencing provides a comprehensive look at a patient's genetic makeup, identifying both common and rare variants. This is useful in research to capture the full spectrum of polymorphisms in metabolic pathways. For example, whole exome sequencing of patients with extreme toxicity phenotypes might uncover rare deleterious mutations in genes like *CES1* or others that are missed by SNP genotyping arrays.
- *Pharmacogenetic Polygenic Risk Modeling:* Researchers are increasingly attempting to create predictive models that incorporate multiple genetic variants. Using statistical methods or machine learning, they combine variants in a weighted manner to predict toxicity risk or drug clearance rates. This requires datasets where genotype and detailed toxicity data are available.

2. Environmental Exposure Assessment

Capturing environmental data is challenging but essential:

- *Biomonitoring:* This involves measuring levels of chemicals, metabolites, or nutrients in biological samples (blood, urine, even tissue) . For example, measuring blood levels of cadmium or lead could directly quantify a patient's exposure to heavy metals. If one wanted to study how heavy metal exposure interacts with genetics to affect chemo toxicity, one could correlate metal levels and genotypes with outcomes.
- *Exposure Surveys and Interviews:* Patients can be surveyed about their lifestyle (diet, exercise, smoking, alcohol) and exposure history (occupation, residential history, use of certain products). While less precise than biomonitoring, surveys can provide data on factors like diet quality or occupational solvent exposure over decades, which might not show up in current biomonitoring.
- *Environmental Databases and Geospatial Analysis:* Linking patients' addresses or regions to environmental data (for example, air pollution indices, water quality reports, toxin release inventory data) is a method to estimate

exposure. Studies have, for instance, used proximity to hazardous waste sites or traffic density as proxies for pollutant exposure. This approach can be combined with genetic data in spatial epidemiology studies (Tatalovich et al., 2024).

3. Integrative Analysis and Statistical Modeling

The heart of gene-environment interaction research lies in integration:

- *Interaction Analysis:* In statistical models (like multivariable regression), an interaction term between a genetic factor and an environmental factor can test if the effect of one depends on the other. For example, a model might look at how *CES1* genotype and alcohol consumption together predict chemotherapy toxicity, including a genotype*alcohol interaction term (Her & Zhu, 2020). A significant interaction suggests the impact of genotype differs by alcohol use status.
- *Stratified Analysis:* Researchers may stratify the cohort by exposure status (e.g., smokers vs non-smokers) and examine genetic effects within each stratum. If a variant shows association with toxicity only in smokers and not in non-smokers, this is evidence of interaction.
- *Bioinformatics and Pathway Analysis:* To handle the vast data from sequencing and environmental measurements, bioinformatics tools help identify pathways that are enriched. For instance, if multiple genes in the same metabolic pathway are found to have variants associated with toxicity in those with a certain exposure, it strengthens a causal story.
- *In Vitro and In Vivo Functional Studies:* While not epidemiological, these are important for mechanism. Cell culture or animal models can be used to test hypotheses from human data. For example, if a particular *CES1* variant is suspected of causing toxicity in the presence of a pollutant, scientists could create cell lines with that variant and expose them to the pollutant and a chemotherapy drug to observe effects. CRISPR-Cas9 gene editing now allows precise introduction of human polymorphisms into cell or animal models to study their functional consequences under controlled "environmental" exposures (Wang et al., 2015).
- *Prospective Clinical Trials:* A future methodology could be trials where patients are stratified or randomized based on genetic testing and perhaps environmental interventions. For instance, a trial could test a genotype-guided dosing strategy vs standard dosing for a chemo drug, or test a detoxification intervention (like giving antioxidants or a drug to upregulate *CES1*) in those with a particular genotype to see if toxicity is reduced.

CHALLENGES AND LIMITATIONS

- *Complexity and Confounding:* Disentangling gene and environment effects is inherently complex. Many exposures correlate with each other (for example, smoking often correlates with alcohol use; diet correlates with socioeconomic status, which correlates with pollution exposure). This makes it difficult to assign cause. Large sample sizes and careful study design are needed to control confounders (Mechanic et al., 2012). Additionally, many small effect factors rather than one big factor might be responsible for toxicity, requiring analysis of multiple variables simultaneously.
- *Reproducibility:* Findings in pharmacogenetics can be inconsistent across studies. A variant might show association in one cohort but not another due to differences in population genetics or environmental backgrounds. For instance, a *CES1* variant might be important in a European cohort (where its allele frequency is higher and maybe the environmental context allows it to manifest) but show no effect in an Asian cohort (where it's nearly absent or overshadowed by other factors). Reproducing gene-environment findings is even more challenging because exposures differ widely by region and time. Collaborative consortia are needed to replicate results in independent populations with careful documentation of exposures.
- *Data Collection Burden:* Genetic data are now relatively easy to collect (a single blood sample can yield a whole genome sequence). But high-quality environmental data over a patient's lifetime is hard. Recall bias (patients may not remember or know what they were exposed to 20 years ago), and the need for longitudinal exposure assessment can limit the quality of data. Some exposures, like medications or supplement use, can change even during the course of chemotherapy, adding more variables.
- *Ethical and Privacy Concerns:* Collecting genetic data raises issues of privacy and data security, ensuring that such sensitive information is protected is paramount. Moreover, if environmental data includes things like occupation or residence, that too could be sensitive (it might inadvertently reveal things like drug use or other personal habits if not handled carefully). Discussions of gene and environment interactions often involve analyses at the population or subgroup level (like communities exposed to pollution). Reporting results that implicate an environmental exposure could have legal or social implications (companies responsible for pollution, etc.). Researchers must navigate these waters responsibly.
- *Clinical Utility vs. Research:* Not all discovered gene-environment interactions will be actionable clinically. There is a threshold of evidence and effect size that typically needs to be met for something to change clinical practice.

Many interactions might be interesting but not strong enough to warrant, say, changing a chemo dose. The challenge is focusing on the most impactful findings and translating those.

Emerging Solutions and Methodologies

To overcome some of these challenges, new tools are being explored:

- *High-throughput in vitro screening:* Using cell lines or organoids with different genotypes to screen for toxicity under various environmental conditions in a high-throughput manner. For example, a panel of human induced pluripotent stem cell-derived hepatocytes each with different enzyme polymorphisms could be tested against a library of pollutants plus a chemotherapy drug to see where toxicity spikes. This could pre-screen potential interactions before investing in large clinical studies.
- *Exposome Research:* The concept of the *exposome* is the totality of exposures an individual faces. Technologies are being developed (like wearable sensors, advanced mass spectrometry for hundreds of chemicals in blood) to characterize the exposome. Combining exposomic data with genomics is a frontier, giving rise to the term "geno-exposomics" or similar.
- *Machine Learning:* Given the complexity, machine learning models might detect patterns of gene-environment interplay that traditional stats miss. These models can handle many variables and interactions, though they require careful validation to ensure findings are not just overfitting noise.
- *International Collaboration:* Forming large cohorts like the UK Biobank or All of Us in the US, which have genetic data and are starting to collect environment and electronic health record data, can provide powerful datasets. Within those, sub-analyses for breast cancer patients receiving chemo could be done to look for patterns of toxicity.
- *Ethical Frameworks:* On the ethical side, establishing clear guidelines for returning genetic findings to patients (especially if they imply something about environment) and consent for how data is used will help maintain trust and allow these studies to proceed. For example, if a study finds a patient has a genetic variant and also finds they have high blood lead levels, should the patient be informed about the lead? Likely yes, but these kinds of scenarios need protocols.

In conclusion, research methodologies to study gene-environment interactions in chemotherapy toxicity are rapidly evolving, blending genomic technologies with environmental health science and advanced analytics. The challenges are significant due to the multifactorial nature of toxicity and the difficulty in measuring the "environment" part, but overcoming these challenges is feasible with interdisciplinary efforts. As data and analytic methods improve, a more comprehensive understanding is anticipated to emerge as research advances, which will directly feed into better clinical guidelines and interventions.

FUTURE DIRECTIONS

Looking ahead, the interplay between *CES1* gene polymorphisms, environmental exposures, and chemotherapy toxicity will be illuminated by new technologies and research paradigms that promise to transform both our understanding and management of these factors. Several future directions are particularly noteworthy:

1. Emerging Research Tools and Technologies

Breakthroughs in biotechnology are providing unprecedented ways to probe gene-environment dynamics. One such tool is CRISPR-Cas9 gene editing, which allows scientists to introduce or correct specific genetic variants in cellular or animal models with pinpoint precision. Using CRISPR, researchers can create isogenic cell lines that differ only at the *CES1* gene (e.g., one line has the G143E variant, another does not) and then expose these cells to chemotherapeutic drugs and various environmental toxins to directly observe interactions. This can definitively establish cause-effect relationships and mechanism (for example, confirming that the G143E variant causes higher intracellular drug levels and more cytotoxicity when an environmental inhibitor is present). Similarly, high-throughput sequencing and *multi-omics approaches* are being employed. Transcriptomics (RNA-seq) can show how gene expression profiles change in response to certain exposures or during chemotherapy, potentially identifying gene networks that are epigenetically regulated by environment. Epigenome sequencing (methylome or chromatin accessibility assays) in patients before and after chemotherapy might reveal persistent changes due to prior exposures that correlate with toxicity outcomes. All these data contribute to more sophisticated models of how *CES1* and other genes are regulated in real time (Zhang et al., 2022).

Another promising area is microbiome research. The gut microbiome, influenced by diet and environment, can modulate drug metabolism (some gut bacteria can inactivate or activate chemo drugs) and also influence inflammation (which might affect toxicity). Future studies may examine whether individuals with certain microbiome compositions have different chemo toxicity profiles and if that interacts with host genetics (Li et al., 2023).

2. New Therapeutic Targets and Interventions

As specific molecular pathways mediating chemotherapy toxicity are identified, novel therapeutic targets for pharmacological intervention may also be revealed. For instance, if a particular *CES1* variant is found to cause the toxic accumulation of a chemotherapeutic metabolite, small-molecule modulators could be developed to adjust *CES1* enzymatic activity. There is growing interest in compounds capable of either inhibiting or enhancing *CES1* function depending on clinical need. One reason alcohol's effect on *CES1* has been studied is to explore whether safe analogs could transiently inhibit *CES1* activity in order to increase the bioavailability of an active prodrug metabolite, or alternatively, whether such inhibition should be avoided to reduce the risk of toxicity (Her & Zhu, 2020). The concept of pharmacological chaperones or enzyme enhancers is also relevant. For example, a drug that stabilizes a structurally impaired *CES1* variant could enhance enzymatic activity in individuals with poor metabolizer genotypes, thereby improving drug clearance and reducing adverse effects.On the flip side, inhibitors might be used to deliberately slow metabolism in ultra-rapid metabolizers to keep drug levels therapeutic. While these are complex to implement in chemo (where timing is critical), they could be adjuvants given alongside chemotherapy.

Another target area is the pathways activated by environmental stress. If, say, oxidative stress from a pollutant is making toxicity worse, the use of strong antioxidants or Nrf2 activators might protect normal tissues during chemo (though caution is warranted to ensure tumors aren't equally protected). Cytoprotective agents (like dexrazoxane used to mitigate anthracycline cardiotoxicity) may be considered in a more personalized way; given only to those who genetically and environmentally are at greatest risk, thereby sparing others unnecessary medication. A concrete future approach: patients who have high predicted risk of anthracycline cardiotoxicity could universally get cardioprotectants or be switched to alternative regimens with similar efficacy but less risk (such as liposomal doxorubicin or non-anthracycline regimens).

It is conceivable that vaccination or chelation therapies for environmental toxicants playing a role. For example, if heavy metal exposure is a known issue for a patient, chelation therapy before starting chemo could reduce the body burden of those metals, potentially improving outcomes (though this is speculative and would need trials).

In terms of cancer therapy, novel drugs might be developed to exploit gene-environment interplay; for instance, targeting a metabolic pathway that's only upregulated in tumors of patients with certain exposure histories, developing therapeutics personalized according to environmental exposures.

3. Precision Medicine and Big Data Integration

Future oncology will likely integrate *big data* from electronic health records, genomics, and environmental sensors to make real-time recommendations. For example an AI-driven system that for each new breast cancer patient, integrates their genomic data (including *CES1* and other pharmacogenes), their medical history, lifestyle factors, neighborhood environmental data (pollution indices, etc.), and even data from wearable devices (such as wearable technology devices detecting heart rate variability or fitness level) and then outputs a personalized treatment protocol. While ambitious, the pieces of this puzzle are being assembled in various research initiatives. The All of Us research program and other large biobanks linking genomic and EHR data will allow discovery of subtle gene-environment interactions by comprehensive computational analysis of thousands of patients. For example, if 100 out of 10000 patients with a specific genotype and living in high-air-pollution areas had severe toxicity, vs only 10 out of 10000 of others, an AI could flag that pattern.

4. Diverse Population Studies

A critical future direction is ensuring research includes diverse populations in terms of ethnicity, geography, and socioeconomic status. Genetic studies in European populations might miss variants prevalent in other groups, and environmental studies in one country might not translate elsewhere. Expanding research to global consortia will capture a fuller range of genetic variation in *CES1* and varied environmental mixtures (for instance, indoor air pollution from cooking smoke is a major exposure in some parts of the world and could be an important factor for patients there). This diversity will improve the robustness and applicability of findings, making personalized approaches inclusive (Kittles, 2013).

5. Policy and Accessibility Issues

As personalized strategies are developed, it is essential to ensure their equitable accessibility across all patient populations. Future efforts must focus on policy changes that support pharmacogenetic and exposure assessments in routine care. This could include guideline updates (e.g., ASCO or ESMO guidelines recommending *CES1* testing in specific scenarios if evidence supports it), insurance coverage for pharmacogenetic panel tests, and funding for clinicians to take detailed exposure histories. On the environmental side, policy implications are broad: recognizing that reducing population exposure to carcinogens and toxins is a form of preventive medicine that could also improve cancer treatment outcomes. Public health policies that clean up air and water, regulate endocrine-disrupting chemicals, and reduce occupational hazards will feed forward into fewer complications during cancer treatment. There is also the ethical policy of who gets access to personalized medicine. It should not be limited to academic centers; community hospitals should benefit too. This might involve creating simplified point-of-care genetic tests (like a rapid *CES1* genotyping kit) that can be used anywhere, or decision support tools that any oncologist can access without needing a specialized pharmacogenomics team.

6. Education and Interdisciplinary Collaboration

Future directions also include educating healthcare providers about gene-environment interplay. Oncologists will need to be comfortable interpreting genetic results and understanding how environment plays a role; something that might be outside the traditional training. Similarly, patients will need education to understand why, for instance, they are being asked about their environment or being offered genetic tests, so they can make informed decisions. Interdisciplinary collaboration between oncologists, pharmacologists, genetic counselors, environmental medicine specialists, and data scientists will likely become standard in designing treatment plans.

7. Monitoring Long-Term Outcomes and Survivorship

Another critical future direction involves assessing how personalized treatment modifications influence long-term clinical outcomes. For example, it remains to be determined whether dose reductions based on genetic risk factors may compromise long-term cure rates. Comprehensive longitudinal data will be necessary to ensure that tailoring chemotherapy to minimize toxicity does not inadvertently reduce therapeutic efficacy. Furthermore, as cancer survivorship extends, understanding the influence of gene-environment interactions on late-onset complications, such as secondary malignancies, cardiac complications in later life, or persistent neuropathy, will be essential for optimizing survivorship care. Individuals with specific genotypic profiles and environmental exposures may require stratified follow-up protocols, customized according to their risk profiles.

In summary, the future of managing chemotherapy toxicity at the intersection of genetics and environment is bright and multifaceted. A continued shift toward precision oncology is anticipated, wherein both genetic and environmental data inform therapeutic decision-making. Advances in technology are expected to enhance our mechanistic understanding of treatment responses; novel interventions may enable the mitigation of toxicity even among high-risk patients; and integrated data infrastructures will support real-time, individualized clinical decision-making. Critically, through equitable policy frameworks and inclusive research efforts, these advancements hold the potential to benefit diverse patient populations, advancing the field toward an era in which breast cancer treatment is not only highly effective but also precisely tailored, with minimal unintended harm.

CONCLUSION

Chemotherapy will likely stay as the cornerstone of breast cancer treatment for the recent future, and thus addressing its toxicity is of paramount importance. This chapter has explored how the interplay between *CES1* gene polymorphisms and environmental exposures contributes to the variability in chemotherapy toxicity observed among breast cancer patients. Several key points emerge from this comprehensive examination:

Firstly, individual genetic makeup, particularly polymorphisms in drug metabolism genes like *CES1*, can significantly effect how chemotherapy drugs are metabolized in the body. *CES1*, being one of the most abundant and active drug-metabolizing enzymes in the liver, plays a crucial role in activating or detoxifying various chemotherapeutic agents (Her & Zhu, 2020). Variants in the *CES1* gene (such as the loss-of-function G143E SNP) can lead to either an accumulation of active drug (increasing toxicity) or insufficient drug activation (potentially reducing efficacy) (Cura et al., 2023). This genetic variability underscores the importance of moving toward *pharmacogenetically guided chemotherapy*, where a patient's genotype informs drug and dose selection to strike the optimal balance between efficacy and safety.

Secondly, no patient exists in a genetic vacuum, environmental exposures and lifestyle factors critically modulate drug responses. Environmental carcinogens like dioxins, organochlorines, and heavy metals not only contribute to breast cancer risk but can also alter gene expression and enzyme activity, thereby impacting chemotherapy metabolism. Lifestyle factors such as diet, alcohol use, and physical activity further shape the body's milieu. For example, chronic alcohol use can inhibit *CES1*, effectively mimicking a poor metabolizer genotype (Her & Zhu, 2020), while a nutritious diet and exercise can bolster overall organ function and perhaps resiliency against side effects. Additionally, exposures like air pollution can induce epigenetic changes that influence how genes like *CES1* function over time (Rider & Carlsten, 2019; Silveyra & Floros, 2012). The gene-environment interplay is complex: It has been witnessed that in some cases environment can exacerbate genetic risks (e.g., a toxic exposure pushing a genetically susceptible patient into severe toxicity), and in other cases, good environmental factors can compensate to a degree for genetic drawbacks.

Thirdly, appreciating these interactions has tangible implications for improving patient care. By integrating genetic testing for polymorphisms (including but not limited to *CES1*) and taking into account environmental and lifestyle factors, clinicians can personalize chemotherapy regimens. This might involve preemptive dose adjustments, enhanced toxicity monitoring, use of alternate drugs, or supportive measures tailored to an individual's risk. The overarching aim is to maximize the therapeutic benefits of chemotherapy (killing cancer cells) while minimizing harm to normal tissues. Personalization also means some patients may safely receive standard or even escalated doses if they are predicted to tolerate them well, potentially improving efficacy for those individuals, while others may avoid life-threatening side effects through dose reduction or prophylactic interventions.

Despite the advances summarized here, challenges remain. The field of pharmacogenomics, especially as it intersects with environmental health, is still growing, more research is needed to validate findings and to discover additional genetic and environmental determinants of toxicity. Not every breast cancer patient who has a certain genotype or exposure will experience toxicity, which means there are likely other modifying factors at play, possibly including tumor-related factors or immune system differences. This highlights the inherent limitations of predictive models while emphasizing their potential for continuous refinement through ongoing research and data integration. The projected future directions suggest a promising landscape. Technological advancements, including CRISPR and high-throughput screening platforms, are expected to enhance our understanding of underlying biological mechanisms. Large-scale data integration and machine learning may yield more accurate predictive algorithms for toxicity. New therapeutic approaches may arise that specifically address gene-environment vulnerabilities, making treatment even safer. Importantly, as personalized medicine becomes standard, it will be crucial to ensure equitable access; all patients, not just those treated at research hospitals, should benefit from genetic testing and tailored therapies. Policy changes, education, and system-level support will be needed to achieve this.

In closing, the interplay between *CES1* polymorphisms and environmental exposures exemplifies the broader theme of how nature and nurture together influence health outcomes. In the realm of breast cancer chemotherapy, unraveling this interplay offers a path to more precise, effective, and tolerable treatment strategies. By continuing to bridge pharmacogenetics with environmental medicine, it can be advanced toward a model of care where each patient's treatment plan is as unique as their own genetic code and life history, thereby optimizing outcomes and ushering in a new era of truly personalized oncology care.

Ultimately, the knowledge gained not only improves management of toxicity but also reinforces a patient-centered approach, acknowledging that each individual's journey with breast cancer is influenced by a constellation of genetic and environmental factors, and that as researchers our job in medicine is to navigate that constellation to guide the patient safely to the best possible outcome.

REFERENCES

Alam, M. N., Shapla, U. M., Shen, H., & Huang, Q. (2021). Linking emerging contaminants exposure to adverse health effects: Crosstalk between epigenome and environment. *Journal of Applied Toxicology*, *41*(6), 878–897. DOI: 10.1002/jat.4092 PMID: 33113590

Aquino, N. B., Sevigny, M. B., Sabangan, J., & Louie, M. C. (2012). The role of cadmium and nickel in estrogen receptor signaling and breast cancer: Metalloestrogens or not? *Journal of Environmental Science and Health. Part C, Environmental Carcinogenesis & Ecotoxicology Reviews*, *30*(3), 189–224. DOI: 10.1080/10590501.2012.705159 PMID: 22970719

Aygüneş, D. D. (2008). *Frequencies of CES1 gene polymorphisms in patients with metastatic breast cancer and retrospective evaluation of their effects on drug response in capecitabine users* (Master's thesis, Ege University).

Bacchiani, G., & Cardinal, D. (2017). Using biomarkers and early prophylactic treatment to prevent cardiotoxicity in cancer patients on chemotherapy: biomarkers: detection and treatment of cardiotoxicity., 9, 250-262. .DOI: 10.24170/9-4-1828

Benoit, L., Koual, M., Tomkiewicz, C., Bats, A.-S., Antignac, J.-P., Coumoul, X., Barouki, R., & Cano-Sancho, G. (2022). Impact of mixtures of persistent organic pollutants on breast cancer aggressiveness. *Environment International*, *170*, 107615. DOI: 10.1016/j.envint.2022.107615 PMID: 36343552

Bratton, M. R., Frigo, D. E., Segar, H. C., Nephew, K. P., McLachlan, J. A., Wiese, T. E., & Burow, M. E. (2012). The organochlorine o,p′-DDT plays a role in coactivator-mediated MAPK crosstalk in MCF-7 breast cancer cells. *Environmental Health Perspectives*, *120*(9), 1291–1296. DOI: 10.1289/ehp.1104296 PMID: 22609851

Byrne, C., Divekar, S. D., Storchan, G. B., Parodi, D. A., & Martin, M. B. (2013). Metals and breast cancer. *Journal of Mammary Gland Biology and Neoplasia*, *18*(1), 63–73. DOI: 10.1007/s10911-013-9273-9 PMID: 23338949

Caetano, A., Silva, D., Martins, P., & De Oliveira Toscano, J. (2020). IMPACT OF PHYSICAL ACTIVITY ON FATIGUE AND QUALITY OF LIFE OF CANCER PATIENTS. *Revista Brasileira de Medicina do Esporte*. https://doi.org/DOI: 10.1590/1517-8692202026062019_0045

Capri, G., Tarenzi, E., Fulfaro, F., & Gianni, L. (1996). The role of taxanes in the treatment of breast cancer. *Seminars in Oncology*, *23*(1, Suppl 2), 68–75. PMID: 8614849

Cha, Y.-J., Jeong, H.-E., Shin, J.-G., Kim, E.-Y., Yu, K.-S., Cho, J.-Y., Yoon, S. H., & Lim, K. S. (2014). Genetic polymorphisms of the carboxylesterase 1 (*CES1*) gene in a Korean population. *Translational and Clinical Pharmacology*, *22*(1), 30–34. DOI: 10.12793/tcp.2014.22.1.30

Crea, F., Giovannetti, E., Zinzani, P., & Danesi, R. (2009). Pharmacologic rationale for early G-CSF prophylaxis in cancer patients and role of pharmacogenetics in treatment optimization. *Critical Reviews in Oncology/Hematology*, *72*(1), 21–44. DOI: 10.1016/j.critrevonc.2008.10.014 PMID: 19111474

Crespi, E., Bottai, G., & Santarpia, L. (2016). Role of inflammation in obesity-related breast cancer. *Current Opinion in Pharmacology*, *31*, 114–122. DOI: 10.1016/j.coph.2016.11.004 PMID: 27889687

Cui, J.-J., Wang, L.-Y., Zhu, T., Gong, W.-J., Zhou, H.-H., Liu, Z.-Q., & Yin, J.-Y. (2017). Gene-gene and gene-environment interactions influence platinum-based chemotherapy response and toxicity in non-small cell lung cancer patients. *Scientific Reports*, *7*(1), 5082. DOI: 10.1038/s41598-017-05246-8 PMID: 28698656

Cura, Y., Sánchez-Martín, A., Márquez-Pete, N., González-Flores, E., Martínez-Martínez, F., Pérez-Ramírez, C., & Jiménez-Morales, A. (2023). Association of single-nucleotide polymorphisms in capecitabine bioactivation pathway with adjuvant therapy safety in colorectal cancer patients. *Pharmaceutics*, *15*(11), 2548. DOI: 10.3390/pharmaceutics15112548 PMID: 38004528

de With, M., Van Doorn, L., Maasland, D., Mulder, T., Hoop, O., Mostert, B., Homs, M., Bouazzaoui, E., Mathijssen, R., Van Schaik, R., & Bins, S. (2023). Capecitabine-induced hand-foot syndrome: A pharmacogenetic study beyond DPYD.. *Biomedicine & pharmacotherapy = Biomedecine & pharmacotherapie*, 159, 114232 . .DOI: 10.1016/j.biopha.2023.114232

du Plessis, M., Fourie, C., Stone, W., & Engelbrecht, A.-M. (2023). The impact of endocrine disrupting compounds and carcinogens in wastewater: Implications for breast cancer. *Biochimie*, *209*, 103–115. DOI: 10.1016/j.biochi.2023.02.006 PMID: 36775066

Elespuru, R., & Fischer, C. (2021). Abstract 2612: Personalized cancer risk and prevention: analysis of risk factors for specific cancers and integration into cancer risk assessment paradigms. *Cancer Research*, *81*(13_Supplement), 2612. Advance online publication. DOI: 10.1158/1538-7445.AM2021-2612

García-González, X., Cortejoso, L., García, M., García-Alfonso, P., Robles, L., Grávalos, C., González-Haba, E., Marta, P., Sanjurjo, M., & López-Fernández, L. (2015). Variants in CDA and ABCB1 are predictors of capecitabine-related adverse reactions in colorectal cancer. *Oncotarget*, *6*(8), 6422–6430. DOI: 10.18632/oncotarget.3289 PMID: 25691056

Gavito-Covarrubias, D., Ramírez-Díaz, I., Guzmán-Linares, J., Limón, I. D., Manuel-Sánchez, D. M., Molina-Herrera, A., Coral-García, M. Á., Anastasio, E., Anaya-Hernández, A., López-Salazar, P., Juárez-Díaz, G., Martínez-Juárez, J., Torres-Jácome, J., Albarado-Ibáñez, A., Martínez-Laguna, Y., Morán, C., & Rubio, K. (2024). Epigenetic mechanisms of particulate matter exposure: Air pollution and hazards on human health. *Frontiers in Genetics*, *14*, 1306600. DOI: 10.3389/fgene.2023.1306600 PMID: 38299096

Georgiadis, P., Bolognesi, C., Palli, D., & Farmer, P. B. (2013). Abstracts of the UKMEG/ECNIS2-sponsored Workshop on Design of Future Molecular Epidemiology Studies and New Biomarkers, Waterloo Conference Centre, London, United Kingdom. November 30, 2012. *Mutagenesis*, *28*(3), e1–e5. DOI: 10.1093/mutage/get011

Gripshover, T., Wahlang, B., Head, K., Young, J., Luo, J., Mustafa, M., Kirpich, I., & Cave, M. (2022). Environmental pollutant, polychlorinated biphenyl 126, alters liver function in a rodent model of alcohol-associated liver disease. *Alcohol, Clinical and Experimental Research*. Advance online publication. DOI: 10.1111/acer.14976 PMID: 36377258

Harnden, K., Deeken, J., Stankowicz, M., Stafford, A., Cocilovo, C., Khromykh, A., Iyer, R., Barnett, S., Lawrence, G., Moeckel, F., Vogt, B., Philips, S., Solares, A., & Edmiston, K. (2019). Clinical pharmacogenomic testing impacts therapy decisions and supportive medication choices in breast cancer. *Journal of Clinical Oncology*, *37*(15_suppl), 569. Advance online publication. DOI: 10.1200/JCO.2019.37.15_suppl.569

He, Y., Wang, X., & Wu, K. (2016). Evaluating breast cancer risk under exposure to environmental estrogen-like chemicals. *Polish Journal of Environmental Studies*, *25*(6), 2239–2249. DOI: 10.15244/pjoes/64282

Her, L., & Zhu, H. J. (2020). Carboxylesterase 1 and precision pharmacotherapy: Pharmacogenetics and nongenetic regulators. *Drug Metabolism and Disposition: the Biological Fate of Chemicals*, *48*(3), 230–244. DOI: 10.1124/dmd.119.089680 PMID: 31871135

Hu, J., & Yu, Y. (2019). Epigenetic response profiles into environmental epigenotoxicant screening and health risk assessment: A critical review. *Chemosphere*, *226*, 259–272. DOI: 10.1016/j.chemosphere.2019.03.096 PMID: 30933735

Hussain, M., Basheer, S., Khalil, A., Haider, Q., Saeed, H., & Faizan, M. (2024). Pharmacogenetic study of CES1 gene and enalapril efficacy. *Journal of Applied Genetics*, *65*(3), 463–471. Advance online publication. DOI: 10.1007/s13353-024-00831-w PMID: 38261266

Hussein, M., & Jensen, A. (2023). Drug-Induced Liver Injury Caused by Capecitabine: A Case Report and a Literature Review. *Case Reports in Oncology*, *16*, 393–399. DOI: 10.1159/000529866 PMID: 37384198

Inbathamizh, L. (2020). Targeting Cytochrome P450 1A1 Enzyme with Crucifer Phytocomponents: An In Silico Approach for Chemopreventive Drug Design against Lung Cancer. *Asian Journal of Pharmaceutics*, *14*(1). Advance online publication. DOI: 10.22377/ajp.v14i1.3508

Iyengar, N. M., Hudis, C. A., & Dannenberg, A. J. (2013). Obesity and inflammation: New insights into breast cancer development and progression. *American Society of Clinical Oncology Educational Book*, *33*(33), 46–51. DOI: 10.14694/EdBook_AM.2013.33.46 PMID: 23714453

Jiang, Y., & Wang, M. (2010). Personalized medicine in oncology: Tailoring the right drug to the right patient. *Biomarkers in Medicine*, *4*(4), 523–533. DOI: 10.2217/bmm.10.66 PMID: 20701441

Joyce, B. T., & Hou, L. (2015). Organic pollutants and telomere length: A new facet of carcinogenesis. *EBioMedicine*, *2*(12), 1854–1855. DOI: 10.1016/j.ebiom.2015.11.046 PMID: 26844257

Kim, H., Min, J., Seo, Y., & Min, K. (2019). Association of Ambient Air Pollution with Increased Liver Enzymes in Korean Adults. *International Journal of Environmental Research and Public Health*, *16*(7), 1213. Advance online publication. DOI: 10.3390/ijerph16071213 PMID: 30987355

Kim, M., Bae, M., Na, H., & Yang, M. (2012). Environmental toxicants-induced epigenetic alterations and their reversers. *Journal of Environmental Science and Health. Part C, Environmental Carcinogenesis & Ecotoxicology Reviews*, *30*(4), 323–367. DOI: 10.1080/10590501.2012.731959 PMID: 23167630

Kittles, R. (2013). Use of GWAS to predict targets associated with cancer in African Americans. *The FASEB Journal*, *27*(S1). Advance online publication. DOI: 10.1096/fasebj.27.1_supplement.460.2

Krol, J., Paepke, S., Jacobs, V., Paepke, D., Euler, U., Kiechle, M., & Harbeck, N. (2006). G-CSF in the Prevention of Febrile Neutropenia in Chemotherapy in Breast Cancer Patients. *Oncology Research and Treatment, 29*(4), 171–178. DOI: 10.1159/000091616 PMID: 16601374

Labourey, J. (2007). Physical activity in the management of cancer-related fatigue induced by oncological treatments.. *Annales de readaptation et de medecine physique: revue scientifique de la Societe francaise de reeducation fonctionnelle de readaptation et de medecine physique*, 50 6, 450-4, 445-9 . .DOI: 10.1016/j.annrmp.2007.03.010

Lee, C., & Riddick, D. (2012). Aryl hydrocarbon receptor-dependence of dioxin's effects on constitutive mouse hepatic cytochromes P450 and growth hormone signaling components. *Canadian Journal of Physiology and Pharmacology, 90*(10), 1354–1363. DOI: 10.1139/y2012-099 PMID: 22978700

Lee, D., Schuetz, J., Lai, A., Burstyn, I., Brooks-Wilson, A., Aronson, K., & Spinelli, J. (2021). Interactions between exposure to polycyclic aromatic hydrocarbons and xenobiotic metabolism genes, and risk of breast cancer. *Breast Cancer (Tokyo, Japan)*. Advance online publication. DOI: 10.1007/s12282-021-01279-0 PMID: 34351578

Li, S., Zhu, S., & Yu, J. (2023). The role of gut microbiota and metabolites in cancer chemotherapy. *Journal of Advanced Research, 64*, 223–235. DOI: 10.1016/j.jare.2023.11.027 PMID: 38013112

Liang, X., Di, L., Song, G., Yan, Y., Wang, C., Jiang, H., & Li, H. (2014). Capecitabine maintenance therapy for XT chemotherapy-sensitive patients with metastatic triple-negative breast cancer.. *Chinese journal of cancer research = Chung-kuo yen cheng yen chiu*, 26 5, 550-7 . .DOI: 10.3978/j.issn.1000-9604.2014.10.02

Longo, R., D'Andrea, M., Sarmiento, R., & Gasparini, G. (2010). Pharmacogenetics in breast cancer: Focus on hormone therapy, taxanes, trastuzumab and bevacizumab. *Expert Opinion on Investigational Drugs, 19*(sup1, Suppl 1), S41–S50. DOI: 10.1517/13543781003732701 PMID: 20374029

Martyniuk, C. J., Mehinto, A. C., & Denslow, N. D. (2020). Organochlorine pesticides: Agrochemicals with potent endocrine-disrupting properties in fish. *Molecular and Cellular Endocrinology, 507*, 110764. DOI: 10.1016/j.mce.2020.110764 PMID: 32112812

Maslarinou, A., Manolopoulos, V. G., & Ragia, G. (2023). Pharmacogenomic-guided dosing of fluoropyrimidines beyond DPYD: Time for a polygenic algorithm? *Frontiers in Pharmacology, 14*, 1184523. Advance online publication. DOI: 10.3389/fphar.2023.1184523 PMID: 37256234

Matsumoto, N., Kubota, Y., Ishida, H., Sekido, M., Ohkuma, R., Ishiguro, T., Hirasawa, Y., Ariizumi, H., Tsunoda, T., Ikusue, T., Kobayashi, K., Hisamatsu, A., Toshima, H., Shimada, K., & Fujita, K. I. (2020). Variants of carboxylesterase 1 have no impact on capecitabine pharmacokinetics and toxicity in capecitabine plus oxaliplatin treated-colorectal cancer patients. *Cancer Chemotherapy and Pharmacology, 85*(6), 1119–1128. DOI: 10.1007/s00280-020-04087-z PMID: 32458030

May, A., Velthuis, M., Travier, N., Bisschop, C., Wall, E., & Peeters, P. (2014). Physical activity during cancer treatment (PACT) study: Short- and long-term effects on fatigue of an 18-week exercise intervention during adjuvant chemotherapy in patients with breast or colon cancer. *Journal of Clinical Oncology, 32*(15_suppl), 9535–9535. DOI: 10.1200/jco.2014.32.15_suppl.9535

Mayer, E. L., & Burstein, H. J. (2016). Chemotherapy for triple-negative breast cancer: Is more better? *Journal of Clinical Oncology, 34*(28), 3369–3371. DOI: 10.1200/JCO.2016.68.4068 PMID: 27551109

McCullough, S. D., Dhingra, R., Fortin, M. C., & Diaz-Sanchez, D. (2017). Air pollution and the epigenome: A model relationship for the exploration of toxicoepigenetics. *Current Opinion in Toxicology, 6*, 18–25. DOI: 10.1016/j.cotox.2017.07.001 PMID: 33869910

Mechanic, L., Simonds, N., Ghazarian, A., Benedicto, C., Schully, S., Ellison, G., & Gillanders, E. (2012). Abstract 46: A review of the gene-environment interaction literature in cancer: What do we know? *Cancer Epidemiology, Biomarkers & Prevention, 21*(11_Supplement), 46–46. DOI: 10.1158/1055-9965.GWAS-46

Merali, Z., Ross, S., & Paré, G. (2014). The pharmacogenetics of carboxylesterases: *CES1* and CES2 genetic variants and their clinical effect. *Drug Metabolism and Drug Interactions, 29*(3), 143–151. DOI: 10.1515/dmdi-2014-0009 PMID: 24988246

Mukherjee, S., Dasgupta, S., Mishra, P. K., & Chaudhury, K. (2021). Air pollution-induced epigenetic changes: Disease development and a possible link with hypersensitivity pneumonitis. *Environmental Science and Pollution Research International, 28*(40), 55981–56002. DOI: 10.1007/s11356-021-16056-x PMID: 34498177

Natarajan, R., Aljaber, D., Au, D., Thai, C., Sanchez, A., Nunez, A., Resto, C., Chavez, T., Jankowska, M. M., Benmarhnia, T., Yang, J.-A., Jones, V., Tomsic, J., McCune, J. S., Sistrunk, C., Doan, S., Serrano, M., Cardiff, R. D., Dietze, E. C., & Seewaldt, V. L. (2020). Environmental exposures during puberty: Window of breast cancer risk and epigenetic damage. *International Journal of Environmental Research and Public Health, 17*(2), 493. DOI: 10.3390/ijerph17020493 PMID: 31941024

National Center for Biotechnology Information. (2024). *CES1 carboxylesterase 1 [Homo sapiens (human)] (Gene ID: 1066)*. NCBI Gene. https://www.ncbi.nlm.nih.gov/gene/1066

Nurgalieva, Z., Liu, C.-C., & Du, X. L. (2011). Chemotherapy use and risk of bone marrow suppression in a large population-based cohort of older women with breast and ovarian cancer. *Medical Oncology (Northwood, London, England)*, *28*(3), 716–725. DOI: 10.1007/s12032-010-9512-5 PMID: 20361359

Palmirotta, R., Carella, C., Silvestris, E., Cives, M., Stucci, S. L., Tucci, M., Lovero, D., & Silvestris, F. (2018). SNPs in predicting clinical efficacy and toxicity of chemotherapy: Walking through the quicksand. *Oncotarget*, *9*(38), 25355–25382. DOI: 10.18632/oncotarget.25256 PMID: 29861877

Panahi, Y., Beiraghdar, F., Amirhamzeh, A., Poursaleh, Z., Saadat, A., & Sahebkar, A. (2016). Environmental toxicant exposure and cancer: The role of epigenetic changes and protection by phytochemicals. *Current Pharmaceutical Design*, *22*(2), 130–140. DOI: 10.2174/1381612822666151112150149 PMID: 26561072

Peng, X., Zheng, J., Liu, T., Zhou, Z., Song, C., Zhang, D., Zhang, X., & Huang, Y. (2025). DNA methylation-based diagnosis and treatment of breast cancer. *Current Cancer Drug Targets*, *25*(1), 26–37. DOI: 10.2174/011568009627897824020416 2353 PMID: 38441008

Qian, Y., & Markowitz, J. S. (2020). Natural products as modulators of *CES1* activity. *Drug Metabolism and Disposition: the Biological Fate of Chemicals*, *48*(10), 993–1007. DOI: 10.1124/dmd.120.000065 PMID: 32591414

Rider, C. F., & Carlsten, C. (2019). Air pollution and DNA methylation: Effects of exposure in humans. *Clinical Epigenetics*, *11*(1), 131. DOI: 10.1186/s13148-019-0713-2 PMID: 31481107

Rochette, L., Guenancia, C., Gudjoncik, A., Hachet, O., Zeller, M., Cottin, Y., & Vergely, C. (2015). Anthracyclines/trastuzumab: New aspects of cardiotoxicity and molecular mechanisms. *Trends in Pharmacological Sciences*, *36*(6), 326–348. DOI: 10.1016/j.tips.2015.03.005 PMID: 25895646

Rofaiel, S., Muo, E. N., & Mousa, S. A. (2010). Pharmacogenetics in breast cancer: Steps toward personalized medicine in breast cancer management. *Pharmacogenomics and Personalized Medicine*, *3*, 129–143. DOI: 10.2147/PGPM.S10789 PMID: 23226048

Shen, S., Sun, Q., Xu, Y., Zhou, Y., Guan, J., Mao, F., Lin, Y., & Wang, X. (2015). Abstract P5-18-06: Trastuzumab can be safely administered concurrently with anthracycline for adjuvant treatment of HER2-positive breast cancer. *Cancer Research, 75*(9_Supplement), P5-18-06. Advance online publication. DOI: 10.1158/1538-7445.SABCS14-P5-18-06

Shimozuma, K., Ohashi, Y., Takeuchi, A., Aranishi, T., Morita, S., Kuroi, K., Ohsumi, S., Makino, H., Katsumata, N., Kuranami, M., Suemasu, K., Watanabe, T., & Hausheer, F. H. (2012). Taxane-induced peripheral neuropathy and health-related quality of life in postoperative breast cancer patients undergoing adjuvant chemotherapy: N-SAS BC 02, a randomized clinical trial. *Supportive Care in Cancer, 20*(12), 3355–3364. DOI: 10.1007/s00520-012-1492-x PMID: 22584733

Silveyra, P., & Floros, J. (2012). Air pollution and epigenetics: Effects on SP-A and innate host defence in the lung. *Swiss Medical Weekly, 142*, w13579. DOI: 10.4414/smw.2012.13579 PMID: 22553125

Sinha, R., Rothman, N., Brown, E., Mark, S., Hoover, R., Caporaso, N., Levander, O., Knize, M., Lang, N., & Kadlubar, F. (1994). Pan-fried meat containing high levels of heterocyclic aromatic amines but low levels of polycyclic aromatic hydrocarbons induces cytochrome P4501A2 activity in humans. *Cancer Research, 54*(23), 6154–6159. PMID: 7954461

Staudigl, C., Seifert, M., Tea, M., Pfeiler, G., Fink-Retter, A., Fritzer, N., & Singer, C. (2012). Abstract P1-15-10: Chemotherapy-Induced Neutropenia in Breast Cancer Patients Receiving Sequential Anthracycline and Taxane Chemotherapy: An institutional experience. *Cancer Research, 72*(24_Supplement), P1-15-10. Advance online publication. DOI: 10.1158/0008-5472.SABCS12-P1-15-10

Stoeva, S., Conev, N., & Marinov, P. (2020). *The role of carboxylesterase enzymes in capecitabine therapy*. Scripta Scientifica Pharmaceutica., DOI: 10.14748/ssp.v6i2.6624

Swagatika, S., & Tomar, R. S. (2016). Modulation of epigenetics by environmental toxic molecules. In *Advances in Molecular Toxicology* (Vol. 10, pp. 361–389). Elsevier., DOI: 10.1016/B978-0-12-804700-2.00008-8

Tatalovich, Z., Chtourou, A., Zhu, L., Dellavalle, C., Hanson, H., Henry, K., & Penberthy, L. (2024). Landscape analysis of environmental data sources for linkage with SEER cancer patients database. *Journal of the National Cancer Institute. Monographs, 2024*(65), 132–144. DOI: 10.1093/jncimonographs/lgae015 PMID: 39102880

Teti, D. (2014). Editorial: Effect of epi-drugs on epigenetic modifications induced by environmental pollutants: Implications for the pathophysiology of cancer and endocrine/metabolic diseases. *Current Genomics*, *15*(6), 419. DOI: 10.2174/138920291506150106145521 PMID: 25646070

VoPham, T., Bertrand, K. A., Jones, R. R., Deziel, N. C., DuPré, N. C., James, P., Liu, Y., Vieira, V. M., Tamimi, R. M., Hart, J. E., Ward, M. H., & Laden, F. Vo-Pham. (2020). Dioxin exposure and breast cancer risk in a prospective cohort study. *Environmental Research*, *186*, 109516. DOI: 10.1016/j.envres.2020.109516 PMID: 32305677

Vu, V., Navalkar, N., & Wei, Y. (2019). Endocrine-disrupting metals in ambient air and female breast cancer incidence in US. *Gynecological Endocrinology*, *35*(12), 1099–1102. DOI: 10.1080/09513590.2019.1622089 PMID: 31142157

Wang, X., Rida, N., Shi, J., Wu, A., Bleske, B., & Zhu, H. (2017). A Comprehensive Functional Assessment of Carboxylesterase 1 Nonsynonymous Polymorphisms. *Drug Metabolism and Disposition: the Biological Fate of Chemicals*, *45*(11), 1149–1155. DOI: 10.1124/dmd.117.077669 PMID: 28838926

Wang, X., Wang, G., Shi, J., Aa, J., Comas, R., Liang, Y., & Zhu, H. (2015). *CES1* genetic variation affects the activation of angiotensin-converting enzyme inhibitors. *The Pharmacogenomics Journal*, *16*(3), 220–230. DOI: 10.1038/tpj.2015.42 PMID: 26076923

Wu, X., & Xiong, H. (2024). The role of pharmacogenetic-based pharmacokinetic analysis in precise breast cancer treatment. *Pharmaceutics*, *16*(11), 1407. DOI: 10.3390/pharmaceutics16111407 PMID: 39598531

Xia, W., Yuan, Z., Wang, S., Zheng, Q., Wu, Z., Zhong, M., Xu, F., Wang, Y. X. S., Zhang, Y., Zhang, L., Shi, Y., Huang, H., Xu, X., & Li, H. (2024). Neoadjuvant pegylated liposomal doxorubicin-containing chemotherapy in combination with trastuzumab and pertuzumab in patients with HER2-positive early breast cancer: A randomized phase II study (METIS). *Journal of Clinical Oncology*, *42*(16_suppl), 596. Advance online publication. DOI: 10.1200/JCO.2024.42.16_suppl.596

Yoshimura, M., Kimura, T., Ishii, M., Ishii, K., Matsuura, T., Geshi, E., Hosokawa, M., & Muramatsu, M. (2008). Functional polymorphisms in carboxylesterase1A2 (CES1A2) gene involves specific protein 1 (Sp1) binding sites. *Biochemical and Biophysical Research Communications*, *369*(3), 939–942. DOI: 10.1016/j.bbrc.2008.02.120 PMID: 18328811

Yüksel, M. K., Öztürk, D., Öztaş, E., Özhan, G., Türker, A. A., Korkmaz, T., Okyar, A., & Kara, Z. P. (2019). Evaluation of the association of SNP in carboxylesterase enzyme (*CES1*) with pharmacokinetic and adverse effects of capecitabine in breast and colorectal cancer patients. *Istanbul Journal of Pharmacy*, *49*(2), 64–69. DOI: 10.26650/IstanbulJPharm.2019.19018

Zarezadeh, M., Saedisomeolia, A., Shekarabi, M., Khorshidi, M., Emami, M., & Müller, D. (2020). The effect of obesity, macronutrients, fasting and nutritional status on drug-metabolizing cytochrome P450s: A systematic review of current evidence on human studies. *European Journal of Nutrition*, *60*(6), 2905–2921. DOI: 10.1007/s00394-020-02421-y PMID: 33141242

Zhang, A., Luo, X., Li, Y., Yan, L., Lai, X., Yang, Q., Zhao, Z., Huang, G., Li, Z., Wu, Q., & Wang, J. (2024). Epigenetic changes driven by environmental pollutants in lung carcinogenesis: A comprehensive review. *Frontiers in Public Health*, *12*, 1420933. Advance online publication. DOI: 10.3389/fpubh.2024.1420933 PMID: 39440184

Zhang, T., Ambrodji, A., Huang, H., Bouchonville, K., Etheridge, A., Schmidt, R., Nunez, J., Temesgen, Z., Innocenti, F., Diasio, R., Largiadèr, C., & Offer, S. (2022). Abstract 5420: DPYD enhancer variant confers increased risk of severe toxicity in 5-FU chemotherapy. *Cancer Research*, *82*(12_Supplement), 5420. Advance online publication. DOI: 10.1158/1538-7445.AM2022-5420

Section 3
Exposome-Driven Insights into Health Disparities and Cancer Prevention

Chapter 6
Toxicogenomics and Pharmacogenomics Research in Health Disparities

Surendra Prakash Gupta
https://orcid.org/0000-0002-4873-6346
Shri Vaishnav Vidhyapeeth Viswavidhayalaya, India

Ankur Bhardwaj
https://orcid.org/0000-0003-0687-8810
Shri Vaishnav Vidhyapeeth Vishwavidyalaya, India

ABSTRACT

In recent years, the fields of toxicogenomics and pharmacogenomics have become increasingly popular as scientists attempt to understand the intricate interactions between genetic variables, environmental exposures, and how these factors affect health outcomes like the onset of diseases and the efficacy of medical treatments. This method has grown in significance for comprehending and resolving health inequalities. Significant racial and ethnic differences in drug response are revealed by combining genetic ancestry and pharmacogenomic data, which can help address health disparities and guide personalized medicine. These fields leverage genetic data to tailor medical treatments, aiming to reduce adverse drug reactions and improve therapeutic efficacy. Understanding these mechanisms are crucial to developing more personalized and effective treatments that account for individual genetic differences and their impact on how people respond to medications. The important developments in the field of omics to comprehend and reduce health disparities are covered in this chapter.

DOI: 10.4018/979-8-3373-5796-6.ch006

Copyright © 2026, IGI Global Scientific Publishing. Copying or distributing in print or electronic forms without written permission of IGI Global Scientific Publishing is prohibited.

1. INTRODUCTION

1.1 Definition of Toxicogenomics (TGx) and Pharmacogenomics (PGx)

TGx and PGx are essential for comprehending and tackling health disparities among at risk populations by customizing medical interventions based on genetic profiles, which enhances health outcomes and fosters health equity. These disciplines examine genetic differences that affect drug efficacy and toxicity, which can differ markedly among various racial and ethnic groups. By integrating these insights into clinical practice, healthcare providers can better address the unique needs of diverse populations, potentially reducing health disparities.

TGx, which integrates toxicology with genomics, has become an essential instrument in health disparities research, providing critical understanding of how environmental factors and genetic predispositions interact to affect health outcomes at both individual and population levels. Through the integration of genomic technologies, conventional drug assessment methodologies, and advanced data analysis techniques, these fields have the potential to significantly impact how new therapeutics are discovered and how clinical populations are understood.

Developments in biological sciences have shed light on both intrinsic and extrinsic elements that influence health and disease, underscoring the necessity for a more holistic and unified approach to research in biomedicine. Numerous factors contribute to the observed differences in health and disease indicators among and within populations, including genetic diversity, geographic context, cultural and psychological influences, behavioral patterns, and the unequal access to resources. These factors interact in complex ways, creating disparities in health outcomes that require multifaceted interventions and a deeper understanding of the underlying mechanisms. A more comprehensive approach that considers the interplay of genetic, environmental, and socioeconomic determinants is crucial for addressing these persistent health disparities and improving the overall well-being of diverse populations (Royal et al., 2021). The Japanese Toxicogenomics Project (TGP) collaborated with the National Institute of Health Sciences, the National Institute of Biomedical Innovation (NIBIO), and numerous pharmaceutical companies to assemble a large array of transcriptome databases. The goal of this project was to develop a toxicogenomics approach, a framework for assessing the safety and toxicity of substances, including drug candidates using the data gathered (Uehara et al., 2010). The initial version of Toxygates, an integrated platform for toxicogenomics data analysis, was released to the general public (Nyström-Persson et al., 2017).

PGx, the study of how an individual's genetic makeup influences their response to drugs, has the potential to play a crucial role in addressing persistent health disparities across racial and ethnic groups. Sickle cell disease, a genetic disorder primarily affecting populations of African, Mediterranean, and Middle Eastern descent, serves as a global prototype for this integrative research. It demonstrates the importance of considering the complex interplay between molecular, epidemiological, and social determinants of health, which collectively contribute to the disproportionate burden of this disease among these populations. This holistic approach is crucial for developing more effective interventions and addressing persistent health disparities. The field of precision medicine, which leverages the analysis of genomic, epigenomic, metabolomic, and microbiome data, has generated interest in exploring the potential role of various biomarkers in explaining racial disparities. PGx examines how genetic differences affect individual responses to drugs, which is essential for precision medicine. It has the potential to either reduce or exacerbate health disparities depending on its implementation (Paetznick & Okoro, 2023). Population PGx emphasizes the importance of understanding genetic variations across different racial and ethnic groups to avoid biases in treatment regimens. This approach can mitigate adverse drug reactions and improve public health outcomes (Jordan et al., 2023). A significant challenge in PGx is the underrepresentation of minority populations in genomic studies, which can lead to health disparities in precision medicine. Increasing diversity in these studies is crucial for developing equitable healthcare solutions (Zhang et al., 2019). Community-engaged PGx, particularly in Indigenous communities, highlights the importance of incorporating cultural values and priorities into research to effectively address health disparities (Claw et al., 2024). Identifying and addressing health disparities at the early stages of PGx research and implementation is vital for achieving equitable health outcomes. This requires a careful examination of the determinants of these disparities and the development of meaningful solutions (Shaaban & Ji, 2023). The integration of TGx and PGx is pivotal in developing personalized medicine approaches aimed at addressing health disparities in vulnerable populations. These fields leverage genetic information to tailor treatments, ensuring that therapies are effective and safe for diverse demographic groups. This personalized approach not only enhances treatment efficacy but also mitigates adverse drug reactions, particularly in populations that have historically been underrepresented in clinical research. Additionally, PGx can be applied more broadly to drug discovery and development, as there is growing evidence that targets that are genomically defined have a higher success rate in clinical development.

1.2 Relevance of Genomics to Health Equity

Genomics extends beyond the traditional focus of genetics, which primarily examines the impact of individual genes or chromosomal changes, to consider the complex interplay between genes, regulatory sequences, and various environmental, social, cultural, and psychosocial factors that can influence an individual's overall health and wellbeing (Hu et al., 2018). This deeper comprehension of the complex nature of genomics has significant ramifications for improving health equity since it emphasizes the necessity of addressing the larger social determinants of health and how they affect the risk of disease and the results of treatment.

The rapid advancements in the field of genomics have opened up new frontiers in the pursuit of personalized and precision medicine, promising to revolutionize healthcare delivery and improve patient outcomes. However, as the potential of genomic technologies becomes increasingly tangible, it is essential to consider their implications for health equity and ensure that the benefits are equitably distributed across diverse populations (Amare et al., 2017). Genomics, as a broader discipline, extends beyond the traditional focus of genetics on individual gene or chromosome changes, and instead examines the complex interactions between genes, regulatory sequences, the environment, and other psychosocial and cultural factors that collectively influence an individual's health (Hu et al., 2018). This holistic approach has the potential to transform the way we understand, prevent, and treat various health conditions, ultimately contributing to the realization of precision public health.

2. TOXICOGENOMICS AND HEALTH DISPARITIES

2.1 Key Concepts in Toxicogenomics

TGx, a rapidly evolving field, combines the principles of toxicology, genomics, and bioinformatics to elucidate the molecular mechanisms underlying chemical-induced biological responses. One of the key concepts in TGx is the use of high-throughput screening techniques to assess the toxicity of a broad range of chemicals. Through the use of techniques like gene expression profiling, proteomics, and metabolomics, scientists can assess how chemicals affect a variety of biological pathways and cellular functions at the same time.

The integration of TGx with conventional drug assessment methodologies has been shown to enhance the ability to predict drug tolerance, identify novel drug targets, and improve the overall efficiency of the drug development process. By leveraging the comprehensive biological data generated through toxicogenomic techniques, researchers can more accurately assess the potential toxicity and efficacy of drug candidates, ultimately leading to the development of safer and more effective pharmaceutical products. The application of TGx to the field of chemical risk assessment has also been a focus of research, with the potential to transform the way toxicity testing and risk assessment are conducted. As described in a report by the National Research Council, the vision for toxicity testing in the 21st century involves a shift from traditional animal-based testing to a greater reliance on high-throughput in vitro screening and computational toxicology (Krewski et al., 2009).

2.2 Genetic Ancestry and Drug Toxicity

In recent years, PGx has attracted a lot of attention as scientists try to understand the intricate relationship between a person's genetic composition and how they react to different medications. The possible impact of genetic heritage on medication toxicity is one component of this field that is especially fascinating. It has long been known that there can be significant variations in the likelihood of certain negative drug reactions among people with different ancestries. This is mostly because single nucleotide polymorphisms, the most prevalent kind of genetic variation in the human genome, can have a significant effect on a drug's pharmacokinetics and pharmacodynamics (Lally et al., 2016).

Researchers have been able to clarify the genetic foundations of these population-specific variations in drug response as our knowledge of the human genome has grown, largely due to programs like the Human Genome Project (McKinnon & Ward, 2003). For example, recent genomics technology has enabled scientists to scan the whole human genome for genetic variations that may affect the way drugs work or work, and many more are likely to emerge in the years to come. Drug toxicity is strongly influenced by genetic heritage; research indicates that Europeans and Americans with mixed ancestry are more likely than East Asians and Oceanians to experience adverse drug-related events. Population-specific pharmacogenomic evaluations are necessary because polygenic risk scores for drug-gene interactions differ among populations.

2.3 Environmental Exposures and Vulnerable Populations

Environmental toxicant exposure is a serious public health issue, especially for vulnerable groups like children, the elderly, and underprivileged communities. These exposures, along with a person's biological predispositions and social vulnerabilities, can have a significant and long-lasting impact on health and well-being throughout their life. This is an issue of increasing importance as scientific advances in toxicogenomics have revealed the complex interplay between genetic factors and environmental exposures, which can amplify health risks for vulnerable populations (Morello-Frosch et al., 2011).

One emerging field that holds promise for understanding and addressing these complex issues is TGx, which explores the interactions between environmental exposures and genetic factors. Recent studies have demonstrated that many environmental pollutants can induce epigenetic modifications, altering gene expression and potentially contributing to disease development (He et al., 2023). Advances in biomedical sciences, including ongoing developments in genomics, proteomics, metabolomics, transcriptomics, nanotechnology, and medical imaging, are providing new quantitative tools for assessing biological response to cumulative environmental exposure, thereby affording expanding opportunities to gain an in-depth understanding of exposure-related events that occur along the pathway from human contact with environmental mixtures to eventual environmentally-induced discomfort, dysfunction, disability, disease, and death (Sexton & Hattis, 2007). These scientific developments underscore the need for a more holistic and equity-focused approach to environmental health policy and practice. By integrating toxicogenomic data with social determinants of health, researchers and policymakers can better identify and mitigate the disproportionate burden of environmental exposures on vulnerable populations. Addressing these complex and multifaceted challenges will require close collaboration and coordination across a diverse range of disciplines, from public health and environmental science to clinical medicine and beyond. For vulnerable populations to be less disproportionately affected by environmental exposures, a thorough understanding of the problems and the implementation of practical solutions will require multidisciplinary teamwork and the integration of expertise from different fields.

2.4 Gene-Environment Interactions in Health Disparities

By studying gene-environment interactions, researchers can unravel disease mechanisms, identify novel genetic variants associated with disease, understand population-level heterogeneity, and inform targeted prevention and treatment strategies. Understanding these interactions will help scientists gain a deeper insight into the complex causes of disease, and thus allow for more targeted and efficient intervention strategies. Furthermore, studying gene-environment interactions can help researchers identify subgroups within populations that are at higher risk for certain conditions, informing public health initiatives and targeted prevention efforts. Ultimately, a comprehensive understanding of how genetic and environmental factors intertwine to influence health is essential for addressing persistent health disparities and improving population-level wellness (Goldenberg et al., 2013). The study's findings demonstrate the variety of individual interpretations of genetic variation, genomic research, and gene-environment interactions, as well as the implications of these interpretations for resolving health disparities. In all focus groups, most participants stated that environmental and social factors contributed more to health disparities than genetics.

2.5 Epigenetic Modifications and Chronic Stress

Anxiety, depression, and post-traumatic stress disorder are among the mental health conditions that are frequently linked to chronic stress. According to recent data, this relationship may be significantly influenced by epigenetic processes like DNA methylation and histone modification. Environmental factors, such as stressful life events, can affect gene expression through epigenetic modifications, which can alter an individual's susceptibility or resilience to stress-related psychopathology over time. These epigenetic modifications may impact the expression of genes related to neurotransmitter systems, stress response, and neural plasticity, ultimately playing a role in the development and progression of mental illnesses. One proposed mechanism by which epigenetic modifications influence depression involves stress-induced changes in chromatin structure within the brain's limbic regions, driving sustained alterations in gene expression that contribute to depressive episodes (Nestler, 2014).

The intricate interplay between epigenetics, the hypothalamic-pituitary-adrenal axis, and early-life stress has been extensively implicated in the development of depression. These studies have highlighted the significant effects of chronic and traumatic stressors occurring at different critical developmental time points, which can lead to long-lasting changes in gene expression and contribute to an individual's vulnerability or resilience to stress-related psychopathologies (Matosin et al., 2017). Preclinical studies have shown a consistent link between the early life environment, DNA methylation changes, and adult stress reactivity and behaviour (Houtepen et al., 2016). The study of epigenetics and its link to chronic stress and psychiatric disorders has significant implications for the field of toxicogenomics, which explores the interactions between environmental exposures, genetic factors, and biological systems.

Exploring the interplay between genetic and environmental factors is particularly relevant in the context of health disparities, where differences in environmental exposures, such as pollution, nutrition, and access to healthcare, as well as differences in genetic factors, may contribute to disparities in disease burden and health outcomes across populations. PGx program implementation necessitates reliable and consistent evidence that can be converted into rules and regulations (Luzum et al. 2021). These can be assembled from PGx resources, including regulatory bodies, networks, consortia, and societies.

2.6 Related Diseases

2.6.1 Air Pollution and Respiratory Diseases

Air pollution is a significant global health concern, with the potential to exacerbate a wide range of respiratory diseases. It is commonly known that air pollutants like particulate matter, O_3, and $(NO)_x$ have a negative impact on lung function and the emergence of chronic respiratory conditions like asthma and COPD. According to several studies, exposure to these air pollutants may exacerbate pre-existing respiratory conditions, increasing the risk of respiratory infections, hospitalization, and lung function. Furthermore, long-term exposure has been linked to the development of new respiratory diseases, underscoring the significant public health burden of air pollution (Balali-Mood et al., 2016). For instance, studies have shown that exposure to air pollutants can interact with certain genes, modulating the expression of specific chronic diseases (Samet, 2020). This suggests that toxicogenomic approaches, which examine the interplay between environmental toxicants and genetic factors, may provide valuable insights into the mechanistic links between air pollution and respiratory diseases. By elucidating how air pollutants influence gene expression and epigenetic changes, researchers can better understand the biological pathways underlying the development and progression of respiratory conditions, ultimately informing more effective prevention and treatment strategies. Surfactant proteins, which play a crucial role in pulmonary host defense, have been identified as a particularly promising target for understanding the relationship between air pollution and respiratory diseases. Previous research has demonstrated that surfactant proteins are subject to epigenetic regulation under various conditions, including exposure to air pollutants (Silveyra & Floros, 2012).

2.6.2 Heavy Metal Exposure and Neurological Disorders

Heavy metal exposure has been increasingly linked to neurological disorders, with PGx providing insights into individual susceptibility and response to these toxicants. According to research, heavy metals like lead, mercury, and cadmium can affect how the brain develops and cause several neurodegenerative diseases through processes like oxidative stress and epigenetic changes. Heavy metals induce oxidative stress, leading to neuronal damage and dysfunction, which is a common pathway in neurodegenerative diseases (Rehman et al., 2021). Exposure to metals like lead can alter gene expression through epigenetic modifications, potentially resulting in cognitive impairments and disorders such as Alzheimer's and Parkinson's disease (Liu et al., 2022). Research indicates that prenatal exposure to heavy metals can lead to developmental delays and long-term neurological issues in children, emphasizing the need for preventive measures (Anesti et al., 2023; Kerna et al., 2024). Focus on heavy metals and their neurotoxic effects is critical, it is also essential to consider the role of other environmental factors and lifestyle choices that may mitigate or exacerbate these risks. Understanding the interplay between genetics and environmental exposures can lead to more effective interventions.

3. PHARMACOGENOMICS AND HEALTH DISPARITIES

3.1 Key Concepts in Pharmacogenomics

By combining genomic methods such as linkage analysis, candidate gene association studies, and genome-wide association studies, physicians can better predict health risks, determine and quantify the dynamics of disease development, and tailor therapeutic protocols to the needs of the individual (Liao & Tsai, 2013).

PGx is particularly important when treating mood disorders, as current psychiatric evaluation and treatment decisions primarily rely on psychiatrists' professional judgment and clinical experience. Genetic markers that influence a person's reaction to psychiatric medications can be found with the use of PGx testing, enabling more individualized and efficient treatment plans. By incorporating pharmacogenomic data into clinical decision-making, medical professionals can minimize the likelihood of adverse reactions, optimize medication selection and dosage, and enhance treatment outcomes for patients with mood disorders. Larger cohort studies and genome-wide association studies have the potential to uncover genetic variables that influence a drug's pharmacology, enabling doctors to customize treatment plans for each patient. Personalized medicine cannot succeed unless precise diagnostic tests are available to identify patients who can benefit from specialized care.

PGx enables the customization of drug therapies based on genetic variations, which can differ significantly among racial and ethnic groups (Jordan et al., 2023). For instance, in oncology, identifying specific PGx variants allows for more effective cancer treatments, reducing the risk of adverse effects and improving patient outcomes (Shriver et al., 2024). Engaging communities, particularly Indigenous populations, in PGx research ensures that their unique genetic and cultural contexts are considered, leading to more relevant health interventions. Community-based approaches can foster trust and improve health outcomes by aligning research with local values and priorities (Claw et al., 2024).

3.2 Genetic Variability in Drug Metabolism

Variability in drug metabolism, a key determinant of therapeutic efficacy and safety, is largely attributed to the genetic diversity observed across different populations. Personalized medicine, which seeks to customize treatment to each patient's distinct genetic profile, is the driving force behind the growth of pharmacogenomics. By enabling more precise dosage, lowering the possibility of adverse effects, and enhancing overall treatment results, this strategy has the potential to completely transform medicine. A person's reaction to a particular medication can be greatly influenced by genetic factors, including differences in the genes encoding transporters, drug targets, and enzymes involved in drug metabolism. These genetic variations may result in differences in how drugs are absorbed, distributed, metabolized, and excreted, which may ultimately impact the drug's pharmacokinetic and pharmacodynamic profiles. In particular, genetic variations can affect the function of drug transporters, which control the flow of drugs into and out of cells, as well as the expression and activity of enzymes involved in drug metabolism. Additionally, genetic variations in drug targets can alter the sensitivity and response to a particular drug (Gupta, 2024).

3.3 Implications for Personalized Medicine

As the field of medicine continues to evolve, the concept of personalized medicine has emerged as a revolutionary approach to healthcare. Instead of using a one-size-fits-all strategy, personalized medicine, sometimes referred to as precision medicine, focuses on adjusting therapeutic and diagnostic procedures to the particular characteristics of each patient. By considering an individual's genetic makeup, lifestyle, and environmental factors, personalized medicine aims to provide more accurate diagnoses, targeted treatments, and improved healthcare outcomes. This personalized approach to medicine has the potential to transform the way we prevent, diagnose, and treat a wide range of medical conditions, from cancer and cardiovascular disease to rare genetic disorders. Personalized medicine holds promise for a future in which healthcare is customized to meet the individual needs of each patient, resulting in more effective and efficient care, through the integration of cutting-edge technology like genome sequencing and data analytics. The key to personalized medicine lies in the ability to harness vast amounts of data generated within the healthcare system, including genetic and genomic information, as well as environmental and regime factors. This thorough comprehension of each person's distinct biological profile enables the creation of more effective and efficient tailored therapies and preventative measures, which eventually improve healthcare results. Targeted therapy is the foundation of contemporary personalized medicine. Having knowledge of the altered pathway and the elements that cause cancer is crucial for targeted therapy. For instance, females with breast cancer who exhibit elevated HER-2 levels are treated with Herceptin.

Apart from genomic data, proteomic data also plays a role in customized medicine. The Human Proteome (HP) Project identifies the profile of every peptide and protein found in clinically healthy individuals and contrasts it with the profile of a diseased individual. The HP Project has become a resource to help clarify biological and molecular activities and enhance disease detection and treatment since it has mapped the protein-based molecular architecture of the human body by defining all 21,000 genes in the known genome.

Metabolomics is a relatively new aspect of personalized medicine that involves the study of tiny molecules or metabolites found in biological systems and cells. Meanwhile, metabolome is a measurement of biological pathways' output, it is frequently thought to be a more accurate indicator of a cell's functional state than other “omics” measurements like proteomics or genomics. The literature has a wealth of information about the potential of personalized medicine. According to one study, advances in fields like routine clinical genomics, artificial intelligence, and large-scale data analysis could lead to personalized medicine revolutionizing healthcare by 2030.

Table 1. Envisioning how PGx affects precision medicine

S.No.	Events	Characteristics	Examples	Area of Interest	Guidelines follow
1	**Genetic Variability in Drug Response**	Different populations have genetic variations affecting drug metabolism, efficacy, and toxicity.	- CYP2C19 polymorphism affecting Clopidogrel response in cardiovascular patients. - TPMT variants affecting Thiopurine toxicity in leukemia treatment.	Pharmacogenetics, Drug Metabolism, Polymorphism	PharmGKB Database, NIH
2	**Personalized Drug Dosing**	Genetic testing helps tailor drug doses to individuals for better efficacy and reduced side effects.	- Warfarin (VKORC1 & CYP2C9) dose adjustments to prevent bleeding risks. - Codeine metabolism (CYP2D6) differences leading to variable pain relief.	Precision Dosing, Therapeutic Window, Biomarkers	FDA, CPIC Guidelines
3	**Adverse Drug Reactions (ADR) Prevention**	Pharmacogenomics helps predict and prevent severe ADRs.	- HLA-B*5701 screening before prescribing Abacavir to prevent hypersensitivity.* - *HLA-B*1502 and Carbamazepine-induced Stevens-Johnson (SJ) Syndrome in Asian individuals.	Drug Safety, Biomarkers, Risk Prediction	Clinical Pharmacogenomics Guidelines
4	**Cancer Pharmacogenomics**	Tumor genetic profiling guides targeted therapy selection.	- Trastuzumab is used to treat HER2-positive breast cancer. - Gefitinib treatment for lung cancer is guided by EGFR mutations.	Targeted Therapy, Biomarker Testing, Companion Diagnostics	NCCN, ASCO Guidelines

continued on following page

Table 1. Continued

S.No.	Events	Characteristics	Examples	Area of Interest	Guidelines follow
5	**Health Disparities in Pharmacogenomics**	Underrepresented populations may lack pharmacogenomic research data, leading to unequal treatment outcomes.	- African American population with different responses to antihypertensive drugs. - Indigenous populations with unique pharmacogenomic profiles.	Genetic Diversity, Clinical Trial Inclusion, Equity in Medicine	FDA, WHO Reports
6	**Regulatory and Ethical Considerations**	Ethical concerns include privacy, data security, and equitable access to genetic testing.	- Direct-to-consumer genetic testing regulations. - Informed consent requirements for pharmacogenomic studies.	Genetic Privacy, Bioethics, Consent in Genomi	FDA, WHO Reports

3.5 Apportionment of Pharmacogenomic Variation

In order to maximize therapeutic efficacy and reduce adverse drug reactions, pharmacogenomics investigates how genetic variation affects the pharmacokinetics and pharmacodynamics of medications (Rollinson et al., 2020). This information allows clinicians to better predict patient responses and tailor drug selection and dosing accordingly, leading to improved treatment outcomes and reduced adverse events (Abdelhalim et al., 2022). The implementation of pharmacogenomic programs is envisaged to provide clinicians with greater certainty of a desired outcome, including the avoidance of underdosing, overdosing, misdosing and adverse drug reactions, which in turn can lead to better health outcomes for patients (McKinnon & Ward, 2003).

3.6 Case Studies: Warfarin Sensitivity and Genetic Variants

Warfarin is a widely used anticoagulant drug, but its clinical use is complicated by the significant variability in individual patient responses. The considerable variability in individual patient response to warfarin anticoagulants complicates its clinical use. The cytochrome P450 2C9 (CYP2C9) and vitamin K epoxide reductase complex subunit 1 genes have polymorphisms that contribute to this variability (Bedewy et al. 2016). Improving patient outcomes, reducing the chance of side effects, and optimizing dosage schedules all depend on an understanding of the genetic influences on warfarin sensitivity. Metabolism and sensitivity to warfarin can be greatly impacted by genetic variations in the CYP2C9 gene. This more powerful S-warfarin enantiomer is metabolized by the main enzyme CYP2C9. This can result in an increased anticoagulant response and a higher risk of bleeding complications. A case study highlighted the significance of genetic testing to guide dosing in these patients by describing a patient with the CYP2C9*3/*4 genotype who needed a low dose of warfarin. Additionally, the VKORC1 gene, which encodes the vitamin K epoxide reductase complex subunit 1, is another key genetic factor influencing warfarin sensitivity. Variants in VKORC1 can affect the enzyme's sensitivity to warfarin, leading to alterations in the anticoagulant response (Lee et al., 2007).

The differences in tamoxifen metabolism between racial groups in patients of breast cancer, highlight the significance of PGx and TGx in comprehending these variations. When it comes to identifying genetic markers that predict drug metabolism and activity, which can vary greatly among ethnic groups, these areas are crucial to optimizing tamoxifen therapy. CYP2D6 is a key enzyme in the metabolism of tamoxifen, which converts it to active metabolites like temazolid. Genetic polymorphisms in CYP2D6 significantly affect the metabolism of tamoxifen. For example, Hispanic populations have a higher prevalence of extensive CYP2D6 metabolisers (EM), resulting in higher levels of endoxifen than non-Hispanic white populations (Rangel et al., 2014). Similarly, in the US and Alaska Native populations, CYP2D6 variation is strongly correlated to endoxifen concentration (Khan et al., 2018). Understanding genetic variation may guide personalized treatment with tamoxifen, improving efficacy and reducing undesirable effects. This is particularly important in understudied populations such as American Indians and Alaska Natives (AIAN) and Asian populations, where specific genetic markers may inform decision-making on treatment.

4. INTEGRATIVE APPROACHES IN GENOMIC RESEARCH

4.1 Combining Toxicogenomics and Pharmacogenomics

The field of genomic research has witnessed remarkable advancements, with the emergence of innovative integrative approaches that have the potential to address pressing health disparities. One such approach is the integration of PGx and TGx, which hold promise in enhancing personalized healthcare and reducing the burden of disease among underserved populations.

The point of delivery into health-care systems, however, presents significant implementation challenges, such as the need to alter current clinical pathways and a significant pharmacogenomics knowledge gap among healthcare professionals as recently a review published in Nature by Pirmohamed, 2023. By using this information, medical practitioners can customize medication regimens and dosages for specific individuals, lowering the possibility of negative drug responses and enhancing treatment results. Similarly, TGx provides important insights into the underlying processes of health inequities by analyzing the connection between genetic variables and an individual's sensitivity to environmental contaminants. Advances in this field can inform public health policies and interventions aimed at mitigating the disproportionate exposure of marginalized communities to environmental hazards. This integrative approach allows researchers to gain deeper insights into the multifaceted nature of health inequities, enabling the design of more targeted and effective interventions to address these persistent challenges. As highlighted in the literature, sickle cell disease serves as a global prototype for this integrative approach, where researchers have leveraged insights from molecular biology, epidemiology, and social determinants to improve treatment and management strategies (Royal et al., 2021).

4.2 Big Data and Multi-Omics in Health Disparities

The rapid advancements in genomics and big data analytics have opened up new frontiers in personalized medicine and public health. Individualizing medical care according to a patient's genetic background, biomarker traits, and additional omics datasets, including transcriptomics, proteomics, and metabolomics, is the idea behind precision medicine. This holistic approach aims to tailor treatments and prevention strategies to individual patients, with the goal of improving health outcomes and reducing health disparities. This approach holds promise in addressing health disparities, as it can enable tailored interventions and therapies that account for individual variability. One particularly promising area within this paradigm is the integration of TGx and PGx. In primary tissues, for example, the biological age of organs (liver, kidneys, etc.) and systems (immune and metabolic systems) can be estimated through molecular profiling employing multi-omics integration, which can also uncover molecular processes of disease progression. Employing multi-omics datasets, researchers can gain deeper insights into the complex interplay between genetics, environment, and health outcomes, especially among underserved and vulnerable populations. The potential of this approach is underscored by recent studies. Big biological datasets have been successfully mined for medical knowledge using integrative data-driven methods, which have found new drug targets and biomarkers. Furthermore, precision public health initiatives driven by big data and predictive analytics can deliver tailored interventions to the right populations at the right time, improving health equity. However, significant challenges remain in translating these research findings into approved medical practices. Despite the potential benefits, challenges such as data integration complexity, high costs, and privacy concerns must be addressed to fully realize the promise of personalized medicine (Desta & Aserese, 2024). Future advancements in technology and methodologies, including the FAIR principles (Findable, Accessible, Interoperable, and Reusable), are essential for enhancing the accessibility and effectiveness of personalized healthcare strategies (Ahmed, 2022). While the integration of these fields offers promising avenues for personalized medicine, it is crucial to remain aware of the ethical implications and potential biases that may arise in data interpretation and application, particularly in underserved populations.

4.3 Role of Precision Medicine in Addressing Disparities

Precision medicine has the potential to significantly address the Social Determinants of Health (SDOH) that contribute to disparities in healthcare outcomes. By integrating SDOH into clinical practice, precision medicine can tailor interventions to individual needs, thereby promoting health equity. SDOH encompasses factors such as socioeconomic status, education, and geographical location, which account for up to 80% of health outcomes (Olden, K. (2024). Disparities in health outcomes are often linked to these determinants, with marginalized groups experiencing worse health due to systemic inequities. Precision medicine can utilize data from diverse populations to identify specific SDOH that affect health outcomes, allowing for targeted interventions (Bhavnani et al., 2023). Algorithms in precision medicine must consider socioeconomic factors, gender, and race to avoid biases and ensure inclusivity. Implementing genomic applications in precision medicine can improve access to preventive care, particularly for underrepresented groups. Addressing SDOH through precision medicine can lead to better health outcomes and reduced morbidity and mortality across various populations.

4.4 Structural Genomics and Drug Binding

The field of structural genomics has revolutionized our understanding of the intricate relationships between genetic variations and their impact on drug efficacy and binding. Advances in the Human Genome Project gave rise to the field of PGx, which has shed light on the genetic variables influencing how each person reacts to drugs (Pilotto et al., 2011). Specifically, pharmacogenomic studies have highlighted the crucial role of genetic variations, such as single nucleotide polymorphisms, in modulating the pharmacokinetics and pharmacodynamics of various drugs (Rollinson et al., 2020). This knowledge has the potential to facilitate a transition from the traditional "one-size-fits-all" approach to a more personalized and precise prescribing paradigm, leading to improved therapeutic outcomes and reduced adverse drug reactions (McKinnon & Ward, 2003). The implementation of pharmacogenomic programs in clinical practice can empower clinicians with greater certainty in predicting the desired therapeutic outcomes, including the avoidance of underdosing, overdosing, misdosing, and adverse drug reactions. This is particularly relevant in the treatment of complex and challenging conditions, such as treatment-resistant schizophrenia, where genetic factors play a significant role in determining the efficacy and safety of antipsychotic medications (Lally et al., 2016). Moreover, the application of structural genomics and pharmacogenomics has been instrumental in the development of targeted therapies, particularly in the field of oncology, where genetic biomarkers have been used to guide the selection of appropriate treatments (Matosin, N., Cruceanu, C., & Binder, E. B. (2017)). One of the key tools in this field is SNPdrug3D, a platform that maps genetic variations affecting drug binding, aiding in the prediction of pharmacogenetic effects and informing drug development. (McKinnon & Ward, 2003). The role of heredity in modifying individual response to drugs has been known for over six decades, but the Human Genome Project and subsequent technical innovations have dramatically accelerated our understanding of this phenomenon (McKinnon & Ward, 2003). SNPdrug3D plays a crucial role in this transition by providing a comprehensive mapping of genetic variations that can influence drug binding and, by extension, pharmacokinetics and pharmacodynamics. This information can be used to inform the development of targeted therapies and guide clinicians in selecting the most appropriate treatment options for individual patients, based on their genetic profiles. The old idea of one disease/one drug is no longer viable due to the quick advancements in the identification of human pharmacogenetic variations and the finding of genes that predispose people to certain diseases.

5. ETHICAL, SOCIAL, AND POLICY IMPLICATIONS

5.1 Data Diversity and Inclusion in Genomic Research

Genomic research has been instrumental in advancing our understanding of human genetics, disease mechanisms, and personalized medicine. However, the field has faced significant challenges in ensuring equitable representation and inclusion of diverse populations. The lack of diversity in genomic datasets has led to biases and gaps in our understanding of genetic variation across different ancestral and geographical backgrounds. This lack of diversity in genomic research represents a significant issue that needs to be addressed to ensure the benefits of genomic advances are equitably distributed and to gain a more comprehensive understanding of human genetic diversity and its implications for health and disease.

One of the primary reasons for the overrepresentation of European ancestry in genomic studies is the preference of researchers for a more homogeneous pool of participants, which can reduce genetic variance and simplify data analysis. However, this approach comes at the cost of excluding the genetic diversity that exists within and across human populations, which is crucial for understanding the full spectrum of human health and disease (Baker, 2019). Furthermore, members of underrepresented groups may face barriers to accessing genomic testing or may be reluctant to participate due to historical mistrust or lack of understanding of the potential benefits of such research. To address these challenges, researchers need to actively engage with diverse communities, tailor their outreach and recruitment strategies, and work to build trust and increase the representation of underrepresented groups in genomic studies (Matshabane et al., 2022). The NIH National Human Genome Research Institute's strategic vision calls for a commitment to the systematic inclusion of ancestrally diverse and underrepresented individuals in major genomic studies. The problem of data inclusiveness and diversity in genomic research is being addressed by programs like the "All of Us" research initiative and the "Global Alliance for Genomics and Health," but more coordinated efforts are required to guarantee that everyone may benefit from these advancements.

5.2 Policy Recommendations for Equitable Genomic Research

As genomic research continues to advance, it is crucial that researchers and policymakers prioritize the ethical and equitable implementation of these technologies. Ensuring diverse participation in genomic studies is essential to guarantee that the benefits of this scientific progress are accessible to all populations, regardless of their background or societal status. Concerted efforts must be made to address the historical and persistent exclusion of marginalized groups, including Indigenous communities, from genomic research endeavors. This is necessary to empower and uplift these underrepresented populations, enabling them to fully participate in and reap the potential rewards of advancements in genomic science.

One key recommendation is for researchers to work closely with Indigenous communities to develop research protocols that align with their cultural values and governance structures. This collaborative approach can help build trust, ensure that research is conducted in an ethical manner, and empower Indigenous peoples to have a greater say in how their genetic data is used. Additionally, funding bodies and scientific institutions should allocate resources to support Indigenous-led research initiatives and capacity building within these communities (Garrison et al., 2019). Another important policy consideration is the need for robust data governance frameworks that protect the privacy and sovereignty of genetic data, particularly for vulnerable populations. Genomic data has immense potential for both individual and community-level benefits, but if not managed responsibly, it can also pose significant risks, such as discrimination and the exploitation of marginalized groups. Policymakers should work closely with diverse stakeholders to develop data governance guidelines that balance the scientific and societal benefits of genomic research with the rights and interests of research participants.

6. BIOETHICAL IMPLICATIONS OF TGx And PGx

The integration of genomics, proteomics, and other high-throughput molecular technologies into toxicology has transformed our understanding of how human and environmental exposures affect human health and the environment. A strong ethical framework is needed to guide the creation and use of these powerful biological tools, given the potential for misuse and the need for responsible innovation (Hoffmann et al., 2023; Carter et al., 2024). These approaches generate huge amounts of data, which requires careful management and poses problems of data ownership, privacy and security (Ormond & Cho, 2014). (Hoffmann et al., 2023; Wolpe & Rommelfanger, 2017). Extensive data sets generated by TGx and PGx studies have the potential to reveal sensitive information about individuals, including their predisposition to certain diseases or adverse effects due to specific environmental exposure. The protection of privacy and confidentiality of individuals in the context of such data-intensive research is paramount, requiring strong data security measures and compliance with ethical guidelines on data sharing and access (McGuire et al., 2008). Proteomic studies, for instance, frequently entail the collection of human tissues, which presents issues with ownership, commercialization, and the possibility of unforeseen consequences. Furthermore, even when data is anonymized, the incorporation of proteomic and genomic information into extensive databases raises the possibility of re-identification of specific individuals. This emphasizes how crucial it is to have strict data protection laws and open lines of communication with study participants. But these developments also bring up important bioethical issues that need careful thought. Fairness, accountability, and the possibility of bias are raised by the growing reliance on algorithms to evaluate massive datasets and automate decision-making procedures (Mittelstadt, 2019). Discriminatory results in risk assessments or clinical interventions can result from algorithmic bias, which can be caused by faulty algorithms or biased training data. The Environmental Genome Project (EGP), for example, seeks to find genetic variations that affect how people react to environmental exposures. Although this could lead to better public health outcomes, there is a chance that underprivileged communities won't benefit from the research, which would exacerbate already-existing health disparities. Although this information can help guide focused interventions, it also presents moral dilemmas regarding the equitable application of such interventions (Calluori et al., 2024). Addressing algorithmic bias requires careful attention to data quality, algorithm design and validation, ensuring that these tools are fair, equitable and do not perpetuate existing health inequalities.

Proteogenomics, which integrates genomic, transcriptomic and proteomic data, poses unique ethical challenges around informed consent. Participants in proteomic studies shall be fully informed of the possible uses of their samples, including the possibility of unexpected findings or data being commercially exploited. Moreover, the use of human samples in proteomic research requires careful consideration of cultural and social norms, especially in international co-operation. Researchers must ensure that sampling procedures are carried out in a manner which respects the rights and dignity of all persons participating in the survey. The bioethical implications of TGx and PGx are complex and multifaceted. These technologies have great potential to advance our understanding of the environment and health at work, but their potential benefits need to be carefully balanced against the risks of discrimination, unfairness and abuse.

7. NAVIGATING THE COMPLEXITIES AND FUTURE DIRECTIONS

This chapter provides a brief overview of the many multi-omics approaches used in human disease research, with an emphasis on the data integration, applicability, difficulties, and future development directions of TGx and PGx. The advancements in the field of genomics over the past few years hold great promises for reshaping healthcare and enhancing methods of disease prevention. Although genomic discoveries have advanced, their implementation in clinical practice and health policy has been slow, particularly in terms of confronting health inequalities. TGx and PGx, two subfields of genomics, hold promise in addressing these disparities, but their impact has been limited by a lack of diversity and inclusion in research and translation to policy.

Diversity and inclusion are critical in genomics research, as genomic factors can have differential impacts across populations. Researchers must prioritize the inclusion of diverse participants from various ancestral and geographical backgrounds to ensure the relevance and accessibility of genomic advancements to all people.

As these fields continue to advance, there are both significant opportunities and persistent challenges in effectively leveraging these approaches to address health disparities. One noteworthy challenge is the need for greater diversity and inclusion in genomics research. Results of toxicogenomics and pharmacogenomics studies must be applicable and useful to all populations, particularly those historically under-represented in biomedical research, and this requires that a more representative sample of participants from different racial, ethnic and socio-economic backgrounds be selected.

Historically, the majority of participants in genomic studies have been of European descent, leading to concerns that findings may not be generalizable to other populations. To address this, initiatives like the NHGRI's Population Architecture using Genomics and Epidemiology, Human Heredity and Health in Africa, and Centers for Common Disease Genomics programs have sought to proactively diversify the genomic data landscape by including more participants from underrepresented racial and ethnic groups. These efforts aim to ensure that the benefits of advancements in TGx and PGx can be equitably distributed and accessible to all communities.

Overcoming barriers to participation from underrepresented groups is crucial, as these populations may face disproportionate burdens from environmental exposures and adverse drug reactions. Racial and ethnic minorities are among the underrepresented groups that frequently face systemic obstacles that deny them access to high-quality healthcare and study participation. It is crucial to address these differences in research participation to guarantee that the conclusions drawn from TGx and PGx studies are useful and applicable to all populations. Another critical obstacle is the complex intersection of genetic, environmental, and social determinants of health. The interplay between these factors can create significant challenges in interpreting and translating research findings into effective interventions. Disentangling the relative contributions of genetics, environmental exposures, and social determinants, such as socioeconomic status, access to healthcare, and cultural beliefs, is crucial for developing targeted strategies to address health disparities.

Another approach to addressing this gap is to foster a comprehensive research agenda that streamlines the translation of genomic discoveries into health practice. This continuum of translation research includes four phases: discovery, evaluation, implementation, and dissemination. Specifically, the discovery phase involves identifying novel genomic markers or targets that could have implications for health and disease. The evaluation phase then assesses the clinical validity and utility of these genomic findings through rigorous study designs. The implementation phase focuses on integrating genomic information into clinical workflows and decision-making, while the dissemination phase ensures that these advances are effectively communicated to healthcare providers, policymakers, and the broader public. This comprehensive approach can help bridge the gap between genomic research and its real-world impact on health disparities. By prioritizing diversity and inclusion throughout this research continuum, researchers and policymakers can ensure that the benefits of TGx and PGx are accessible to all populations, ultimately reducing health disparities.

8. CONCLUSION

The emerging fields of TGx and PGx, which explore the complex interplay between genetic makeup and an individual's responses to drugs and chemical exposures, hold immense promise to revolutionize healthcare delivery and combat long standing health disparities. By harnessing the power of genomic technologies, these disciplines can enable more personalized, targeted, and effective interventions that better address the unique needs and characteristics of individuals from diverse backgrounds. This holds immense promise for reducing the burden of disease and promoting greater health equity across populations, as tailored treatments and preventive strategies become more accessible and responsive to the genetic and environmental factors that contribute to health disparities.

TGx, the study of how genetic variation influences an individual's susceptibility to toxic substances, has the potential to transform pre-clinical drug development and post-market safety surveillance. By identifying genetic markers that predispose individuals to adverse drug reactions or environmental toxicities, toxicogenomic approaches can facilitate the design of safer and more tailored therapies, reducing the risk of harmful side effects. As described in Accelerating Drug Discovery, the integration of toxicogenomics in the drug discovery process can lead to the prospective identification of true responders, ultimately saving healthcare resources and restoring consumer trust. Likewise, the secret to more individualized and successful treatment plans lie in pharmacogenomics, the study of how genetic variables affect a person's reaction to drugs. Pharmacogenomic insights can help doctors choose the best drugs and dosage plans for each patient by clarifying the genetic foundations of drug metabolism and target engagement, reducing the chance of therapy failure or side events.

REFERENCES

Abdelhalim, H., Berber, A., Lodi, M., Jain, R., Nair, A., Pappu, A., Patel, K., Venkat, V., Venkatesan, C., Wable, R., Dinatale, M., Fu, A., Iyer, V., Kalove, I., Kleyman, M., Koutsoutis, J., Menna, D., Paliwal, M., Patel, N., & Ahmed, Z. (2022). Artificial Intelligence, Healthcare, Clinical Genomics, and Pharmacogenomics Approaches in Precision Medicine. *Frontiers in Genetics*, *13*, 929736. Advance online publication. DOI: 10.3389/fgene.2022.929736 PMID: 35873469

Ahmed, Z. (2022). Multi-omics strategies for personalized and predictive medicine: Past, current, and future translational opportunities. *Emerging Topics in Life Sciences*, *2*(2), 215–225. DOI: 10.1042/ETLS20210244 PMID: 35234253

Amare, A. T., Schubert, K. O., & Baune, B. T. (2017). Pharmacogenomics in the treatment of mood disorders: Strategies and Opportunities for personalized psychiatry. *The EPMA Journal*, *3*(3), 211–227. DOI: 10.1007/s13167-017-0112-8 PMID: 29021832

Anesti, O., Papaioannou, N., Gabriel, C., Karakoltzidis, A., Dzhedzheia, V., Petridis, I., Stratidakis, A., Dickinson, M., Horvat, M., Snoj Tratnik, J., Tsatsakis, A., Karakitsios, S., & Sarigiannis, D. A. (2023). An exposome connectivity paradigm for the mechanistic assessment of the effects of prenatal and early life exposure to metals on neurodevelopment. *Frontiers in Public Health*, *10*, 871218. Advance online publication. DOI: 10.3389/fpubh.2022.871218 PMID: 36699871

Baker, B. (2019). Tackling the Lack of Diversity in Human Genome Collection. *Bioscience*, biz067. Advance online publication. DOI: 10.1093/biosci/biz067

Balali-Mood, M., Ghorani-Azam, A., & Riahi-Zanjani, B. (2016). Effects of air pollution on human health and practical measures for prevention in Iran. *Journal of Research in Medical Sciences : the Official Journal of Isfahan University of Medical Sciences*, *1*(1), 65. DOI: 10.4103/1735-1995.189646 PMID: 27904610

Bedewy, A. M. L., Showeta, S., Mostafa, M. H., & Kandil, L. S. (2016). The Influence of CYP2C9 and VKORC1 Gene Polymorphisms on the Response to Warfarin in Egyptians. *Indian Journal of Hematology & Blood Transfusion : An Official Journal of Indian Society of Hematology and Blood Transfusion*, *2*(2), 328–336. DOI: 10.1007/s12288-016-0725-4 PMID: 29622878

Bhavnani, S. K., Zhang, W., Bao, D., Raji, M., Ajewole, V., Hunter, R., Kuo, Y.-F., Schmidt, S., Pappadis, M. R., Smith, E., Bokov, A., Reistetter, T., Visweswaran, S., & Downer, B. (2023). *Subtyping Social Determinants of Health in*All of Us*: Network Analysis and Visualization Approach.* https://doi.org/DOI: 10.1101/2023.01.27.23285125

Calluori, S., Heimke, K. K., Caga-anan, C., Kaufman, D., Mechanic, L. E., & McAllister, K. A. (2024). Ethical, Legal, and Social Implications of Gene-Environment Interaction Research. *Genetic Epidemiology, 1*. Advance online publication. DOI: 10.1002/gepi.22591 PMID: 39315585

Carter, B. J., Jafry, M. Z., Siddiqi, A. D., Rogova, A., Liaw, W., & Reitzel, L. R. (2024). Incorporation of social determinants of health into health care practice: A strategy to address health disparities. In *Comprehensive Precision Medicine* (pp. 363–382). Elsevier., DOI: 10.1016/B978-0-12-824010-6.00016-2

Claw, K. G., Dorr, C. R., & Woodahl, E. L. (2024). Implementing community-engaged pharmacogenomics in Indigenous communities. *Nature Communications*, *1*(1), 920. Advance online publication. DOI: 10.1038/s41467-024-45032-5 PMID: 38296967

Desta, G. M., & Aserese, M. B. (2024). *Revolutionizing Personalized Medicine: Synergy with Multi-Omics Data Generation, Main Hurdles, and Future Perspectives.* https://doi.org/DOI: 10.20944/preprints202409.0196.v1

Garrison, N. A., Hudson, M., Ballantyne, L. L., Garba, I., Martinez, A., Taualii, M., Arbour, L., Caron, N. R., & Rainie, S. C. (2019). Genomic Research Through an Indigenous Lens: Understanding the Expectations. *Annual Review of Genomics and Human Genetics*, *1*(1), 495–517. DOI: 10.1146/annurev-genom-083118-015434 PMID: 30892943

Goldenberg, A. J., Hartmann, C. D., Morello, L., Brooks, S., Colón-Zimmermann, K., & Marshall, P. A. (2013). Gene–environment interactions and health inequalities: Views of underserved communities. *Journal of Community Genetics*, *4*(4), 425–434. DOI: 10.1007/s12687-013-0143-3 PMID: 23494820

Gupta, S. P. (2024). Mathematical models in drug target analysis: pharmacokinetic and pharmacodynamic approach. In *Futuristic Trends in Contemporary Mathematics & Applications Volume 3 Book 4* (pp. 123–133). Iterative International Publisher, Selfypage Developers Pvt Ltd. DOI: 10.58532/V3BBCM4P2CH3

He, X., Liu, J., & Li, G. (2023). Editorial: Role of epigenetics in environmental pollution associated diseases. *Frontiers in Genetics*, *14*, 1266714. Advance online publication. DOI: 10.3389/fgene.2023.1266714 PMID: 37600665

Hoffmann, S. A., Diggans, J., Densmore, D., Dai, J., Knight, T., Leproust, E., Boeke, J. D., Wheeler, N., & Cai, Y. (2023). Safety by design: Biosafety and biosecurity in the age of synthetic genomics. *iScience*, *3*(3), 106165. DOI: 10.1016/j.isci.2023.106165 PMID: 36895643

Houtepen, L. C., Vinkers, C. H., Carrillo-Roa, T., Hiemstra, M., van Lier, P. A., Meeus, W., Branje, S., Heim, C. M., Nemeroff, C. B., Mill, J., Schalkwyk, L. C., Creyghton, M. P., Kahn, R. S., Joëls, M., Binder, E. B., & Boks, M. P. M. (2016). Genome-wide DNA methylation levels and altered cortisol stress reactivity following childhood trauma in humans. *Nature Communications*, *1*(1), 10967. Advance online publication. DOI: 10.1038/ncomms10967 PMID: 26997371

Hu, J., Yu, L., Modanloo, S., Zhou, Y., & Yang, Y. (2018). A theoretical framework for interaction of nursing discipline with genetics and genomics. *International Journal of Nursing Sciences*, *4*(4), 336–342. DOI: 10.1016/j.ijnss.2018.08.004 PMID: 31406845

Jordan, I. K., Sharma, S., & Mariño-Ramírez, L. (2023). Population Pharmacogenomics for Health Equity. *Genes*, *10*(10), 1840. DOI: 10.3390/genes14101840 PMID: 37895188

Kerna, N. A., Holets, H. M., Anderson, I. I. J.II, Flores, J. V., Pruitt, K. D., McKee, D., Carsrud, N. D. V., Ngwu, D. C., Nnake, I., Chawla, S., Nwokorie, U., Azi, C. I., Jomsky, B. M., Ukachukwu, C. A., Odefemi, O. F., Egli, A., Obi, M. O., & Ikokwu, O. D. (2024). Heavy Metals and Human Health: From Neurological Disorders to Developmental Delays. *European Journal of Ecology. Biology and Agriculture*, *3*(3), 152–184. DOI: 10.59324/ejeba.2024.1(3).12

Khan, B. A., Robinson, R., Fohner, A. E., Muzquiz, L. I., Schilling, B. D., Beans, J. A., Olnes, M. J., Trawicki, L., Frydenlund, H., Laukes, C., Beatty, P., Phillips, B., Nickerson, D., Howlett, K., Dillard, D. A., Thornton, T. A., Thummel, K. E., & Woodahl, E. L. (2018). Cytochrome P450 Genetic Variation Associated with Tamoxifen Biotransformation in American Indian and Alaska Native People. *Clinical and Translational Science*, *3*(3), 312–321. DOI: 10.1111/cts.12542 PMID: 29436156

Krewski, D., Andersen, M. E., Mantus, E., & Zeise, L. (2009). Toxicity Testing in the 21st Century: Implications for Human Health Risk Assessment. *Risk Analysis*, *4*(4), 474–479. DOI: 10.1111/j.1539-6924.2008.01150.x PMID: 19144067

Lally, J., Gaughran, F., Timms, P., & Curran, S. (2016). Treatment-resistant schizophrenia: Current insights on the pharmacogenomics of antipsychotics. *Pharmacogenomics and Personalized Medicine*, *9*, 117–129. DOI: 10.2147/PGPM.S115741 PMID: 27853387

Lee, S.-Y., Nam, M.-H., Kim, J. S., & Kim, J.-W. (2007). A Case Report of a Patient Carrying CYP2C9*3/4 Genotype with Extremely Low Warfarin Dose Requirement. *Journal of Korean Medical Science*, *3*(3), 557. DOI: 10.3346/jkms.2007.22.3.557 PMID: 17596671

Liao, W.-L., & Tsai, F.-J. (2013). Personalized medicine: A paradigm shift in healthcare. *Biomedicine (Taipei)*, *2*(2), 66–72. DOI: 10.1016/j.biomed.2012.12.005

Liu, M., Liu, R., Wang, R., Ba, Y., Yu, F., Deng, Q., & Huang, H. (2022). Lead-induced neurodevelopmental lesion and epigenetic landscape: Implication in neurological disorders. *Journal of Applied Toxicology*, *9*(9), 1256–1271. DOI: 10.1002/jat.4419 PMID: 36433892

Luzum, J. A., Petry, N., Taylor, A. K., Van Driest, S. L., Dunnenberger, H. M., & Cavallari, L. H. (2021). Moving Pharmacogenetics Into Practice: It's All About the Evidence! *Clinical Pharmacology &amp. Therapeutics*, *3*(3), 649–661. DOI: 10.1002/cpt.2327 PMID: 34101169

Matshabane, O. P., Whitted, C. G., & Koehly, L. M. (2022). Addressing diversity and inclusion challenges in global neuro-psychiatric and behavioral genomics research. *Frontiers in Genetics*, *13*, 1021649. Advance online publication. DOI: 10.3389/fgene.2022.1021649 PMID: 36583023

McGuire, A. L., Caulfield, T., & Cho, M. K. (2008). Research ethics and the challenge of whole-genome sequencing. *Nature Reviews. Genetics*, *2*(2), 152–156. DOI: 10.1038/nrg2302 PMID: 18087293

McKinnon, R. A., & Ward, M. B. (2003). The Emergence of Pharmacogenomics. *Journal of Pharmacy Practice and Research*, 2(2), 133–137. DOI: 10.1002/jppr2003332133

Mittelstadt, B. (2019). The Ethics of Biomedical 'Big Data' Analytics. Philosophy &amp. *Philosophy & Technology*, *1*(1), 17–21. DOI: 10.1007/s13347-019-00344-z

Nestler, E. J. (2014). Epigenetic Mechanisms of Depression. *JAMA Psychiatry*, *4*(4), 454. DOI: 10.1001/jamapsychiatry.2013.4291 PMID: 24499927

Nyström-Persson, J., Natsume-Kitatani, Y., Igarashi, Y., Satoh, D., & Mizuguchi, K. (2017). Interactive Toxicogenomics: Gene set discovery, clustering and analysis in Toxygates. *Scientific Reports*, *1*(1), 1390. Advance online publication. DOI: 10.1038/s41598-017-01500-1 PMID: 28469246

Olden, K. (2024). Social determinants of health: How social and environmental factors affect human health. In *Comprehensive Precision Medicine* (pp. 355–362). Elsevier., DOI: 10.1016/B978-0-12-824010-6.00007-1

Ormond, K. E., & Cho, M. K. (2014). Translating Personalized Medicine Using New Genetic Technologies in Clinical Practice: The Ethical Issues. *Personalized Medicine*, *2*(2), 211–222. DOI: 10.2217/pme.13.104 PMID: 25221608

Paetznick, C., & Okoro, O. (2023). The Intersection between Pharmacogenomics and Health Equity: A Case Example. *Pharmacy (Basel, Switzerland)*, *6*(6), 186. DOI: 10.3390/pharmacy11060186 PMID: 38133461

Pilotto, A., Panza, F., & Seripa, D. (2011). Pharmacogenetics in Geriatric Medicine: Challenges and Opportunities for Clinical Practice. *Current Drug Metabolism*, *7*(7), 621–634. DOI: 10.2174/138920011796504545 PMID: 21495974

Pirmohamed, M. (2023). Pharmacogenomics: Current status and future perspectives. *Nature Reviews. Genetics*, *6*(6), 350–362. DOI: 10.1038/s41576-022-00572-8 PMID: 36707729

Rangel, L. B. A., Taraba, J. L., Frei, C. R., Smith, L., Rodriguez, G., & Kuhn, J. G. (2014). Pharmacogenomic diversity of tamoxifen metabolites and estrogen receptor genes in Hispanics and non-Hispanic whites with breast cancer. *Breast Cancer Research and Treatment*, *3*(3), 571–580. DOI: 10.1007/s10549-014-3191-4 PMID: 25395315

Rehman, Q., Rehman, K., & Akash, M. S. H. (2021). Heavy Metals and Neurological Disorders: From Exposure to Preventive Interventions. In *Emerging Contaminants and Associated Treatment Technologies* (pp. 69–87). Springer International Publishing. http://dx.doi.org/DOI: 10.1007/978-3-030-66376-6_4

Rollinson, V., Turner, R., & Pirmohamed, M. (2020). Pharmacogenomics for Primary Care: An Overview. *Genes*, *11*(11), 1337. DOI: 10.3390/genes11111337 PMID: 33198260

Royal, C. D. M., Babyak, M., Shah, N., Srivatsa, S., Stewart, K. A., Tanabe, P., Wonkam, A., & Asnani, M. (2021). Sickle cell disease is a global prototype for integrative research and healthcare. *Advanced Genetics*, *1*(1), e10037. Advance online publication. DOI: 10.1002/ggn2.10037 PMID: 36618444

Samet, J. M. (2020). Air Pollution: Adverse Effects and Disease Burden. In *Health of People, Health of Planet and Our Responsibility* (pp. 63–78). Springer International Publishing. http://dx.doi.org/DOI: 10.1007/978-3-030-31125-4_6

Sexton, K., & Hattis, D. (2007). Assessing Cumulative Health Risks from Exposure to Environmental Mixtures—Three Fundamental Questions. *Environmental Health Perspectives*, *5*(5), 825–832. DOI: 10.1289/ehp.9333 PMID: 17520074

Shaaban, S., & Ji, Y. (2023). Pharmacogenomics and health disparities, are we helping? *Frontiers in Genetics*, *14*, 1099541. Advance online publication. DOI: 10.3389/fgene.2023.1099541 PMID: 36755573

Shriver, S. P., Adams, D., McKelvey, B. A., McCune, J. S., Miles, D., Pratt, V. M., Ashcraft, K., McLeod, H. L., Williams, H., & Fleury, M. E. (2024). Overcoming Barriers to Discovery and Implementation of Equitable Pharmacogenomic Testing in Oncology. *Journal of Clinical Oncology*, *10*(10), 1181–1192. DOI: 10.1200/JCO.23.01748 PMID: 38386947

Silveyra, P., & Floros, J. (2012). Air pollution and epigenetics: Effects on SP-A and innate host defence in the lung. *Swiss Medical Weekly*. Advance online publication. DOI: 10.4414/smw.2012.13579 PMID: 22553125

Uehara, T., Ono, A., Maruyama, T., Kato, I., Yamada, H., Ohno, Y., & Urushidani, T. (2010). The Japanese toxicogenomics project: Application of toxicogenomics. *Molecular Nutrition &amp. Food Research*, 2(2), 218–227. DOI: 10.1002/mnfr.200900169 PMID: 20041446

Zhang, H., De, T., Zhong, Y., & Perera, M. A. (2019). The Advantages and Challenges of Diversity in Pharmacogenomics: Can Minority Populations Bring Us Closer to Implementation? *Clinical Pharmacology &amp. Therapeutics*, 2(2), 338–349. DOI: 10.1002/cpt.1491 PMID: 31038731

Chapter 7
Exposome Insights to Action A Unified Call for Cancer Prevention, and a Vision for Precision Prevention

Merve Saide Uzunoglu
https://orcid.org/0000-0001-9115-9305
University of Health Sciences Türkiye, Turkey

Sümeyya Çapuk
https://orcid.org/0000-0003-3883-1419
Faculty of Medicine, Adiyaman University, Turkey

Aylin Seher Uzunoglu
https://orcid.org/0000-0003-0065-180X
University of Health Sciences Türkiye, Turkey

Sevgi Kalkanli Taş
https://orcid.org/0000-0001-5288-6040
Faculty of Medicine, University of Health Sciences Türkiye, Turkey

ABSTRACT

Cancer exposomics moves from data acquisition to actionable interventions through a multi-step, integrative approach that spans precise exposure assessment, mechanistic insight generation, and the translation the results into targeted prevention and treatment strategies. Comprehensive exposure assessment is performed by capturing external environmental factors and internal exposures using advanced tools

DOI: 10.4018/979-8-3373-5796-6.ch007

Copyright © 2026, IGI Global Scientific Publishing. Copying or distributing in print or electronic forms without written permission of IGI Global Scientific Publishing is prohibited.

which is accomplished by combining traditional methods with omic technologies, metabolomics, genomics, transcriptomics, and proteomics to elucidate the pathways by which environmental exposures modulate disease risk and progression. Cancer exposomics its ethical dimensions demand rigorous protections around consent, privacy, and responsible communication. This chapter explores the translational potential of exposomic science, emphasizing its ability to shape personalized cancer prevention strategies. It considers ethical, legal, and societal implications (ELSI), the role of public and community engagement, and culminates with a unified, multilevel call to action for cancer prevention.

INTRODUCTION

The exposome is a term used to describe the overall environmental exposures, both external and internal, that an individual experiences from conception to death, including exogenous agents, such as pollutants, diet, radiation, and chemicals, as well as endogenous processes, such as metabolism, inflammation, and the microbiome. Most conventional epidemiological studies have underestimated the multidimensionality of exposures by examining one or a few carcinogens. By contrast, cancer exposomics is a comprehensive approach that incorporates various modern tools of analytic technology and omics research, such as genomics, epigenomics, transcriptomics, proteomics, and metabolomics, to describe the dynamic interaction of environmental factors and biological responses that contribute to the process of carcinogenesis (Bessonneau & Rudel, 2019). The integration of nanotechnology into environmental monitoring provides innovative approaches to understanding the exposome. Nanoparticle-based sensors are being developed to detect environmental toxins with high sensitivity and specificity, thereby enabling real-time monitoring of hazardous exposures (Justino et al., 2017; Koedrith et al., 2015). This technological advancement opens a new pathway for personalized public health interventions by allowing for the timely identification and mitigation of exposure risks based on individual profiles and environmental data (Yarima et al., 2020).

The idea behind cancer exposomics and environmental factors that cause cancer is that harmful exposures, whether they are chemical, physical, or biological, build up over time and cause molecular changes that lead to the main signs of cancer. This approach with many parts emerged concerning because it has been shown that gene-environment interactions are very important for determining the risk of getting cancer. By combining data on environmental exposure with sensitive molecular biomarkers and advanced data analytics, we have been able to better identify early events in carcinogenesis better. This gives us a chance to intervene and prevent cancer early on (Herceg et al., 2018).

As exposome research aims to map the totality of environmental influences on cancer risk, it raises significant ethical considerations regarding participant rights, data management, and the potential consequences of findings. The ethical challenges involve ensuring participant autonomy, making informed consent crucial, as participants must understand the nature of the research and the potential risks associated with the use of their data in large-scale studies (Safarlou et al., 2023). The use of big data and biomonitoring raises concerns about the confidentiality of personal health information, requiring robust data protection measures (D'Adamo et al., 2021). Ethical dilemmas arise when research findings may not lead to actionable health interventions, potentially causing distress among participants who receive ambiguous results. There is a risk of bias in exposome research, which could exacerbate health disparities if certain populations are underrepresented in studies (Lewis et al., 2020; Safarlou et al., 2023).

To fully realize the transformative potential of exposome research in cancer prevention, it is essential to foster collaboration among scientists, ethicists, policymakers, and communities. This collaboration must be grounded in transparency, trust, and shared commitment to equity and public benefit. By addressing ethical concerns proactively and inclusively, we can ensure that science advances responsibly while maximizing its societal impact.This chapter also explores the translational potential of exposomic science, emphasizing its ability to shape personalized cancer prevention strategies while concluding with a multi-level call to action, spanning individual, institutional, and policy levels, and a forward-looking vision for precision prevention that integrates ethical integrity with scientific innovation. It considers ethical, legal, and societal implications (ELSI), the role of public and community engagement, and culminates with a unified, multilevel call to action for cancer prevention.

THE CONCEPT AND EVOLUTION OF CANCER EXPOSOMICS

Cancer exposomics is based on the concept that the traditional risk assessment model based on genotype and targeted exposure, does not cover the complete etiological picture of cancer occurrence. Alternatively, risk for cancer is considered on the basis of lifelong exposures that influence cellular homeostasis and thus regulate fundamental biological processes. The exposome includes exogenous agents (air pollutants, pesticides, radiation, industrial chemicals, dietary mutagens) and endogenous factors (metabolic by-products, inflammation, oxidative stress), with the combination resulting in a molecular signature that contributes to tumorigenesis (Patierno, 2020; Young et al., 2024; Sharif & Ooi, 2024).

Exposomics has changed from being a theoretical framework to being used in real-world research over the past ten years. Biological samples can now be tested for thousands of chemicals and their metabolites using advanced high-resolution mass spectrometry, nuclear magnetic resonance spectroscopy, and omics platforms that are becoming more and more integrated. These technologies make it possible to find and count biomarkers that show both recent and long-term exposures without bias (Balcells et al., 2023; Neveu et al., 2019). When combined with traditional epidemiologic methods, this large amount of molecular data gives a full picture of the outside and inside factors that lead to cancer (Juarez et al., 2018; Wan et al., 2025). Exposomics is transitioning from data collection to actionable interventions. The translational goals of exposomics focus on leveraging these insights to inform public health policies and personalized medicine strategies.

MEASURING THE EXPOSOME: OMICS TECHNOLOGIES AND DATA INTEGRATION

A key challenge inherent in cancer exposomics is the accurate measurement of an individual's complete exposure history. New methods like exposome-wide association studies (ExWAS) have made it easier to combine different types of exposure data with molecular profiles. These methods use multi-omics technologies to create detailed exposure maps and then connect these maps to disease outcomes (Balcells et al., 2023; Juarez et al., 2018). Researchers can now use high-resolution analytical platforms to test blood, urine, and tissue samples for chemical signatures with unprecedented sensitivity and specificity. This allows them to keep track of environmental chemicals, dietary components, and even microbial metabolites that build up over time (Mckeon et al., 2021).

Furthermore, emerging databases such as Exposome-Explorer consolidate comprehensive information on exposure biomarkers, including those related to dietary patterns and pollutant exposures. These curated repositories facilitate the identification of candidate biomarkers whose levels correlate with cancer risk and help to elucidate the mechanistic underpinnings of exposure-related carcinogenesis (Neveu et al., 2019). Integration of these databases with advanced bioinformatics and statistical modeling enables the construction of hazard indices, which help quantify the overall burden of carcinogenic exposures at the population level (Balcells et al., 2023; Mckeon et al., 2021).

Bioinformatics tools and machine learning methods are fundamental to the analysis of exposomics data, serving to integrate, reduce, and interpret complex, high-dimensional datasets that span multiple types of exposures and biological responses. These computational approaches enable researchers to concurrently analyze vast numbers of environmental, genetic, and clinical variables, thus uncovering patterns and associations that are critical for designing targeted health interventions (Alemu et al., 2025; Bocato et al., 2019; Chang et al., 2024).

At the data preprocessing and integration stage, bioinformatics platforms combine information from various omics sources such as genomics, metabolomics, proteomics, and others with exposome data collected via high-resolution mass spectrometry and wearable sensors. This integration improves data quality and enables the mapping of metabolic and proteomic pathways affected by environmental exposures (Cheung et al. 2020; Wan et al., 2025). By harmonizing these diverse datasets, researchers gain a comprehensive view of how exposures influence molecular mechanisms and disease processes.

Machine learning is employed to manage the inherent complexity of exposomics research. Its algorithms, ranging from classical methods like decision trees, random forests, and support vector machines to advanced deep neural network ensembles and ensemble methods like XGBoost, are used for variable selection, pattern recognition, and predictive modeling (Bocato et al., 2019; Chang et al., 2024). These techniques facilitate the identification of potential biomarkers and exposure profiles that are predictive of disease risk, thus enabling personalized health interventions.

One key role for machine learning is the detection of non-linear and interactive effects among multiple exposures, which traditional statistical methods might miss. Approaches such as structured linear mixed models, Bayesian kernel machine regression, and nonparametric regression are utilized to discern complex exposure and exposure interactions (Alemu et al., 2025). By enabling the integration of large-scale, multidimensional datasets and facilitating rigorous, statistically sound analyses, bioinformatics and machine learning tools underpin the development of precision public health strategies and personalized medicine approaches. This integration leads to improved early detection, better patient stratification, and more effective intervention strategies, ultimately enhancing overall health outcomes (Sarigiannis et al., 2025; Wan et al., 2025)

ENVIRONMENTAL INFLUENCES ON CARCINOGENESIS

Environmental influences on carcinogenesis encompass a broad array of extrinsic and intrinsic factors that disrupt normal cellular and tissue homeostasis. Among the major environmental carcinogens are chemical agents such as polycyclic aromatic hydrocarbons (PAHs), aromatic amines, heavy metals (arsenic, chromium), and persistent organic pollutants, all of which are known to induce DNA damage, promote oxidative stress, and disrupt cell signaling pathways. In addition, radiation (ultraviolet and ionizing) and certain fibrous materials such as asbestos are established environmental risk factors that contribute to the development of cancers such as skin cancer, mesothelioma, and lung cancer (Patierno, 2020).

Dietary factors also play a significant role in carcinogenesis. Exposure to mutagenic food components, consumption of food contaminated with environmental chemicals, and exposure to dietary patterns that promote metabolic dysfunction (such as high-fat, low-fiber diets) have all been implicated in increasing cancer risk. These dietary mechanisms often act through the induction of chronic, low-grade inflammation, oxidative stress, and epigenetic alterations, which collectively contribute to tumor initiation and promotion. Likewise, lifestyle factors such as tobacco use, alcohol consumption, and sedentary behavior further compound exposure risks, with smoking, being responsible for nearly 30% of all cancers globally (Jaiswara et al., 2021; Patierno, 2020). High-fat, low-fiber diets contribute to metabolic dysfunction, leading to obesity-driven inflammation. This inflammation is characterized by proinflammatory cytokines and altered adipokine levels, promoting chronic, low-grade inflammation and oxidative stress, which are significant factors in carcinogenesis (Jaiswara et al., 2021).

Importantly, environmental exposures are not isolated but rather have synergistic or antagonistic interactions with each other. The overall cancer risk of an individual is determined not simply by the presence of a single carcinogen, but rather by the cumulative and often simultaneous effects of multiple exposures. This recognition has spurred the need for integrative models that account for complex exposure mixtures and dynamic interactions over time (Patierno, 2020).

Carcinogenesis is a complex and multistep process that arises when genetic predisposition interacts with external environmental factors. These environmental exposures can initiate or promote tumor formation through direct DNA damage, metabolic activation into electrophilic intermediates that bind nucleic acids, chronic inflammatory responses, epigenetic modifications, genotoxicity, and chronic inflammation, leading to cancer. Over recent decades, numerous studies based on molecular biology, epidemiology, and toxicology have established that a spectrum of exposures, including infectious agents, airborne pollutants, dietary toxins and cooking by-products, ionizing and ultraviolet radiation, as well as occupational chemicals, play major roles in cancer development (Agboola et al., 2024; Ajayi & Ogunjobi, 2024; Sharma et al., 2015).

Location is a crucial factor in human health, affecting our environment and our lived experiences. Geospatial science, using tools like geographic information systems (GIS), helps understand, analyze, and visualize environmental features based on location and aids in epidemiologic studies by integrating methods and tools to assess environmental exposures and spatially analyze the distribution of carcinogenic agents and their correlation with health outcomes. It is particularly useful in environmental epidemiology due to its ability to model geographically varying exposures. GIS tools like mapping and spatial cluster analyses are used for descriptive epidemiology, allowing visualization of environmental exposure distribution, identifying disproportionately impacted areas, and highlighting temporal trends (VoPham et al., 2024). The integration of GIS in environmental epidemiology enhances the understanding of exposure patterns and disease incidence, facilitating targeted public health interventions. GIS is utilized to create exposure and disease maps, revealing spatial patterns of chemical exposure and disease occurrence, which aids in risk assessment (Jarup, 2004). GIS-EpiLink tool links environmental and health data, allowing epidemiologists to analyze proximity to pollution sources as a proxy for exposure, thus enhancing epidemiological research capabilities (Zhan et al., 2006).

Integrating neighborhood environment data into Geographic Information and Experimentation (GxE) research can improve risk predictions for disease and health outcomes. However, geospatial measures pose unique privacy challenges. New tools and approaches are needed to maximize the benefits of geospatial data while protecting participants' privacy. High-resolution geomarker assessment tools have become available, but more work is needed to develop and apply them with appropriate privacy protections. Geospatial data containing protected health information (PHI) is often collected without explicit informed consent and lacks consistent messaging from institutional review boards. A reproducible, standardized, and decentralized resource is needed for secure, efficient, automated, and reproducible linkage of geomarkers to PHI (Calluori et al., 2025).

Current GIS-based studies employ a range of advanced spatial technologies and exposure models to assess environmental carcinogen exposures and their impact on human health. One primary approach involves the development of GIS-based metrics that incorporate detailed industrial emission inventories, atmospheric dispersion simulations, and residential proximity data. For example, Coudon et al. (2019) developed and validated a metric to assess long-term exposure to airborne pollutants like dioxins and cadmium. Their approach integrates annual emissions data from over 2500 industrial sources across multiple French regions and calibrates against urban dispersion models such as SIRANE using statistical measures (e.g., weighted kappa and R^2). This method addresses spatial–temporal variability and reduces exposure misclassification in epidemiologic studies, particularly those investigating cancer outcomes like breast cancer.

Another prominent line of inquiry uses GIS to perform risk mapping that aggregates multiple pollutant measures obtained through environmental monitoring. Rovira et al. (2021) demonstrated this by constructing a hazard index based on soil, vegetation, and air data for various carcinogenic compounds, including heavy metals, PAHs, and PCDD/Fs, to estimate human health risks near industrial complexes. Their work integrates self-organizing maps and Monte Carlo simulations within a GIS framework to account for the complexities in pollutant mixtures and highlight exposure disparities among socioeconomically distinct groups.

Further, GIS-based research has expanded into evaluating the impact of the built environment. Studies like those by Wang et al. (2019) employ spatial clustering and geographical detector methods to investigate the association between urban spatial factors such as the presence of industrial parks, traffic density, and urban–rural gradients and lung cancer incidence. Their work underscores the role of nuanced urban planning and land use characteristics in modulating exposure levels and subsequent health risks.

Citizen science initiatives focused on mitigating indoor radon concentrations exemplify a community-driven approach to environmental health (Stanifer et al., 2022) Such endeavors aim to enhance environmental health literacy and empower individuals, particularly in low-income populations, to engage in testing and addressing radon levels in their homes. The emphasis on citizen science reflects an understanding that socioeconomic disparities can significantly influence access to radon testing and mitigation (Naidu et al., 2013; Stanifer et al., 2022).

Current GIS-based studies in environmental epidemiology integrate detailed emission inventories, advanced dispersion models, multimodal geospatial datasets, and sophisticated spatial statistical techniques. These methods collectively enable the precise characterization of exposure to complex mixtures of carcinogenic pollutants and provide critical insights for public health and urban planning interventions aimed at reducing cancer risk.

PREVENTIVE STRATEGIES AND REGULATORY INTERVENTIONS

Understanding the environmental origins of cancer has led to comprehensive preventive strategies at multiple levels, ranging from individual behavioral changes to broad regulatory policies. Vaccination campaigns directed at preventing infections with oncogenic viruses such as HPV and HBV have proven to be highly effective in reducing the incidence of cervical and liver cancers (Agboola et al., 2024).

Regulatory oversight has also played a critical role in lowering exposure levels to harmful pollutants. In many urban areas, standards for ambient air pollutants including PM2.5, NO_X, and VOCs have been tightened to reduce the global burden of lung cancer and related diseases (Ali et al., 2020; Espina et al., 2015). Likewise, efforts to improve indoor air quality by promoting cleaner cooking fuels and better ventilation are particularly crucial in regions where traditional biomass or coal burning remains common (Gbemudu, 2023). Occupational health standards are designed to protect workers from chronic exposure to industrial carcinogens such as benzene, vinyl chloride, and asbestos. These standards typically require the use of engineering controls, personal protective equipment, and regular health monitoring to detect early signs of carcinogen-induced damage (Birkett et al., 2019; Ajayi & Ogunjobi, 2024; Talibov et al., 2017).

Over 60% of rural counties in the United States face a significant deficit in oncologists, leading to delays in diagnoses and increasing the incidence of late-stage cancer mortality (Gummadi et al., 2014). The lack of accessible cancer care not only exacerbates health disparities but also reflects broader systemic issues in the healthcare delivery model. The identification of "cancer care deserts," which are areas with limited access to cancer-related healthcare services, can be effectively achieved through the utilization of geospatial tools and GIS. These tools allow for the visual representation of cancer service availability, demographic factors, and healthcare infrastructure.

Geospatial analysis can reveal correlations between cancer care availability and factors such as population density, socioeconomic status, and historical healthcare access. By mapping areas where oncologists are scarce and juxtaposing this with data on cancer incidence and mortality (Stanifer et al., 2022), health officials can locate potential interventions. Moreover, the identification of such geographic disparities enables targeted resource allocation, such as the establishment of telemedicine hubs, which can provide oncological consultations remotely, and the training of community health workers to assist in tasks like biopsy collection and patient navigation (Naidu et al., 2013).

Despite the potential for geospatial tools to inform cancer care interventions, significant ethical challenges arise, particularly when the target populations are historically marginalized groups. Medical distrust rooted in historical exploitation and systemic inequities can hinder the effectiveness of healthcare initiatives in these communities. For instance, marginalized populations may view intervention efforts as top-down impositions rather than collaborative partnerships, resulting in skepticism and resistance.

To address these ethical challenges, adopting a participatory approach is required. Engaging community members in the decision-making process regarding the development and implementation of cancer care strategies not only enhances trust but also ensures that interventions are culturally sensitive and tailored to community needs. Such collaborative frameworks emphasize the importance of transparency, informed consent, and the consideration of local values in healthcare delivery.

MOLECULAR MECHANISMS MEDIATING ENVIRONMENTAL CARCINOGENESIS

At the molecular level, environmental carcinogens initiate a series of events that culminate in the malignant transformation of cells. One key mechanism is direct DNA damage, which may result in mutations if cellular repair processes are overwhelmed or defective. Genotoxic compounds such as PAHs form DNA adducts that interfere with normal replication and transcription processes. If these adducts are not efficiently repaired, they can produce mutations that predispose cells to oncogenic transformation (Patierno, 2020).

In addition to direct DNA damage, many environmental exposures induce oxidative stress, leading to the generation of ROS and reactive nitrogen species. These molecules cause extensive damage not only to DNA but also to proteins and lipids, thereby contributing to genomic instability which is a hallmark of cancer. Chronic inflammation, which is frequently fueled by persistent exposures to environmental stressors, represents another critical pathway. Inflammatory mediators such as cytokines, chemokines, and growth factors create a tumor-promoting microenvironment by facilitating processes such as cell proliferation, angiogenesis, and immune evasion (Gonda et al., 2009; Patierno, 2020).

Environmental exposures also perturb cellular signaling pathways. Aberrant activation of pathways such as NF-κB and STAT3 by exogenous agents can lead to heightened cell survival, proliferation, and resistance to apoptosis. In parallel, these pathways stimulate the secretion of inflammatory mediators that perpetuate the cycle of chronic inflammation, a key driver of tumor progression. Furthermore, many carcinogens influence cellular metabolism, shifting energy production towards glycolysis even in the presence of oxygen (the Warburg effect) to meet the demands of rapidly proliferating tumor cells (Akl & Ahmed, 2024; Patierno, 2020).

EPIGENETIC REGULATION IN EXPOSOME-INDUCED TUMORIGENESIS

A rapidly expanding body of literature has illuminated the critical role of epigenetic mechanisms in mediating the effects of environmental exposures on carcinogenesis. Epigenetic alterations, such as DNA methylation, histone modifications, and regulation by noncoding RNAs, offer a mechanistic link between environmental exposures and alterations in gene expression without modifying the underlying DNA sequence. These modifications are not only pivotal in tumorigenesis but are often reversible, thereby presenting potential targets for early detection and therapeutic intervention (Olmedosuarez et al., 2022).

Environmental agents can induce stable epigenetic signatures or "fingerprints" that serve as biomarkers of exposure. Pollutants and dietary factors may alter the methylation status of tumor suppressor genes or oncogenes, thereby predisposing cells to malignant transformation. In addition, alterations in the expression of histone-modifying enzymes have been observed in exposure-related cancers, contributing to chromatin remodeling that facilitates or hinders the transcription of genes critical for cell cycle regulation and apoptosis (Herceg et al., 2018).

Recent studies have highlighted the role of noncoding RNAs, including microRNAs (miRNAs) and long noncoding RNAs (lncRNAs), as essential regulators of gene expression in response to environmental factors. These molecules can modulate immune responses, influence cell proliferation, and contribute to tumor metabolism, further linking environmental exposures to cancer development. miRNAs may be downregulated or upregulated by exposure to chemical carcinogens, subsequently impacting pathways that govern cellular proliferation and immune surveillance (Gavito-Covarrubias et al., 2024; Olmedosuarez et al., 2022).

The interplay between genetic polymorphisms in detoxification genes, such as GSTP1, and susceptibility to environmental carcinogens highlights the importance of understanding individual risk factors in cancer prevention strategies. Studies indicate that variations in GSTP1, along with other glutathione S-transferase (GST) genes, have been directly linked to alterations in cancer risk, particularly in pediatric populations exposed to pollutants (Gutiérrez-Camino et al., 2017; Smith, 2010). Research has shown that individuals with the GSTP1 Ile105Val variant display impaired benzene metabolism, compounded by environmental exposure from traffic emissions, significantly elevating the risk of leukemia in susceptible adolescents (D'Andrea & Reddy, 2013; Filippini et al., 2015). Integrating genetic screening with public health outreach can enhance community awareness regarding the risks associated with environmental exposures. Educational initiatives aimed at informing families of environmental health risks, coupled with advocacy for policy changes concerning traffic emissions reduction, could lead to cumulative benefits for public health in these high-risk populations (Gutiérrez-Camino et al., 2017; Smith, 2010).

CASE STUDIES: CANCER EXPOSOMICS IN DIFFERENT TUMOR TYPES

Cancer exposomics is not confined to a single cancer type but has been applied across a wide spectrum of malignancies. Breast cancer exposomics examines how environmental xenobiotics, dietary carcinogens, and lifestyle-related factors such as exposure to endocrine-disrupting chemicals interact with the breast tissue micro-environment. Epidemiological data indicate that non-genetic factors may account for as much as 70–95% of breast cancer risk, with migration studies revealing that populations adopting Western lifestyles experience marked increases in incidence (Neagu et al., 2024).

Lung cancer is another area where exposomics has provided critical insights. Environmental pollutants including fine particulate matter (PM2.5), nitrogen dioxide (NO2), volatile organic compounds (VOCs), and diesel exhaust are being studied within an exposomics framework to better understand lung cancer risk. By integrating satellite monitoring data, emission inventories, and high-throughput molecular analyses, researchers have constructed hazard indices that predict lung cancer risk at the population level based on zip code–level environmental exposures. These studies highlight the significant burden of environmental carcinogens and underscore the need for precision public health approaches that target high-risk regions (Mckeon et al., 2021).

Colorectal cancer (CRC) has similarly been linked to exposures from dietary chemicals, pesticides, and other environmental agents that disrupt gut microbiota composition and promote chronic inflammation. Exposomic studies of CRC aim to capture the cumulative lifetime exposures that contribute to metabolic dysfunction and inflammatory pathways that drive tumorigenesis. These analyses suggest that exposures beginning in early life play a critical role in setting the stage for later carcinogenic events (Murphy et al., 2024).

Cutaneous squamous cell carcinoma (SCC) also exemplifies the potential of cancer exposomics. While ultraviolet (UV) radiation remains the principal cause of SCC, other exposures such as environmental pollution, water and food contaminants, and even lifestyle stressors have been identified as contributing factors. Multi-center case–control studies are now applying comprehensive exposome assessments to better delineate the contributions of these varied exposures to skin cancer risk, thereby informing targeted prevention strategies (Navarrobielsa et al., 2023).

School-based disparities in cancer education significantly impact students' understanding and engagement with cancer-related health issues. These disparities are influenced by various factors, including socioeconomic status, educational attainment, and regional health literacy. Addressing these disparities through targeted educational interventions can enhance cancer literacy and potentially reduce cancer incidence and mortality rates. Individuals with lower educational attainment experience higher cancer mortality rates. For instance, lung cancer accounts for over half of the mortality rate difference between those with less than a high school education and those with a Bachelor's degree or higher (Withrow et al., 2021). Programs like the Cancer Health Education Curriculum (CHEC) in Milwaukee have demonstrated significant improvements in cancer knowledge and health behaviors among high school students (O'Connell et al., 2023). A brief educational intervention in Kentucky resulted in a notable increase in cancer literacy among middle and high school students, suggesting that integrating cancer education into curricula can drive positive health behavior changes (Hudson et al., 2021). Engaging underrepresented minority students in STEM-focused programs, such as the Youth Enjoy Science program, emphasizes the importance of disparities education in fostering a diverse cancer workforce and addressing health inequities(Omoijuanfo et al., 2022).

African American communities in the United States experience approximately 1.5-fold higher exposure to industrial pollutants compared to white populations due largely to historical patterns of residential segregation that concentrated these communities in urban industrial zones. Residential segregation, stemming from policies like redlining and discriminatory zoning, ensured that African Americans were confined to neighborhoods that are proximal to industrial areas emitting elevated levels of toxic air contaminants. These urban settings have become enduring "pollution riskscapes" where facilities that once operated under less-stringent regulations continue to operate with outdated emission controls and exemptions, often maintained by grandfather clauses (Ard, 2016). The resultant spatial clustering forces African Americans into environments with persistently high ambient exposure to hazardous pollutants, which cumulatively increases their overall health risks (Ard et al., 2016).

IMPLICATIONS FOR PUBLIC HEALTH AND PREVENTIVE STRATEGIES

The integration of cancer exposomics into public health practice holds tremendous promise for improving cancer prevention, early detection, and individualized intervention strategies. By quantifying the cumulative burden of exposures, it is possible to identify high-risk individuals and populations before morphological changes occur. This predictive capacity supports the development of early intervention and chemoprevention programs that may modify risk trajectories and reduce cancer incidence (Patierno, 2020).

Primary prevention measures such as reducing environmental exposures through regulatory policies, improving air quality standards, and promoting healthier dietary practices can be informed by exposome-wide data. Moreover, the identification of biomarkers of exposure and early effect can aid in the implementation of screening programs that detect subtle molecular changes indicative of early carcinogenic events. In this way, cancer exposomics bridges the gap between epidemiological data and clinical practice, fostering multidisciplinary strategies that target modifiable risk factors (Juarezet al., 2022).

Additionally, the ability to stratify individuals based on their cumulative environmental exposure burden offers a new avenue for precision public health. Such stratification is especially valuable in regions where environmental pollution is concentrated, allowing for targeted interventions that reduce overall cancer burden in vulnerable communities. By coupling exposomic data with health outcomes and demographic information, public health authorities can design and implement interventions that have maximal impact on population health (Patierno, 2020).

The concept of chemoprevention further expands the role of exposomics in cancer control. Chemopreventive agents, including dietary polyphenols, vitamins, and other bioactive compounds, can be deployed to counteract the adverse molecular effects induced by environmental exposures. Given that many epigenetic modifications are reversible, strategies that employ demethylating agents or histone deacetylase inhibitors may be effective in restoring normal gene expression in early-stage lesions, thereby halting progression to invasive cancer (Herceg et al., 2018).

CHALLENGES AND FUTURE DIRECTIONS IN CANCER EXPOSOMICS

Despite the significant advances in characterizing the cancer exposome, several challenges remain. One major hurdle is the inherent complexity of exposure mixtures and the dynamic nature of environmental interactions over a lifetime. Measuring low-level exposures with high temporal resolution remains technically demanding, and the potential for confounding by co-exposures complicates the causal inference of specific risk factors. There is also the challenge of harmonizing data across diverse omics platforms and ensuring reproducibility across studies (Juarez et al., 2018).

Future directions in cancer exposomics include the refinement of high-throughput analytical techniques that enable more precise quantification of chemical exposures and the integration of longitudinal cohort data with omics datasets. The development of sophisticated machine learning algorithms that can process and analyze these large-scale datasets is a promising avenue for unraveling the complex gene–environment interactions that underlie carcinogenesis. Furthermore, collaborative efforts among epidemiologists, toxicologists, molecular biologists, and data scientists will be essential for translating exposomic findings into actionable public health interventions (Herceg et al., 2018; Juarez et al., 2022a).

Translational research in cancer exposomics is expected to lead to the discovery of novel biomarkers that reflect not just individual exposures but also the biological responses to these exposures. Changes in the epigenome that occur in response to specific environmental agents may serve as early indicators of cellular stress and transformation. These biomarkers can then be incorporated into routine screening programs, potentially allowing for cancer interception strategies that halt the progression of pre-malignant lesions before they become clinically apparent (Olmedosuarez et al., 2022).

The emerging field of exposomics also offers potential to refine risk assessment models. Current models that rely solely on genetic susceptibility or self-reported exposure histories are inherently limited. Integrative exposomic approaches, by contrast, can provide quantitative measures of exposure that are linked to biological outcomes, thereby enhancing the precision of risk prediction. Such refined models have the potential to guide personalized prevention strategies and to inform regulatory decisions regarding environmental pollutants (Patierno, 2020).

Moreover, the interplay between the exposome and the microbiome adds an additional layer of complexity. Microbial communities within the human body not only modulate inflammatory and immune responses but also interact with environmental chemicals—altering their bioavailability and toxicity. The gut microbiota can metabolize dietary carcinogens, sometimes activating pro-carcinogens into their active forms or in other cases detoxifying harmful compounds. Understanding these interactions requires an integrative approach that considers the exposome, the microbiome, and host genetics simultaneously, which is increasingly being addressed by multi-omics studies (Bessonneau et al., 2020; Juarez et al., 2018).

TRANSLATIONAL APPLICATIONS: FROM EXPOSOMICS TO INTERVENTION

The ultimate goal of cancer exposomics is to translate molecular insights into effective cancer prevention and therapeutic interventions. By providing an in-depth understanding of the molecular mechanisms by which environmental exposures induce carcinogenesis, exposomics can help identify "windows of opportunity" for intervention. If certain epigenetic modifications are consistently observed following exposure to a specific pollutant, interventions aimed at reversing these modifications may be effective in reducing cancer risk. Clinical trials exploring demethylating agents or histone deacetylase inhibitors in populations with defined exposure histories represent one avenue for such translational research (Herceg et al., 2018).

Beyond chemoprevention, cancer exposomics has implications for public health policy. Regulatory agencies can use data from exposomic studies to more accurately assess the carcinogenic potential of chemical mixtures and to set exposure limits that better reflect the cumulative burden of exposures. This evidence-based approach to environmental risk management could lead to stricter controls on industrial emissions, improved food safety standards, and more rigorous monitoring of air and water quality, ultimately reducing the overall incidence of environmentally induced cancers (Patierno, 2020).

Furthermore, the integration of exposomic data into clinical practice promises to usher in an era of precision prevention. By combining genetic risk profiles with detailed environmental exposure histories, clinicians may eventually be able to provide individualized recommendations for lifestyle modifications, early screening, and even targeted pharmacological interventions. Such precision prevention strategies could significantly reduce the burden of cancer at both the individual and population levels (Juarez et al., 2022).

Challenges in implementation, however, remain. The enormous complexity of exposomic data necessitates robust computational infrastructure and interdisciplinary collaboration. It is essential to establish standardized protocols for sample collection, data processing, and analysis to ensure that findings are reproducible and generalizable across different populations and contexts. Moving forward, continued investment in exposomic research, along with the development of international consortia and data-sharing initiatives, will be critical for overcoming these barriers and fully realizing the promise of cancer exposomics.

ETHICAL, LEGAL, AND SOCIETAL IMPLICATIONS (ELSI) IN CANCER EXPOSOMICS

Cancer exposomics, which integrates high-throughput molecular technologies with comprehensive environmental exposure assessments, inherently raises complex ethical, societal, and policy dimensions that must be addressed to ensure research integrity and public benefit (Juarez et al., 2018).

Cancer exposomics research that integrates genetic/epigenetic information with environmental exposure data poses several nuanced ELSI challenges that require precise attention. One of the primary issues is informed consent and adolescent autonomy. The inherent complexity of gene–environment data means that consent processes must go beyond mere formality and instead ensure that participants fully understand the scientific and personal implications of the research. This is particularly challenging when engaging adolescent populations, who are in a developmental phase where decision-making capacities are still evolving (Calluori et al., 2025; Kuther & Posada, 2004). Consent procedures must carefully balance respect for emerging autonomy with the need for protective parental involvement, ensuring that adolescents are neither overburdened by technical details nor insufficiently informed about potential risks, uncertainties, and long-term impacts. Tailored communication and educational strategies are critical to achieving an ethically robust consent process for these younger populations. Researchers are encouraged to create environments that respect adolescents' opinions, fostering their involvement in the consent process (Calluori et al., 2025; Lind et al., 2003; Vega et al., 2024).

Developmental psychology suggests that adolescents possess the capacity to make informed decisions, advocating for their rights to participate in research (Kuther & Posada, 2004). A hybrid consent model, combining caregiver consent with opportunities for adolescents to opt-in or opt-out, can enhance their autonomy while ensuring protection (Overbeek et al., 2024).

Health disparities and social justice further complicate the ethical landscape in cancer exposomics. The distribution of both environmental exposures and genetic predispositions is non-uniform, with marginalized communities often disproportionately burdened by adverse exposures. This imbalance necessitates that research designs not only document these differences but actively work toward mitigating them through integrating environmental justice principles and social determinants of health. Such an approach ensures that the benefits of research, including advanced diagnostic techniques, are equitably distributed and that the research does not inadvertently reinforce existing inequities (Calluori et al., 2025).

Ethically, cancer exposomics challenges traditional conceptions of informed consent and privacy because it involves the collection and analysis of extremely sensitive molecular data, including genomics, epigenomics, metabolomics, and proteomics, which may reveal not only an individual's current health status but also predispositions to future diseases. Rigorous informed consent processes are necessary to ensure that participants understand both the scope and potential consequences of sharing such data (Rodriguez et al., 2013; Safarlou et al., 2023). Moreover, there is a moral obligation to protect participant privacy and prevent misuse of data, particularly given the risk that biobank samples and associated molecular profiles might be repurposed for unintended forensic or commercial applications (Safarlou et al., 2023). The integration of complex omics with environmental data increases the potential for both re-identification of participants and subsequent discrimination in various contexts such as employment and insurance. Current legal protections are not comprehensive, statutes like the Genetic Information Nondiscrimination Act (GINA) do not cover epigenomic nuances or environmental data. Consequently, there is a pressing need for stringent privacy safeguards, transparent disclosure of data-sharing protocols, and robust consent processes that fully inform participants of the potential risks associated with data security, re-identification, and misuse (Calluori et al., 2025). Researchers therefore must adopt a cautious approach, ensuring that both individual privacy and community-level harms are mitigated by detailed internal protocols and oversight mechanisms (Safarlou et al., 2023).

A related ethical concern stems from the "molecularization" of disease, wherein the focus on complex biomarker signatures could potentially devalue patients' subjective illness experiences and create challenging thresholds for clinical action. This redefinition of disease in molecular terms may inadvertently narrow healthcare interventions by privileging precise biomarker-defined conditions over more holistic understanding of patient well-being (Dupras et al., 2019; Safarlou et al., 2023). Alongside these issues, researchers grapple with the ethical dilemma of result disclosure. There exists uncertainty regarding which findings should be imparted to participants, only those with clear clinical actionability, or also preliminary data that might empower lifestyle changes while avoiding undue psychological or behavioral harm (Safarlou et al., 2023).

Societal dimensions of cancer exposomics center on environmental justice and the recognition that exposure to hazardous agents is often unequally distributed across populations. For instance, historically marginalized and low-income communities, such as many Latino populations facing rapid demographic shifts, may experience disproportionately high exposures and consequently endure greater cancer risks (Juarez et al., 2022). These disparities call for a broader incorporation of social determinants into exposome research. The integration of sociomarkers, factors like socioeconomic status, neighborhood conditions, and collective stressors, helps to situate molecular data within the lived realities of affected communities, thereby preventing a reductionist view that overlooks broader systemic injustices (Senier et al., 2017).

Collectively, these challenges underscore the intertwined nature of informed consent (particularly when considering adolescent empowerment), social and health equity, robust data protection, and the imperative for participatory models that ensure communities are both informed and engaged. Addressing these ELSI issues requires multidisciplinary collaboration, updated legal frameworks, and a commitment to community engagement to guide cancer exposomics research towards equitable and just outcomes (Calluori et al., 2025; Safarlou et al., 2023).

UNIFIED CALL TO ACTION AND VISION FOR PRECISION PREVENTION

The science of cancer exposomics necessitates a collaborative, multisectoral approach to effectively address the complexities of environmental exposures and their impact on health. This call to action involves educators, policymakers, urban planners, geneticists, clinicians, and communities working together to enhance understanding and mitigate cancer risks associated with the exposome.

Cancer exposomics, defined as the comprehensive study of the totality of environmental exposures and their impact on cancer risk, inherently demands an urgent, multisectoral, and multilevel response due to the complex interplay between diverse exposures over the life course and the multiple pathways involved in carcinogenesis (VoPham et al., 2024). The integration of external factors, ranging from physical and chemical agents in our natural, built, and social environments, to internal biological responses measured by multi-omics technologies demands coordinated action across educational, regulatory, urban planning, clinical, and community domains (Calluori et al., 2025).

Educators play a fundamental role in this response, as they are responsible for disseminating interdisciplinary knowledge and training the next generation of experts who can navigate both the technical aspects of geospatial modeling and the biological nuances of gene-environment interactions. By incorporating exposomic principles and advanced measurement techniques, educational programs can nurture future researchers and public health professionals equipped to tackle these multifactorial challenges (Calluori et al., 2025; VoPham et al., 2024).

Policymakers are equally indispensable. They must develop, implement, and enforce evidence-based regulations that mitigate hazardous environmental exposures. Given that exposomic research provides insights into cumulative lifetime exposures, policy decisions that integrate geospatial exposure evidence can more effectively target risk factors at the population level. Policymakers can develop regulations that limit harmful exposures, informed by exposomic research, to protect public health (Parker, 2014; VoPham et al., 2024). Regulatory frameworks informed by such research not only reduce exposure to carcinogens like air pollution and toxic chemical mixtures but also ensure that interventions consider social determinants of health and environmental justice, thereby protecting vulnerable populations (Calluori et al., 2025; Juarez et al., 2014; VoPham et al., 2024).

Urban planners contribute critically by leveraging geospatial science to design healthier built environments. By carefully planning urban spaces that increase green zones, reduce industrial pollutant exposure, and promote sustainable transportation networks, urban planners can effectively lower the population's exposure to cancer risk factors (Miller, 2014; VoPham et al., 2024). Their designs can promote healthier environments by considering factors like air quality and access to green spaces, which influence exposure levels This multisectoral design approach also involves optimizing residential geocoding and spatial risk assessments, ensuring that interventions are both precise and locally relevant (Juarez et al., 2014; VoPham et al., 2024).

Geneticists and clinicians can utilize exposomic data to personalize treatment and prevention strategies, recognizing the interplay between genetics and environmental factors (Wright & Hanson, 2022). This integration is pivotal for understanding individual susceptibilities and the mechanistic pathways by which environmental exposures potentiate cancer development. Clinicians, informed by personalized geospatial exposure profiles, can tailor screening protocols and therapeutic interventions, thereby moving toward precision prevention and treatment strategies that consider both genetic predisposition and environmental risk factors. This dual focus improves early detection and healthcare outcomes while contributing to overall population health management (Juarez et al., 2014). Communities themselves are indispensable to this multisectoral response. Engaging local populations in exposomic research can empower them to advocate for healthier environments and policies that address specific local exposures (Wan et al., 2025).Active community engagement ensures that interventions are culturally appropriate, locally tailored, and address the social realities that contribute to unequal exposure burdens. By participating in exposure assessment and advocacy efforts, communities help identify critical local needs and empower policy and design decisions that lead to healthier environments. This inclusive approach to community involvement not only legitimizes the research process but also ensures that the benefits of cancer prevention strategies are equitably distributed across diverse populations (Malecki et al., 2022).

Consequently, the science of cancer exposomics requires an urgent and inclusive call to action that mobilizes an interconnected network of educators, policymakers, urban planners, geneticists, clinicians, and communities. This multisectoral strategy is essential to translate complex, integrative data on environmental exposures into effective public health policies and personalized clinical interventions, thereby reducing cancer risk and promoting health equity at every societal level (Calluori et al., 2025; Parker, 2014). While the focus on exposomics is critical, it is also essential to recognize that not all environmental exposures are preventable, and some individuals may remain at risk due to socioeconomic factors or genetic predispositions. This highlights the need for ongoing research and support systems to address these disparities.

CONCLUSION

Cancer exposomics and the study of environmental influences on carcinogenesis represent a transformative approach to understanding the origins of cancer. By integrating data on lifelong exposures with advanced molecular analyses, this field provides a comprehensive framework for elucidating the complex interplay between environmental agents and biological systems. From direct DNA damage to oxidative stress, chronic inflammation, and epigenetic dysregulation, the molecular underpinnings of environmentally induced carcinogenesis are multifaceted and dynamic. These insights are critical not only for improving our understanding of cancer etiology but also for the development of innovative prevention, early detection, and treatment strategies.

The integration of multi-omics data into exposomic studies is already reshaping risk assessment models and providing new biomarkers that serve as early indicators of carcinogenic exposures. As these approaches continue to evolve, they are expected to play an increasingly important role in precision public health, enabling interventions that are tailored to an individual's cumulative exposure burden and molecular susceptibility. Ultimately, the promise of cancer exposomics lies in its potential to bridge the gap between environmental risk factors and clinical outcomes, thereby paving the way for a proactive rather than reactive approach to cancer management.

The role of ELSI factors in cancer exposomics research is crucial for ensuring equitable access and benefits for diverse populations. ELSI considerations address the systemic barriers that hinder participation from underrepresented groups, thereby promoting inclusivity and enhancing the relevance of research outcomes across different demographics. While ELSI factors play a pivotal role in promoting equity in cancer exposomics research, challenges remain. For instance, the persistent underrepresentation of certain ethnic groups in clinical trials continues to hinder the development of tailored interventions, suggesting that more robust strategies are needed to overcome these barriers (García-Cárdenas et al., 2024; Langley et al., 2023). Collaborative actions involving regulatory bodies can promote equitable representation, ensuring that research findings are applicable to a broader population.

The journey toward fully characterizing the cancer exposome is complex, yet it holds unparalleled promise for transforming how we perceive, prevent, and treat cancer. With collaborative interdisciplinary efforts and continued technological innovations, the integration of exposomic data into clinical practice may soon enable us to intercept carcinogenic processes at their earliest stages, thereby reducing the overall incidence and impact of cancer in society.

REFERENCES

Agboola, O. O., Emmanuel, A. O., Sabina, C. E., Anejo-Okopi, J., Naomi, A. I., Ene, U. I., & Olowoyo, J. O. (2024). Occurrence of Carcinogens and their Potential Effects on Human Health – A Review. *UMYU Scientifica Journal*, *3*(1), 129–143. DOI: 10.56919/usci.2431.015

Ajayi, R. O., & Ogunjobi, T. T. (2024). *Environmental Exposures and Cancer Risk: A Comprehensive Review*. Deleted Journal., DOI: 10.47852/bonviewMEDIN42023598

Akl, M. M., & Ahmed, A. (2024). Exploring the interplay between the warburg effect and glucolipotoxicity in cancer development: A novel perspective on cancer etiology. *Advanced Pharmaceutical Bulletin*, *14*(3), 705–713. DOI: 10.34172/apb.2024.049 PMID: 39494260

Alemu, R., Sharew, N. T., Arsano, Y. Y., Ahmed, M., Tekola-Ayele, F., Mersha, T. B., & Amare, A. T. (2025). Multi-omics approaches for understanding gene-environment interactions in noncommunicable diseases: Techniques, translation, and equity issues. *Human Genomics*, *19*(1), 8. DOI: 10.1186/s40246-025-00718-9 PMID: 39891174

Ali, M. U., Lin, S., Yousaf, B., Abbas, Q., Munir, M. M., Rashid, A., Zheng, C., Kuang, X., & Wong, M. H. (2020). Pollution characteristics, mechanism of toxicity and health effects of the ultrafine particles in the indoor environment: Current status and future perspectives. *Critical Reviews in Environmental Science and Technology*, *52*(3), 436–473. DOI: 10.1080/10643389.2020.1831359

Ard, K. (2016). By all measures: An examination of the relationship between segregation and health risk from air pollution. *Population and Environment*, *38*(1), 1–20. DOI: 10.1007/s11111-015-0251-6

Ard, K., Colen, C., Becerra, M., & Velez, T. (2016). Two Mechanisms: The Role of Social Capital and Industrial Pollution Exposure in Explaining Racial Disparities in Self-Rated Health. *International Journal of Environmental Research and Public Health*, *13*(10), 1025. DOI: 10.3390/ijerph13101025 PMID: 27775582

Balcells, C., Xu, Y., Gil-Solsona, R., Maitre, L., Gago-Ferrero, P., & Keun, H. C. (2023). Blurred lines: Crossing the boundaries between the chemical exposome and the metabolome. *Current Opinion in Chemical Biology*, *78*, 102407. DOI: 10.1016/j.cbpa.2023.102407 PMID: 38086287

Bessonneau, V., & Rudel, R. A. (2019). Mapping the Human Exposome to Uncover the Causes of Breast Cancer. *International Journal of Environmental Research and Public Health*, *17*(1), 189. DOI: 10.3390/ijerph17010189 PMID: 31892107

Birkett, N., Al-Zoughool, M., Bird, M., Baan, R. A., Zielinski, J., & Krewski, D. (2019). Overview of biological mechanisms of human carcinogens. *Journal of Toxicology and Environmental Health. Part B, Critical Reviews*, *22*(7-8), 288–359. DOI: 10.1080/10937404.2019.1643539 PMID: 31631808

Bocato, M. Z., Bianchi Ximenez, J. P., Hoffmann, C., & Barbosa, F. (2019). An overview of the current progress, challenges, and prospects of human biomonitoring and exposome studies. *Journal of Toxicology and Environmental Health. Part B, Critical Reviews*, *22*(5-6), 131–156. DOI: 10.1080/10937404.2019.1661588 PMID: 31543064

Calluori, S., Heimke, K. K., Caga-Anan, C., Kaufman, D., Mechanic, L. E., & McAllister, K. A. (2025). Ethical, Legal, and Social Implications of Gene-Environment Interaction Research. *Genetic Epidemiology*, *49*(1), e22591. DOI: 10.1002/gepi.22591 PMID: 39315585

Chang, L., Ewald, J., Hui, F., Bayen, S., & Xia, J. (2024). A data-centric perspective on exposomics data analysis. *Exposome*, *4*(1), osae005. Advance online publication. DOI: 10.1093/exposome/osae005

Cheung, A. C., Walker, D. I., Juran, B. D., Miller, G. W., & Lazaridis, K. N. (2020). Studying the Exposome to Understand the Environmental Determinants of Complex Liver Diseases. *Hepatology (Baltimore, Md.)*, *71*(1), 352–362. DOI: 10.1002/hep.31028 PMID: 31701542

Coudon, T., Danjou, A. M. N., Faure, E., Praud, D., Severi, G., Mancini, F. R., Salizzoni, P., & Fervers, B. (2019). Development and performance evaluation of a GIS-based metric to assess exposure to airborne pollutant emissions from industrial sources. *Environmental Health : A Global Access Science Source*, *18*(1), 8. DOI: 10.1186/s12940-019-0446-x PMID: 30683108

D'Adamo, G. L., Widdop, J. T., & Giles, E. M. (2021). The future is now? Clinical and translational aspects of "Omics" technologies. *Immunology and Cell Biology*, *99*(2), 168–176. DOI: 10.1111/imcb.12404 PMID: 32924178

D'Andrea, M. A., & Reddy, G. K. (2013). Health effects of benzene exposure among children following a flaring incident at the british petroleum refinery in texas city. *Pediatric Hematology and Oncology*, *31*(1), 1–10. DOI: 10.3109/08880018.2013.831511 PMID: 24088183

Dupras, C., Saulnier, K. M., & Joly, Y. (2019). Epigenetics, ethics, law and society: A multidisciplinary review of descriptive, instrumental, dialectical and reflexive analyses. *Social Studies of Science*, *49*(5), 785–810. DOI: 10.1177/0306312719866007 PMID: 31366289

Espina, C., Straif, K., Friis, S., Kogevinas, M., Saracci, R., Vainio, H., & Schüz, J. (2015). European Code against Cancer 4th Edition: Environment, occupation and cancer. Cancer Epidemiology, 39, S84–S92. DOI: 10.1016/j.canep.2015.03.017

Filippini, T., Heck, J. E., Malagoli, C., Giovane, C. D., & Vinceti, M. (2015). A review and meta-analysis of outdoor air pollution and risk of childhood leukemia. *Journal of Environmental Science and Health. Part C, Environmental Carcinogenesis & Ecotoxicology Reviews, 33*(1), 36–66. DOI: 10.1080/10590501.2015.1002999 PMID: 25803195

García-Cárdenas, J. M., Indacochea, A., Pesantez-Coronel, D., Terán-Navas, M., Aleaga, A., Armendáriz-Castillo, I., Peña Zúñiga, L., Morán-Erazo, C., Chávez-Vélez, E., Pérez-Villa, A., López-Cortés, A., & Guerrero, S. (2024). Toward Equitable Precision Oncology: Monitoring Racial and Ethnic Inclusion in Genomics and Clinical Trials. *JCO Precision Oncology, 8*(8), e2300398. DOI: 10.1200/PO.23.00398 PMID: 38662980

Gavito-Covarrubias, D., Ramírez-Díaz, I., Guzmán-Linares, J., Limón, I. D., Manuel-Sánchez, D. M., Molina-Herrera, A., Coral-García, M. Á., Anastasio, E., Anaya-Hernández, A., López-Salazar, P., Juárez-Díaz, G., Martínez-Juárez, J., Torres-Jácome, J., Albarado-Ibáñez, A., Martínez-Laguna, Y., Morán, C., & Rubio, K. (2024). Epigenetic mechanisms of particulate matter exposure: Air pollution and hazards on human health. *Frontiers in Genetics, 14*, 1306600. DOI: 10.3389/fgene.2023.1306600 PMID: 38299096

Gbemudu, B. A. (2023). Environmental risk factors in lung and skin cancer. SSRN Electronic Journal. DOI: 10.2139/ssrn.4579295

Gonda, T. A., Tu, S., & Wang, T. C. (2009). Chronic inflammation, the tumor microenvironment and carcinogenesis. *Cell Cycle (Georgetown, Tex.), 8*(13), 2005–2013. DOI: 10.4161/cc.8.13.8985 PMID: 19550141

Gummadi, J., Bhatt, D. L., Adusumilli, S., Devabhaktuni, V., Acosta, W., & Kumar, A. (2014). Interpolation techniques for modeling and estimating indoor radon concentrations in ohio: Comparative study. Environmental Progress &Amp. *Environmental Progress & Sustainable Energy, 34*(1), 169–177. DOI: 10.1002/ep.11937

Gutiérrez-Camino, Á., Martín-Guerrero, I., & García-Orad, Á. (2017). Genetic susceptibility in childhood acute lymphoblastic leukemia. *Medical Oncology (Northwood, London, England), 34*(10), 179. Advance online publication. DOI: 10.1007/s12032-017-1038-7 PMID: 28905228

Herceg, Z., Ghantous, A., Wild, C. P., Sklias, A., Casati, L., Duthie, S. J., Fry, R., Issa, J. P., Kellermayer, R., Koturbash, I., Kondo, Y., Lepeule, J., Lima, S. C. S., Marsit, C. J., Rakyan, V., Saffery, R., Taylor, J. A., Teschendorff, A. E., Ushijima, T., & Hernandez-Vargas, H. (2018). Roadmap for investigating epigenome deregulation and environmental origins of cancer. *International Journal of Cancer, 142*(5), 874–882. DOI: 10.1002/ijc.31014 PMID: 28836271

Hudson, L., Samons, K. M., Dicken, H., Prichard, C., Weiss, L. T., Edward, J., Vanderpool, R. C., & Vanderford, N. L. (2021). A Brief Educational Intervention Enhances Basic Cancer Literacy Among Kentucky Middle and High School Students. *Journal of Cancer Education, 36*(4), 735–740. DOI: 10.1007/s13187-020-01696-3 PMID: 31989408

Jaiswara, P. K., Sonker, P., & Kumar, A. (2021). *Immune Response and Oxidative Stress in Obesity-Induced Cancer*. Springer., DOI: 10.1007/978-981-16-1846-8_6

Jarup, L. (2004). Health and environment information systems for exposure and disease mapping, and risk assessment. *Environmental Health Perspectives, 112*(9), 995–997. DOI: 10.1289/ehp.6736 PMID: 15198919

Juarez, P. D., Hood, D. B., Song, M. A., & Ramesh, A. (2022). Applying an Exposome-wide Association Study (ExWAS) Approach to Latino Cancer Disparities. In Ramirez, A. G. (Ed.), *et al., Advancing the Science of Cancer in Latinos: Building Collaboration for Action* (pp. 17–32). Springer.

Juarez, P. D., & Matthews-Juarez, P. (2018). Applying an Exposome-Wide (ExWAS) Approach to Cancer Research. *Frontiers in Oncology, 8*, 313. DOI: 10.3389/fonc.2018.00313 PMID: 30211112

Juarez, P. D., Matthews-Juarez, P., Hood, D. B., Im, W., Levine, R. S., Kilbourne, B. J., Langston, M. A., Al-Hamdan, M. Z., Crosson, W. L., Estes, M. G., Estes, S. M., Agboto, V. K., Robinson, P., Wilson, S., & Lichtveld, M. Y. (2014). The public health exposome: A population-based, exposure science approach to health disparities research. *International Journal of Environmental Research and Public Health, 11*(12), 12866–12895. DOI: 10.3390/ijerph111212866 PMID: 25514145

Justino, C. I., Duarte, A. C., & Rocha-Santos, T. (2017). Recent progress in biosensors for environmental monitoring: A review. *Sensors (Basel), 17*(12), 2918. DOI: 10.3390/s17122918 PMID: 29244756

Koedrith, P., Thasiphu, T., Weon, J., Boonprasert, R., Tuitemwong, K., & Tuitemwong, P. (2015). Recent trends in rapid environmental monitoring of pathogens and toxicants: potential of nanoparticle-based biosensor and applications. The Scientific World Journal, 2015(1). DOI: 10.1155/2015/510982

Kuther, T. L., & Posada, M. (2004). Children and adolescents' capacity to provide informed consent for participation in research. *Advances in Psychology Research, 32*, 163–173. PMID: 16986221

Langley, B., Talas, S., El-Shakankery, K. H., & Michie, C. (2023). Improving Inclusivity, Equity, and Diversity in Oncology Clinical Trials: A European Perspective. DOI: 10.33590/emjoncol/10303428

Lewis, C. M.Jr, McCall, L. I., Sharp, R. R., & Spicer, P. G. (2020). Ethical priority of the most actionable system of biomolecules: The metabolome. *American Journal of PhysicalAnthropology, 171*(2), 177–181. DOI: 10.1002/ajpa.23943 PMID: 31643083

Lind, C., Anderson, B., & Oberle, K. (2003). Ethical issues in adolescent consent for research. *Nursing Ethics, 10*(5), 504–511. DOI: 10.1191/0969733003ne632oa PMID: 14529117

Malecki, K. M. C., Nikodemova, M., Schultz, A. A., LeCaire, T. J., Bersch, A. J., Cadmus-Bertram, L., Engelman, C. D., Hagen, E., McCulley, L., Palta, M., Rodriguez, A., Sethi, A. K., Walsh, M. C., Nieto, F. J., & Peppard, P. E. (2022). The Survey of the Health of Wisconsin (SHOW) Program: An Infrastructure for Advancing Population Health. *Frontiers in Public Health, 10*, 818777. DOI: 10.3389/fpubh.2022.818777 PMID: 35433595

McKeon, T. P., Hwang, W. T., Ding, Z., Tam, V., Wileyto, P., Glanz, K., & Penning, T. M. (2021). Environmental exposomics and lung cancer risk assessment in the Philadelphia metropolitan area using ZIP code-level hazard indices. *Environmental Science and Pollution Research International, 28*(24), 31758–31769. DOI: 10.1007/s11356-021-12884-z PMID: 33611735

Miller, G. W. (2014). *Staging the Exposome: A Vision for International Collaboration.*, DOI: 10.1016/B978-0-12-417217-3.00007-0

Murphy, C. C., & Zaki, T. A. (2024). Changing epidemiology of colorectal cancer - birth cohort effects and emerging risk factors. *Nature Reviews. Gastroenterology & Hepatology, 21*(1), 25–34. DOI: 10.1038/s41575-023-00841-9 PMID: 37723270

Naidu, S. C., Manolakos, P. T., & Hopkins, T. (2013). Environmental justice in ohio. *The Review of Radical Political Economics, 45*(3), 384–399. DOI: 10.1177/0486613412470094

Navarro-Bielsa, A., Gracia-Cazaña, T., Almagro, M., De la Fuente-Meira, S., Flórez, Á., Yélamos, O., Montero-Vilchez, T., González-Cruz, C., Diago, A., Abadías-Granado, I., Fuentelsaz, V., Colmenero, M., Bañuls, J., Arias-Santiago, S., Buendía-Eisman, A., Almenara-Blasco, M., Gil-Pallares, P., & Gilaberte, Y. (2023). The Influence of the Exposome in the Cutaneous Squamous Cell Carcinoma, a Multicenter Case-Control Study. *Cancers (Basel), 15*(22), 5376. DOI: 10.3390/cancers15225376 PMID: 38001636

Neagu, A. N., Jayaweera, T., Corrice, L., Johnson, K., & Darie, C. C. (2024). Breast Cancer Exposomics. *Life (Basel, Switzerland), 14*(3), 402. DOI: 10.3390/life14030402 PMID: 38541726

Neveu, V., Nicolas, G., Salek, R. M., Wishart, D. S., & Scalbert, A. (2019). Exposome-Explorer 2.0: An update incorporating candidate dietary biomarkers and dietary associations with cancer risk. *Nucleic Acids Research, 48*, gkz1009. Advance online publication. DOI: 10.1093/nar/gkz1009 PMID: 31724701

O'Connell, K. A., Stolley, M. R., Berg, D., & Kerschner, A. (2023). Cancer health education in high schools: A qualitative analysis of student gains. *Cancer Epidemiology, Biomarkers & Prevention, 32*(12, Supplement), A072. DOI: 10.1158/1538-7755.DISP23-A072

Olmedo-Suárez, M. Á., Ramírez-Díaz, I., Pérez-González, A., Molina-Herrera, A., Coral-García, M. Á., Lobato, S., Sarvari, P., Barreto, G., & Rubio, K. (2022). Epigenetic Regulation in Exposome-Induced Tumorigenesis: Emerging Roles of ncRNAs. *Biomolecules, 12*(4), 513. DOI: 10.3390/biom12040513 PMID: 35454102

Omoijuanfo, E.-O., Williams, J. T., Qua, K., Cullen, J., Trapl, E. S., Owusu, C., Junk, D. J., & Berger, N. A. (2022). Disparities Education Strategies in the Case Comprehensive Cancer Center STEM Focused Youth Enjoy Science Program. *Journal of STEM Outreach, 5*(2). Advance online publication. DOI: 10.15695/jstem/v5i2.07 PMID: 36200123

Overbeek, G., Finkenauer, C., Alink, L. R. A., Leijten, P., Branje, S., Schrama, W., & Schenk, J. (2024). Caregiver Consent in Research on Minors: Towards an Inclusive, Hybrid Approach Running Head: Consent Approaches in Human Behavior Research. DOI: 10.31234/osf.io/k8muz

Parker, L. (2014). *The Impact of the Environment on Cancer Genomics*. Academic Press., DOI: 10.1016/B978-0-12-396967-5.00026-8

Patierno, S. R. (2020). Environmental Factors. In *Abeloff's Clinical Oncology* (pp. 139–153.e2). Elsevier. DOI: 10.1016/B978-0-323-47674-4.00010-4

Rodriguez, L. L., Brooks, L. D., Greenberg, J. H., & Green, E. D. (2013). Research ethics. The complexities of genomic identifiability. *Science*, *339*(6117), 275–276. DOI: 10.1126/science.1234593 PMID: 23329035

Rovira, J., Nadal, M., Schuhmacher, M., & Domingo, J. L. (2021). Environmental impact and human health risks of air pollutants near a large chemical/petrochemical complex: Case study in Tarragona, Spain. *The Science of the Total Environment*, *787*, 147550. DOI: 10.1016/j.scitotenv.2021.147550 PMID: 33991912

Safarlou, C. W., Jongsma, K. R., Vermeulen, R., & Bredenoord, A. L. (2023). The ethical aspects of exposome research: A systematic review. *Exposome*, *3*(1), osad004. Advance online publication. DOI: 10.1093/exposome/osad004 PMID: 37745046

Sarigiannis, D., Karakitsios, S., Anesti, O., Stem, A., Valvi, D., Sumner, S. C. J., Chatzi, L., Snyder, M. P., Thompson, D. C., & Vasiliou, V. (2025). Advancing translational exposomics: Bridging genome, exposome and personalized medicine. *Human Genomics*, *19*(1), 48. DOI: 10.1186/s40246-025-00761-6 PMID: 40307849

Senier, L., Brown, P., Shostak, S., & Hanna, B. (2017). The Socio-Exposome: Advancing Exposure Science and Environmental Justice in a Post-Genomic Era. *Environmental Sociology*, *3*(2), 107–121. DOI: 10.1080/23251042.2016.1220848 PMID: 28944245

Sharif, R., & Ooi, T. C. (2024). Understanding exposomes and its relation with cancer risk in Malaysia based on epidemiological evidence: A narrative review. *Genes and Environment : the Official Journal of the Japanese Environmental Mutagen Society*, *46*(1), 5. Advance online publication. DOI: 10.1186/s41021-024-00300-0 PMID: 38326915

Sharma, A., Kishore, D., & Singh, B. (2015). Environmental and anthropogenic carcinogens and their carcinogenic effects on humans. *Journal of Biomedical and Pharmaceutical Research*, *4*(2). http://www.jbpr.in/index.php/jbpr/article/view/405/0

Smith, M. T. (2010). Advances in understanding benzene health effects and susceptibility. *Annual Review of Public Health*, *31*(1), 133–148. DOI: 10.1146/annurev.publhealth.012809.103646 PMID: 20070208

Stanifer, S., Hoover, A., Rademacher, K., Rayens, M. K., Haneberg, W. C., & Hahn, E. J. (2022). Citizen science approach to home radon testing, environmental health literacy and efficacy. *Citizen Science: Theory and Practice*, *7*(1), 26. Advance online publication. DOI: 10.5334/cstp.472 PMID: 36845873

Talibov, M., Salmelin, R., Lehtinen-Jacks, S., & Auvinen, A. (2017). Estimation of occupational cosmic radiation exposure among airline personnel: Agreement between a job-exposure matrix, aggregate, and individual dose estimates. *American Journal of Industrial Medicine*, *60*(4), 386–393. DOI: 10.1002/ajim.22705 PMID: 28262960

Vega Vega, P., Miranda Castillo, C., & Vargas Celis, I. (2024). Consideraciones claves en el proceso de asentimiento en niños, niñas y adolescentes: Revisión integrativa [Key considerations in the process of assent in children and adolescents: an integrative review]. *Andes Pediatrica : Revista Chilena de Pediatria*, *95*(1), 91–106. DOI: 10.32641/andespediatr.v95i1.4968 PMID: 38587349

VoPham, T., White, A. J., & Jones, R. R. (2024). Geospatial Science for the Environmental Epidemiology of Cancer in the Exposome Era. *Cancer Epidemiology, Biomarkers & Prevention*, *33*(4), 451–460. DOI: 10.1158/1055-9965.EPI-23-1237 PMID: 38566558

Wan, M., Simonin, E. M., Johnson, M., Zhang, X., Lin, X., Gao, P., Patel, C. J., Yousuf, A. M. M., Hong, X., Wang, X., Sampath, V., & Nadeau, K. C. (2025). Exposomics: A review of methodologies, applications, and future directions in molecular medicine. *EMBO Molecular Medicine*, *17*(4), 599–608. Advance online publication. DOI: 10.1038/s44321-025-00191-w PMID: 39870881

Wang, L., Sun, W., Zhou, K., Zhang, M., & Bao, P. (2019). Spatial Analysis of Built Environment Risk for Respiratory Health and Its Implication for Urban Planning: A Case Study of Shanghai. *International Journal of Environmental Research and Public Health*, *16*(8), 1455. DOI: 10.3390/ijerph16081455 PMID: 31022924

Withrow, D. R., Freedman, N. D., Gibson, J. T., Yu, M., Nápoles, A. M., Berrington de Gonzalez, A., & Shiels, M. S. (2021). Leading cancers contributing to educational disparities in cancer mortality in the US, 2017. *Cancer Causes & Control*, *32*(11), 1193–1196. DOI: 10.1007/s10552-021-01471-9 PMID: 34244895

Wright, R. O., & Hanson, H. A. (2022). A tipping point in cancer epidemiology: Embracing a life course exposomic framework. *Trends in Cancer*, *8*(4), 280–282. DOI: 10.1016/j.trecan.2022.01.016 PMID: 35181274

Yarima, A., Ali, R. S., Abdullahi, A. A., & Idris, Z. I. (2020). Nanotechnology: Review on emerging techniques in remediating water and soil pollutions. *Journal of Applied Science & Environmental Management*, *24*(5), 933–941. DOI: 10.4314/jasem.v24i5.31

Young, A. S., Mullins, C. E., Sehgal, N., Vermeulen, R., Kolijn, P. M., Vlaanderen, J., Rahman, M. L., Birmann, B. M., Barupal, D. K., Lan, Q., Rothman, N., & Walker, D. I. (2024). The Need for a Cancer Exposome Atlas: A Scoping Review. *JNCI Cancer Spectrum*, *9*(1), pkae122. Advance online publication. DOI: 10.1093/jncics/pkae122 PMID: 39700422

Zhan, F. B., Brender, J. D., Han, Y., Suarez, L., & Langlois, P. H. (2006). GIS-EpiLink: A Spatial Search Tool for Linking Environmental and Health Data. *Journal of Medical Systems*, *30*(5), 405–412. DOI: 10.1007/s10916-006-9027-y PMID: 17069004

Zhang, Y., Yin, X., & Zheng, X. (2023). The relationship between pm2.5 and the onset and exacerbation of childhood asthma: A short communication. *Frontiers in Pediatrics*, *11*, 1191852. Advance online publication. DOI: 10.3389/fped.2023.1191852 PMID: 37593445

Compilation of References

Abate-Shen, C., & de Almeida, F. N. (2022). Establishment of the LNCaP cell line – the dawn of an era for prostate cancer research. *Cancer Research*, *82*(9), 1689–1691. DOI: 10.1158/0008-5472.CAN-22-1065 PMID: 35502546

Abdelhalim, H., Berber, A., Lodi, M., Jain, R., Nair, A., Pappu, A., Patel, K., Venkat, V., Venkatesan, C., Wable, R., Dinatale, M., Fu, A., Iyer, V., Kalove, I., Kleyman, M., Koutsoutis, J., Menna, D., Paliwal, M., Patel, N., & Ahmed, Z. (2022). Artificial Intelligence, Healthcare, Clinical Genomics, and Pharmacogenomics Approaches in Precision Medicine. *Frontiers in Genetics*, *13*, 929736. Advance online publication. DOI: 10.3389/fgene.2022.929736 PMID: 35873469

Agboola, O. O., Emmanuel, A. O., Sabina, C. E., Anejo-Okopi, J., Naomi, A. I., Ene, U. I., & Olowoyo, J. O. (2024). Occurrence of Carcinogens and their Potential Effects on Human Health – A Review. *UMYU Scientifica Journal*, *3*(1), 129–143. DOI: 10.56919/usci.2431.015

Aguayo, F., Muñoz, J. P., Perez-Dominguez, F., Carrillo-Beltrán, D., Oliva, C., Calaf, G. M., Blanco, R., & Nuñez-Acurio, D. (2020). High-risk human papillomavirus and tobacco smoke interactions in epithelial carcinogenesis. *Cancers (Basel)*, *12*(8), 2201. DOI: 10.3390/cancers12082201 PMID: 32781676

Ahmed, Z. (2022). Multi-omics strategies for personalized and predictive medicine: Past, current, and future translational opportunities. *Emerging Topics in Life Sciences*, *2*(2), 215–225. DOI: 10.1042/ETLS20210244 PMID: 35234253

Ahn, C., & Jeung, E. B. (2023). Endocrine-Disrupting Chemicals and Disease End-points. *International Journal of Molecular Sciences*, *24*(6), 5342. DOI: 10.3390/ijms24065342 PMID: 36982431

Ai, J., Wang, Y., Dar, J. A., Liu, J., Liu, L., Nelson, J. B., & Wang, Z. (2009). HDAC6 regulates androgen receptor hypersensitivity and nuclear localization via modulating Hsp90 acetylation in castration-resistant prostate cancer. *Molecular Endocrinology (Baltimore, Md.)*, *23*(12), 1963–1972. DOI: 10.1210/me.2009-0188 PMID: 19855091

Aimola, P., Carmignani, M., Volpe, A. R., Di Benedetto, A., Claudio, L., Waalkes, M. P., van Bokhoven, A., Tokar, E. J., & Claudio, P. P. (2012). Cadmium Induces p53-Dependent Apoptosis in Human Prostate Epithelial Cells. *PLoS One*, *7*(3), e33647. DOI: 10.1371/journal.pone.0033647 PMID: 22448262

Aitken, J. B., Naumovski, N., Curry, B., Grupen, C. G., Gibb, Z., & Aitken, R. J. (2015). Characterization of an L-amino acid oxidase in equine spermatozoa. *Biology of Reproduction*, *92*(5), 125. DOI: 10.1095/biolreprod.114.126052 PMID: 25740544

Aitken, R. J. (2020). *The male is significantly implicated as the cause of unexplained infertility*. Sem Reprod Med. DOI: 10.1055/s-0040-1718941

Ajayi, R. O., & Ogunjobi, T. T. (2024). *Environmental Exposures and Cancer Risk: A Comprehensive Review*. Deleted Journal., DOI: 10.47852/bonviewMEDIN42023598

Akl, M. M., & Ahmed, A. (2024). Exploring the interplay between the warburg effect and glucolipotoxicity in cancer development: A novel perspective on cancer etiology. *Advanced Pharmaceutical Bulletin*, *14*(3), 705–713. DOI: 10.34172/apb.2024.049 PMID: 39494260

Alam, M. N., Shapla, U. M., Shen, H., & Huang, Q. (2021). Linking emerging contaminants exposure to adverse health effects: Crosstalk between epigenome and environment. *Journal of Applied Toxicology*, *41*(6), 878–897. DOI: 10.1002/jat.4092 PMID: 33113590

Alavanja, M. C., Ross, M. K., & Bonner, M. R. (2013). Increased cancer burden among pesticide applicators and others due to pesticide exposure. *CA: a Cancer Journal for Clinicians*, *63*(2), 120–142. DOI: 10.3322/caac.21170 PMID: 23322675

Alexandrov, L. B., Kim, J., Haradhvala, N. J., Huang, M. N., Tian, N. G., Wu, Y., Boot, A., Covington, K. R., Gordenin, D. A., Bergstrom, E. N., Islam, S. M., Lopez-Bigas, N., Klimczak, L. J., McPherson, J. R., Morganella, S., Sabarinathan, R., Wheeler, D. A., & Mustonen, V. (2020, February). PCAWG Mutational Signatures Working Group; Getz G, Rozen SG, Stratton MR; PCAWG Consortium. The repertoire of mutational signatures in human cancer. [Erratum in: Nature. 2023 Feb;614] [7948] [:E41. doi: 10.1038/s41586-022-05600-5]. *Nature*, *578*(7793), 94–101. DOI: 10.1038/s41586-020-1943-3 PMID: 32025018

Ali, M. U., Lin, S., Yousaf, B., Abbas, Q., Munir, M. M., Rashid, A., Zheng, C., Kuang, X., & Wong, M. H. (2020). Pollution characteristics, mechanism of toxicity and health effects of the ultrafine particles in the indoor environment: Current status and future perspectives. *Critical Reviews in Environmental Science and Technology*, *52*(3), 436–473. DOI: 10.1080/10643389.2020.1831359

Al-Kafaji, G., Al-Naieb, Z. T., & Bakhiet, M. (2016). Increased oncogenic microRNA-18a expression in the peripheral blood of patients with prostate cancer: A potential novel non-invasive biomarker. *Oncology Letters*, *11*(2), 1201–1206. DOI: 10.3892/ol.2015.4014 PMID: 26893719

Alonso-Magdalena, P., S. Morimoto, C. Ripoll, E. Fuentes, & A. Nadal. (2011). The Estrogenic Effect of Bisphenol A Disrupts Pancreatic β-Cell Function in Vivo & Induces Insulin Resistance. *Aging Cell*, 10 (1), 19–30. https,//DOI: 10.1111/j.1474-9726.2010.00633.x

Alwadi, D., Felty, Q., Yoo, C., Roy, D., & Deoraj, A. (2023a). Endocrine Disrupting Chemicals Influence Hub Genes Associated with Aggressive Prostate Cancer. *International Journal of Molecular Sciences*, *24*(4), 3191. Advance online publication. DOI: 10.3390/ijms24043191 PMID: 36834602

Amare, A. T., Schubert, K. O., & Baune, B. T. (2017). Pharmacogenomics in the treatment of mood disorders: Strategies and Opportunities for personalized psychiatry. *The EPMA Journal*, *3*(3), 211–227. DOI: 10.1007/s13167-017-0112-8 PMID: 29021832

Andra, S. S., Austin, C., Wright, R. O., & Arora, M. (2015). Reconstructing pre-natal and early childhood exposure to multi-class organic chemicals using teeth: Towards a retrospective temporal exposome. *Environment International*, *83*, 137–145. DOI: 10.1016/j.envint.2015.05.010 PMID: 26134987

Anesti, O., Papaioannou, N., Gabriel, C., Karakoltzidis, A., Dzhedzheia, V., Petridis, I., Stratidakis, A., Dickinson, M., Horvat, M., Snoj Tratnik, J., Tsatsakis, A., Karakitsios, S., & Sarigiannis, D. A. (2023). An exposome connectivity paradigm for the mechanistic assessment of the effects of prenatal and early life exposure to metals on neurodevelopment. *Frontiers in Public Health*, *10*, 871218. Advance online publication. DOI: 10.3389/fpubh.2022.871218 PMID: 36699871

Anway, M. D., Cupp, A. S., Uzumcu, M., & Skinner, M. K. (2005). Epigenetic transgenerational actions of endocrine disruptors and male fertility. *Science*, *308*(5727), 1466–1469. DOI: 10.1126/science.1108190 PMID: 15933200

Anway, M. D., Leathers, C., & Skinner, M. K. (2006). Endocrine disruptor vinclozolin induced epigenetic transgenerational adult-onset disease. *Endocrinology, 147*(12), 5515–5523. DOI: 10.1210/en.2006-0640 PMID: 16973726

Appenzeller, B. M. R., Chadeau-Hyam, M., & Aguilar, L. (2020). Skin exposome science in practice: Current evidence on hair biomonitoring and future perspectives. *Journal of the European Academy of Dermatology and Venereology, 34*(S4, Suppl. 4), 26–30. DOI: 10.1111/jdv.16640 PMID: 32677066

Aquino, N. B., Sevigny, M. B., Sabangan, J., & Louie, M. C. (2012). The role of cadmium and nickel in estrogen receptor signaling and breast cancer: Metalloestrogens or not? *Journal of Environmental Science and Health. Part C, Environmental Carcinogenesis & Ecotoxicology Reviews, 30*(3), 189–224. DOI: 10.1080/10590501.2012.705159 PMID: 22970719

Arbuckle, T. E., Liang, C. L., Morisset, A. S., Fisher, M., Weiler, H., Cirtiu, C. M., Legrand, M., Davis, K., Ettinger, A. S., & Fraser, W. D. (2016). MIREC Study Group. Maternal and fetal exposure to cadmium, lead, manganese and mercury: The MIREC study. *Chemosphere, 163*, 270–282. DOI: 10.1016/j.chemosphere.2016.08.023 PMID: 27540762

Ard, K. (2016). By all measures: An examination of the relationship between segregation and health risk from air pollution. *Population and Environment, 38*(1), 1–20. DOI: 10.1007/s11111-015-0251-6

Ard, K., Colen, C., Becerra, M., & Velez, T. (2016). Two Mechanisms: The Role of Social Capital and Industrial Pollution Exposure in Explaining Racial Disparities in Self-Rated Health. *International Journal of Environmental Research and Public Health, 13*(10), 1025. DOI: 10.3390/ijerph13101025 PMID: 27775582

Arora, M., & Austin, C. (2013). Teeth as a Biomarker of Past Chemical Exposure. *Current Opinion in Pediatrics, 25*(2), 261–267. Advance online publication. DOI: 10.1097/MOP.0b013e32835e9084 PMID: 23429707

Arzuaga, X., Reiterer, G., Majkova, Z., Kilgore, M. W., Toborek, M., & Hennig, B. (2007). PPARα ligands reduce PCB-induced endothelial activation: Possible interactions in inflammation and atherosclerosis. *Cardiovascular Toxicology, 7*(4), 264–272. DOI: 10.1007/s12012-007-9005-8 PMID: 17955387

Asmuss, M., L. H. F. Mullenders, A. P. M. Eker, & A. Hartwig. (2000). Differential Effects of Toxic Metal Compounds on the Activities of Fpg & XPA, Two Zinc-Finger Proteins Involved in DNA Repair. *Carcinogenesis*, 21 (11), 2097–2104. https,//. DOI: 10.1093/carcin/21.11.2097

Athinarayanan, S., Dhanakodi, K., Rajamanickam, A.T., Sanjaygandhi, A., & Athinarayanan, S., (2025). Review on Advancements and Challenges in Cervical Cancer Diagnosis. *Communications on Applied Nonlinear Analysis, 32*(9), 2324–2336. DOI: 10.52783/cana.v32.4518

Athinarayanan, S., & Srinath, M. V. (2012). Cervical cell for Thinprep image enhancement using morphological segmentation. *International Journal of Management. IT and Engineering, 2*(4), 284–295.

Athinarayanan, S., Srinath, M. V., & Kavitha, R. (2017). Multi class cervical cancer classification by using ERSTCM, EMSD & CFE methods-based texture features and fuzzy logic-based hybrid kernel support vector machine classifier. *IOSR Journal of Computer Engineering, 19*(1), 23–34. DOI: 10.9790/0661-1901042334

Audouze, K., & Grandjean, P. (2011). Application of computational systems biology to explore environmental toxicity hazards. *Environmental Health Perspectives, 119*(12), 1754–1759. DOI: 10.1289/ehp.1103533 PMID: 21846611

Aygüneş, D. D. (2008). *Frequencies of CES1 gene polymorphisms in patients with metastatic breast cancer and retrospective evaluation of their effects on drug response in capecitabine users* (Master's thesis, Ege University).

Bacchiani, G., & Cardinal, D. (2017). Using biomarkers and early prophylactic treatment to prevent cardiotoxicity in cancer patients on chemotherapy: biomarkers: detection and treatment of cardiotoxicity., 9, 250-262. .DOI: 10.24170/9-4-1828

Baev, A. Y., Vinokurov, A. Y., Potapova, E. V., Dunaev, A. V., Angelova, P. R., & Abramov, A. Y. (2024). Mitochondrial Permeability Transition, Cell Death and Neurodegeneration. *Cells, 13*(7), 648. DOI: 10.3390/cells13070648 PMID: 38607087

Baker, B. (2019). Tackling the Lack of Diversity in Human Genome Collection. *Bioscience*, biz067. Advance online publication. DOI: 10.1093/biosci/biz067

Balali-Mood, M., Ghorani-Azam, A., & Riahi-Zanjani, B. (2016). Effects of air pollution on human health and practical measures for prevention in Iran. *Journal of Research in Medical Sciences : the Official Journal of Isfahan University of Medical Sciences, 1*(1), 65. DOI: 10.4103/1735-1995.189646 PMID: 27904610

Balbo, S., Turesky, R. J., & Villalta, P. W. (2014). DNA adductomics. *Chemical Research in Toxicology, 27*(3), 356–366. DOI: 10.1021/tx4004352 PMID: 24437709

Balcells, C., Xu, Y., Gil-Solsona, R., Maitre, L., Gago-Ferrero, P., & Keun, H. C. (2023). Blurred lines: Crossing the boundaries between the chemical exposome and the metabolome. *Current Opinion in Chemical Biology, 78*, 102407. DOI: 10.1016/j.cbpa.2023.102407 PMID: 38086287

Barabási, A. L., Gulbahce, N., & Loscalzo, J. (2011). Network medicine: A network-based approach to human disease. *Nature Reviews. Genetics*, *12*(1), 56–68. DOI: 10.1038/nrg2918 PMID: 21164525

Bartucci, M., Ferrari, A. C., Kim, I. Y., Ploss, A., Yarmush, M., & Sabaawy, H. E. (2016). Personalized medicine approaches in prostate cancer employing patient derived 3D organoids and humanized mice. *Frontiers in Cell and Developmental Biology*, *4*(JUN). Advance online publication. DOI: 10.3389/fcell.2016.00064 PMID: 27446916

Basanta, D., Strand, D. W., Lukner, R. B., Franco, O. E., Cliffel, D. E., Ayala, G. E., Hayward, S. W., & Anderson, A. R. A. (2009). The role of TGF-β mediated tumor-stroma interactions in prostate cancer progression: An integrative approach. *Cancer Research*, *69*(17), 7111. DOI: 10.1158/0008-5472.CAN-08-3957 PMID: 19706777

Bedewy, A. M. L., Showeta, S., Mostafa, M. H., & Kandil, L. S. (2016). The Influence of CYP2C9 and VKORC1 Gene Polymorphisms on the Response to Warfarin in Egyptians. *Indian Journal of Hematology & Blood Transfusion : An Official Journal of Indian Society of Hematology and Blood Transfusion*, *2*(2), 328–336. DOI: 10.1007/s12288-016-0725-4 PMID: 29622878

Bellinger, P. (2020, June). Functional Overreaching in Endurance Athletes: A Necessity or Cause for Concern? *Sports Medicine (Auckland, N.Z.)*, *50*(6), 1059–1073. DOI: 10.1007/s40279-020-01269-w PMID: 32064575

Ben-Levy, R., Hooper, S., Wilson, R., Paterson, H. F., & Marshall, C. J. (1998). Nuclear export of the stress-activated protein kinase p38 mediated by its substrate MAPKAP kinase-2. *Current Biology*, *8*(19), 1049–1057. DOI: 10.1016/S0960-9822(98)70442-7 PMID: 9768359

Benoit, L., Koual, M., Tomkiewicz, C., Bats, A.-S., Antignac, J.-P., Coumoul, X., Barouki, R., & Cano-Sancho, G. (2022). Impact of mixtures of persistent organic pollutants on breast cancer aggressiveness. *Environment International*, *170*, 107615. DOI: 10.1016/j.envint.2022.107615 PMID: 36343552

Bergman, A., Heindel, J. J., Kasten, T., Kidd, K. A., Jobling, S., Neira, M., Zoeller, R. T., Becher, G., Bjerregaard, P., Bornman, R., Brandt, I., Kortenkamp, A., Muir, D., Drisse, M.-N. B., Ochieng, R., Skakkebaek, N. E., Byléhn, A. S., Iguchi, T., Toppari, J., & Woodruff, T. J. (2013). The impact of endocrine disruption: A consensus statement on the state of the science. *Environmental Health Perspectives*, *121*(4), A104–A106. DOI: 10.1289/ehp.1205448 PMID: 23548368

Beshiri, M., Agarwal, S., Yin, J. J., & Kelly, K. (2023). Prostate organoids: emerging experimental tools for translational research. In *Journal of Clinical Investigation* (Vol. 133, Issue 10). American Society for Clinical Investigation. https://doi.org/ DOI: 10.1172/JCI169616

Bessonneau, V., & Rudel, R. A. (2019). Mapping the Human Exposome to Uncover the Causes of Breast Cancer. *International Journal of Environmental Research and Public Health, 17*(1), 189. DOI: 10.3390/ijerph17010189 PMID: 31892107

Bhan, A., Soleimani, M., & Mandal, S. S. (2017). Long Noncoding RNA and Cancer: A New Paradigm. *Cancer Research, 77*(15), 3965–3981. DOI: 10.1158/0008-5472. CAN-16-2634 PMID: 28701486

Bhavnani, S. K., Zhang, W., Bao, D., Raji, M., Ajewole, V., Hunter, R., Kuo, Y.-F., Schmidt, S., Pappadis, M. R., Smith, E., Bokov, A., Reistetter, T., Visweswaran, S., & Downer, B. (2023). *Subtyping Social Determinants of Health in*All of Us*: Network Analysis and Visualization Approach.* https://doi.org/DOI: 10.1101/2023.01.27.23285125

Bhowmik, A., Das, S., Bhattacharjee, A., Choudhury, B., Naiding, M., Deka, S., Ghosh, S. K., & Choudhury, Y. (2015). MDM2 and TP53 polymorphisms as predictive markers for head and neck cancer in Northeast Indian population: Effect of gene-gene and gene-environment interactions. *Asian Pacific Journal of Cancer Prevention : APJCP, 16*(14), 5767–5772. DOI: 10.7314/APJCP.2015.16.14.5767 PMID: 26320449

Bian, X., Wang, W., Abudurexiti, M., Zhang, X., Ma, W., Shi, G., Du, L., Xu, M., Wang, X., Tan, C., Sun, H., He, X., Zhang, C., Zhu, Y., Zhang, M., Ye, D., & Wang, J. (2024a). Integration Analysis of Single-Cell Multi-Omics Reveals Prostate Cancer Heterogeneity. *Advancement of Science, 11*(18), 2305724. DOI: 10.1002/ advs.202305724 PMID: 38483933

Bilancio, A., Bontempo, P., Di Donato, M., Conte, M., Giovannelli, P., Altucci, L., Migliaccio, A., & Castoria, G. (2017). Bisphenol A induces cell cycle arrest in primary and prostate cancer cells through EGFR/ERK/p53 signaling pathway activation. *Oncotarget, 8*(70), 115620–115631. DOI: 10.18632/oncotarget.23360 PMID: 29383186

Birkett, N., Al-Zoughool, M., Bird, M., Baan, R. A., Zielinski, J., & Krewski, D. (2019). Overview of biological mechanisms of human carcinogens. *Journal of Toxicology and Environmental Health. Part B, Critical Reviews, 22*(7-8), 288–359. DOI: 10.1080/10937404.2019.1643539 PMID: 31631808

Blake, B. E., & Fenton, S. E. (2020). Early life exposure to per- and polyfluoroalkyl substances (PFAS) and latent health outcomes: A review including the placenta as a target tissue and possible driver of peri- and postnatal effects. *Toxicology, 443,* 152565. DOI: 10.1016/j.tox.2020.152565 PMID: 32861749

Bloom, M. S., Fujimoto, V. Y., Steuerwald, A. J., Cheng, G., Browne, R. W., & Parsons, P. J. (2012). Background exposure to toxic metals in women adversely influences pregnancy during in vitro fertilization (IVF). *Reproductive Toxicology (Elmsford, N.Y.), 34*(3), 471–481. DOI: 10.1016/j.reprotox.2012.06.002 PMID: 22732149

Blum, B. C., Lin, W., Lawton, M. L., Liu, Q., Kwan, J., Turcinovic, I., Hekman, R., Hu, P., & Emili, A. (2022). Multiomic Metabolic Enrichment Network Analysis Reveals Metabolite–Protein Physical Interaction Subnetworks Altered in Cancer. *Molecular & Cellular Proteomics, 21*(1), 100189. DOI: 10.1016/j.mcpro.2021.100189 PMID: 34933084

Boas, M., U. Feldt-Rasmussen, & K. M. Main. (2006). Thyroid Effects of Endocrine Disrupting Chemicals. *Molecular & Cellular Endocrinology,* 254–255, 31–40. https,//.DOI: 10.1016/j.mce.2006.04.010

Bocato, M. Z., Bianchi Ximenez, J. P., Hoffmann, C., & Barbosa, F. (2019). An overview of the current progress, challenges, and prospects of human biomonitoring and exposome studies. *Journal of Toxicology and Environmental Health. Part B, Critical Reviews, 22*(5-6), 131–156. DOI: 10.1080/10937404.2019.1661588 PMID: 31543064

Bohacek, J., & Mansuy, I. M. (2015). Molecular insights into transgenerational non-genetic inheritance of acquired behaviours. *Nature Reviews. Genetics, 16*(11), 641–652. DOI: 10.1038/nrg3964 PMID: 26416311

Brann, D. W., K. Dh&apani, C. Wakade, V. B. Mahesh, & M. M. Khan. (2015). Estrogen & Its Receptors, An Overview Focused on Estrogen-Mediated Neuroprotection in the Context of Alzheimer's Disease. *Frontiers in Neuroendocrinology,* 35, 124–140. https,//.DOI: 10.1016/j.yfrne.2014.11.006

Bratton, M. R., Frigo, D. E., Segar, H. C., Nephew, K. P., McLachlan, J. A., Wiese, T. E., & Burow, M. E. (2012). The organochlorine o,p′-DDT plays a role in coactivator-mediated MAPK crosstalk in MCF-7 breast cancer cells. *Environmental Health Perspectives, 120*(9), 1291–1296. DOI: 10.1289/ehp.1104296 PMID: 22609851

Bray, F., Jemal, A., Grey, N., Ferlay, J., & Forman, D. (2012). Global cancer transitions according to the Human Development Index (2008–2030): A population-based study. *The Lancet. Oncology, 13*(8), 790–801. DOI: 10.1016/S1470-2045(12)70211-5 PMID: 22658655

Brown, E. A., Chain, F. J. J., Zhan, A., MacIsaac, H. J., & Cristescu, M. E. (2016). Early detection of aquatic invaders using metabarcoding reveals a high number of non-indigenous species in Canadian ports. *Diversity & Distributions, 22*(10), 1045–1059. DOI: 10.1111/ddi.12465

Buchanan, D. L., Ohsako, S., Tohyama, C., Cooke, P. S., & Iguchi, T. (2002). Dioxin Inhibition of Estrogen-Induced Mouse Uterine Epithelial Mitogenesis Involves Changes in Cyclin and Transforming Growth Factor-β Expression. *Toxicological Sciences, 66*(1), 62–68. DOI: 10.1093/toxsci/66.1.62 PMID: 11861973

Buoso, E., M. Masi, M. Racchi, & E. Corsini. (2020). Endocrine-Disrupting Chemicals' (EDCs) Effects on Tumour Microenvironment & Cancer Progression, Emerging Contribution of RACK1. International *Journal of Molecular Sciences,* 21 (23), 9229. https,//.DOI: 10.3390/ijms21239229

Burris-Hiday, S. D., & Scott, E. E. (2021). Steroidogenic Cytochrome P450 17A1 Structure and Function. *Molecular and Cellular Endocrinology, 528,* 111261. DOI: 10.1016/j.mce.2021.111261 PMID: 33781841

Byrne, C., Divekar, S. D., Storchan, G. B., Parodi, D. A., & Martin, M. B. (2013). Metals and breast cancer. *Journal of Mammary Gland Biology and Neoplasia, 18*(1), 63–73. DOI: 10.1007/s10911-013-9273-9 PMID: 23338949

Caetano, A., Silva, D., Martins, P., & De Oliveira Toscano, J. (2020). IMPACT OF PHYSICAL ACTIVITY ON FATIGUE AND QUALITY OF LIFE OF CANCER PATIENTS. *Revista Brasileira de Medicina do Esporte.* https://doi.org/DOI: 10.1590/1517-8692202026062019_0045

Cai, H., Zhang, B., Ahrenfeldt, J., Joseph, J. V., Riedel, M., Gao, Z., Thomsen, S. K., Christensen, D. S., Bak, R. O., Hager, H., Vendelbo, M. H., Gao, X., Birkbak, N., & Thomsen, M. K. (2024). CRISPR/Cas9 model of prostate cancer identifies Kmt2c deficiency as a metastatic driver by Odam/Cabs1 gene cluster expression. *Nature Communications, 15*(1), 2088. Advance online publication. DOI: 10.1038/s41467-024-46370-0 PMID: 38453924

Calderon-Gierszal, E. L., & Prins, G. S. (2015). Directed Differentiation of Human Embryonic Stem Cells into Prostate Organoids In Vitro and its Perturbation by Low-Dose Bisphenol A Exposure. *PLoS One, 10*(7), e0133238. DOI: 10.1371/journal.pone.0133238 PMID: 26222054

Calder, P. C., Carr, A. C., Gombart, A. F., & Eggersdorfer, M. (2020). Optimal nutritional status for a well-functioning immune system is an important factor to protect against viral infections. *Nutrients, 12*(4), 1181. DOI: 10.3390/nu12041181 PMID: 32340216

Calluori, S., Heimke, K. K., Caga-anan, C., Kaufman, D., Mechanic, L. E., & McAllister, K. A. (2024). Ethical, Legal, and Social Implications of Gene-Environment Interaction Research. *Genetic Epidemiology, 1*. Advance online publication. DOI: 10.1002/gepi.22591 PMID: 39315585

Capri, G., Tarenzi, E., Fulfaro, F., & Gianni, L. (1996). The role of taxanes in the treatment of breast cancer. *Seminars in Oncology*, *23*(1, Suppl 2), 68–75. PMID: 8614849

Carpenter, D. O. (2006). Polychlorinated Biphenyls (PCBs), Routes of Exposure & Effects on Human Health. *Reviews on Environmental Health,* 21 (1), 1–23. https,//. DOI: 10.1515/REVEH.2006.21.1.1

Carter, B. J., Jafry, M. Z., Siddiqi, A. D., Rogova, A., Liaw, W., & Reitzel, L. R. (2024). Incorporation of social determinants of health into health care practice: A strategy to address health disparities. In *Comprehensive Precision Medicine* (pp. 363–382). Elsevier., DOI: 10.1016/B978-0-12-824010-6.00016-2

Casals-Casas, C., & Desvergne, B. (2011). Endocrine disruptors: From endocrine to metabolic disruption. *Annual Review of Physiology*, *73*(1), 135–162. DOI: 10.1146/annurev-physiol-012110-142200 PMID: 21054169

Casati, L. (2013). Epigenetics and PCBs. *Endocrine Disruptors (Austin, Tex.)*, *1*(1), e27347. DOI: 10.4161/endo.27347

Castillo-Fernandez, J., Herrera-Puerta, E., Demond, H., Clark, S. J., Hanna, C. W., Hemberger, M., & Kelsey, G. (2020). Increased transcriptome variation and localised DNA methylation changes in oocytes from aged mice revealed by parallel single-cell analysis. *Aging Cell, 19*(12), e13278. DOI: 10.1111/acel.13278 PMID: 33201571

Cebrià, F., Kobayashi, C., Umesono, Y., Nakazawa, M., Mineta, K., Ikeo, K., Gojobori, T., Itoh, M., Taira, M., Sánchez Alvarado, A., & Agata, K. (2002). FGFR-related gene nou-darake restricts brain tissues to the head region of planarians. *Nature, 419*(6907), 620–624. DOI: 10.1038/nature01042 PMID: 12374980

Chang, L., Ewald, J., Hui, F., Bayen, S., & Xia, J. (2024). A data-centric perspective on exposomics data analysis. *Exposome*, *4*(1), osae005. Advance online publication. DOI: 10.1093/exposome/osae005

Cha, Y.-J., Jeong, H.-E., Shin, J.-G., Kim, E.-Y., Yu, K.-S., Cho, J.-Y., Yoon, S. H., & Lim, K. S. (2014). Genetic polymorphisms of the carboxylesterase 1 (*CES1*) gene in a Korean population. *Translational and Clinical Pharmacology*, *22*(1), 30–34. DOI: 10.12793/tcp.2014.22.1.30

Chen, Z., & Lu, W. (2015). Roles of ubiquitination and SUMOylation on prostate cancer: Mechanisms and clinical implications. *International Journal of Molecular Sciences*, *16*(3), 4560–4580. DOI: 10.3390/ijms16034560 PMID: 25734985

Cheong, A., Zhang, X., Cheung, Y. Y., Tang, W. Y., Chen, J., Ye, S. H., Medvedovic, M., Leung, Y. K., Prins, G. S., & Ho, S. M. (2016). DNA methylome changes by estradiol benzoate and bisphenol A links early-life environmental exposures to prostate cancer risk. *Epigenetics*, *11*(9), 674–689. DOI: 10.1080/15592294.2016.1208891 PMID: 27415467

Chervona, Y., & Costa, M. (2012). Histone modifications and cancer: Biomarkers of prognosis? *American Journal of Cancer Research*, *2*(5), 589–597. PMID: 22957310

Cheung, A. C., Walker, D. I., Juran, B. D., Miller, G. W., & Lazaridis, K. N. (2020). Studying the Exposome to Understand the Environmental Determinants of Complex Liver Diseases. *Hepatology (Baltimore, Md.)*, *71*(1), 352–362. DOI: 10.1002/hep.31028 PMID: 31701542

Cho, E., Allemang, A., Audebert, M., Chauhan, V., Dertinger, S., Hendriks, G., Marchetti, F., Minocherhomji, S., Pfuhler, S., Roberts, D. J., Trenz, K., & Yauk, C. L. (2023). Oxidative DNA damage leading to chromosomal aberrations and mutations. *OECD Series on Adverse Outcome Pathways*, *29*. Advance online publication. DOI: 10.1787/2415170X

Choi, K. Y. G., Wu, B. C., Lee, A. H. Y., Baquir, B., & Hancock, R. E. W. (2020). Utilizing Organoid and Air-Liquid Interface Models as a Screening Method in the Development of New Host Defense Peptides. *Frontiers in Cellular and Infection Microbiology*, *10*, 534019. DOI: 10.3389/fcimb.2020.00228 PMID: 32509598

Chopra, M., & Schrenk, D. (2011). Dioxin toxicity, aryl hydrocarbon receptor signaling, and apoptosis—Persistent pollutants affect programmed cell death. *Critical Reviews in Toxicology*, *41*(4), 292–320. DOI: 10.3109/10408444.2010.524635 PMID: 21323611

Choudhary, V., Kaddour-Djebbar, I., Lakshmikanthan, V., Ghazaly, T., Thangjam, G. S., Sreekumar, A., Lewis, R. W., Mills, I. G., Bollag, W. B., & Kumar, M. V. (2011). Novel Role of Androgens in Mitochondrial Fission and Apoptosis. *Molecular Cancer Research*, *9*(8), 1067–1077. DOI: 10.1158/1541-7786.MCR-10-0445 PMID: 21724752

Chung, H. Y., Kim, J. H., Han, I. H., & Ryu, J. S. (2020). Polarization of M2 Macrophages by Interaction between Prostate Cancer Cells Treated with Trichomonas vaginalis and Adipocytes. *Korean Journal of Parasitology, 58*(3), 217–227. DOI: 10.3347/kjp.2020.58.3.217 PMID: 32615735

Claw, K. G., Dorr, C. R., & Woodahl, E. L. (2024). Implementing community-engaged pharmacogenomics in Indigenous communities. *Nature Communications, 1*(1), 920. Advance online publication. DOI: 10.1038/s41467-024-45032-5 PMID: 38296967

Coffey, K., & Robson, C. N. (2012). Regulation of the androgen receptor by post-translational modifications. *The Journal of Endocrinology, 215*(2), 221–237. DOI: 10.1530/JOE-12-0238 PMID: 22872761

Coffey, K., Rogerson, L., Ryan-Munden, C., Alkharaif, D., Stockley, J., Heer, R., Sahadevan, K., O'Neill, D., Jones, D., Darby, S., Staller, P., Mantilla, A., Gaughan, L., & Robson, C. N. (2013). The lysine demethylase, KDM4B, is a key molecule in androgen receptor signalling and turnover. *Nucleic Acids Research, 41*(8), 4433–4446. DOI: 10.1093/nar/gkt106 PMID: 23435229

Conteduca, V., Hess, J., Yamada, Y., Ku, S. Y., & Beltran, H. (2021). Epigenetics in prostate cancer: Clinical implications. *Translational Andrology and Urology, 10*(7), 3104–3116. DOI: 10.21037/tau-20-1339 PMID: 34430414

Copp, A. J., Stanier, P., & Greene, N. D. (2013). Neural tube defects: Recent advances, unsolved questions, and controversies. *Lancet Neurology, 12*(8), 799–810. DOI: 10.1016/S1474-4422(13)70110-8 PMID: 23790957

Corn, P. G. (2012). The tumor microenvironment in prostate cancer: Elucidating molecular pathways for therapy development. *Cancer Management and Research, 4*(1), 183. DOI: 10.2147/CMAR.S32839 PMID: 22904640

Corti, M., Lorenzetti, S., Ubaldi, A., Zilli, R., & Marcoccia, D. (2022). Endocrine Disruptors and Prostate Cancer. *International Journal of Molecular Sciences, 23*(3), 1216. DOI: 10.3390/ijms23031216 PMID: 35163140

Corton, J. C., & Lapinskas, P. J. (2005). Peroxisome Proliferator-Activated Receptors: Mediators of Phthalate Ester-Induced Effects in the Male Reproductive Tract? *Toxicological Sciences, 83*(1), 4–17. DOI: 10.1093/toxsci/kfi011 PMID: 15496498

Coudon, T., Danjou, A. M. N., Faure, E., Praud, D., Severi, G., Mancini, F. R., Salizzoni, P., & Fervers, B. (2019). Development and performance evaluation of a GIS-based metric to assess exposure to airborne pollutant emissions from industrial sources. *Environmental Health : A Global Access Science Source, 18*(1), 8. DOI: 10.1186/s12940-019-0446-x PMID: 30683108

Craighead, J. E., & Gibbs, A. R. (2008). *Asbestos and Its Diseases* (Craighead, J. E., & Gibbs, A. R., Eds.). Oxford University Press. Print DOI: 10.1093/acprof:oso/9780195178692.001.0001

Crea, F., Giovannetti, E., Zinzani, P., & Danesi, R. (2009). Pharmacologic rationale for early G-CSF prophylaxis in cancer patients and role of pharmacogenetics in treatment optimization. *Critical Reviews in Oncology/Hematology*, *72*(1), 21–44. DOI: 10.1016/j.critrevonc.2008.10.014 PMID: 19111474

Crea, F., Sun, L., Mai, A., Chiang, Y. T., Farrar, W. L., Danesi, R., & Helgason, C. D. (2012). The emerging role of histone lysine demethylases in prostate cancer. *Molecular Cancer*, *11*(1), 52. DOI: 10.1186/1476-4598-11-52 PMID: 22867098

Crespi, E., Bottai, G., & Santarpia, L. (2016). Role of inflammation in obesity-related breast cancer. *Current Opinion in Pharmacology*, *31*, 114–122. DOI: 10.1016/j.coph.2016.11.004 PMID: 27889687

Cross, A. J., Leitzmann, M. F., Gail, M. H., Hollenbeck, A. R., Schatzkin, A., & Sinha, R. (2007). A Prospective Study of Red and Processed Meat Intake in Relation to Cancer Risk. *PLoS Medicine*, *4*(12), e325. DOI: 10.1371/journal.pmed.0040325 PMID: 18076279

Crumbaker, M., Khoja, L., & Joshua, A. M. (2017). AR Signaling and the PI3K Pathway in Prostate Cancer. *Cancers (Basel)*, *9*(4), 34. DOI: 10.3390/cancers9040034 PMID: 28420128

Cui, H., Zhang, W., Zhang, L., Qu, Y., Xu, Z., Tan, Z., Yan, P., Tang, M., Yang, C., Wang, Y., Chen, L., Xiao, C., Zou, Y., Liu, Y., Zhang, L., Yang, Y., Yao, Y., Li, J., Liu, Z., & Zhang, B. (2024). Risk factors for prostate cancer: An umbrella review of prospective observational studies and mendelian randomization analyses. *PLoS Medicine*, *21*(3), e1004362. Advance online publication. DOI: 10.1371/journal.pmed.1004362 PMID: 38489391

Cui, J.-J., Wang, L.-Y., Zhu, T., Gong, W.-J., Zhou, H.-H., Liu, Z.-Q., & Yin, J.-Y. (2017). Gene-gene and gene-environment interactions influence platinum-based chemotherapy response and toxicity in non-small cell lung cancer patients. *Scientific Reports*, *7*(1), 5082. DOI: 10.1038/s41598-017-05246-8 PMID: 28698656

Cura, Y., Sánchez-Martín, A., Márquez-Pete, N., González-Flores, E., Martínez-Martínez, F., Pérez-Ramírez, C., & Jiménez-Morales, A. (2023). Association of single-nucleotide polymorphisms in capecitabine bioactivation pathway with adjuvant therapy safety in colorectal cancer patients. *Pharmaceutics*, *15*(11), 2548. DOI: 10.3390/pharmaceutics15112548 PMID: 38004528

D'Adamo, G. L., Widdop, J. T., & Giles, E. M. (2021). The future is now? Clinical and translational aspects of "Omics" technologies. *Immunology and Cell Biology*, *99*(2), 168–176. DOI: 10.1111/imcb.12404 PMID: 32924178

D'Andrea, M. A., & Reddy, G. K. (2013). Health effects of benzene exposure among children following a flaring incident at the british petroleum refinery in texas city. *Pediatric Hematology and Oncology*, *31*(1), 1–10. DOI: 10.3109/08880018.2013.831511 PMID: 24088183

Damaschke, N. A., Yang, B., Bhusari, S., Svaren, J. P., & Jarrard, D. F. (2013). Epigenetic susceptibility factors for prostate cancer with aging. *The Prostate*, *73*(16), 1721–1730. DOI: 10.1002/pros.22716 PMID: 23999928

Darbre, P. D., & P. W. Harvey. (2008). Paraben Esters, Review of Recent Studies of Endocrine Toxicity, Absorption, Esterase & Human Exposure, & Discussion of Potential Human Health Risks. *Journal of Applied Toxicology,* 28 (5), 561–578. https,//.DOI: 10.1002/jat.1358

Das, R., Sjöström, M., Shrestha, R., Yogodzinski, C., Egusa, E. A., Chesner, L. N., Chen, W. S., Chou, J., Dang, D. K., Swinderman, J. T., Ge, A., Hua, J. T., Kabir, S., Quigley, D. A., Small, E. J., Ashworth, A., Feng, F. Y., & Gilbert, L. A. (2021). An integrated functional and clinical genomics approach reveals genes driving aggressive metastatic prostate cancer. *Nature Communications*, *12*(1), 4601. Advance online publication. DOI: 10.1038/s41467-021-24919-7 PMID: 34326322

De Coster, S., & Van Larebeke, N. (2012). Endocrine-Disrupting Chemicals: Associated Disorders and Mechanisms of Action. *Journal of Environmental and Public Health, 713696*, 1–52. Advance online publication. DOI: 10.1155/2012/713696 PMID: 22991565

De Marzo, A. M., Platz, E. A., Sutcliffe, S., Xu, J., Grönberg, H., Drake, C. G., Nakai, Y., Isaacs, W. B., & Nelson, W. G. (2007). Inflammation in prostate carcinogenesis. *Nature Reviews. Cancer*, *7*(4), 256–269. DOI: 10.1038/nrc2090 PMID: 17384581

de With, M., Van Doorn, L., Maasland, D., Mulder, T., Hoop, O., Mostert, B., Homs, M., Bouazzaoui, E., Mathijssen, R., Van Schaik, R., & Bins, S. (2023). Capecitabine-induced hand-foot syndrome: A pharmacogenetic study beyond DPYD.. *Biomedicine & pharmacotherapy = Biomedecine & pharmacotherapie*, 159, 114232 . .DOI: 10.1016/j.biopha.2023.114232

Dehm, S. M., & Tindall, D. J. (2011). Alternatively Spliced Androgen Receptor Variants. *Endocrine-Related Cancer*, *18*(5), R183–R196. DOI: 10.1530/ERC-11-0141 PMID: 21778211

Desta, G. M., & Aserese, M. B. (2024). *Revolutionizing Personalized Medicine: Synergy with Multi-Omics Data Generation, Main Hurdles, and Future Perspectives*. https://doi.org/DOI: 10.20944/preprints202409.0196.v1

Di Donato, M., Cernera, G., Giovannelli, P., Galasso, G., Bilancio, A., Migliaccio, A., & Castoria, G. (2017). Recent advances on bisphenol-A and endocrine disruptor effects on human prostate cancer. *Molecular and Cellular Endocrinology*, *457*, 35–42. DOI: 10.1016/j.mce.2017.02.045 PMID: 28257827

Diamanti-Kandarakis, E., Bourguignon, J. P., Giudice, L. C., Hauser, R., Prins, G. S., Soto, A. M., Zoeller, R. T., & Gore, A. C. (2009). Endocrine-disrupting chemicals: An endocrine society scientific statement. *Endocrine Reviews*, *30*(4), 293–342. DOI: 10.1210/er.2009-0002 PMID: 19502515

Doherty, L. F., Bromer, J. G., Zhou, Y., Aldad, T. S., & Taylor, H. S. (2010). In Utero Exposure to Diethylstilbestrol (DES) or Bisphenol-A (BPA) Increases EZH2 Expression in the Mammary Gl&, An Epigenetic Mechanism Linking Endocrine Disruptors to Breast Cancer. *Hormones & Cancer*, 1 (3), 146–155. https,//DOI: 10.1007/s12672-010-0015-9

Dolinoy, D. C., Huang, D., & Jirtle, R. L. (2007). Maternal Nutrient Supplementation Counteracts Bisphenol A-Induced DNA Hypomethylation in Early Development. *Proceedings of the National Academy of Sciences*, 104 (32), 13056–13061. https,// DOI: 10.1073/pnas.0703739104

Donkin, I., & Barrès, R. (2018). Sperm epigenetics and influence of environmental factors. *Molecular Metabolism*, *14*, 1–11. DOI: 10.1016/j.molmet.2018.02.006 PMID: 29525406

du Plessis, M., Fourie, C., Stone, W., & Engelbrecht, A.-M. (2023). The impact of endocrine disrupting compounds and carcinogens in wastewater: Implications for breast cancer. *Biochimie*, *209*, 103–115. DOI: 10.1016/j.biochi.2023.02.006 PMID: 36775066

Dupras, C., Saulnier, K. M., & Joly, Y. (2019). Epigenetics, ethics, law and society: A multidisciplinary review of descriptive, instrumental, dialectical and reflexive analyses. *Social Studies of Science*, *49*(5), 785–810. DOI: 10.1177/0306312719866007 PMID: 31366289

Durairajanayagam, D., Agarwal, A., & Ong, C. (2015). Causes, effects and molecular mechanisms of testicular heat stress. *Reproductive Biomedicine Online*, *30*(1), 14–27. DOI: 10.1016/j.rbmo.2014.09.018 PMID: 25456164

Edson, M. A., Nagaraja, A. K., & Matzuk, M. M. (2009). The mammalian ovary from genesis to revelation. *Endocrine Reviews, 30*(6), 624–712. DOI: 10.1210/er.2009-0012 PMID: 19776209

Elespuru, R., & Fischer, C. (2021). Abstract 2612: Personalized cancer risk and prevention: analysis of risk factors for specific cancers and integration into cancer risk assessment paradigms. *Cancer Research, 81*(13_Supplement), 2612. Advance online publication. DOI: 10.1158/1538-7445.AM2021-2612

Ellem, S. J., De-Juan-Pardo, E. M., & Risbridger, G. P. (2014). In vitro modeling of the prostate cancer microenvironment. In *Advanced Drug Delivery Reviews* (Vol. 79, pp. 214–221). Elsevier B.V., DOI: 10.1016/j.addr.2014.04.008

Erlandsson, A., Carlsson, J., Lundholm, M., Fält, A., Andersson, S. O., Andrén, O., & Davidsson, S. (2018). M2 macrophages and regulatory T cells in lethal prostate cancer. *The Prostate, 79*(4), 363–369. DOI: 10.1002/pros.23742 PMID: 30500076

Espina, C., Straif, K., Friis, S., Kogevinas, M., Saracci, R., Vainio, H., & Schüz, J. (2015). European Code against Cancer 4th Edition: Environment, occupation and cancer. Cancer Epidemiology, 39, S84–S92. DOI: 10.1016/j.canep.2015.03.017

European Chemicals Agency. (2013). *Nonylphenol and nonylphenol ethoxylates restricted under*. REACHUS.

European Chemicals Agency. (2017). Bisphenol A added to the Candidate List for authorisation. *ECHA*. https://echa.europa.eu/-/bisphenol

European Chemicals Agency. (2020). Phthalates: DEHP, DBP, BBP and DIBP. *ECHA*. https://echa.europa.eu/hot-topics/phthalates

European Commission. (2004). Directive 2004/248/EC, Banning Atrazine in the EU. Official Journal of the European Union. https,//eur-lex.europa.eu/legal-content/EN/TXT/

European Food Safety Authority. (2018). Risks for Animal & Human Health Related to the Presence of Dioxins & Dioxin-like PCBs in Feed & Food. EFSA Journal 16 (11), e05333. https,//.DOI: 10.2903/j.efsa.2018.5333

Fatma Karaman, E., Caglayan, M., Sancar-Bas, S., Ozal-Coskun, C., Arda-Pirincci, P., & Ozden, S. (2019). Global and region-specific post-transcriptional and post-translational modifications of bisphenol A in human prostate cancer cells. *Environmental Pollution, 255*, 113318. DOI: 10.1016/j.envpol.2019.113318 PMID: 31610501

Feil, R., & Fraga, M. F. (2012). Epigenetics and the environment: Emerging patterns and implications. *Nature Reviews. Genetics*, *13*(2), 97–109. DOI: 10.1038/nrg3142 PMID: 22215131

Feinberg, A. P., Koldobskiy, M. A., & Göndör, A. (2016). Epigenetic modulators, modifiers and mediators in cancer aetiology and progression. *Nature Reviews. Genetics*, *17*(5), 284–299. DOI: 10.1038/nrg.2016.13 PMID: 26972587

Feng, J., & Yang, W. (2012). Effects of particulate air pollution on cardiovascular health: A population health risk assessment. *PLoS One*, *7*(3), e33385. DOI: 10.1371/journal.pone.0033385 PMID: 22432017

Ferro, M., Ungaro, P., Cimmino, A., Lucarelli, G., Busetto, G. M., Cantiello, F., Damiano, R., & Terracciano, D. (2017). Epigenetic signature: A new player as predictor of clinically significant prostate cancer (PCa) in patients on active surveillance (AS). In International Journal of Molecular Sciences (Vol. 18, Issue 6). MDPI AG. https://doi.org/DOI: 10.3390/ijms18061146

Filippini, T., Heck, J. E., Malagoli, C., Giovane, C. D., & Vinceti, M. (2015). A review and meta-analysis of outdoor air pollution and risk of childhood leukemia. *Journal of Environmental Science and Health. Part C, Environmental Carcinogenesis & Ecotoxicology Reviews*, *33*(1), 36–66. DOI: 10.1080/10590501.2015.1002999 PMID: 25803195

Foley, R., Marignol, L., Keane, J. P., Lynch, T. H., & Hollywood, D. (2011). Androgen hypersensitivity in prostate cancer: Molecular perspectives on androgen deprivation therapy strategies. *The Prostate*, *71*(5), 550–557. DOI: 10.1002/pros.21266 PMID: 20945429

Frew, P. M., Fisher, A. K., Basket, M. M., Chung, Y., Schamel, J., Weiner, J. L., Mullen, J., Omer, S. B., & Orenstein, W. A. (2016). Changes in childhood immunization decisions in the United States: Results from 2012 & 2014 National Parental Surveys. *Vaccine*, *34*(46), 5689–5696. DOI: 10.1016/j.vaccine.2016.08.001 PMID: 27720447

Fullston, T., Teague, E. M. C. O., Palmer, N. O., Deblasio, M. J., Mitchell, M., Corbett, M., Print, C. G., Owens, J. A., & Lane, M. (2013). Paternal obesity initiates metabolic disturbances in two generations of mice with incomplete penetrance to the F2 generation and alters the transcriptional profile of testis and sperm microRNA content. *The FASEB Journal*, *27*(10), 4226–4243. DOI: 10.1096/fj.12-224048 PMID: 23845863

Gao, D., Vela, I., Sboner, A., Iaquinta, P. J., Karthaus, W. R., Gopalan, A., Dowling, C., Wanjala, J. N., Undvall, E. A., Arora, V. K., Wongvipat, J., Kossai, M., Ramazanoglu, S., Barboza, L. P., Di, W., Cao, Z., Zhang, Q. F., Sirota, I., Ran, L., & Chen, Y. (2014). Organoid cultures derived from patients with advanced prostate cancer. *Cell, 159*(1), 176–187. DOI: 10.1016/j.cell.2014.08.016 PMID: 25201530

Gao, H., Chen, X., Cai, Q., Shang, Z., & Niu, Y. (2018). Increased KIF4a expression is a potential prognostic factor in prostate cancer. *Oncology Letters*, *15*(5), 7941–7947. DOI: 10.3892/ol.2018.8322 PMID: 29725481

Gao, M., Li, H., Dang, F., Chen, L., Liu, X., & Gao, J. (2020). Induction of proliferative and mutagenic activity by benzo(a)pyrene in PC-3 cells via JAK2/STAT3 pathway. *Mutation Research. Fundamental and Molecular Mechanisms of Mutagenesis*, *821*, 111720. DOI: 10.1016/j.mrfmmm.2020.111720 PMID: 32841893

Gao, S., Chen, S., Han, D., Wang, Z., Li, M., Han, W., Besschetnova, A., Liu, M., Zhou, F., Barrett, D., Luong, M. P., Owiredu, J., Liang, Y., Ahmed, M., Petricca, J., Patalano, S., Macoska, J. A., Corey, E., Chen, S., & Cai, C. (2020). Chromatin binding of FOXA1 is promoted by LSD1-mediated demethylation in prostate cancer. *Nature Genetics*, *52*(10), 1011–1017. DOI: 10.1038/s41588-020-0681-7 PMID: 32868907

Gao, W., Wang, Y., Yu, S., Wang, Z., Ma, T., Chan, A. M. L., Chiu, P. K. F., Ng, C. F., Wu, D., & Chan, F. L. (2022). Endothelial nitric oxide synthase (eNOS)-NO signaling axis functions to promote the growth of prostate cancer stem-like cells. *Stem Cell Research & Therapy*, *13*(1), 188. Advance online publication. DOI: 10.1186/s13287-022-02864-6 PMID: 35526071

Garcia-Bermudez, J., & Birsoy, K. (2016). Drugging ACAT1 for Cancer Therapy. *Molecular Cell*, *64*(5), 856–857. DOI: 10.1016/j.molcel.2016.11.023 PMID: 27912096

García-Cárdenas, J. M., Indacochea, A., Pesantez-Coronel, D., Terán-Navas, M., Aleaga, A., Armendáriz-Castillo, I., Peña Zúñiga, L., Morán-Erazo, C., Chávez-Vélez, E., Pérez-Villa, A., López-Cortés, A., & Guerrero, S. (2024). Toward Equitable Precision Oncology: Monitoring Racial and Ethnic Inclusion in Genomics and Clinical Trials. *JCO Precision Oncology*, *8*(8), e2300398. DOI: 10.1200/PO.23.00398 PMID: 38662980

García-González, X., Cortejoso, L., García, M., García-Alfonso, P., Robles, L., Grávalos, C., González-Haba, E., Marta, P., Sanjurjo, M., & López-Fernández, L. (2015). Variants in CDA and ABCB1 are predictors of capecitabine-related adverse reactions in colorectal cancer. *Oncotarget*, *6*(8), 6422–6430. DOI: 10.18632/oncotarget.3289 PMID: 25691056

Garofoli, M., Maiorano, B. A., Bruno, G., Giordano, G., Di Tullio, P., Maselli, F. M., Landriscina, M., & Conteduca, V. (2024). Androgen receptor, PARP signaling, and tumor microenvironment: The 'perfect triad' in prostate cancer? *Therapeutic Advances in Medical Oncology*, *16*, 17588359241258444. DOI: 10.1177/17588359241258443 PMID: 38887656

Garrison, N. A., Hudson, M., Ballantyne, L. L., Garba, I., Martinez, A., Taualii, M., Arbour, L., Caron, N. R., & Rainie, S. C. (2019). Genomic Research Through an Indigenous Lens: Understanding the Expectations. *Annual Review of Genomics and Human Genetics*, *1*(1), 495–517. DOI: 10.1146/annurev-genom-083118-015434 PMID: 30892943

Gavito-Covarrubias, D., Ramírez-Díaz, I., Guzmán-Linares, J., Limón, I. D., Manuel-Sánchez, D. M., Molina-Herrera, A., Coral-García, M. Á., Anastasio, E., Anaya-Hernández, A., López-Salazar, P., Juárez-Díaz, G., Martínez-Juárez, J., Torres-Jácome, J., Albarado-Ibáñez, A., Martínez-Laguna, Y., Morán, C., & Rubio, K. (2024). Epigenetic mechanisms of particulate matter exposure: Air pollution and hazards on human health. *Frontiers in Genetics*, *14*, 1306600. DOI: 10.3389/fgene.2023.1306600 PMID: 38299096

Gbemudu, B. A. (2023). Environmental risk factors in lung and skin cancer. SSRN Electronic Journal. DOI: 10.2139/ssrn.4579295

Georgiadis, P., Bolognesi, C., Palli, D., & Farmer, P. B. (2013). Abstracts of the UKMEG/ECNIS2-sponsored Workshop on Design of Future Molecular Epidemiology Studies and New Biomarkers, Waterloo Conference Centre, London, United Kingdom. November 30, 2012. *Mutagenesis*, *28*(3), e1–e5. DOI: 10.1093/mutage/get011

Ghalehbandi, S., Yuzugulen, J., Pranjol, M. Z. I., & Pourgholami, M. H. (2023). The role of VEGF in cancer-induced angiogenesis and research progress of drugs targeting VEGF. *European Journal of Pharmacology*, *949*, 175586. DOI: 10.1016/j.ejphar.2023.175586 PMID: 36906141

Gluckman, P. D., Hanson, M. A., Buklijas, T., Low, F. M., & Beedle, A. S. (2009). Epigenetic mechanisms that underpin metabolic and cardiovascular diseases. *Nature Reviews. Endocrinology*, *5*(7), 401–408. DOI: 10.1038/nrendo.2009.102 PMID: 19488075

Goldenberg, A. J., Hartmann, C. D., Morello, L., Brooks, S., Colón-Zimmermann, K., & Marshall, P. A. (2013). Gene–environment interactions and health inequalities: Views of underserved communities. *Journal of Community Genetics*, *4*(4), 425–434. DOI: 10.1007/s12687-013-0143-3 PMID: 23494820

Gómez-Acebo, I., Dierssen-Sotos, T., Fernandez-Navarro, P., Palazuelos, C., Moreno, V., Aragonés, N., Castaño-Vinyals, G., Jiménez-Monleón, J. J., Ruiz-Cerdá, J. L., Pérez-Gómez, B., Ruiz-Dominguez, J. M., Molero, J. A., Pollán, M., Kogevinas, M., & Llorca, J. (2017). Risk Model for Prostate Cancer Using Environmental and Genetic Factors in the Spanish Multi-Case-Control (MCC). *Scientific Reports*, *7*(1), 8994. Advance online publication. DOI: 10.1038/s41598-017-09386-9 PMID: 28827750

Gómez-Olarte, S., Mailänder, V., Castro-Neves, J., Stojanovska, V., Schumacher, A., Meyer, N., & Zenclussen, A. C. (2024). The ENDOMIX perspective: How everyday chemical mixtures impact human health and reproduction by targeting the immune system. *Biology of Reproduction*, *111*(6), 1170–1187. DOI: 10.1093/biolre/ioae142 PMID: 39446589

Gonda, T. A., Tu, S., & Wang, T. C. (2009). Chronic inflammation, the tumor microenvironment and carcinogenesis. *Cell Cycle (Georgetown, Tex.)*, *8*(13), 2005–2013. DOI: 10.4161/cc.8.13.8985 PMID: 19550141

Goodson, W. H.III, Lowe, L., Carpenter, D. O., Gilbertson, M., Manaf Ali, A., Lopez de Cerain Salsamendi, A., & Pavanello, S. (2015). Assessing the carcinogenic potential of low-dose exposures to chemical mixtures in the environment: The challenge ahead. *Carcinogenesis*, *36*(Suppl_1), S254–S296.

Gore, A. C., V. A. Chappell, S. E. Fenton, J. A. Flaws, A. Nadal, G. S. Prins, J. Toppari, & R. T. Zoeller. (2015). Executive Summary to EDC-2, The Endocrine Society's Second Scientific Statement on Endocrine-Disrupting Chemicals. *Endocrine Reviews,* 36 (6), 593–602. https,//.DOI: 10.1210/er.2015-1093

Gore, A. C., Chappell, V. A., Fenton, S. E., Flaws, J. A., Nadal, A., Prins, G. S., Toppari, J., & Zoeller, R. T. (2015). EDC-2: The Endocrine Society's second scientific statement on endocrine-disrupting chemicals. *Endocrine Reviews*, *36*(6), 1–150. DOI: 10.1210/er.2015-1010

Gou, Z., Li, J., Liu, J., & Yang, N. (2024). The hidden messengers: Cancer associated fibroblasts—derived exosomal miRNAs as key regulators of cancer malignancy. *Frontiers in Cell and Developmental Biology*, *12*, 1378302. DOI: 10.3389/fcell.2024.1378302 PMID: 38694824

Goyal, T., Mitra, P., Singh, P., Sharma, S., Purohit, P., & Sharma, P. (2022). Effect of occupational co-exposure to lead and cadmium on selected immunomodulatory cytokines. *Toxicology and Industrial Health*, *38*(1), 1–10. DOI: 10.1177/07482337211019172 PMID: 34874211

Granata, I., & Barboro, P. (2024). Identification of Molecular Markers Associated with Prostate Cancer Subtypes: An Integrative Bioinformatics Approach. *Biomolecules, 14*(1), 87. DOI: 10.3390/biom14010087 PMID: 38254687

Grandjean, P., E. W. & E. Budtz-Jorgensen, F. Nielsen, K. Molbak, P. Weihe, & C. Heilmann. (2012). Serum Vaccine Antibody Concentrations in Children Exposed to Perfluorinated Compounds. *JAMA*, 307 (4), 391–397. https,//.DOI: 10.1001/jama.2011.2034

Gray, L. E. Jr., J. Ostby, E. Monosson, & W. R. Kelce. (2000). Developmental Effects of an Environmental Anti&rogen, The Fungicide Vinclozolin Alters Sex Differentiation of the Male Rat. *Toxicology & Applied Pharmacology,* 164 (2), 294–305. https,//.DOI: 10.1006/taap.2000.9021

Greco, T., Poole, E. M., Young, A. C., & Alexander, J. K. (2024). Application of the Bayesian network theory in clinical trial data: Severity shift in spasticity numeric rating scale in patients with multiple sclerosis. *Multiple Sclerosis and Related Disorders, 83*, 105466. DOI: 10.1016/j.msard.2024.105466 PMID: 38310831

Gripshover, T., Wahlang, B., Head, K., Young, J., Luo, J., Mustafa, M., Kirpich, I., & Cave, M. (2022). Environmental pollutant, polychlorinated biphenyl 126, alters liver function in a rodent model of alcohol-associated liver disease. *Alcohol, Clinical and Experimental Research.* Advance online publication. DOI: 10.1111/acer.14976 PMID: 36377258

Grivennikov, S. I., Greten, F. R., & Karin, M. (2010). Immunity, inflammation, and cancer. *Cell, 140*(6), 883–899. DOI: 10.1016/j.cell.2010.01.025 PMID: 20303878

Grun, F., & B. Blumberg. (2006). Environmental Obesogens, Organotins & Endocrine Disruption via Nuclear Receptor Signaling. *Molecular & Cellular Endocrinology*, 254, 32–38. https,//.DOI: 10.1016/j.mce.2006.03.018

Grypari, I. M., Tzelepi, V., & Gyftopoulos, K. (2023). DNA Damage Repair Pathways in Prostate Cancer: A Narrative Review of Molecular Mechanisms, Emerging Biomarkers and Therapeutic Targets in Precision Oncology. *International Journal of Molecular Sciences, 24*(14), 11418. DOI: 10.3390/ijms241411418 PMID: 37511177

Gummadi, J., Bhatt, D. L., Adusumilli, S., Devabhaktuni, V., Acosta, W., & Kumar, A. (2014). Interpolation techniques for modeling and estimating indoor radon concentrations in ohio: Comparative study. Environmental Progress &Amp. *Environmental Progress & Sustainable Energy, 34*(1), 169–177. DOI: 10.1002/ep.11937

Guo, T., Meng, X., Liu, X., Wang, J., Yan, S., Zhang, X., Wang, M., Ren, S., & Huang, Y. (2023). Associations of phthalates with prostate cancer among the US population. *Reproductive Toxicology (Elmsford, N.Y.)*, *116*, 108337. Advance online publication. DOI: 10.1016/j.reprotox.2023.108337 PMID: 36646329

Gupta, S. P. (2024). Mathematical models in drug target analysis: pharmacokinetic and pharmacodynamic approach. In *Futuristic Trends in Contemporary Mathematics & Applications Volume 3 Book 4* (pp. 123–133). Iterative International Publisher, Selfypage Developers Pvt Ltd. DOI: 10.58532/V3BBCM4P2CH3

Gutiérrez-Camino, Á., Martín-Guerrero, I., & García-Orad, Á. (2017). Genetic susceptibility in childhood acute lymphoblastic leukemia. *Medical Oncology (Northwood, London, England)*, *34*(10), 179. Advance online publication. DOI: 10.1007/s12032-017-1038-7 PMID: 28905228

Halliwell, B. (2007). Oxidative stress and neurodegeneration: Where are we now? *Journal of Neurochemistry*, *97*(6), 1634–1658. DOI: 10.1111/j.1471-4159.2006.03907.x PMID: 16805774

Hamanaka, R. B., & Mutlu, G. M. (2018). Particulate matter air pollution: Effects on the cardiovascular system. *Frontiers in Endocrinology*, *9*, 680. DOI: 10.3389/fendo.2018.00680 PMID: 30505291

Harnden, K., Deeken, J., Stankowicz, M., Stafford, A., Cocilovo, C., Khromykh, A., Iyer, R., Barnett, S., Lawrence, G., Moeckel, F., Vogt, B., Philips, S., Solares, A., & Edmiston, K. (2019). Clinical pharmacogenomic testing impacts therapy decisions and supportive medication choices in breast cancer. *Journal of Clinical Oncology*, *37*(15_suppl), 569. Advance online publication. DOI: 10.1200/JCO.2019.37.15_suppl.569

Harper, D. M., & DeMars, L. R. (2017). HPV vaccines–a review of the first decade. *Gynecologic Oncology*, *146*(1), 196–204. DOI: 10.1016/j.ygyno.2017.04.004 PMID: 28442134

Harris, A. E., Metzler, V. M., Lothion-Roy, J., Varun, D., Woodcock, C. L., Haigh, D. B., Endeley, C., Haque, M., Toss, M. S., Alsaleem, M., Persson, J. L., Gudas, L. J., Rakha, E., Robinson, B. D., Khani, F., Martin, L. M., Moyer, J. E., Brownlie, J., Madhusudan, S., & Jeyapalan, J. N. (2022). Exploring anti-androgen therapies in hormone dependent prostate cancer and new therapeutic routes for castration resistant prostate cancer. *Frontiers in Endocrinology*, *13*, 1006101. DOI: 10.3389/fendo.2022.1006101 PMID: 36263323

Hartley, A., & Ahmad, I. (2022). The role of PPARγ in prostate cancer development and progression. *British Journal of Cancer, 128*(6), 940–945. DOI: 10.1038/s41416-022-02096-8 PMID: 36510001

Hayes, T. B., Collins, A., Lee, M., Mendoza, M., Noriega, N., Stuart, A. A., & Vonk, A. (2002). Hermaphroditic, Demasculinized Frogs after Exposure to the Herbicide Atrazine at Low Ecologically Relevant Doses. *Proceedings of the National Academy of Sciences*, 99 (8), 5476–5480. https,//DOI: 10.1073/pnas.082121499

Hebert, J. R., Hurley, T. G., Olendzki, B. C., Teas, J., Ma, Y., & Hampl, J. S. (1998). *Nutritional and Socioeconomic Factors in Relation to Prostate Cancer Mortality: a Cross-National Study*. https://academic.oup.com/jnci/article/90/21/1637/2520516

Heery, D. M., Kalkhoven, E., Hoare, S., & Parker, M. G. (1997). A signature motif in transcriptional co-activators mediates binding to nuclear receptors. *Nature, 387*(6634), 733–736. DOI: 10.1038/42750 PMID: 9192902

Herbst, A. L., R. J. Kurman, R. E. Scully, & D. C. Poskanzer. (1972). Clear-Cell Adenocarcinoma of the Vagina & Cervix in Girls, A Registry Report. *New Engl & Journal of Medicine*, 287 (25), 1259–1264. https,//DOI: 10.1056/NEJM197212212872501

Herceg, A. G., Wild, C. P., Sklias, A., Casati, L., Duthie, S. J., Fry, R., Issa, J.-P., Kellermayer, R., Koturbash, I., Kondo, Y., Lepeule, J., Lima, S. C. S., Marsit, C. J., Rakyan, V., Saffery, R., Taylor, J. A., Teschendorff, A. E., Ushijima, T., Vineis, P., & Hernandez, H. (2018). Vargas Roadmap for investigating epigenome deregulation and environmental origins of cancer. *International Journal of Cancer, 142*(5), 874–882. DOI: 10.1002/ijc.31014 PMID: 28836271

Her, L., & Zhu, H. J. (2020). Carboxylesterase 1 and precision pharmacotherapy: Pharmacogenetics and nongenetic regulators. *Drug Metabolism and Disposition: the Biological Fate of Chemicals, 48*(3), 230–244. DOI: 10.1124/dmd.119.089680 PMID: 31871135

Hess-Wilson, J. K., Webb, S. L., Daly, H. K., Leung, Y. K., Boldison, J., Comstock, C. E. S., Sartor, M. A., Ho, S. M., & Knudsen, K. E. (2007). Unique Bisphenol A Transcriptome in Prostate Cancer: Novel Effects on ERβ Expression That Correspond to Androgen Receptor Mutation Status. *Environmental Health Perspectives, 115*(11), 1646–1653. DOI: 10.1289/ehp.10283 PMID: 18007998

He, X., Liu, J., & Li, G. (2023). Editorial: Role of epigenetics in environmental pollution associated diseases. *Frontiers in Genetics, 14*, 1266714. Advance online publication. DOI: 10.3389/fgene.2023.1266714 PMID: 37600665

He, Y., Wang, X., & Wu, K. (2016). Evaluating breast cancer risk under exposure to environmental estrogen-like chemicals. *Polish Journal of Environmental Studies*, *25*(6), 2239–2249. DOI: 10.15244/pjoes/64282

Hiatt, R. A., & Brody, J. G. (2018). Environmental Determinants of Breast Cancer. *Annual Review of Public Health*, *1*(39), 113–133. DOI: 10.1146/annurev-publhealth-040617-014101 PMID: 29328875

Hockley, S. L., Arlt, V. M., Brewer, D., Te Poele, R., Workman, P., Giddings, I., & Phillips, D. H. (2007). AHR- and DNA-damage-mediated gene expression responses induced by benzo(a)pyrene in human cell lines. *Chemical Research in Toxicology*, *20*(12), 1797–1810. DOI: 10.1021/tx700252n PMID: 17944540

Hodgson, M. C., Shen, H. C., Hollenberg, A. N., & Balk, S. P. (2008). Structural basis for nuclear receptor corepressor recruitment by antagonist-liganded androgen receptor. *Molecular Cancer Therapeutics*, *7*(10), 3187–3194. DOI: 10.1158/1535-7163.MCT-08-0461 PMID: 18852122

Hoffmann, S. A., Diggans, J., Densmore, D., Dai, J., Knight, T., Leproust, E., Boeke, J. D., Wheeler, N., & Cai, Y. (2023). Safety by design: Biosafety and biosecurity in the age of synthetic genomics. *iScience*, *3*(3), 106165. DOI: 10.1016/j.isci.2023.106165 PMID: 36895643

Home - HEAP. (n.d.). Retrieved 14 April 2025, from https://heap-exposome.eu/?utm_source=chatgpt.com

Ho, S. M., Johnson, A., Tarapore, P., Janakiram, V., Zhang, X., & Leung, Y. K. (2012). Environmental epigenetics and its implication on disease risk and health outcomes. *ILAR Journal*, *53*(3-4), 289–305. DOI: 10.1093/ilar.53.3-4.289 PMID: 23744968

Hotchkiss, A. K., C. V. Rider, C. R. Blystone, V. S. Wilson, P. C. Hartig, G. T. Ankley, P. M. Foster, C. L. Gray, & L. E. Gray. (2008). Fifteen Years after 'Wingspread'—Environmental Endocrine Disrupters & Human & Wildlife Health, Where We Are Today & Where We Need to Go. *Toxicological Sciences*, 105 (2), 235–259. https,//.DOI: 10.1093/toxsci/kfn030

Houtepen, L. C., Vinkers, C. H., Carrillo-Roa, T., Hiemstra, M., van Lier, P. A., Meeus, W., Branje, S., Heim, C. M., Nemeroff, C. B., Mill, J., Schalkwyk, L. C., Creyghton, M. P., Kahn, R. S., Joëls, M., Binder, E. B., & Boks, M. P. M. (2016). Genome-wide DNA methylation levels and altered cortisol stress reactivity following childhood trauma in humans. *Nature Communications*, *1*(1), 10967. Advance online publication. DOI: 10.1038/ncomms10967 PMID: 26997371

Hou, Y., Li, S., Xia, L., Yang, Q., Zhang, L., Zhang, X., Liu, H., Huo, R., Cao, G., Huang, C., Tian, X., Sun, L., Cao, D., Zhang, M., Zhang, Q., & Tang, N. (2021). Associations of urinary phenolic environmental estrogens exposure with blood glucose levels and gestational diabetes mellitus in Chinese pregnant women. *The Science of the Total Environment*, *754*, 142085. DOI: 10.1016/j.scitotenv.2020.142085 PMID: 32898782

Huang, Y., X. Chen, Z. Wang, W. Li, & H. Zhang. (2021). Bisphenol A Exposure Confers Chemoresistance to Tamoxifen, Doxorubicin, & Cisplatin in ER-Positive Breast Cancer Cells. *Journal of Cancer Therapeutics*, 12 (4), 301–312. https,//

Huang, N., Gao, Y., Zhang, M., Guo, L., Qin, L., Liao, S., & Wang, H. (2022). METTL3-Mediated m6A RNA Methylation of ZBTB4 Interferes with Trophoblast Invasion and Maybe Involved in RSA. *Frontiers in Cell and Developmental Biology*, *10*, 10. DOI: 10.3389/fcell.2022.894810 PMID: 35774226

Hudson, L., Samons, K. M., Dicken, H., Prichard, C., Weiss, L. T., Edward, J., Vanderpool, R. C., & Vanderford, N. L. (2021). A Brief Educational Intervention Enhances Basic Cancer Literacy Among Kentucky Middle and High School Students. *Journal of Cancer Education*, *36*(4), 735–740. DOI: 10.1007/s13187-020-01696-3 PMID: 31989408

Hu, J., Yu, L., Modanloo, S., Zhou, Y., & Yang, Y. (2018). A theoretical framework for interaction of nursing discipline with genetics and genomics. *International Journal of Nursing Sciences*, *4*(4), 336–342. DOI: 10.1016/j.ijnss.2018.08.004 PMID: 31406845

Hu, J., & Yu, Y. (2019). Epigenetic response profiles into environmental epigenotoxicant screening and health risk assessment: A critical review. *Chemosphere*, *226*, 259–272. DOI: 10.1016/j.chemosphere.2019.03.096 PMID: 30933735

Humphrey, K. M., Pandey, S., Martin, J., Hagoel, T., Grand'Maison, A., & Ohm, J. E. (2018). Establishing a role for environmental toxicant exposure induced epigenetic remodeling in malignant transformation. *Seminars in Cancer Biology*, *57*, 86–94. DOI: 10.1016/j.semcancer.2018.11.002 PMID: 30453042

Hunt, P. A., Koehler, K. E., Susiarjo, M., Hodges, C. A., Ilagan, A., Voigt, R. C., Thomas, S., Thomas, B. F., & Hassold, T. J. (2003, April 1). Bisphenol A Exposure Causes Meiotic Aneuploidy in the Female Mouse. *Current Biology*, *13*(7), 546–553. DOI: 10.1016/S0960-9822(03)00189-1 PMID: 12676084

Hussain, M., Basheer, S., Khalil, A., Haider, Q., Saeed, H., & Faizan, M. (2024). Pharmacogenetic study of CES1 gene and enalapril efficacy. *Journal of Applied Genetics*, *65*(3), 463–471. Advance online publication. DOI: 10.1007/s13353-024-00831-w PMID: 38261266

Hussein, M., & Jensen, A. (2023). Drug-Induced Liver Injury Caused by Capecitabine: A Case Report and a Literature Review. *Case Reports in Oncology*, *16*, 393–399. DOI: 10.1159/000529866 PMID: 37384198

Huttunen, J., Aaltonen, N., Helminen, L., Rilla, K., & Paakinaho, V. (2024). EP300/CREBBP acetyltransferase inhibition limits steroid receptor and FOXA1 signaling in prostate cancer cells. *Cellular and Molecular Life Sciences : CMLS*, *81*(1), 1–21. DOI: 10.1007/s00018-024-05209-z PMID: 38564048

Hu, W. Y., Shi, G., Hu, D.-P., Nelles, J. L., & Prins, G. S. (2011). Actions of Estrogens and Endocrine Disrupting Chemicals on Human Prostate Stem/Progenitor Cells and Prostate Cancer Risk. *Molecular and Cellular Endocrinology*, *354*(1–2), 63–73. DOI: 10.1016/j.mce.2011.08.032 PMID: 21914459

Hu, Y., Tanriverdi, F., MacColl, G. S., & Bouloux, P. M. (2003). Kallmann syndrome: Molecular pathogenesis. *The International Journal of Biochemistry & Cell Biology*, *35*(8), 1157–1162. DOI: 10.1016/S1357-2725(02)00395-3 PMID: 12757752

Hwang, G. C., Wankowicz, J., Zhang, S. A. M., Liu, Z., Cibulskis, D., Gaviola, C., Ghazikhanian, G. C., Mc, V., Kay, R. R., Bubley, G. J., Carter, S. L., Balk, S. P., Hahn, W. C., Taplin, M.-E., & Van Allen, E. M. (2017). Genomic resistance patterns to second-generation androgen blockade in paired tumor biopsies of metastatic castration-resistant prostate cancer. *JCO Precision Oncology*, (1), 1–11. DOI: 10.1200/PO.17.00140 PMID: 32913968

IARC. (2012). Asbestos (Chrysotile, Amosite, Crocidolite, Tremolite, Actinolite and Anthophyllite). *IARC Monographs on the Evaluation of Carcinogenic Risks to Humans*, *100*, C.

Imamura, Y., & Sadar, M. D. (2016). Androgen receptor targeted therapies in castration-resistant prostate cancer: Bench to clinic. *International Journal of Urology*, *23*(8), 654–665. DOI: 10.1111/iju.13137 PMID: 27302572

Imir, O. B., Kaminsky, A. Z., Zuo, Q. Y., Liu, Y. J., Singh, R., Spinella, M. J., Irudayaraj, J., Hu, W. Y., Prins, G. S., & Erdogan, Z. M. (2021). Per- and Polyfluoroalkyl Substance Exposure Combined with High-Fat Diet Supports Prostate Cancer Progression. *Nutrients*, *13*(11), 3902. Advance online publication. DOI: 10.3390/nu13113902 PMID: 34836157

Inbathamizh, L. (2020). Targeting Cytochrome P450 1A1 Enzyme with Crucifer Phytocomponents: An In Silico Approach for Chemopreventive Drug Design against Lung Cancer. *Asian Journal of Pharmaceutics, 14*(1). Advance online publication. DOI: 10.22377/ajp.v14i1.3508

Ioannidis, J. P., Loy, E. Y., Poulton, R., & Chia, K. S. (2009). *Sci. Transl. Med.* 1, 7ps8.Wild, C.P. (2005). Complementing the genome with an 'exposome': The outstanding challenge of environmental exposure measurement in molecular epidemiology. *Cancer Epidemiology, Biomarkers & Prevention, 14*, 1847–1850.

Iyengar, N. M., Hudis, C. A., & Dannenberg, A. J. (2013). Obesity and inflammation: New insights into breast cancer development and progression. *American Society of Clinical Oncology Educational Book, 33*(33), 46–51. DOI: 10.14694/EdBook_AM.2013.33.46 PMID: 23714453

Jaiswara, P. K., Sonker, P., & Kumar, A. (2021). *Immune Response and Oxidative Stress in Obesity-Induced Cancer*. Springer., DOI: 10.1007/978-981-16-1846-8_6

Jarup, L. (2004). Health and environment information systems for exposure and disease mapping, and risk assessment. *Environmental Health Perspectives, 112*(9), 995–997. DOI: 10.1289/ehp.6736 PMID: 15198919

Jayshree, R. S., Sreenivas, A., Tessy, M., & Krishna, S. (2009). Cell intrinsic & extrinsic factors in cervical carcinogenesis. *The Indian Journal of Medical Research, 130*(3), 286–295. PMID: 19901438

Jiang, L., Khawaja, H., Tahsin, S., Clarkson, T. A., Miranti, C. K., & Zohar, Y. (2024). Microfluidic-based human prostate-cancer-on-chip. *Frontiers in Bioengineering and Biotechnology, 12*, 1302223. Advance online publication. DOI: 10.3389/fbioe.2024.1302223 PMID: 38322789

Jiang, Y., & Wang, M. (2010). Personalized medicine in oncology: Tailoring the right drug to the right patient. *Biomarkers in Medicine, 4*(4), 523–533. DOI: 10.2217/bmm.10.66 PMID: 20701441

Jirtle, R. L., & Skinner, M. K. (2007). Environmental epigenomics and disease susceptibility. *Nature Reviews. Genetics, 8*(4), 253–262. DOI: 10.1038/nrg2045 PMID: 17363974

Jöckel, K. H., Ahrens, W., Jahn, I., Pohlabeln, H., & Bolm-AudorfF, U. (1998). Occupational risk factors for lung cancer: A case-control study in West Germany. *International Journal of Epidemiology, 27*(4), 549–560. DOI: 10.1093/ije/27.4.549 PMID: 9758106

Joehanes, R., Just, A. C., Marioni, R. E., Pilling, L. C., Reynolds, L. M., Mandaviya, P. R., Guan, W., Xu, T., Elks, C. E., Aslibekyan, S., Moreno-Macias, H., Smith, J. A., Brody, J. A., Dhingra, R., Yousefi, P., Pankow, J. S., Kunze, S., Shah, S. H., McRae, A. F., & London, S. J. (2016). Epigenetic Signatures of Cigarette Smoking. *Circulation: Cardiovascular Genetics, 9*(5), 436–447. DOI: 10.1161/CIRCGENETICS.116.001506 PMID: 27651444

Joensen, U. N., Bossi, R., Leffers, H., Jensen, A. A., Skakkebaek, N. E., & Jorgensen, N. (2009). Do perfluoroalkyl compounds impair human semen quality? *Environmental Health Perspectives, 117*(6), 923–927. DOI: 10.1289/ehp.0800517 PMID: 19590684

Jordan, I. K., Sharma, S., & Mariño-Ramírez, L. (2023). Population Pharmacogenomics for Health Equity. *Genes, 10*(10), 1840. DOI: 10.3390/genes14101840 PMID: 37895188

Joubert, B. R., Felix, J. F., Yousefi, P., Bakulski, K. M., Just, A. C., Breton, C., & London, S. J. (2016). DNA methylation in newborns and maternal smoking in pregnancy: Genome-wide consortium meta-analysis. *American Journal of Human Genetics, 98*(4), 680–696.

Joyce, B. T., & Hou, L. (2015). Organic pollutants and telomere length: A new facet of carcinogenesis. *EBioMedicine, 2*(12), 1854–1855. DOI: 10.1016/j.ebiom.2015.11.046 PMID: 26844257

Juarez, P. D., Hood, D. B., Song, M. A., & Ramesh, A. (2022). Applying an Exposome-wide Association Study (ExWAS) Approach to Latino Cancer Disparities. In Ramirez, A. G. (Ed.), *et al., Advancing the Science of Cancer in Latinos: Building Collaboration for Action* (pp. 17–32). Springer.

Juarez, P. D., & Matthews-Juarez, P. (2018). Applying an Exposome-Wide (ExWAS) Approach to Cancer Research. *Frontiers in Oncology, 8*, 313. DOI: 10.3389/fonc.2018.00313 PMID: 30211112

Juarez, P. D., Matthews-Juarez, P., Hood, D. B., Im, W., Levine, R. S., Kilbourne, B. J., Langston, M. A., Al-Hamdan, M. Z., Crosson, W. L., Estes, M. G., Estes, S. M., Agboto, V. K., Robinson, P., Wilson, S., & Lichtveld, M. Y. (2014). The public health exposome: A population-based, exposure science approach to health disparities research. *International Journal of Environmental Research and Public Health, 11*(12), 12866–12895. DOI: 10.3390/ijerph111212866 PMID: 25514145

Justino, C. I., Duarte, A. C., & Rocha-Santos, T. (2017). Recent progress in biosensors for environmental monitoring: A review. *Sensors (Basel), 17*(12), 2918. DOI: 10.3390/s17122918 PMID: 29244756

Kahn, L. G., Philippat, C., Nakayama, S. F., Slama, R., & Trasande, L. (2020). Endocrine-disrupting chemicals: implications for human health. In *The Lancet Diabetes and Endocrinology* (Vol. 8, Issue 8, pp. 703–718). Lancet Publishing Group. DOI: 10.1016/S2213-8587(20)30129-7

Kamada, S., Takeiwa, T., Ikeda, K., Horie-Inoue, K., & Inoue, S. (2020). Long Non-coding RNAs Involved in Metabolic Alterations in Breast and Prostate Cancers. *Frontiers in Oncology*, *10*, 593200. DOI: 10.3389/fonc.2020.593200 PMID: 33123488

Karthaus, W. R., Chan, J., Setty, M., Love, J. R., Zaidi, S., Choo, Z., Persad, S., LaClair, J., Lawrence, K. E., Chaudhary, O., Xu, T., Masilionis, I., Mazutis, L., Chaligne, R., Pe'er, D., & Sawyers, C. L. (2021). Reversal of lineage plasticity in RB1/TP53-deleted prostate cancer through FGFR and Janus kinase inhibition. *BioRxiv*, 2021.11.01.466615. DOI: 10.1101/2021.11.01.466615

Kassotis, C. D., Vandenberg, L. N., Demeneix, B. A., Porta, M., Slama, R., & Trasande, L. (2020). Endocrine-disrupting chemicals: economic, regulatory, and policy implications. In *The Lancet Diabetes and Endocrinology* (Vol. 8, Issue 8, pp. 719–730). Lancet Publishing Group. https://doi.org/DOI: 10.1016/S2213-8587(20)30128-5

Kaupang, Å., Paulsen, S. M., Steindal, C. C., Ravna, A. W., Sylte, I., Halvorsen, T. G., Thoresen, G. H., & Hansen, T. V. (2002). Structural basis for antagonist-mediated recruitment of nuclear co-repressors by PPARalpha. *Nature*, *415*(6873), 229–236. DOI: 10.1038/415813a PMID: 11845213

Kelly, M., Connolly, L., & Dean, M. (2020). Public awareness and risk perceptions of endocrine disrupting chemicals: A qualitative study. *International Journal of Environmental Research and Public Health*, *17*(21), 1–16. DOI: 10.3390/ijerph17217778 PMID: 33114266

Kerna, N. A., Holets, H. M., Anderson, I. I. J.II, Flores, J. V., Pruitt, K. D., McKee, D., Carsrud, N. D. V., Ngwu, D. C., Nnake, I., Chawla, S., Nwokorie, U., Azi, C. I., Jomsky, B. M., Ukachukwu, C. A., Odefemi, O. F., Egli, A., Obi, M. O., & Ikokwu, O. D. (2024). Heavy Metals and Human Health: From Neurological Disorders to Developmental Delays. *European Journal of Ecology. Biology and Agriculture*, *3*(3), 152–184. DOI: 10.59324/ejeba.2024.1(3).12

Khan, B. A., Robinson, R., Fohner, A. E., Muzquiz, L. I., Schilling, B. D., Beans, J. A., Olnes, M. J., Trawicki, L., Frydenlund, H., Laukes, C., Beatty, P., Phillips, B., Nickerson, D., Howlett, K., Dillard, D. A., Thornton, T. A., Thummel, K. E., & Woodahl, E. L. (2018). Cytochrome P450 Genetic Variation Associated with Tamoxifen Biotransformation in American Indian and Alaska Native People. *Clinical and Translational Science*, *3*(3), 312–321. DOI: 10.1111/cts.12542 PMID: 29436156

Khan, M. M., Mohsen, M. T., Malik, M. Z., Bagabir, S. A., Alkhanani, M. F., Haque, S., Serajuddin, M., & Bharadwaj, M. (2022). Identification of Potential Key Genes in Prostate Cancer with Gene Expression, Pivotal Pathways and Regulatory Networks Analysis Using Integrated Bioinformatics Methods. *Genes*, *13*(4), 655. DOI: 10.3390/genes13040655 PMID: 35456461

Khatiwada, P., Rimal, U., Han, Z., & Shemshedini, L. (2024). MDM2 regulates the stability of AR, AR-V7, and TM4SF3 proteins in prostate cancer. *Endocrine Oncology*, *4*(1). Advance online publication. DOI: 10.1530/EO-23-0017 PMID: 38410785

Khurana, N., & Sikka, S. C. (2018). Targeting Crosstalk between Nrf-2, NF-κB and Androgen Receptor Signaling in Prostate Cancer. *Cancers (Basel)*, *10*(10), 352. DOI: 10.3390/cancers10100352 PMID: 30257470

Kim, H. M., & Kang, J. S. (2021). Metabolomic Studies for the Evaluation of Toxicity Induced by Environmental Toxicants on Model Organisms. *Metabolites*, *11*(8), 485. DOI: 10.3390/metabo11080485 PMID: 34436425

Kim, H., Min, J., Seo, Y., & Min, K. (2019). Association of Ambient Air Pollution with Increased Liver Enzymes in Korean Adults. *International Journal of Environmental Research and Public Health*, *16*(7), 1213. Advance online publication. DOI: 10.3390/ijerph16071213 PMID: 30987355

Kim, M., Bae, M., Na, H., & Yang, M. (2012). Environmental toxicants-induced epigenetic alterations and their reversers. *Journal of Environmental Science and Health. Part C, Environmental Carcinogenesis & Ecotoxicology Reviews*, *30*(4), 323–367. DOI: 10.1080/10590501.2012.731959 PMID: 23167630

Kitamura, S., T. Kato, M. Iida, N. Jinno, T. Suzuki, S. Ohta, N. Fujimoto, & H. Hanada. (2005). Anti-Thyroid Hormonal Activity of Tetrabromobisphenol A, a Flame Retardant, & Its Metabolites in Vitro. Environmental Health Perspectives 113 (4), 478–483. https,//.DOI: <ALIGNMENT.qj></ALIGNMENT>10.1289/ehp.7558

Kittles, R. (2013). Use of GWAS to predict targets associated with cancer in African Americans. *The FASEB Journal*, *27*(S1). Advance online publication. DOI: 10.1096/fasebj.27.1_supplement.460.2

Kiyama, R. (2016). Endocrine disruptor actions through receptor crosstalk. *Environmental Biotechnology, 12*(1), 1–16. DOI: 10.14799/ebms262

Kleinstreuer, N. C., Harris, M. A., Wambaugh, J. F., Judson, R. S., Richard, A. M., Setzer, R. W., Rastogi, S., Martin, M. T., Reif, D. M., Sipes, N. S., Thomas, R. S., Simmons, S. O., Deshpande, A. V., Levin, E. D., Houck, K. A., Shah, I., Shah, R. R., Knudsen, T. B., & Knudsen, D.. (2016). A predictive framework for androgen receptor activity from ToxCast in vitro and computational modeling. *Chemical Research in Toxicology, 30*(6), 946–964. DOI: 10.1021/acs.chemrestox.5b00419 PMID: 27933809

Kleinstreuer, N. C., Hoffmann, S., Alépée, N., Allen, D., Ashikaga, T., Casey, W., Clouet, E., Cluzel, M., Desprez, B., Gellatly, N., Göbel, C., Kern, P. S., Klaric, M., Kühnl, J., Martinozzi-Teissier, S., Mewes, K., Miyazawa, M., Strickland, J., van Vliet, E., & Petersohn, D. (2018). Non-animal methods to predict skin sensitization (II): An assessment of defined approaches. *Critical Reviews in Toxicology, 48*(5), 359–374. DOI: 10.1080/10408444.2018.1429386 PMID: 29474122

Klinge, C. M. (2009). Estrogen Regulation of MicroRNA Expression. *Current Genomics* 10 (3), 169–183. https,//.DOI: 10.2174/138920209788185289

Klukovich, R., Nilsson, E., Sadler-Riggleman, I., Beck, D., Xie, Y., Yan, W., & Skinner, M. K. (2019). Environmental Toxicant Induced Epigenetic Transgenerational Inheritance of Prostate Pathology and Stromal-Epithelial Cell Epigenome and Transcriptome Alterations: Ancestral Origins of Prostate Disease. *Scientific Reports, 9*(1), 2209. Advance online publication. DOI: 10.1038/s41598-019-38741-1 PMID: 30778168

Knudson, A. G.Jr. (1971). Mutation and cancer: Statistical study of retinoblastoma. *Proceedings of the National Academy of Sciences of the United States of America, 68*(4), 820–823. DOI: 10.1073/pnas.68.4.820 PMID: 5279523

Kodanch, S. M., Mukherjee, S., Prabhu, N. B., Kabekkodu, S. P., Bhat, S. K., & Rai, P. S. (2024). Altered mitochondrial homeostasis on bisphenol-A exposure and its association in developing polycystic ovary syndrome: A comprehensive review. *Reproductive Toxicology (Elmsford, N.Y.), 130*, 108700. DOI: 10.1016/j.reprotox.2024.108700 PMID: 39181417

Koedrith, P., Thasiphu, T., Weon, J., Boonprasert, R., Tuitemwong, K., & Tuitemwong, P. (2015). Recent trends in rapid environmental monitoring of pathogens and toxicants: potential of nanoparticle-based biosensor and applications. The Scientific World Journal, 2015(1). DOI: 10.1155/2015/510982

Koistinen, H., Künnapuu, J., & Jeltsch, M. (2021). KLK3 in the Regulation of Angiogenesis—Tumorigenic or Not? *International Journal of Molecular Sciences*, *22*(24), 13545. DOI: 10.3390/ijms222413545 PMID: 34948344

Kokai, D., Stanic, B., Tesic, B., Samardzija Nenadov, D., Pogrmic-Majkic, K., Fa Nedeljkovic, S., & Andric, N. (2022). Dibutyl phthalate promotes angiogenesis in EA.hy926 cells through estrogen receptor-dependent activation of ERK1/2, PI3K-Akt, and NO signaling pathways. *Chemico-Biological Interactions*, *366*, 110174. DOI: 10.1016/j.cbi.2022.110174 PMID: 36089060

Korbas, M., & Tracy, C. (2012). Chemical Form Matters: Differential Accumulation of Mercury Following Inorganic and Organic Mercury Exposures in Zebrafish Larvae. *ACS Chemical Biology*, *7*(2), 411–420. DOI: 10.1021/cb200287c PMID: 22026432

Kortenkamp, A., Martin, O., Evans, R., Orton, F., McKinlay, R., Rosivatz, E., & Faust, M. (2012). Response to A critique of the European Commission Document, "State of the Art Assessment of Endocrine Disruptors" by Rhomberg and colleagues – letter to the editor. *Critical Reviews in Toxicology*, *42*(9), 787–789. DOI: 10.3109/10408444.2012.712943 PMID: 22900988

Krauss, R. S., & Hong, M. (2016). Gene–environment Interactions and the etiology of birth defects. *Current Topics in Developmental Biology*, *116*, 569–580. DOI: 10.1016/bs.ctdb.2015.12.010 PMID: 26970642

Krawetz, S. A., Kruger, A., Lalancette, C., Tagett, R., Anton, E., Draghici, S., & Diamond, M. P. (2011). A survey of small RNAs in human sperm. *Human Reproduction (Oxford, England)*, *26*(12), 3401–3412. DOI: 10.1093/humrep/der329 PMID: 21989093

Krewski, D., Andersen, M. E., Mantus, E., & Zeise, L. (2009). Toxicity Testing in the 21st Century: Implications for Human Health Risk Assessment. *Risk Analysis*, *4*(4), 474–479. DOI: 10.1111/j.1539-6924.2008.01150.x PMID: 19144067

Krieger, N. (2007). Theories for social epidemiology in the 21st century: An ecosocial perspective. *International Journal of Epidemiology*, *30*(4), 668–677. DOI: 10.1093/ije/30.4.668 PMID: 11511581

Krol, J., Paepke, S., Jacobs, V., Paepke, D., Euler, U., Kiechle, M., & Harbeck, N. (2006). G-CSF in the Prevention of Febrile Neutropenia in Chemotherapy in Breast Cancer Patients. *Oncology Research and Treatment*, *29*(4), 171–178. DOI: 10.1159/000091616 PMID: 16601374

Kulkarni, P., Dasgupta, P., Bhat, N. S., Hashimoto, Y., Saini, S., Shahryari, V., Yamamura, S., Shiina, M., Tanaka, Y., Dahiya, R., & Majid, S. (2020). Role of the PI3K/Akt pathway in cadmium induced malignant transformation of normal prostate epithelial cells. *Toxicology and Applied Pharmacology*, *409*, 115308. DOI: 10.1016/j.taap.2020.115308 PMID: 33129824

Kuo, C. H., Yang, S. N., Kuo, P. L., & Hung, C. H. (2012). Immunomodulatory effects of environmental endocrine disrupting chemicals. *The Kaohsiung Journal of Medical Sciences*, *28*(7, SUPPL.), S37–S42. DOI: 10.1016/j.kjms.2012.05.008 PMID: 22871600

Kuther, T. L., & Posada, M. (2004). Children and adolescents' capacity to provide informed consent for participation in research. *Advances in Psychology Research*, *32*, 163–173. PMID: 16986221

Labourey, J. (2007). Physical activity in the management of cancer-related fatigue induced by oncological treatments.. *Annales de readaptation et de medecine physique: revue scientifique de la Societe francaise de reeducation fonctionnelle de readaptation et de medecine physique*, 50 6, 450-4, 445-9 . .DOI: 10.1016/j.annrmp.2007.03.010

Lally, J., Gaughran, F., Timms, P., & Curran, S. (2016). Treatment-resistant schizophrenia: Current insights on the pharmacogenomics of antipsychotics. *Pharmacogenomics and Personalized Medicine*, *9*, 117–129. DOI: 10.2147/PGPM.S115741 PMID: 27853387

Landrigan, P. J., Fuller, R., Acosta, N. J. R., Adeyi, O., Arnold, R., Basu, N., Balde, A. B., Bertollini, R., Bose-O'Reilly, S., Boufford, J. I., Breysse, P. N., Chiles, T., Mahidol, C., Coll-Seck, A. M., Cropper, M. L., Fobil, J., Fuster, V., Greenstone, M., Haines, A., & Zhong, M. (2018). The Lancet Commission on pollution and health. *Lancet*, *391*(10119), 462–512. DOI: 10.1016/S0140-6736(17)32345-0 PMID: 29056410

Langley, B., Talas, S., El-Shakankery, K. H., & Michie, C. (2023). Improving Inclusivity, Equity, and Diversity in Oncology Clinical Trials: A European Perspective. DOI: 10.33590/emjoncol/10303428

Latonen, L., Afyounian, E., Jylhä, A., Nättinen, J., Aapola, U., Annala, M., Kivinummi, K. K., Tammela, T. T. L., Beuerman, R. W., Uusitalo, H., Nykter, M., & Visakorpi, T. (2018). Integrative proteomics in prostate cancer uncovers robustness against genomic and transcriptomic aberrations during disease progression. *Nature Communications*, *9*(1), 1176. Advance online publication. DOI: 10.1038/s41467-018-03573-6 PMID: 29563510

Launonen, K. M., Varis, V., Aaltonen, N., Niskanen, E. A., Varjosalo, M., Paakinaho, V., & Palvimo, J. J. (2024). Central role of SUMOylation in the regulation of chromatin interactions and transcriptional outputs of the androgen receptor in prostate cancer cells. *Nucleic Acids Research, 52*(16), 9519–9535. DOI: 10.1093/nar/gkae653 PMID: 39106160

Laury, A. R., Zheng, S., Aho, N., Fallegger, R., Hänninen, S., Saez-Rodriguez, J., Tanevski, J., Youssef, O., Tang, J., & Carpén, O. M. (2024). Opening the Black Box: Spatial Transcriptomics and the Relevance of Artificial Intelligence–Detected Prognostic Regions in High-Grade Serous Carcinoma. *Modern Pathology, 37*(7), 100508. DOI: 10.1016/j.modpat.2024.100508 PMID: 38704029

Lee, C., & Riddick, D. (2012). Aryl hydrocarbon receptor-dependence of dioxin's effects on constitutive mouse hepatic cytochromes P450 and growth hormone signaling components. *Canadian Journal of Physiology and Pharmacology, 90*(10), 1354–1363. DOI: 10.1139/y2012-099 PMID: 22978700

Lee, D., Schuetz, J., Lai, A., Burstyn, I., Brooks-Wilson, A., Aronson, K., & Spinelli, J. (2021). Interactions between exposure to polycyclic aromatic hydrocarbons and xenobiotic metabolism genes, and risk of breast cancer. *Breast Cancer (Tokyo, Japan)*. Advance online publication. DOI: 10.1007/s12282-021-01279-0 PMID: 34351578

Lee, S.-Y., Nam, M.-H., Kim, J. S., & Kim, J.-W. (2007). A Case Report of a Patient Carrying CYP2C9*3/4 Genotype with Extremely Low Warfarin Dose Requirement. *Journal of Korean Medical Science, 3*(3), 557. DOI: 10.3346/jkms.2007.22.3.557 PMID: 17596671

Lei, S., Zheng, R., Zhang, S., Wang, S., Chen, R., Sun, K., Zeng, H., Zhou, J., & Wei, W. (2020). Global patterns of breast cancer incidence and mortality: A population-based cancer registry data analysis from 2000 to 2020. [Lond]. *Cancer Communications, 41*(11), 1183–1194. DOI: 10.1002/cac2.12207 PMID: 34399040

Lemen, J. R., Title, A. M., Akin, D. J., Boerner, P. F., Chou, C., Drake, J. F., Duncan, D. W., Edwards, C. G., Friedlaender, F. M., Heyman, G. F., Hurlburt, N. E., Katz, N. L., Kushner, G. D., Levay, M., Lindgren, R. W., Mathur, D. P., McFeaters, E. L., Mitchell, S., Rehse, R. A., & Waltham, N. (2012). The *Atmospheric Imaging Assembly* (AIA) on the *Solar Dynamics Observatory* (SDO). *Solar Physics, 275*(1-2), 17–40. DOI: 10.1007/s11207-011-9776-8

Leng, L., Chen, X., Li, C. P., Luo, X. Y., & Tang, N. J. (2014). 2,3,7,8-Tetrachlorodibezo-p-dioxin exposure and prostate cancer: A meta-analysis of cohort studies. *Public Health, 128*(3), 207–213. DOI: 10.1016/j.puhe.2013.10.006 PMID: 24461260

Lerro, C. C., Beane Freeman, L. E., DellaValle, C. T., Andreotti, G., Hofmann, J. N., Koutros, S., Parks, C. G., Shrestha, S., Alavanja, M. C. R., Blair, A., Lubin, J. H., Sandler, D. P., & Ward, M. H. (2021). Pesticide exposure and incident thyroid cancer among male pesticide applicators in agricultural health study. *Environment International, 146*, 106187. DOI: 10.1016/j.envint.2020.106187 PMID: 33126065

Levine, H., Jørgensen, N., Martino-Andrade, A., Mendiola, J., Weksler-Derri, D., Mindlis, I., Pinotti, R., & Swan, S. H. (2017). Temporal trends in sperm count: A systematic review and meta-regression analysis. *Human Reproduction Update, 23*(6), 646–659. DOI: 10.1093/humupd/dmx022 PMID: 28981654

Lewandowska, A. M., Rudzki, M., Rudzki, S., Lewandowski, T., & Laskowska, B. (2018). Environmental risk factors for cancer-review paper. *Annals of Agricultural and Environmental Medicine, 26*(1), 1–7. DOI: 10.26444/aaem/94299 PMID: 30922021

Lewis, C. M.Jr, McCall, L. I., Sharp, R. R., & Spicer, P. G. (2020). Ethical priority of the most actionable system of biomolecules: The metabolome. *American Journal of Physical Anthropology, 171*(2), 177–181. DOI: 10.1002/ajpa.23943 PMID: 31643083

Li, A. P., Q. Zhang, & Z. Q. Liu. (2017). Endocrine Disruptors Accelerate Alzheimer's Disease Pathology via Aβ & Tau Regulation. *Neurotoxicology*, 65, 56–66. https,//.

Liang, X., Di, L., Song, G., Yan, Y., Wang, C., Jiang, H., & Li, H. (2014). Capecitabine maintenance therapy for XT chemotherapy-sensitive patients with metastatic triple-negative breast cancer.. *Chinese journal of cancer research = Chung-kuo yen cheng yen chiu*, 26 5, 550-7 . .DOI: 10.3978/j.issn.1000-9604.2014.10.02

Liang, Y., Chu, P. H., Tian, L., Ho, K. F., Ip, M. S. M., & Mak, J. C. W. (2022). Targeting mitochondrial permeability transition pore ameliorates PM2.5-induced mitochondrial dysfunction in airway epithelial cells. *Environmental Pollution, 295*, 118720. Advance online publication. DOI: 10.1016/j.envpol.2021.118720 PMID: 34953947

Liao, W.-L., & Tsai, F.-J. (2013). Personalized medicine: A paradigm shift in healthcare. *Biomedicine (Taipei), 2*(2), 66–72. DOI: 10.1016/j.biomed.2012.12.005

Li, D., Chang, B., & Huang, Q. (2025). Using XBGoost, an interpretable machine learning model, for diagnosing prostate cancer in patients with PSA <20 ng/ml based on the PSAMR indicator. *Scientific Reports, 15*(1), 1532. DOI: 10.1038/s41598-025-85963-7 PMID: 39789130

Liew, S. L., Anglin, J. M., Banks, N. W., Sondag, M., Ito, K. L., Kim, H., Chan, J., Ito, J., Jung, C., Khoshab, N., Lefebvre, S., Nakamura, W., Saldana, D., Schmiesing, A., Tran, C., Vo, D., Ard, T., Heydari, P., Kim, B., & Stroud, A. (2018). A large, open-source dataset of stroke anatomical brain images and manual lesion segmentations. *Scientific Data*, *5*(1), 1–11. DOI: 10.1038/sdata.2018.11 PMID: 29461514

Li, J., & Bluth, M. H. (2011). Pharmacogenomics of drug metabolizing enzymes and transporters: Implications for cancer therapy. *Pharmacogenomics and Personalized Medicine*, *4*(1), 11. DOI: 10.2147/PGPM.S18861 PMID: 23226051

Li, K., Wang, Q., Tang, X., Akakuru, O. U., Li, R., Wang, Y., Zhang, R., Jiang, Z., & Yang, Z. (2024). Advances in Prostate Cancer Biomarkers and Probes. In *Cyborg and Bionic Systems* (Vol. 5). American Association for the Advancement of Science., DOI: 10.34133/cbsystems.0129

Lind, C., Anderson, B., & Oberle, K. (2003). Ethical issues in adolescent consent for research. *Nursing Ethics*, *10*(5), 504–511. DOI: 10.1191/0969733003ne632oa PMID: 14529117

Lin, S., Chai, Y., Zheng, X., & Xu, X. (2024). The role of HIF in angiogenesis, lymphangiogenesis, and tumor microenvironment in urological cancers. *Molecular Biology Reports*, *51*(1), 1–13. DOI: 10.1007/s11033-023-08931-2 PMID: 38085375

Lin, Z., & Chou, W. C. (2022). Machine Learning and Artificial Intelligence in Toxicological Sciences. *Toxicological Sciences*, *189*(1), 7–19. DOI: 10.1093/toxsci/kfac075 PMID: 35861448

Li, Q., Wang, Y., Chen, J., Zeng, K., Wang, C., Guo, X., Hu, Z., Hu, J., Liu, B., Xiao, J., & Zhou, P. (2024). Machine learning based androgen receptor regulatory gene-related random forest survival model for precise treatment decision in prostate cancer. *Heliyon*, *10*(17), e37256. DOI: 10.1016/j.heliyon.2024.e37256 PMID: 39296076

Li, S., Kang, Y., & Zeng, Y. (2024). Targeting tumor and bone microenvironment: Novel therapeutic opportunities for castration-resistant prostate cancer patients with bone metastasis. *Biochimica et Biophysica Acta. Reviews on Cancer*, *1879*(1), 189033. Advance online publication. DOI: 10.1016/j.bbcan.2023.189033 PMID: 38040267

Li, S., Zhu, S., & Yu, J. (2023). The role of gut microbiota and metabolites in cancer chemotherapy. *Journal of Advanced Research*, *64*, 223–235. DOI: 10.1016/j.jare.2023.11.027 PMID: 38013112

Liu, C., Yang, J., Fu, W., Qi, S., Wang, C., Quan, C., & Yang, K. (2014). Coactivation of the PI3K/Akt and ERK signaling pathways in PCB153-induced NF-κB activation and caspase inhibition. *Toxicology and Applied Pharmacology*, *277*(3), 270–278. DOI: 10.1016/j.taap.2014.03.027 PMID: 24726520

Liu, M., Liu, R., Wang, R., Ba, Y., Yu, F., Deng, Q., & Huang, H. (2022). Lead-induced neurodevelopmental lesion and epigenetic landscape: Implication in neurological disorders. *Journal of Applied Toxicology*, *9*(9), 1256–1271. DOI: 10.1002/jat.4419 PMID: 36433892

Liu, Q., Harvey, C. T., Geng, H., Xue, C., Chen, V., Beer, T. M., & Qian, D. Z. (2013). Malate dehydrogenase 2 confers docetaxel resistance via regulations of JNK signaling and oxidative metabolism. *The Prostate*, *73*(10), 1028–1037. DOI: 10.1002/pros.22650 PMID: 23389923

Liu, Y., Asnani, A., Zou, L., Bentley, V. L., Yu, M., Wang, Y., Dellaire, G., Sarkar, K. S., Dai, M., Chen, H. H., Sosnovik, D. E., Shin, J. T., Haber, D. A., Berman, J. N., Chao, W., & Peterson, R. T. (2014). Visnagin protects against doxorubicin-induced cardiomyopathy through modulation of mitochondrial malate dehydrogenase. *Science Translational Medicine*, *6*(266). Advance online publication. DOI: 10.1126/scitranslmed.3010189 PMID: 25504881

Liu, Y., Horn, J. L., Banda, K., Goodman, A. Z., Lim, Y., Jana, S., Arora, S., Germanos, A. A., Wen, L., Hardin, W. R., Yang, Y. C., Coleman, I. M., Tharakan, R. G., Cai, E. Y., Uo, T., Pillai, S. P. S., Corey, E., Morrissey, C., Chen, Y., & Hsieh, A. C. (2019). The androgen receptor regulates a druggable translational regulon in advanced prostate cancer. *Science Translational Medicine*, *11*(503), eaaw4993. Advance online publication. DOI: 10.1126/scitranslmed.aaw4993 PMID: 31366581

Liu, Z., Hu, M., Yang, Y., Du, C., Zhou, H., Liu, C., Chen, Y., Fan, L., Ma, H., Gong, Y., & Xie, Y. (2022). An overview of PROTACs: A promising drug discovery paradigm. *Molecular Biomedicine*, *3*(1), 46. DOI: 10.1186/s43556-022-00112-0 PMID: 36536188

Li, Y., Zhou, T., Liu, Z., Zhu, X., Wu, Q., Meng, C., & Deng, Q. (2025). Air pollution and prostate cancer: Unraveling the connection through network toxicology and machine learning. *Ecotoxicology and Environmental Safety*, *292*, 117966. Advance online publication. DOI: 10.1016/j.ecoenv.2025.117966 PMID: 40022828

Li, Z., Schieber, J., & Pedersen, P. K. (2021). On the origin and significance of composite particles in mudstones: Examples from the Cenomanian Dunvegan Formation. *Sedimentology*, *68*(2), 737–754. DOI: 10.1111/sed.12801

Loehr, A., Hussain, A., Patnaik, A., Bryce, A. H., Castellano, D., Font, A., Shapiro, J., Zhang, J., Sautois, B., Vogelzang, N. J., Chatta, G., Courtney, K., Harzstark, A., Ricci, F., Despain, D., Watkins, S., King, C., Nguyen, M., Simmons, A. D., & Abida, W. (2023). Emergence of BRCA Reversion Mutations in Patients with Metastatic Castration-resistant Prostate Cancer After Treatment with Rucaparib. *European Urology*, *83*(3), 200–209. DOI: 10.1016/j.eururo.2022.09.010 PMID: 36243543

Longo, R., D'Andrea, M., Sarmiento, R., & Gasparini, G. (2010). Pharmacogenetics in breast cancer: Focus on hormone therapy, taxanes, trastuzumab and bevacizumab. *Expert Opinion on Investigational Drugs*, *19*(sup1, Suppl 1), S41–S50. DOI: 10.1517/13543781003732701 PMID: 20374029

Loomis, D., Grosse, Y., Lauby-Secretan, B., El Ghissassi, F., Bouvard, V., Benbrahim-Tallaa, L., Guha, N., Baan, R., Mattock, H., & Straif, K. (2013). International Agency for Research on Cancer Monograph Working Group IARC. The carcinogenicity of outdoor air pollution. *The Lancet. Oncology*, *14*(13), 1262–1263. DOI: 10.1016/S1470-2045(13)70487-X PMID: 25035875

López, J., Añazco-Guenkova, A. M., Monteagudo-García, Ó., & Blanco, S. (2022). Epigenetic and Epitranscriptomic Control in Prostate Cancer. *Genes*, *13*(2), 378. DOI: 10.3390/genes13020378 PMID: 35205419

Luccio-Camelo, D. C., & Prins, G. S. (2011). Disruption of androgen receptor signaling in males by environmental chemicals. *The Journal of Steroid Biochemistry and Molecular Biology*, *127*(1–2), 74–82. DOI: 10.1016/j.jsbmb.2011.04.004 PMID: 21515368

Luo, J., Chen, Z., Qiao, Y., Tien, J. C.-Y., Young, E., Mannan, R., Mahapatra, S., He, T., Eyunni, S., Zhang, Y., Zheng, Y., Su, F., Cao, X., Wang, R., Cheng, Y., Seri, R., George, J., Shahine, M., Miner, S. J., . . . Chinnaiyan, A. M. (2024). p300/CBP degradation is required to disable the active AR enhanceosome in prostate cancer. BioRxiv, 2024.03.29.587346. https://doi.org/DOI: 10.1101/2024.03.29.587346

Luzum, J. A., Petry, N., Taylor, A. K., Van Driest, S. L., Dunnenberger, H. M., & Cavallari, L. H. (2021). Moving Pharmacogenetics Into Practice: It's All About the Evidence! *Clinical Pharmacology &amp. Therapeutics*, *3*(3), 649–661. DOI: 10.1002/cpt.2327 PMID: 34101169

Maeda, K., Habara, M., Kawaguchi, M., Matsumoto, H., Hanaki, S., Masaki, T., Sato, Y., Matsuyama, H., Kunieda, K., Nakagawa, H., & Shimada, M. (2022). FKBP51 and FKBP52 regulate androgen receptor dimerization and proliferation in prostate cancer cells. *Molecular Oncology*, *16*(4), 940–956. DOI: 10.1002/1878-0261.13030 PMID: 34057812

Maertens, A., E. W. Golden, R. Pizzi, & K. Kannan. (2021). Bisphenol S, F, & Other Analogues in the Environment, Overlooked Endocrine Disruptors & 'Regrettable Substitutions' in Consumer Products. *Environmental Science & Technolog,y* 55 (22), 3569–3579. https,//.DOI: 10.1021/acs.est.0c06095

Maffini, M. V., B. S. Rubin, C. Sonnenschein, & A. M. Soto. (2006). Endocrine Disruptors & Reproductive Health, The Case of Bisphenol-A. *Molecular & Cellular Endocrinology,* 254–255, 179–186. https,//.DOI: 10.1016/j.mce.2006.04.033

Malecki, K. M. C., Nikodemova, M., Schultz, A. A., LeCaire, T. J., Bersch, A. J., Cadmus-Bertram, L., Engelman, C. D., Hagen, E., McCulley, L., Palta, M., Rodriguez, A., Sethi, A. K., Walsh, M. C., Nieto, F. J., & Peppard, P. E. (2022). The Survey of the Health of Wisconsin (SHOW) Program: An Infrastructure for Advancing Population Health. *Frontiers in Public Health, 10*, 818777. DOI: 10.3389/fpubh.2022.818777 PMID: 35433595

Manzar, N., Khan, U. K., Goel, A., Carskadon, S., Gupta, N., Palanisamy, N., & Ateeq, B. (2024). An integrative proteomics approach identifies tyrosine kinase KIT as a therapeutic target for SPINK1-positive prostate cancer. *iScience, 27*(3), 108794. Advance online publication. DOI: 10.1016/j.isci.2024.108794 PMID: 38384854

Marcon, A., Pesce, G., Calciano, L., Bellisario, V., Dharmage, S. C., Garcia-Aymerich, J., Gislasson, T., Heinrich, J., Holm, M., Janson, C., Jarvis, D., Leynaert, B., Matheson, M. C., Pirina, P., Svanes, C., Villani, S., Zuberbier, T., Minelli, C., & Accordini, S. (2018). Trends in smoking initiation in Europe over 40 years: A retrospective cohort study. *PLoS One, 13*(8), e0201881. Advance online publication. DOI: 10.1371/journal.pone.0201881 PMID: 30133533

Marczylo, E. L., Amoako, A. A., Konje, J. C., Gant, T. W., & Marczylo, T. H. (2012). Smoking induces differential miRNA expression in human spermatozoa: A potential transgenerational epigenetic concern? *Epigenetics, 7*(5), 432–439. DOI: 10.4161/epi.19794 PMID: 22441141

Marquez, J., Ángel, J., Sandoval, C., Erb, H. H. H., Polishchuk, N., Stasyk, O., Gur Kahya, U. ˇ., Weigel, M. M., Dubrovska, A., & Dresden-Rossendorf, H.-Z. (2024). Glutamine Metabolism and Prostate Cancer. *Cancers (Basel), 16*(16), 2871. DOI: 10.3390/cancers16162871 PMID: 39199642

Martyniuk, C. J., Mehinto, A. C., & Denslow, N. D. (2020). Organochlorine pesticides: Agrochemicals with potent endocrine-disrupting properties in fish. *Molecular and Cellular Endocrinology, 507*, 110764. DOI: 10.1016/j.mce.2020.110764 PMID: 32112812

Maslarinou, A., Manolopoulos, V. G., & Ragia, G. (2023). Pharmacogenomic-guided dosing of fluoropyrimidines beyond DPYD: Time for a polygenic algorithm? *Frontiers in Pharmacology, 14*, 1184523. Advance online publication. DOI: 10.3389/fphar.2023.1184523 PMID: 37256234

Matshabane, O. P., Whitted, C. G., & Koehly, L. M. (2022). Addressing diversity and inclusion challenges in global neuro-psychiatric and behavioral genomics research. *Frontiers in Genetics, 13*, 1021649. Advance online publication. DOI: 10.3389/fgene.2022.1021649 PMID: 36583023

Matsumoto, N., Kubota, Y., Ishida, H., Sekido, M., Ohkuma, R., Ishiguro, T., Hirasawa, Y., Ariizumi, H., Tsunoda, T., Ikusue, T., Kobayashi, K., Hisamatsu, A., Toshima, H., Shimada, K., & Fujita, K. I. (2020). Variants of carboxylesterase 1 have no impact on capecitabine pharmacokinetics and toxicity in capecitabine plus oxaliplatin treated-colorectal cancer patients. *Cancer Chemotherapy and Pharmacology, 85*(6), 1119–1128. DOI: 10.1007/s00280-020-04087-z PMID: 32458030

May, A., Velthuis, M., Travier, N., Bisschop, C., Wall, E., & Peeters, P. (2014). Physical activity during cancer treatment (PACT) study: Short- and long-term effects on fatigue of an 18-week exercise intervention during adjuvant chemotherapy in patients with breast or colon cancer. *Journal of Clinical Oncology, 32*(15_suppl), 9535–9535. DOI: 10.1200/jco.2014.32.15_suppl.9535

Mayer, E. L., & Burstein, H. J. (2016). Chemotherapy for triple-negative breast cancer: Is more better? *Journal of Clinical Oncology, 34*(28), 3369–3371. DOI: 10.1200/JCO.2016.68.4068 PMID: 27551109

McCullough, S. D., Dhingra, R., Fortin, M. C., & Diaz-Sanchez, D. (2017). Air pollution and the epigenome: A model relationship for the exploration of toxicoepigenetics. *Current Opinion in Toxicology, 6*, 18–25. DOI: 10.1016/j.cotox.2017.07.001 PMID: 33869910

McGirt, L. Y., Jia, P., Baerenwald, D. A., Duszynski, R. J., Dahlman, K. B., Zic, J. A., Zwerner, J. P., Hucks, D., Dave, U., Zhao, Z., & Eischen, C. M. (2015). Whole-genome sequencing reveals oncogenic mutations in mycosis fungoides. *Blood, 126*(4), 508–519. DOI: 10.1182/blood-2014-11-611194 PMID: 26082451

McGuire, A. L., Caulfield, T., & Cho, M. K. (2008). Research ethics and the challenge of whole-genome sequencing. *Nature Reviews. Genetics, 2*(2), 152–156. DOI: 10.1038/nrg2302 PMID: 18087293

McKeon, T. P., Hwang, W. T., Ding, Z., Tam, V., Wileyto, P., Glanz, K., & Penning, T. M. (2021). Environmental exposomics and lung cancer risk assessment in the Philadelphia metropolitan area using ZIP code-level hazard indices. *Environmental Science and Pollution Research International, 28*(24), 31758–31769. DOI: 10.1007/s11356-021-12884-z PMID: 33611735

McKinnon, R. A., & Ward, M. B. (2003). The Emergence of Pharmacogenomics. *Journal of Pharmacy Practice and Research, 2*(2), 133–137. DOI: 10.1002/jppr2003332133

Mechanic, L., Simonds, N., Ghazarian, A., Benedicto, C., Schully, S., Ellison, G., & Gillanders, E. (2012). Abstract 46: A review of the gene-environment interaction literature in cancer: What do we know? *Cancer Epidemiology, Biomarkers & Prevention, 21*(11_Supplement), 46–46. DOI: 10.1158/1055-9965.GWAS-46

Mediwala, S. N., Sun, H., Szafran, A. T., Hartig, S. M., Sonpavde, G., Hayes, T. G., Thiagarajan, P., Mancini, M. A., & Marcelli, M. (2013). The activity of the androgen receptor variant AR-V7 is regulated by FOXO1 in a PTEN-PI3K-AKT-dependent way. *The Prostate, 73*(3), 267–277. DOI: 10.1002/pros.22566 PMID: 22821817

Meeker, J. D., S. Sathyanarayana, & S. H. Swan. (2009). Phthalates & Other Additives in Plastics, Human Exposure & Associated Health Outcomes. Philosophical Transactions of the Royal Society B, *Biological Sciences*, 364 (1526), 2097–2113. https,//.DOI: 10.1098/rstb.2008.0268

Mehrpour, O., Karrari, P., Zamani, N., Tsatsakis, A. M., & Abdollahi, M. (2014). Occupational exposure to pesticides and consequences on male semen and Fertility: A review. *Toxicology Letters, 230*(2), 146–156. DOI: 10.1016/j.toxlet.2014.01.029 PMID: 24487096

Meng, L., Zheng, Y., Liu, H., & Fan, D. (2024). The tumor microenvironment: A key player in multidrug resistance in cancer. *Oncologie, 26*(1), 41–58. DOI: 10.1515/oncologie-2023-0459

Merali, Z., Ross, S., & Paré, G. (2014). The pharmacogenetics of carboxylesterases: *CES1* and CES2 genetic variants and their clinical effect. *Drug Metabolism and Drug Interactions, 29*(3), 143–151. DOI: 10.1515/dmdi-2014-0009 PMID: 24988246

Miller, G. W. (2014). *Staging the Exposome: A Vision for International Collaboration.*, DOI: 10.1016/B978-0-12-417217-3.00007-0

Miller, G. W., & Jones, D. P. (2014). The nature of nurture: Refining the definition of the exposome. *Toxicological Sciences, 137*(1), 1–2. DOI: 10.1093/toxsci/kft251 PMID: 24213143

Mishra, R., Haldar, S., Suchanti, S., & Bhowmick, N. A. (2019). Epigenetic changes in fibroblasts drive cancer metabolism and differentiation. *Endocrine-Related Cancer, 26*(12), R673–R688. DOI: 10.1530/ERC-19-0347 PMID: 31627186

Mittal, R., Woo, F. W., Castro, C. S., Cohen, M. A., Karanxha, J., Mittal, J., Chhibber, T., & Jhaveri, V. M. (2019). Organ-on-chip models: Implications in drug discovery and clinical applications. In *Journal of Cellular Physiology* (Vol. 234, Issue 6, pp. 8352–8380). Wiley-Liss Inc. https://doi.org/DOI: 10.1002/jcp.27729

Mittelstadt, B. (2019). The Ethics of Biomedical 'Big Data' Analytics. Philosophy &amp. *Philosophy & Technology, 1*(1), 17–21. DOI: 10.1007/s13347-019-00344-z

Miura, R., Ikeda-Araki, A., Ishihara, T., Miyake, K., Miyashita, C., Nakajima, T., Kobayashi, S., Ishizuka, M., Kubota, T., & Kishi, R. (2021). Effect of prenatal exposure to phthalates on epigenome-wide DNA methylations in cord blood and implications for fetal growth: The Hokkaido Study on Environment and Children's Health. *The Science of the Total Environment, 783*, 147035. DOI: 10.1016/j.scitotenv.2021.147035 PMID: 33872906

Modica, R., Benevento, E., & Colao, A. (2023). Endocrine-disrupting chemicals (EDCs) and cancer: New perspectives on an old relationship. *Journal of Endocrinological Investigation, 46*(4), 667–677. DOI: 10.1007/s40618-022-01983-4 PMID: 36526827

Moldogazieva, N. T., Mokhosoev, I. M., & Terentiev, A. A. (2020). Metabolic Heterogeneity of Cancer Cells: An Interplay between HIF-1, GLUTs, and AMPK. *Cancers (Basel), 12*(4), 862. DOI: 10.3390/cancers12040862 PMID: 32252351

Montoya-Novoa, I., Gardeazábal-Torbado, J. L., Alegre-Martí, A., Fuentes-Prior, P., & Estébanez-Perpiñá, E. (2024). Androgen receptor post-translational modifications and their implications for pathology. *Biochemical Society Transactions, 52*(4), 1673–1694. DOI: 10.1042/BST20231082 PMID: 38958586

Moreno, V., Bosch, F. X., Muñoz, N., Meijer, C. J., Shah, K. V., Walboomers, J. M., Herrero, R., & Franceschi, S. (2002). Effect of oral contraceptives on risk of cervical cancer in women with human papillomavirus infection: The IARC multicentric case-control study. *Lancet, 359*(9312), 1085–1092. DOI: 10.1016/S0140-6736(02)08150-3 PMID: 11943255

Morgan, M., Deoraj, A., Felty, Q., & Roy, D. (2017). Environmental estrogen-like endocrine disrupting chemicals and breast cancer. *Molecular and Cellular Endocrinology, 457*, 89–102. DOI: 10.1016/j.mce.2016.10.003 PMID: 27717745

Mukherjee, S., Dasgupta, S., Mishra, P. K., & Chaudhury, K. (2021). Air pollution-induced epigenetic changes: Disease development and a possible link with hypersensitivity pneumonitis. *Environmental Science and Pollution Research International, 28*(40), 55981–56002. DOI: 10.1007/s11356-021-16056-x PMID: 34498177

Mukhopadhyay, S., Huang, H. Y., Lin, Z., Ranieri, M., Li, S., Sahu, S., Liu, Y., Ban, Y., Guidry, K., Hu, H., Lopez, A., Sherman, F., Tan, Y. J., Lee, Y. T., Armstrong, A. P., Dolgalev, I., Sahu, P., Zhang, T., Lu, W., & Neel, B. G. (2023). Genome-Wide CRISPR Screens Identify Multiple Synthetic Lethal Targets That Enhance KRASG12C Inhibitor Efficacy. *Cancer Research, 83*(24), 4095–4111. DOI: 10.1158/0008-5472.CAN-23-2729 PMID: 37729426

Murphy, C. C., & Zaki, T. A. (2024). Changing epidemiology of colorectal cancer - birth cohort effects and emerging risk factors. *Nature Reviews. Gastroenterology & Hepatology, 21*(1), 25–34. DOI: 10.1038/s41575-023-00841-9 PMID: 37723270

Mustieles, V., & M. F. Fern&ez. (2020). Bisphenol A Shapes Children's Brain & Behavior, Toward an Integrated Neurotoxicity Assessment Including Human Data. *Environmental Health*, 19, 66. https,//.DOI: 10.1186/s12940-020-00620-y

Na, A. Y., Choi, S., Yang, E., Liu, K. H., Kim, S., Jung, H. J., Choe, Y., Ha, Y. S., Kwon, T. G., Lee, J. N., & Lee, S. (2021). Characterization of novel progression factors in castration-resistant prostate cancer based on global comparative proteome analysis. *Cancers (Basel), 13*(14), 3432. Advance online publication. DOI: 10.3390/cancers13143432 PMID: 34298646

Naidu, S. C., Manolakos, P. T., & Hopkins, T. (2013). Environmental justice in ohio. *The Review of Radical Political Economics, 45*(3), 384–399. DOI: 10.1177/0486613412470094

Narayanan, D. L., Saladi, R. N., & Fox, J. L. (2010). Ultraviolet radiation and skin cancer. *International Journal of Dermatology, 49*(9), 978–986. DOI: 10.1111/j.1365-4632.2010.04474.x PMID: 20883261

Nargund, V. H. (2015). Effects of psychological stress on male fertility. *Nature Reviews. Urology, 12*(7), 373–382. DOI: 10.1038/nrurol.2015.112 PMID: 26057063

Natarajan, R., Aljaber, D., Au, D., Thai, C., Sanchez, A., Nunez, A., Resto, C., Chavez, T., Jankowska, M. M., Benmarhnia, T., Yang, J.-A., Jones, V., Tomsic, J., McCune, J. S., Sistrunk, C., Doan, S., Serrano, M., Cardiff, R. D., Dietze, E. C., & Seewaldt, V. L. (2020). Environmental exposures during puberty: Window of breast cancer risk and epigenetic damage. *International Journal of Environmental Research and Public Health, 17*(2), 493. DOI: 10.3390/ijerph17020493 PMID: 31941024

National Center for Biotechnology Information. (2024). *CES1 carboxylesterase 1 [Homo sapiens (human)] (Gene ID: 1066)*. NCBI Gene. https://www.ncbi.nlm.nih.gov/gene/1066

Navarro-Bielsa, A., Gracia-Cazaña, T., Almagro, M., De la Fuente-Meira, S., Flórez, Á., Yélamos, O., Montero-Vilchez, T., González-Cruz, C., Diago, A., Abadías-Granado, I., Fuentelsaz, V., Colmenero, M., Bañuls, J., Arias-Santiago, S., Buendía-Eisman, A., Almenara-Blasco, M., Gil-Pallares, P., & Gilaberte, Y. (2023). The Influence of the Exposome in the Cutaneous Squamous Cell Carcinoma, a Multicenter Case-Control Study. *Cancers (Basel)*, *15*(22), 5376. DOI: 10.3390/cancers15225376 PMID: 38001636

Neagu, A. N., Jayaweera, T., Corrice, L., Johnson, K., & Darie, C. C. (2024). Breast Cancer Exposomics. *Life (Basel, Switzerland)*, *14*(3), 402. DOI: 10.3390/life14030402 PMID: 38541726

Nemmiche, S., & Guiraud, P. (2016). Cadmium-induced oxidative damages in the human BJAB cells correlate with changes in intracellular trace elements levels and zinc transporters expression. *In Vitro*, *37*, 169–177. DOI: 10.1016/j.tiv.2016.09.014 PMID: 27647474

Nestler, E. J. (2014). Epigenetic Mechanisms of Depression. *JAMA Psychiatry*, *4*(4), 454. DOI: 10.1001/jamapsychiatry.2013.4291 PMID: 24499927

Nevedomskaya, E., & Haendler, B. (2022). From Omics to Multi-Omics Approaches for In-Depth Analysis of the Molecular Mechanisms of Prostate Cancer. In *International Journal of Molecular Sciences* (Vol. 23, Issue 11). MDPI. https://doi.org/ DOI: 10.3390/ijms23116281

Neveu, V., Nicolas, G., Salek, R. M., Wishart, D. S., & Scalbert, A. (2019). Exposome-Explorer 2.0: An update incorporating candidate dietary biomarkers and dietary associations with cancer risk. *Nucleic Acids Research*, *48*, gkz1009. Advance online publication. DOI: 10.1093/nar/gkz1009 PMID: 31724701

Newbold, R. R. (2004). Lessons Learned from Perinatal Exposure to Diethylstilbestrol. *Toxicology & Applied Pharmacology,* 199 (2), 142–150. https,//.DOI: 10.1016/j.taap.2003.12.028

Nientiedt, C., Budczies, J., Endris, V., Kirchner, M., Schwab, C., Jurcic, C., Behnisch, R., Hoveida, S., Lantwin, P., Kaczorowski, A., Geisler, C., Dieffenbacher, S., Falkenbach, F., Franke, D., Görtz, M., Heller, M., Himmelsbach, R., Pecqueux, C., Rath, M., & Duensing, S. (2022). Mutations in TP53 or DNA damage repair genes define poor prognostic subgroups in primary prostate cancer. *Urologic Oncology*, *40*(1), 8.e11–8.e18. DOI: 10.1016/j.urolonc.2021.06.024 PMID: 34325986

Nilsson, E. E., Sadler-Riggleman, I., & Skinner, M. K. (2018). Environmentally induced epigenetic transgenerational inheritance of disease. In Environmental Epigenetics (Vol. 4, Issue 2, pp. 1–13). Oxford University Press. https://doi.org/DOI: 10.1093/eep/dvy016

Nilsson, C., Hessman, E., Sjöblom, H., Dencker, A., Jangsten, E., Mollberg, M., Patel, H., Sparud-Lundin, C., Wigert, H., & Begley, C. (2018). Definitions, measurements and prevalence of fear of childbirth: A systematic review. *BMC Pregnancy and Childbirth, 18*(1), 28. DOI: 10.1186/s12884-018-1659-7 PMID: 29329526

Nilsson, E. E., & Skinner, M. K. (2015). Environmentally Induced Epigenetic Transgenerational Inheritance of Reproductive Disease. *Biology of Reproduction, 93*(6), 145. DOI: 10.1095/biolreprod.115.134817 PMID: 26510870

Nock, N. L., Liu, X., Cicek, M. S., Li, L., Macarie, F., Rybicki, B. A., Plummer, S. J., MacLennan, G. T., Casey, G., & Witte, J. S. (2006). Polymorphisms in polycyclic aromatic hydrocarbon metabolism and conjugation genes, interactions with smoking and prostate cancer risk. *Cancer Epidemiology, Biomarkers & Prevention, 15*(4), 756–761. DOI: 10.1158/1055-9965.EPI-05-0826 PMID: 16614120

Nurgalieva, Z., Liu, C.-C., & Du, X. L. (2011). Chemotherapy use and risk of bone marrow suppression in a large population-based cohort of older women with breast and ovarian cancer. *Medical Oncology (Northwood, London, England), 28*(3), 716–725. DOI: 10.1007/s12032-010-9512-5 PMID: 20361359

Nyström-Persson, J., Natsume-Kitatani, Y., Igarashi, Y., Satoh, D., & Mizuguchi, K. (2017). Interactive Toxicogenomics: Gene set discovery, clustering and analysis in Toxygates. *Scientific Reports, 1*(1), 1390. Advance online publication. DOI: 10.1038/s41598-017-01500-1 PMID: 28469246

O'Connell, K. A., Stolley, M. R., Berg, D., & Kerschner, A. (2023). Cancer health education in high schools: A qualitative analysis of student gains. *Cancer Epidemiology, Biomarkers & Prevention, 32*(12, Supplement), A072. DOI: 10.1158/1538-7755.DISP23-A072

O'Connell, S. G., Kincl, L. D., & Anderson, K. A. (2014). Silicone wristbands as personal passive samplers. *Environmental Science & Technology, 48*(6), 3327–3335. DOI: 10.1021/es405022f PMID: 24548134

Olmedo-Suárez, M. Á., Ramírez-Díaz, I., Pérez-González, A., Molina-Herrera, A., Coral-García, M. Á., Lobato, S., Sarvari, P., Barreto, G., & Rubio, K. (2022). Epigenetic Regulation in Exposome-Induced Tumorigenesis: Emerging Roles of ncRNAs. *Biomolecules, 12*(4), 513. DOI: 10.3390/biom12040513 PMID: 35454102

Omoijuanfo, E.-O., Williams, J. T., Qua, K., Cullen, J., Trapl, E. S., Owusu, C., Junk, D. J., & Berger, N. A. (2022). Disparities Education Strategies in the Case Comprehensive Cancer Center STEM Focused Youth Enjoy Science Program. *Journal of STEM Outreach*, *5*(2). Advance online publication. DOI: 10.15695/jstem/v5i2.07 PMID: 36200123

Ormond, K. E., & Cho, M. K. (2014). Translating Personalized Medicine Using New Genetic Technologies in Clinical Practice: The Ethical Issues. *Personalized Medicine*, *2*(2), 211–222. DOI: 10.2217/pme.13.104 PMID: 25221608

Ostermeier, G. C., & Krawetz, S. A. (2005). *Spermatozoal RNAs as surrogate markers of paternal exposure*. Surrogate.

Overbeek, G., Finkenauer, C., Alink, L. R. A., Leijten, P., Branje, S., Schrama, W., & Schenk, J. (2024). Caregiver Consent in Research on Minors: Towards an Inclusive, Hybrid Approach Running Head: Consent Approaches in Human Behavior Research. DOI: 10.31234/osf.io/k8muz

Paetznick, C., & Okoro, O. (2023). The Intersection between Pharmacogenomics and Health Equity: A Case Example. *Pharmacy (Basel, Switzerland)*, *6*(6), 186. DOI: 10.3390/pharmacy11060186 PMID: 38133461

Palmer, J. R., Wise, L. A., Hatch, E. E., Troisi, R., Titus-Ernstoff, L., Strohsnitter, W. C., Kaufman, R. H., Herbst, A. L., Noller, K. L., Hyer, M., Hoover, R. N., Robboy, S. J., Cowan, C. M., Adam, E., Gibson-Chambers, J., Hartge, P., & Strohsnitter, W. C. (2006). Prenatal diethylstilbestrol exposure and risk of ectopic pregnancy, miscarriage, and premature birth. *Obstetrics and Gynecology*, *107*(5), 101–110.

Palmirotta, R., Carella, C., Silvestris, E., Cives, M., Stucci, S. L., Tucci, M., Lovero, D., & Silvestris, F. (2018). SNPs in predicting clinical efficacy and toxicity of chemotherapy: Walking through the quicksand. *Oncotarget*, *9*(38), 25355–25382. DOI: 10.18632/oncotarget.25256 PMID: 29861877

Panahi, Y., Beiraghdar, F., Amirhamzeh, A., Poursaleh, Z., Saadat, A., & Sahebkar, A. (2016). Environmental toxicant exposure and cancer: The role of epigenetic changes and protection by phytochemicals. *Current Pharmaceutical Design*, *22*(2), 130–140. DOI: 10.2174/1381612822666151112150149 PMID: 26561072

Pandiri, A. R., Auerbach, S. S., Stevens, J. L., & Blomme, E. A. G. (2024). Toxicogenomics approaches to address toxicity and carcinogenicity in the liver. *Toxicologic Pathology*, *51*(7–8), 470–481. DOI: 10.1177/01926233241227942 PMID: 38288963

Park, J., Lee, H., Lee, S., & Lee, H. (2022). Interventions on Reducing Exposure to Endocrine Disrupting Chemicals in Human Health Care Context: A Scoping Review. In *Risk Management and Healthcare Policy* (Vol. 15, pp. 779–791). Dove Medical Press Ltd. https://doi.org/DOI: 10.2147/RMHP.S358561

Parker, L. (2014). *The Impact of the Environment on Cancer Genomics*. Academic Press., DOI: 10.1016/B978-0-12-396967-5.00026-8

Patel, C. J., Bhattacharya, J., & Butte, A. J. (2010). An environment-wide association study (EWAS) on type 2 diabetes mellitus. *PLoS One*, *5*(5), e10746. DOI: 10.1371/journal.pone.0010746 PMID: 20505766

Patierno, S. R. (2020). Environmental Factors. In *Abeloff's Clinical Oncology* (pp. 139–153.e2). Elsevier. DOI: 10.1016/B978-0-323-47674-4.00010-4

Paul, K. B., J. M. Hedge, R. Bansal, R. T. Zoeller, R. Peter, & M. J. DeVito. (2010). Developmental Triclosan Exposure Decreases Maternal, Fetal, & Neonatal Thyroxine Levels in Rats. *Environmental Toxicology & Chemistry*, 29 (2), 284–291. https,//DOI: 10.1002/etc.21

Peng, X., Zheng, J., Liu, T., Zhou, Z., Song, C., Zhang, D., Zhang, X., & Huang, Y. (2025). DNA methylation-based diagnosis and treatment of breast cancer. *Current Cancer Drug Targets*, *25*(1), 26–37. DOI: 10.2174/0115680096278978240204162353 PMID: 38441008

Pereira, S. A., & Antunes, A. M. M. (2019). Special issue 'Adductomics: Elucidating the environmental causes of disease'. *High-Throughput*, *8*(3), 17. Advance online publication. DOI: 10.3390/ht8030017 PMID: 31370290

Peretz, J., & J. A. Flaws. (2014). Endocrine Disruptors & Female Reproductive Health. Endocrinology & *Metabolism Clinics of North America*, 43 (1), 133–146. https,//.DOI: 10.1016/j.ecl.2013.09.005

Perry, A. S., Watson, R. W. G., Lawler, M., & Hollywood, D. (2010). The epigenome as a therapeutic target in prostate cancer. In Nature Reviews Urology (Vol. 7, Issue 12, pp. 668–680). https://doi.org/DOI: 10.1038/nrurol.2010.185

Pilotto, A., Panza, F., & Seripa, D. (2011). Pharmacogenetics in Geriatric Medicine: Challenges and Opportunities for Clinical Practice. *Current Drug Metabolism*, *7*(7), 621–634. DOI: 10.2174/138920011796504545 PMID: 21495974

Pirmohamed, M. (2023). Pharmacogenomics: Current status and future perspectives. *Nature Reviews. Genetics*, *6*(6), 350–362. DOI: 10.1038/s41576-022-00572-8 PMID: 36707729

Plummer, F., Manea, L., Trepel, D., & McMillan, D. (2015). Screening for anxiety disorders with the GAD-7 and GAD-2: A systematic review and diagnostic meta analysis. *General Hospital Psychiatry, 39*, 24–31. DOI: 10.1016/j.genhosppsych.2015.11.005 PMID: 26719105

Plummer, M., Herrero, R., Franceschi, S., Meijer, C. J., Snijders, P., Bosch, F. X., de Sanjosé, S., & Muñoz, N. (2003). Smoking and cervical cancer: Pooled analysis of the IARC multi-centric case–control study. *Cancer Causes & Control, 14*(9), 805–814. DOI: 10.1023/B:CACO.0000003811.98261.3e PMID: 14682438

Portugal, J., Mansilla, S., & Piña, B. (2022). Perspectives on the Use of Toxicogenomics to Assess Environmental Risk. *Frontiers in Bioscience (Landmark Edition), 27*(10), 294. Advance online publication. DOI: 10.31083/j.fbl2710294 PMID: 36336867

Prakash, P., Verma, S., & Gupta, S. (2024). Risk factors influencing chronic inflammation in neoplastic transition to prostate cancer. *Journal of Translational Genetics and Genomics, 8*(4), 312–327. DOI: 10.20517/jtgg.2024.52

Prins, G. S. (2008). Endocrine disruptors and prostate cancer risk. *Endocrine-Related Cancer, 15*(3), 649–656. DOI: 10.1677/ERC-08-0043 PMID: 18524946

Prins, G. S., Ye, S. H., Birch, L., Zhang, X., Cheong, A., Lin, H., Calderon-Gierszal, E., Groen, J., Hu, W. Y., Ho, S. M., & Van Breemen, R. B. (2017). Prostate Cancer Risk and DNA Methylation Signatures in Aging Rats following Developmental BPA Exposure: A Dose-Response Analysis. *Environmental Health Perspectives, 125*(7), 077007. Advance online publication. DOI: 10.1289/EHP1050 PMID: 28728135

Priyadarshini, E., Parambil, A. M., Rajamani, P., Ponnusamy, V. K., & Chen, Y. H. (2023). Exposure, toxicological mechanism of endocrine disrupting compounds and future direction of identification using nano-architectonics. *Environmental Research, 225*, 115577. DOI: 10.1016/j.envres.2023.115577 PMID: 36871939

Puca, L., Bareja, R., Prandi, D., Shaw, R., Benelli, M., Karthaus, W. R., Hess, J., Sigouros, M., Donoghue, A., Kossai, M., Gao, D., Cyrta, J., Sailer, V., Vosoughi, A., Pauli, C., Churakova, Y., Cheung, C., Deonarine, L. D., McNary, T. J., & Beltran, H. (2018). Patient derived organoids to model rare prostate cancer phenotypes. *Nature Communications, 9*(1), 2404. Advance online publication. DOI: 10.1038/s41467-018-04495-z PMID: 29921838

Puca, L., Vlachostergios, P. J., & Beltran, H. (2019). Neuroendocrine Differentiation in Prostate Cancer: Emerging Biology, Models, and Therapies. *Cold Spring Harbor Perspectives in Medicine, 9*(2), a030593. DOI: 10.1101/cshperspect.a030593 PMID: 29844220

Qian, Y., & Markowitz, J. S. (2020). Natural products as modulators of *CES1* activity. *Drug Metabolism and Disposition: the Biological Fate of Chemicals*, *48*(10), 993–1007. DOI: 10.1124/dmd.120.000065 PMID: 32591414

Quagliariello, V., Rossetti, S., Cavaliere, C., Di Palo, R., Lamantia, E., Castaldo, L., Nocerino, F., Ametrano, G., Cappuccio, F., Malzone, G., Montanari, M., Vanacore, D., Romano, F. J., Piscitelli, R., Iovane, G., Pepe, M. F., Berretta, M., D'Aniello, C., Perdonà, S., & Facchini, G. (2017). Metabolic syndrome, endocrine disruptors and prostate cancer associations: Biochemical and pathophysiological evidences. *Oncotarget*, *8*(18), 30606–30616. DOI: 10.18632/oncotarget.16725 PMID: 28389628

Querol Cano, L., Lavery, D. N., & Bevan, C. L. (2013). Mini-review: Foldosome regulation of androgen receptor action in prostate cancer. *Molecular and Cellular Endocrinology*, *369*(1–2), 52–62. DOI: 10.1016/j.mce.2013.01.023 PMID: 23395916

Rajdeo, P., Aronow, B., & Surya Prasath, V. B. (2024). Deep learning-based multimodal spatial transcriptomics analysis for cancer. *Advances in Cancer Research*, *163*, 1–38. DOI: 10.1016/bs.acr.2024.08.001 PMID: 39271260

Ralph, J. L., Orgebin-Crist, M. C., Lareyre, J. J., & Nelson, C. C. (2003a). Disruption of androgen regulation in the prostate by the environmental contaminant hexachlorobenzene. In *Environmental Health Perspectives* (Vol. 111, Issue 4, pp. 461–466). Public Health Services, US Dept of Health and Human Services. DOI: 10.1289/ehp.5919

Ramamoorthy, T., Nath, A., Singh, S., Mathew, S., Pant, A., Sheela, S., Kaur, G., Sathishkumar, K., & Mathur, P. (2024). Assessing the global impact of ambient air pollution on cancer incidence and mortality: A comprehensive meta-analysis. *JCO Global Oncology*, *10*(10), e2300427. DOI: 10.1200/GO.23.00427 PMID: 38513187

Rangel, L. B. A., Taraba, J. L., Frei, C. R., Smith, L., Rodriguez, G., & Kuhn, J. G. (2014). Pharmacogenomic diversity of tamoxifen metabolites and estrogen receptor genes in Hispanics and non-Hispanic whites with breast cancer. *Breast Cancer Research and Treatment*, *3*(3), 571–580. DOI: 10.1007/s10549-014-3191-4 PMID: 25395315

Rao, X., Zhong, J., Brook, R. D., & Rajagopalan, S. (2018). Effect of particulate matter air pollution on cardiovascular oxidative stress pathways. *Antioxidants & Redox Signaling*, *28*(9), 797–818. DOI: 10.1089/ars.2017.7394 PMID: 29084451

Rappaport, S. M. (2011). Implications of the exposome for exposure science. *Journal of Exposure Science & Environmental Epidemiology*, *21*(1), 5–9. DOI: 10.1038/jes.2010.50 PMID: 21081972

Rappaport, S. M., & Smith, M. T. (2010). Epidemiology. Environment and disease risks. *Science, 330*(6003), 460–461. DOI: 10.1126/science.1192603 PMID: 20966241

Rathkopf, D. E., Smith, M. R., Ryan, C. J., Berry, W. R., Shore, N. D., Liu, G., Higano, C. S., Alumkal, J. J., Hauke, R., Tutrone, R. F., Saleh, M., Maneval, E. C., Thomas, S., Ricci, D. S., Yu, M. K., de Boer, C. J., Trinh, A., Kheoh, T., Bandekar, R., & Antonarakis, E. S. (2017). Androgen receptor mutations in patients with castration-resistant prostate cancer treated with apalutamide. *Annals of Oncology : Official Journal of the European Society for Medical Oncology, 28*(9), 2264–2271. DOI: 10.1093/annonc/mdx283 PMID: 28633425

Regnier, S. M., & R. M. Sargis. (2014). Adipocytes under Assault, Environmental Disruption of Adipose Physiology. *Biochimica et Biophysica Acta — Molecular Basis of Disease*, 1842 (3), 520–533. https,//.DOI: 10.1016/j.bbadis.2013.08.001

Rehman, Q., Rehman, K., & Akash, M. S. H. (2021). Heavy Metals and Neurological Disorders: From Exposure to Preventive Interventions. In *Emerging Contaminants and Associated Treatment Technologies* (pp. 69–87). Springer International Publishing. http://dx.doi.org/DOI: 10.1007/978-3-030-66376-6_4

Ren, S., He, K., & Girshick, R. (2015). Faster R-CNN: Towards Real-Time Object Detection with Region Proposal Networks. *Advances in Neural Information Processing Systems, 28*, 91–99.

Ren, X., McHale, C. M., Skibola, C. F., Smith, A. H., Smith, M. T., & Zhang, L. (2011). An emerging role for epigenetic dysregulation in arsenic toxicity and carcinogenesis. *Environmental Health Perspectives, 119*(1), 11–19. DOI: 10.1289/ehp.1002114 PMID: 20682481

Rhomberg, L. R., & Goodman, J. E. (2012). Low-dose effects and nonmonotonic dose-responses of endocrine disrupting chemicals: Has the case been made? *Regulatory Toxicology and Pharmacology, 64*(1), 130–133. DOI: 10.1016/j.yrtph.2012.06.015 PMID: 22750031

Richmond, A. S., Boysen, G. A., Hudson, D. L., Gurung, R. A. R., Naufel, K. Z., Neufeld, G., Landrum, R. E., Dunn, D. S., & Beers, M. (2021). The Introductory Psychology Census: A national study. *Scholarship of Teaching and Learning in Psychology, 7*(3), 163–180. DOI: 10.1037/stl0000277

Richmond, D., Sibthorp, J., Gookin, J., Annarella, S., & Ferri, S. (2018). Complementing classroom learning through outdoor adventure education: Out-of-school-time experiences that make a difference. *Journal of Adventure Education and Outdoor Learning, 18*(1), 36–52. DOI: 10.1080/14729679.2017.1324313

Rider, C. F., & Carlsten, C. (2019). Air pollution and DNA methylation: Effects of exposure in humans. *Clinical Epigenetics, 11*(1), 131. DOI: 10.1186/s13148-019-0713-2 PMID: 31481107

Riley, R. D., Higgins, J. P., & Deeks, J. J. (2011). Interpretation of random effects meta-analyses. *BMJ (Clinical Research Ed.), 10*(feb10 2), 342–549. DOI: 10.1136/bmj.d549 PMID: 21310794

Risdon, E. N., Chau, C. H., Price, D. K., Sartor, O., & Figg, W. D. (2020). PARP Inhibitors and Prostate Cancer: To Infinity and Beyond BRCA. *The Oncologist, 26*(1), e115–e129. DOI: 10.1634/theoncologist.2020-0697 PMID: 32790034

Rochester, J. R. (2013). Bisphenol A & Human Health, A Review of the Literature. *Reproductive Toxicology (Elmsford, N.Y.), 42*, 132–155. DOI: 10.1016/j.reprotox.2013.08.008 PMID: 23994667

Rochette, L., Guenancia, C., Gudjoncik, A., Hachet, O., Zeller, M., Cottin, Y., & Vergely, C. (2015). Anthracyclines/trastuzumab: New aspects of cardiotoxicity and molecular mechanisms. *Trends in Pharmacological Sciences, 36*(6), 326–348. DOI: 10.1016/j.tips.2015.03.005 PMID: 25895646

Rodriguez, L. L., Brooks, L. D., Greenberg, J. H., & Green, E. D. (2013). Research ethics. The complexities of genomic identifiability. *Science, 339*(6117), 275–276. DOI: 10.1126/science.1234593 PMID: 23329035

Rofaiel, S., Muo, E. N., & Mousa, S. A. (2010). Pharmacogenetics in breast cancer: Steps toward personalized medicine in breast cancer management. *Pharmacogenomics and Personalized Medicine, 3*, 129–143. DOI: 10.2147/PGPM.S10789 PMID: 23226048

Rollinson, V., Turner, R., & Pirmohamed, M. (2020). Pharmacogenomics for Primary Care: An Overview. *Genes, 11*(11), 1337. DOI: 10.3390/genes11111337 PMID: 33198260

Ronsmans, S., Sørig Hougaard, K., Nawrot, T. S., Plusquin, M., Huaux, F., Jesús Cruz, M., Moldovan, H., Verpaele, S., Jayapala, M., Tunney, M., Humblet-Baron, S., Dirven, H., Cecilie Nygaard, U., Lindeman, B., Duale, N., Liston, A., Flachs, E. M., Kastaniegaard, K., Ketzel, M., & Yserbyt, J. (2022). The EXIMIOUS project—Mapping exposure-induced immune effects: Connecting the exposome and the immunome. *Environmental Epidemiology (Philadelphia, Pa.), 6*(1), e193. DOI: 10.1097/EE9.0000000000000193 PMID: 35169671

Roux, P. P., & Blenis, J. (2004). ERK and p38 MAPK-Activated Protein Kinases: A Family of Protein Kinases with Diverse Biological Functions. *Microbiology and Molecular Biology Reviews : MMBR, 68*(2), 320–344. DOI: 10.1128/MMBR.68.2.320-344.2004 PMID: 15187187

Rovira, J., Nadal, M., Schuhmacher, M., & Domingo, J. L. (2021). Environmental impact and human health risks of air pollutants near a large chemical/petrochemical complex: Case study in Tarragona, Spain. *The Science of the Total Environment, 787*, 147550. DOI: 10.1016/j.scitotenv.2021.147550 PMID: 33991912

Royal, C. D. M., Babyak, M., Shah, N., Srivatsa, S., Stewart, K. A., Tanabe, P., Wonkam, A., & Asnani, M. (2021). Sickle cell disease is a global prototype for integrative research and healthcare. *Advanced Genetics, 1*(1), e10037. Advance online publication. DOI: 10.1002/ggn2.10037 PMID: 36618444

Ruan, Y., Fang, X., Guo, T., Liu, Y., Hu, Y., Wang, X., Hu, Y., Gao, L., Li, Y., Pi, J., & Xu, Y. (2022). Metabolic reprogramming in the arsenic carcinogenesis. *Ecotoxicology and Environmental Safety, 229*, 113098. DOI: 10.1016/j.ecoenv.2021.113098 PMID: 34952379

Rubin, B. S. (2011). Bisphenol A, An Endocrine Disruptor with Widespread Exposure & Multiple Effects. *Journal of Steroid Biochemistry & Molecular Biology,* 127 (1–2), 27–34. https,//DOI: 10.1016/j.jsbmb.2011.05.002

Rudel, R. A., J. M. Gray, C. L. Engel, T. W. Rawsthorne, R. E. Dodson, J. M. Ackerman, J. Rizzo, J. L. Nudelman, & J. G. Brody. (2011). Food Packaging & Bisphenol A & Bis(2-ethylhexyl) Phthalate Exposure, Findings from a Dietary Intervention. *Environmental Health Perspectives,* 119 (7), 914–920. https,//.DOI: 10.1289/ehp.1003170

Ruggeri, R. M., Minuti, A., Gianì, F., Masto, R., Romano, D., Aliquò, F., Campennì, A., Campo, S., Cannavò, S., & D'Ascola, A. (2025). Polychlorinated Biphenyls (PCBS)-induced oxidative stress and inflammation in human thyrocytes: Involvement of AhR and NRF-2/HO-1 pathway. *Endocrine, 87*(1), 252–261. Advance online publication. DOI: 10.1007/s12020-024-04005-w PMID: 39174753

Rusiecki, J. A., Beane Freeman, L. E., Bonner, M. R., Alexander, M., Chen, L., Andreotti, G., Barry, K. H., Moore, L. E., Byun, H. M., Kamel, F., Alavanja, M., Hoppin, J. A., & Baccarelli, A. (2017). High pesticide exposure events and DNA methylation among pesticide applicators in the agricultural health study. *Environmental and Molecular Mutagenesis, 58*(1), 19–29. DOI: 10.1002/em.22067 PMID: 27996157

Ruttkies, C., Schymanski, E. L., Wolf, S., Hollender, J., & Neumann, S. (2016). MetFrag relaunched: Incorporating strategies beyond in silico fragmentation. *Journal of Cheminformatics, 8*(1), 1–16. DOI: 10.1186/s13321-016-0115-9 PMID: 26834843

Ryeom, S. W., Paul, D., & Goodenough, D. A. (2000). Truncation mutants of the tight junction protein ZO-1 disrupt corneal epithelial cell morphology. *Molecular Biology of the Cell, 11*(5), 1687–1696. DOI: 10.1091/mbc.11.5.1687 PMID: 10793144

Sadar, M. D., & Gleave, M. E. (2000). Ligand-independent Activation of the Androgen Receptor by the Differentiation Agent Butyrate in Human Prostate Cancer Cells 1. In *CANCER RESEARCH* (Vol. 60).

Safarlou, C. W., Jongsma, K. R., Vermeulen, R., & Bredenoord, A. L. (2023). The ethical aspects of exposome research: A systematic review. *Exposome, 3*(1), osad004. Advance online publication. DOI: 10.1093/exposome/osad004 PMID: 37745046

Sagiv, S. K., Bruno, J. L., Baker, J. M., Palzes, V., Kogut, K., Rauch, S., Gunier, R., Mora, A. M., Reiss, A. L., & Eskenazi, B. (2019). "Prenatal exposure to organophosphate pesticides and functional neuroimaging in adolescents living in proximity to pesticide application;" *Proceedings of the National Academy of Sciences of the United States of America*. DOI: DOI: 10.1073/pnas.1903940116

Saha, D., Dang, H. X., Zhang, M., Quigley, D. A., Feng, F. Y., & Maher, C. A. (2024). Single cell-transcriptomic analysis informs the lncRNA landscape in metastatic castration resistant prostate cancer. *NPJ Genomic Medicine, 9*(1), 14. Advance online publication. DOI: 10.1038/s41525-024-00401-3 PMID: 38396008

Sakhvidi, M. J. Z., Knobel, P., Bauwelinck, M., de Keijzer, C., Boll, L. M., Spano, G., & Dadvand, P. (2022). Greenspace exposure and children behavior: A systematic review. *The Science of the Total Environment, 824*, 153608. DOI: 10.1016/j.scitotenv.2022.153608 PMID: 35134416

Sakuma, K., Kitamura, A., Malins, A., Kurikami, H., Machida, M., Mori, K., Tada, K., Kobayashi, T., Tawara, Y., & Tosaka, H. (2017). Characteristics of radio-cesium transport and discharge between different basins near to the Fukushima Dai-ichi Nuclear Power Plant after heavy rainfall events. *Journal of Environmental Radioactivity, 169-170*, 137–150. DOI: 10.1016/j.jenvrad.2016.12.006 PMID: 28161603

Salian, S., Doshi, T., & Vanage, G. (2009). Impairment in protein expression profile of testicular steroid receptor coregulators in male rat offspring perinatally exposed to Bisphenol A. *Life Sciences, 85*(1–2), 11–18. DOI: 10.1016/j.lfs.2009.04.005 PMID: 19379760

Samet, J. M. (2020). Air Pollution: Adverse Effects and Disease Burden. In *Health of People, Health of Planet and Our Responsibility* (pp. 63–78). Springer International Publishing. http://dx.doi.org/DOI: 10.1007/978-3-030-31125-4_6

Santos-Pereira, M., Pereira, S. C., Rebelo, I., Spadella, M. A., Oliveira, P. F., & Alves, M. G. (2023). Decoding the Influence of Obesity on Prostate Cancer and Its Transgenerational Impact. In Nutrients (Vol. 15, Issue 23). Multidisciplinary Digital Publishing Institute (MDPI). https://doi.org/DOI: 10.3390/nu15234858

Sardar, S., McNair, C. M., Ravindranath, L., Chand, S. N., Yuan, W., Bogdan, D., Welti, J., Sharp, A., Ryan, N. K., Schiewer, M. J., DeArment, E. G., Janas, T., Su, X. A., Butler, L. M., de Bono, J. S., Frese, K., Brooks, N., Pegg, N., Knudsen, K. E., & Shafi, A. A. (2024). AR coactivators, CBP/p300, are critical mediators of DNA repair in prostate cancer. BioRxiv, 2024.05.07.592966. DOI: 10.1101/2024.05.07.592966

Sarigiannis, D., Karakitsios, S., Anesti, O., Stem, A., Valvi, D., Sumner, S. C. J., Chatzi, L., Snyder, M. P., Thompson, D. C., & Vasiliou, V. (2025). Advancing translational exposomics: Bridging genome, exposome and personalized medicine. *Human Genomics*, *19*(1), 48. DOI: 10.1186/s40246-025-00761-6 PMID: 40307849

Sarkar, A., Paul, A., Banerjee, T., Maji, A., Saha, S., Bishayee, A., & Maity, T. K. (2023). Therapeutic advancements in targeting BCL-2 family proteins by epigenetic regulators, natural, and synthetic agents in cancer. *European Journal of Pharmacology*, *944*, 175588. DOI: 10.1016/j.ejphar.2023.175588 PMID: 36791843

Sassi, A., & You, L. (2024). Microfluidics-Based Technologies for the Assessment of Castration-Resistant Prostate Cancer. In *Cells* (Vol. 13, Issue 7). Multidisciplinary Digital Publishing Institute (MDPI). https://doi.org/DOI: 10.3390/cells13070575

Schuler, M. S., & Rose, S. (2017). Targeted Maximum Likelihood Estimation for Causal Inference in Observational Studies. *American Journal of Epidemiology*, *185*(1), 65–73. DOI: 10.1093/aje/kww165 PMID: 27941068

Schulz, H., Abdelfattah, F., Heinrich, A., Melnik, D., Sandt, V., Krüger, M., Wehland, M., Hoffmann, P., Cortés-Sánchez, J. L., Evert, M., Evert, K., & Grimm, D. (2025). Omics Investigations of Prostate Cancer Cells Exposed to Simulated Microgravity Conditions. *Biomolecules*, *15*(2), 303. DOI: 10.3390/biom15020303 PMID: 40001606

Schwarzenbach, H., Alix-Panabières, C., Müller, I., Letang, N., Vendrell, J. P., Rebillard, X., & Pantel, K. (2009). Cell-free tumor DNA in blood plasma as a marker for circulating tumor cells in prostate cancer. *Clinical Cancer Research*, *15*(3), 1032–1038. DOI: 10.1158/1078-0432.CCR-08-1910 PMID: 19188176

Segovia-Mendoza, M., Nava-Castro, K. E., Palacios-Arreola, M. I., Garay-Canales, C., & Morales-Montor, J. (2020). How microplastic components influence the immune system and impact on children health: Focus on cancer. *Birth Defects Research*, *112*(17), 1341–1361. DOI: 10.1002/bdr2.1779 PMID: 32767490

Sender, R., Fuchs, S., & Milo, R. (2016). Are We really vastly outnumbered? revisiting the ratio of bacterial to host cells in humans. *Cell*, *164*(3), 337–340. DOI: 10.1016/j.cell.2016.01.013 PMID: 26824647

Senier, L., Brown, P., Shostak, S., & Hanna, B. (2017). The Socio-Exposome: Advancing Exposure Science and Environmental Justice in a Post-Genomic Era. *Environmental Sociology*, *3*(2), 107–121. DOI: 10.1080/23251042.2016.1220848 PMID: 28944245

Sermondade, N., Dupont, C., Faure, C., Boubaya, M., Cédrin-Durnerin, I., Chavatte-Palmer, P., Sifer, C., & Lévy, R. (2013). Body mass index is not associated with sperm–zona pellucida binding ability in subfertile males. *Asian Journal of Andrology*, *15*(5), 626–629. DOI: 10.1038/aja.2013.10 PMID: 23770940

Sexton, K., & Hattis, D. (2007). Assessing Cumulative Health Risks from Exposure to Environmental Mixtures—Three Fundamental Questions. *Environmental Health Perspectives*, *5*(5), 825–832. DOI: 10.1289/ehp.9333 PMID: 17520074

Shaaban, S., & Ji, Y. (2023). Pharmacogenomics and health disparities, are we helping? *Frontiers in Genetics*, *14*, 1099541. Advance online publication. DOI: 10.3389/fgene.2023.1099541 PMID: 36755573

Shafi, A. A., Yen, A. E., & Weigel, N. L. (2013). Androgen receptors in hormone-dependent and castration-resistant prostate cancer. *Pharmacology & Therapeutics*, *140*(3), 223–238. DOI: 10.1016/j.pharmthera.2013.07.003 PMID: 23859952

Sharif, R., & Ooi, T. C. (2024). Understanding exposomes and its relation with cancer risk in Malaysia based on epidemiological evidence: A narrative review. *Genes and Environment : the Official Journal of the Japanese Environmental Mutagen Society*, *46*(1), 5. Advance online publication. DOI: 10.1186/s41021-024-00300-0 PMID: 38326915

Sharma, A., Kishore, D., & Singh, B. (2015). Environmental and anthropogenic carcinogens and their carcinogenic effects on humans. *Journal of Biomedical and Pharmaceutical Research*, *4*(2). http://www.jbpr.in/index.php/jbpr/article/view/405/0

Sharma, R., Suravarjhula, L., Banerjee, M., Kumar, G., & Kumar, N. (2023). Chimeric antigen receptor T-cell therapy in cancer: A critical review. *Current Drug Research Reviews*, *15*(3), 241–261. DOI: 10.2174/2589977515666230220092125 PMID: 36825696

Shen, S., Sun, Q., Xu, Y., Zhou, Y., Guan, J., Mao, F., Lin, Y., & Wang, X. (2015). Abstract P5-18-06: Trastuzumab can be safely administered concurrently with anthracycline for adjuvant treatment of HER2-positive breast cancer. *Cancer Research*, *75*(9_Supplement), P5-18-06. Advance online publication. DOI: 10.1158/1538-7445. SABCS14-P5-18-06

Shih, C., Tomita, N. L., Yanick, X., Reguera, Á. H., Fleisch, E., & Kowatsch, T. (2019). Breeze: Smartphone-based Acoustic Real-time Detection of Breathing Phases for a Gamified Biofeedback Breathing Training. *Proceedings of the ACM on Interactive, Mobile, Wearable and Ubiquitous Technologies*, *3*(4), 152. Advance online publication. DOI: 10.1145/3369835

Shimozuma, K., Ohashi, Y., Takeuchi, A., Aranishi, T., Morita, S., Kuroi, K., Ohsumi, S., Makino, H., Katsumata, N., Kuranami, M., Suemasu, K., Watanabe, T., & Hausheer, F. H. (2012). Taxane-induced peripheral neuropathy and health-related quality of life in postoperative breast cancer patients undergoing adjuvant chemotherapy: N-SAS BC 02, a randomized clinical trial. *Supportive Care in Cancer*, *20*(12), 3355–3364. DOI: 10.1007/s00520-012-1492-x PMID: 22584733

Shin, H. J., Hua, J. T., & Li, H. (2023). Recent advances in understanding DNA methylation of prostate cancer. *Frontiers in Oncology*, *13*, 1182727. DOI: 10.3389/fonc.2023.1182727 PMID: 37234978

Shorning, B. Y., Dass, M. S., Smalley, M. J., & Pearson, H. B. (2020). The PI3K-AKT-mTOR Pathway and Prostate Cancer: At the Crossroads of AR, MAPK, and WNT Signaling. *International Journal of Molecular Sciences*, *21*(12), 4507. DOI: 10.3390/ijms21124507 PMID: 32630372

Shriver, S. P., Adams, D., McKelvey, B. A., McCune, J. S., Miles, D., Pratt, V. M., Ashcraft, K., McLeod, H. L., Williams, H., & Fleury, M. E. (2024). Overcoming Barriers to Discovery and Implementation of Equitable Pharmacogenomic Testing in Oncology. *Journal of Clinical Oncology*, *10*(10), 1181–1192. DOI: 10.1200/JCO.23.01748 PMID: 38386947

Silkina, M. O., Razumovskaya, A. V., Nikulin, S. V., Tonevitsky, A. G., & Alekseev, B. Y. (2023). Assessing the Efficacy of Anti-Cancer Drugs on Organoid Models Derived from Prostate Cancer. *Doklady. Biochemistry and Biophysics*, *513*(S1, Suppl 1), S96–S99. Advance online publication. DOI: 10.1134/S1607672923700692 PMID: 38337100

Silveyra, P., & Floros, J. (2012). Air pollution and epigenetics: Effects on SP-A and innate host defence in the lung. *Swiss Medical Weekly*, *142*, w13579. DOI: 10.4414/smw.2012.13579 PMID: 22553125

Singh, A. V., Bhardwaj, P., Laux, P., Pradeep, P., Busse, M., Luch, A., Hirose, A., Osgood, C. J., & Stacey, M. W. (2024). AI and ML-based risk assessment of chemicals: Predicting carcinogenic risk from chemical-induced genomic instability. *Frontiers in Toxicology*, *6*, 1461587. DOI: 10.3389/ftox.2024.1461587 PMID: 39659701

Singh, D. D. (2024). Epigenetic Mechanisms of Endocrine-Disrupting Chemicals in Breast Cancer and Their Impact on Dietary Intake. *Journal of Xenobiotics*, *15*(1), 1. DOI: 10.3390/jox15010001 PMID: 39846533

Singh, G., Trehan, S., Singh, A., Goswami, K., Farooq, A., Antil, P., Puri, P., Bector, G., Jain, A., Azhar, W., Singh, G., Trehan, S., Singh, A., Goswami, K., Farooq, A., Antil, P., Puri, P., Bector, G., Jain, A., & Azhar, W. (2024). Aryl Hydrocarbon Receptor Signaling in Prostate Cancer Therapy: A Review of Implications for Anti-androgen Treatment Strategies and Resistance. *Cureus*, *16*(7). Advance online publication. DOI: 10.7759/cureus.65247 PMID: 39184676

Singh, P., Lanman, N. A., Kendall, H. L. R., Wilson, L., Long, R., Franco, O. E., Buskin, A., Miles, C. G., Hayward, S. W., Heer, R., & Robson, C. N. (2023). Human prostate organoid generation and the identification of prostate development drivers using inductive rodent tissues. *Development (Cambridge, England)*, *150*(13), dev201328. Advance online publication. DOI: 10.1242/dev.201328 PMID: 37376888

Singh, V. K., Pal, R., Srivastava, P., Misra, G., Shukla, Y., & Sharma, P. K. (2021). Exposure of androgen mimicking environmental chemicals enhances proliferation of prostate cancer (LNCaP) cells by inducing AR expression and epigenetic modifications. *Environmental Pollution*, *272*, 116397. Advance online publication. DOI: 10.1016/j.envpol.2020.116397 PMID: 33433340

Sinha, R., Rothman, N., Brown, E., Mark, S., Hoover, R., Caporaso, N., Levander, O., Knize, M., Lang, N., & Kadlubar, F. (1994). Pan-fried meat containing high levels of heterocyclic aromatic amines but low levels of polycyclic aromatic hydrocarbons induces cytochrome P4501A2 activity in humans. *Cancer Research*, *54*(23), 6154–6159. PMID: 7954461

Skakkebaek, N. E., Rajpert-De Meyts, E., Buck Louis, G. M., Toppari, J., Andersson, A. M., Eisenberg, M. L., Jensen, T. K., Jørgensen, N., Swan, S. H., Sapra, K. J., Ziebe, S., Priskorn, L., & Juul, A. (2016). Male Reproductive Disorders and Fertility Trends: Influences of Environment and Genetic Susceptibility. *Physiological Reviews*, *96*(1), 55–97. DOI: 10.1152/physrev.00017.2015 PMID: 26582516

Skinner, M. K. (2014). Endocrine Disruptor Induction of Epigenetic Transgenerational Inheritance of Disease. *Molecular & Cellular Endocrinology*, 398 (1–2), 4–12. https,//.DOI: 10.1016/j.mce.2014.07.019

Smith, S. (2021). Can Relational Feed-Forward Enhance Students' Cognitive and Affective Responses to Assessment? Teaching and Learning Inquiry: The *ISSOTL Journal*. ISSN 2167-4787 DOI: DOI: 10.20343/teachlearninqu.9.2.18

Smith, E. N., Romero, C., Donovan, B., Herter, R., Paunesku, D., Cohen, G. L., Dweck, C. S., & Gross, J. J. (2018). Emotion theories and adolescent well-being: Results of an online intervention. *Emotion (Washington, D.C.)*, *18*(6), 781–788. DOI: 10.1037/emo0000379 PMID: 29265838

Smith, M. T. (2010). Advances in understanding benzene health effects and susceptibility. *Annual Review of Public Health*, *31*(1), 133–148. DOI: 10.1146/annurev.publhealth.012809.103646 PMID: 20070208

Snow, J. S. (1855). Cholera. The Commonwealth Fund; New York: 1936. On the mode of transmission of cholera.

Snyder, L. B., Neklesa, T. K., Willard, R. R., Gordon, D. A., Pizzano, J., Vitale, N., Robling, K., Dorso, M. A., Moghrabi, W., Landrette, S., Gedrich, R., Lee, S. H., Taylor, I. C. A., & Houston, J. G. (2025). Preclinical Evaluation of Bavdegalutamide (ARV-110), a Novel PROteolysis TArgeting Chimera Androgen Receptor Degrader. *Molecular Cancer Therapeutics*, *24*(4), 511–522. DOI: 10.1158/1535-7163.MCT-23-0655 PMID: 39670468

Solecki, R., Kortenkamp, A., Bergman, A., Chahoud, I., Degen, G. H., Dietrich, D., Greim, H., Hakansson, H., Hass, U., Husoy, T., Jacobs, M., Jobling, S., Mantovani, A., Marx-Stoelting, P., Piersma, A., Ritz, V., Slama, R., Stahlmann, R., van den Berg, M., & Boobis, A. R. (2017). Scientific principles for the identification of endocrine-disrupting chemicals: A consensus statement. *Archives of Toxicology*, *91*(2), 1001–1006. DOI: 10.1007/s00204-016-1866-9 PMID: 27714423

Soto, A. M., & Sonnenschein, C. (2010). Environmental causes of cancer: Endocrine disruptors as carcinogens. In *Nature Reviews Endocrinology* (Vol. 6, Issue 7, pp. 363–370). DOI: 10.1038/nrendo.2010.87

Soubry, A., Hoyo, C., Butt, C. M., Fieuws, S., Price, T. M., Murphy, S. K., & Stapleton, H. M. (2017). Human exposure to flame-retardants is associated with aberrant DNA methylation at imprinted genes in sperm. *Environmental Epigenetics, 13*(1). Advance online publication. DOI: 10.1093/eep/dvx003 PMID: 29492305

Sreekumar, A., & Saini, S. (2022). Role of MicroRNAs in Neuroendocrine Prostate Cancer. *Non-Coding RNA, 8*(2), 25. DOI: 10.3390/ncrna8020025 PMID: 35447888

St. John, J., Powell, K., Katie Conley-LaComb, M., & Chinni, S. R. (2012). TMPRSS2-ERG Fusion Gene Expression in Prostate Tumor Cells and Its Clinical and Biological Significance in Prostate Cancer Progression. *Journal of Cancer Science & Therapy, 4*(4), 94. DOI: 10.4172/1948-5956.1000119 PMID: 23264855

Stanifer, S., Hoover, A., Rademacher, K., Rayens, M. K., Haneberg, W. C., & Hahn, E. J. (2022). Citizen science approach to home radon testing, environmental health literacy and efficacy. *Citizen Science: Theory and Practice, 7*(1), 26. Advance online publication. DOI: 10.5334/cstp.472 PMID: 36845873

Staudigl, C., Seifert, M., Tea, M., Pfeiler, G., Fink-Retter, A., Fritzer, N., & Singer, C. (2012). Abstract P1-15-10: Chemotherapy-Induced Neutropenia in Breast Cancer Patients Receiving Sequential Anthracycline and Taxane Chemotherapy: An institutional experience. *Cancer Research, 72*(24_Supplement), P1-15-10. Advance online publication. DOI: 10.1158/0008-5472.SABCS12-P1-15-10

Steegers-Theunissen, R. P., Twigt, J., Pestinger, V., & Sinclair, K. D. (2013). The periconceptional period, reproduction and long-term health of offspring: The importance of one-carbon metabolism. *Human Reproduction Update, 19*(6), 640–655. DOI: 10.1093/humupd/dmt041 PMID: 23959022

Steroid 5 alpha-reductase 2 enzyme variants, biomass exposure and tobacco use in Mexican patients with prostate cancer. (n.d.). Retrieved 14 April 2025, from https://www.spandidos-publications.com/10.3892/ol.2020.12124?utm_source=chatgpt.com

Stevenson, G. P., & A. C. Gore. (2017). Endocrine Disruptors & Kisspeptin Signaling. *Frontiers in Endocrinology,* 8, 1–9. https,//.DOI: 10.3389/fendo.2017.00007

Stoeva, S., Conev, N., & Marinov, P. (2020). *The role of carboxylesterase enzymes in capecitabine therapy*. Scripta Scientifica Pharmaceutica., DOI: 10.14748/ssp.v6i2.6624

Stouder, C., & Paoloni-Giacobino, A. (2010). Transgenerational effects of the endocrine disruptor vinclozolin on the methylation pattern of imprinted genes in the mouse sperm. *Reproduction (Cambridge, England)*, *139*(2), 373–379. DOI: 10.1530/REP-09-0340 PMID: 19887539

Sulik, K. K. (2005). Genesis of alcohol-induced craniofacial dysmorphism. [Maywood]. *Experimental Biology and Medicine (Maywood, N.J.)*, *230*(6), 366–375. DOI: 10.1177/15353702-0323006-04 PMID: 15956766

Swagatika, S., & Tomar, R. S. (2016). Modulation of epigenetics by environmental toxic molecules. In *Advances in Molecular Toxicology* (Vol. 10, pp. 361–389). Elsevier., DOI: 10.1016/B978-0-12-804700-2.00008-8

Swanton, C., McGranahan, N., Starrett, G. J., & Harris, R. S. (2015). APOBEC Enzymes: Mutagenic Fuel for Cancer Evolution and Heterogeneity. *Cancer Discovery*, *5*(7), 704–712. DOI: 10.1158/2159-8290.CD-15-0344 PMID: 26091828

Talibov, M., Salmelin, R., Lehtinen-Jacks, S., & Auvinen, A. (2017). Estimation of occupational cosmic radiation exposure among airline personnel: Agreement between a job-exposure matrix, aggregate, and individual dose estimates. *American Journal of Industrial Medicine*, *60*(4), 386–393. DOI: 10.1002/ajim.22705 PMID: 28262960

Tan, K., & Naylor, M. J. (2022). The Influence of Modifiable Factors on Breast and Prostate Cancer Risk and Disease Progression. *Frontiers in Physiology*, *13*, 840826. DOI: 10.3389/fphys.2022.840826 PMID: 35330933

Tatalovich, Z., Chtourou, A., Zhu, L., Dellavalle, C., Hanson, H., Henry, K., & Penberthy, L. (2024). Landscape analysis of environmental data sources for linkage with SEER cancer patients database. *Journal of the National Cancer Institute. Monographs*, *2024*(65), 132–144. DOI: 10.1093/jncimonographs/lgae015 PMID: 39102880

Teti, D. (2014). Editorial: Effect of epi-drugs on epigenetic modifications induced by environmental pollutants: Implications for the pathophysiology of cancer and endocrine/metabolic diseases. *Current Genomics*, *15*(6), 419. DOI: 10.2174/1389202915061501061455 21 PMID: 25646070

Thakur, I. S., & Roy, D. (2020). Environmental DNA and RNA as records of human exposome, including biotic/abiotic exposures and its implications in the assessment of the role of environment in chronic diseases. In International Journal of Molecular Sciences (Vol. 21, Issue 14, pp. 1–15). MDPI AG. https://doi.org/DOI: 10.3390/ijms21144879

Thompson, P. A., Khatami, M., Baglole, C. J., Sun, J., Harris, S. A., Moon, E. Y., Al-Mulla, F., Al-Temaimi, R., Brown, D. G., Colacci, A. M., Mondello, C., Raju, J., Ryan, E. P., Woodrick, J., Ivana Scovassi, A., Singh, N., Vaccari, M., Roy, R., Forte, S., & Bisson, W. H. (2015). Environmental immune disruptors, inflammation and cancer risk. *Carcinogenesis, 36*(Suppl 1), S232–S253. DOI: 10.1093/carcin/bgv038 PMID: 26106141

Tilghman, S. L., M. R. Bratton, H. C. Segar, E. C. Martin, L. V. Rhodes, & M. Li. (2012). Endocrine Disruptor Regulation of MicroRNA Expression in Breast Carcinoma Cells. *PLoS ONE,* 7 (3), e32754. https,//.DOI: 10.1371/journal.pone.0032754

Torres-Cuevas, I., García Miralles, E., Ribelles Llop, M., & Marqués Martínez, L. (2021, February). Flipped Classroon en prácticas de ciencias de la salud. In IN-RED 2020: VI Congreso de Innovación Educativa y Docencia en Red (pp. 184-192). Editorial Universitat Politècnica de València.

Trasande, L., Attina, T. M., & Blustein, J. (2012). Association between Urinary Bisphenol A & Obesity Prevalence in Children & Adolescents. *Journal of the American Medical Association, 308*(11), 1114–1121. DOI: 10.1001/2012.jama.11461 PMID: 22990270

Trudeau, V. L., Iguchi, T., Di Donato, M., Maradonna, F., & Carnevali, O. (2018). Lipid Metabolism Alteration by Endocrine Disruptors in Animal Models: An Overview. *Frontiers in Endocrinology, 9,* 654. DOI: 10.3389/fendo.2018.00654 PMID: 30467492

Trummer, O., Langsenlehner, U., Krenn-Pilko, S., Pieber, T. R., Obermayer-Pietsch, B., Gerger, A., Renner, W., & Langsenlehner, T. (2016). Vitamin D and prostate cancer prognosis: A Mendelian randomization study. *World Journal of Urology, 34*(4), 607–611. DOI: 10.1007/s00345-015-1646-9 PMID: 26209090

Truong, L. K., Mosewich, A. D., Holt, C. J., Le, C. Y., Miciak, M., & Whittaker, J. L. (2020). Psychological, social and contextual factors across recovery stages following a sport-related knee injury: A scoping review. *British Journal of Sports Medicine, 54*(19), 1149–1156. DOI: 10.1136/bjsports-2019-101206 PMID: 32060141

Turner, A. I., Smyth, N., Hall, S. J., Torres, S. J., Hussein, M., Jayasinghe, S. U., Ball, K., & Clow, A. J. (2020). Psychological stress reactivity and future health and disease outcomes: A systematic review of prospective evidence. *Psychoneuroendocrinology, 114,* 104599. DOI: 10.1016/j.psyneuen.2020.104599 PMID: 32045797

Tyser, R. C., Mahammadov, E., Nakanoh, S., Vallier, L., Scialdone, A., & Srinivas, S. (2021). Single-cell transcriptomic characterization of a gastrulating human embryo. *Nature, 600*(7888), 285–289. DOI: 10.1038/s41586-021-04158-y PMID: 34789876

U.S. Consumer Product Safety Commission. (2022). Final Rule, Prohibition of Children's Toys & Child Care Articles Containing Specified Phthalates. CPSC. https,//www.federalregister.gov/documents/2022/01/26/2022-01563/prohibition-of-childrens-toys-&-child-care-articles-containing-specified-phthalates

U.S. Environmental Protection Agency. (2014). Action Plan, Nonylphenol & Nonylphenol Ethoxylates (NP/NPEs*). EPA.* https,//www.epa.gov/sites/default/files/2015-09/documents/rin2070-za09_np-npe_action_plan_final_2010-08-18.pdf

U.S. Environmental Protection Agency. (2020). Polychlorinated Biphenyls (PCBs) Manufacturing, Processing, Distribution in Commerce, and Use Prohibitions. EPA. https://www.epa.gov/pcbs

U.S. Environmental Protection Agency. (2021). Atrazine ecological risk assessments. *EPA*. https://www.epa.gov/ingredients-used-pesticide-products/atrazine

U.S. Food & Drug Administration. (2022). Bisphenol A (BPA), Use in Food Contact Applications. *FDA*. https,//www.fda.gov/food/food-additives-petitions/bisphenol-bpa-use-food-contact-application

Ueda, T., Mawji, N. R., Bruchovsky, N., & Sadar, M. D. (2002). Ligand-independent activation of the androgen receptor by interleukin-6 and the role of steroid receptor coactivator-1 in prostate cancer cells. *The Journal of Biological Chemistry*, *277*(41), 38087–38094. DOI: 10.1074/jbc.M203313200 PMID: 12163482

Uehara, T., Ono, A., Maruyama, T., Kato, I., Yamada, H., Ohno, Y., & Urushidani, T. (2010). The Japanese toxicogenomics project: Application of toxicogenomics. *Molecular Nutrition &amp. Food Research*, *2*(2), 218–227. DOI: 10.1002/mnfr.200900169 PMID: 20041446

United Nations Environment Programme. (2019). DDT — A Global Review. *Stockholm Convention Secretariat*. https,//www.unep.org/resources/report/ddt-global-review

United Nations Environment Programme. (2019). Polychlorinated Biphenyls (PCBs*). Stockholm Convention.*https://www.pops.int/TheConvention/ThePOPs/TheNewPOPs/tabid/2511/Default.aspx

Unno, K., Roh, M., Yoo, Y. A., Al-Shraideh, Y., Wang, L., Nonn, L., Abdulkadir, S. A., Unno, K., Roh, M., Yoo, Y. A., Al-Shraideh, Y., Wang, L., Nonn, L., & Abdulkadir, S. A. (2017). Modeling African American prostate adenocarcinoma by inducing defined genetic alterations in organoids. *Oncotarget*, *8*(31), 51264–51276. DOI: 10.18632/oncotarget.17230 PMID: 28881646

Urade, R., Chou, C. K., Chou, H. L., Chen, B. H., Wang, T. N., Tsai, E. M., Hung, C. T., Wu, S. J., & Chiu, C. C. (2023). Phthalate derivative DEHP disturbs the anti-proliferative effect of camptothecin in human lung cancer cells by attenuating DNA damage and activating Akt/NF-κB signaling pathway. *Environmental Toxicology*, *38*(2), 332–342. DOI: 10.1002/tox.23686 PMID: 36394428

Urdinguio, R. G., Bayón, G. F., Dmitrijeva, M., Toraño, E. G., Bravo, C., Fraga, M. F., Bassas, L., Larriba, S., & Fernández, A. F. (2015). Aberrant DNA methylation patterns of spermatozoa in men with unexplained infertility. *Human Reproduction (Oxford, England)*, *30*(5), 1014–1028. DOI: 10.1093/humrep/dev053 PMID: 25753583

Vaiserman, A. (2014). Early-life Exposure to Endocrine Disrupting Chemicals and Later-life Health Outcomes: An Epigenetic Bridge? *Aging and Disease*, *5*(6), 419. DOI: 10.14336/ad.2014.0500419 PMID: 25489493

van Dessel, L. F., van Riet, J., Smits, M., Zhu, Y., Hamberg, P., van der Heijden, M. S., Bergman, A. M., van Oort, I. M., de Wit, R., Voest, E. E., Steeghs, N., Yamaguchi, T. N., Livingstone, J., Boutros, P. C., Martens, J. W. M., Sleijfer, S., Cuppen, E., Zwart, W., van de Werken, H. J. G., & Lolkema, M. P. (2019). The genomic landscape of metastatic castration-resistant prostate cancers reveals multiple distinct genotypes with potential clinical impact. *Nature Communications*, *10*(1), 5251. Advance online publication. DOI: 10.1038/s41467-019-13084-7 PMID: 31748536

Van Hée, V. F., Labar, D., Dehon, G., Grasso, D., Grégoire, V., Muccioli, G. G., Frédérick, R., & Sonveaux, P. (2017). *Radiosynthesis and validation of (±)-[18 F]-3-fluoro-2-hydroxypropionate ([18 F]-FLac) as a PET tracer of lactate to monitor MCT1-dependent lactate uptake in tumors*. www.impactjournals.com/oncotarget

Van Hemelryk, A., Mout, L., Erkens-Schulze, S., French, P. J., van Weerden, W. M., & van Royen, M. E. (2021). Modeling prostate cancer treatment responses in the organoid era: 3D environment impacts drug testing. *Biomolecules*, *11*(11), 1572. DOI: 10.3390/biom11111572 PMID: 34827570

Van Hemelryk, A., Tomljanovic, I., de Ridder, C. M. A., Stuurman, D. C., Teubel, W. J., Erkens-Schulze, S., Verhoef, E. I., Remmers, S., Mahes, A. J., van Leenders, G. J. L. H., van Royen, M. E., van de Werken, H. J. G., Grudniewska, M., Jenster, G. W., & van Weerden, W. M. (2022). Patient-Derived Xenografts and Organoids Recapitulate Castration-Resistant Prostate Cancer with Sustained Androgen Receptor Signaling. *Cells*, *11*(22), 3632. DOI: 10.3390/cells11223632 PMID: 36429059

Vandenberg, L. N., Colborn, T., Hayes, T. B., Heindel, J. J., Jacobs, D. R.Jr, Lee, D.-K., Shioda, T., Soto, A. M., vom Saal, F. S., Welshons, W. V., Zoeller, R. T., & Myers, J. P. (2012). Hormones and Endocrine-Disrupting Chemicals: Low-Dose Effects and Nonmonotonic Dose Responses. *Endocrine Reviews, 33*(3), 378–455. DOI: 10.1210/er.2011-1050 PMID: 22419778

Vargesson, N. (2013). Thalidomide embryopathy: An enigmatic challenge. *ISRN Dev Biol, 2013*, 1–18. DOI: 10.1155/2013/241016

Varnai, R., Koskinen, L. M., Mäntylä, L. E., Szabo, I., Fitzgerald, L. M., & Sipeky, C. (2019). Pharmacogenomic Biomarkers in Docetaxel Treatment of Prostate Cancer: From Discovery to Implementation. *Genes, 10*(8), 599. DOI: 10.3390/genes10080599 PMID: 31398933

Vazquez, J. P., Pulido, E. G., & Aparicio, L. M. A. (2012). Cytokine and endocrine signaling in prostate cancer. *Medical Oncology (Northwood, London, England), 29*(3), 1956–1963. DOI: 10.1007/s12032-011-0036-4 PMID: 21858553

Vega Vega, P., Miranda Castillo, C., & Vargas Celis, I. (2024). Consideraciones claves en el proceso de asentimiento en niños, niñas y adolescentes: Revisión integrativa [Key considerations in the process of assent in children and adolescents: an integrative review]. *Andes Pediatrica : Revista Chilena de Pediatria, 95*(1), 91–106. DOI: 10.32641/andespediatr.v95i1.4968 PMID: 38587349

Vermeulen, R., Schymanski, E. L., Barabasi, A.-L., & Miller, G. W. (2020). The exposome and health: Where chemistry meets biology. *Science, 367*(6476), 392–396. DOI: 10.1126/science.aay3164 PMID: 31974245

Villalta, P. W., & Balbo, S. (2017). The Future of DNA Adductomic Analysis. *International Journal of Molecular Sciences, 18*(9), 1870. DOI: 10.3390/ijms18091870 PMID: 32962318

Villeneuve, D. L., Crump, D., Garcia-Reyero, N., Hecker, M., Hutchinson, T. H., LaLone, C. A., Landesmann, B., Lettieri, T., Munn, S., Nepelska, M., Ottinger, M. A., Vergauwen, L., Whelan, M., Embry, M. R., Belanger, S. E., Leonard, M., Schirmer, K., Tanguay, R., & Truong, L.. (2014). Adverse outcome pathway development I: Strategies and principles. *Toxicological Sciences, 142*(2), 312–320. DOI: 10.1093/toxsci/kfu199 PMID: 25466378

Vineis, P., Avendano-Pabon, M., Barros, H., Bartley, M., Carmeli, C., Carra, L., Chadeau-Hyam, M., Costa, G., Delpierre, C., D'Errico, A., Fraga, S., Giles, G., Goldberg, M., Kelly-Irving, M., Kivimaki, M., Lepage, B., Lang, T., Layte, R., MacGuire, F., & Zins, M. (2020). Special Report: The Biology of Inequalities in Health: The Lifepath Consortium. *Frontiers in Public Health, 8*, 118. DOI: 10.3389/fpubh.2020.00118 PMID: 32478023

VoPham, T., Bertrand, K. A., Jones, R. R., Deziel, N. C., DuPré, N. C., James, P., Liu, Y., Vieira, V. M., Tamimi, R. M., Hart, J. E., Ward, M. H., & Laden, F.Vo-Pham. (2020). Dioxin exposure and breast cancer risk in a prospective cohort study. *Environmental Research, 186*, 109516. DOI: 10.1016/j.envres.2020.109516 PMID: 32305677

VoPham, T., White, A. J., & Jones, R. R. (2024). Geospatial Science for the Environmental Epidemiology of Cancer in the Exposome Era. *Cancer Epidemiology, Biomarkers & Prevention, 33*(4), 451–460. DOI: 10.1158/1055-9965.EPI-23-1237 PMID: 38566558

Vrijheid, M., Casas, M., Gascon, M., Valvi, D., & Nieuwenhuijsen, M. (2016). Environmental pollutants and child health-A review of recent concerns. *International Journal of Hygiene and Environmental Health, 219*(4-5), 331–342. DOI: 10.1016/j.ijheh.2016.05.001 PMID: 27216159

Vrijheid, M., Slama, R., Robinson, O., Chatzi, L., Coen, M., van den Hazel, P., Thomsen, C., Wright, J., Athersuch, T. J., Avellana, N., Basagaña, X., Brochot, C., Bucchini, L., Bustamante, M., Carracedo, A., Casas, M., Estivill, X., Fairley, L., van Gent, D., & Nieuwenhuijsen, M. J. (2014). The human early-life exposome (HELIX): Project rationale and design. *Environmental Health Perspectives, 122*(6), 535–544. DOI: 10.1289/ehp.1307204 PMID: 24610234

Vu, V., Navalkar, N., & Wei, Y. (2019). Endocrine-disrupting metals in ambient air and female breast cancer incidence in US. *Gynecological Endocrinology, 35*(12), 1099–1102. DOI: 10.1080/09513590.2019.1622089 PMID: 31142157

Waddell, A. R., Huang, H., & Liao, D. (2021a). CBP/p300: Critical Co-Activators for Nuclear Steroid Hormone Receptors and Emerging Therapeutic Targets in Prostate and Breast Cancers. *Cancers (Basel), 13*(12), 2872. DOI: 10.3390/cancers13122872 PMID: 34201346

Waddington, C. H. (2012). The epigenotype. 1942. *International Journal of Epidemiology, 41*(1), 10–13. DOI: 10.1093/ije/dyr184 PMID: 22186258

Waltering, K. K., Helenius, M. A., Sahu, B., Manni, V., Linja, M. J., Jänne, O. A., & Visakorpi, T. (2009). Increased expression of androgen receptor sensitizes prostate cancer cells to low levels of androgens. *Cancer Research, 69*(20), 8141–8149. DOI: 10.1158/0008-5472.CAN-09-0919 PMID: 19808968

Wan, M., Simonin, E. M., Johnson, M. M., Zhang, X., Lin, X., Gao, P., Patel, C. J., Yousuf, A., Snyder, M. P., Hong, X., Wang, X., Sampath, V., & Nadeau, K. C. (2025). Exposomics: a review of methodologies, applications, and future directions in molecular medicine. In *EMBO Molecular Medicine*. Springer Science and Business Media Deutschland GmbH. https://doi.org/DOI: 10.1038/s44321-025-00191-w

Wang, K., & Zhao, Z. pharmacotherapy, W. J.-B. &, & 2019, undefined. (n.d.). Bisphenol A induces apoptosis, oxidative stress and inflammatory response in colon and liver of mice in a mitochondria-dependent manner. *ElsevierK Wang, Z Zhao, W JiBiomedicine & Pharmacotherapy, 2019•Elsevier*. Retrieved 3 April 2025, from https://www.sciencedirect.com/science/article/pii/S0753332219323017

Wang, H., Liu, B., Chen, H., Xu, P., Xue, H., & Yuan, J. (2023). Dynamic changes of DNA methylation induced by benzo(a)pyrene in cancer. *Genes and Environment : the Official Journal of the Japanese Environmental Mutagen Society, 45*(1), 21. DOI: 10.1186/s41021-023-00278-1 PMID: 37391844

Wang, L., Sun, W., Zhou, K., Zhang, M., & Bao, P. (2019). Spatial Analysis of Built Environment Risk for Respiratory Health and Its Implication for Urban Planning: A Case Study of Shanghai. *International Journal of Environmental Research and Public Health, 16*(8), 1455. DOI: 10.3390/ijerph16081455 PMID: 31022924

Wang, Q., Huang, J., Yang, M., & Deng, X. (2017). MEHP Exposure Impairs Sperm DNA Integrity & Chromatin Structure in Rats. *Reproductive Toxicology (Elmsford, N.Y.), 74*, 28–35.

Wang, X., Hu, Z., Jin, Y., Yang, M., Zhang, Z., Zhou, X., Qiu, S., & Zou, X. (2024). Exploring the relationships between exposure levels of bisphenols and phthalates and prostate cancer occurrence. *Journal of Hazardous Materials, 474*, 134736. Advance online publication. DOI: 10.1016/j.jhazmat.2024.134736 PMID: 38815394

Wang, X., Rida, N., Shi, J., Wu, A., Bleske, B., & Zhu, H. (2017). A Comprehensive Functional Assessment of Carboxylesterase 1 Nonsynonymous Polymorphisms. *Drug Metabolism and Disposition: the Biological Fate of Chemicals, 45*(11), 1149–1155. DOI: 10.1124/dmd.117.077669 PMID: 28838926

Wang, X., Wang, G., Shi, J., Aa, J., Comas, R., Liang, Y., & Zhu, H. (2015). *CES1* genetic variation affects the activation of angiotensin-converting enzyme inhibitors. *The Pharmacogenomics Journal, 16*(3), 220–230. DOI: 10.1038/tpj.2015.42 PMID: 26076923

Wang, Y. N., Zeng, Z. L., Lu, J. H., Wang, Y., Liu, Z. X., He, M. M., Zhao, Q., Wang, Z., Li, T., Lu, Y., Wu, Q., Yu, K., Wang, F., Pu, H.-Y., Li, B., Jia, W., shi, M., Xie, D., Kang, T., & Xu, R. (2018). CPT1A-mediated fatty acid oxidation promotes colorectal cancer cell metastasis by inhibiting anoikis. *Oncogene, 37*(46), 6025–6040. DOI: 10.1038/s41388-018-0384-z PMID: 29995871

Welshons, W. V., K. A. Thayer, B. M. Judy, J. A. Taylor, E. M. Curran, & F. S. vom Saal. (2006). Large Effects from Small Exposures. I. Mechanisms for Endocrine-Disrupting Chemicals with Estrogenic Activity. *Environmental Health Perspectives*, 114 (1), 98–105. https,//.DOI: 10.1289/ehp.7300

Weng, J.-R., M. Hager, & D. C. Christiani. (2010). Low-Dose BPA Exposure Induces Epigenetic Changes & Gene Expression Alterations in MCF-7 Breast Cancer Cells. *Environmental Research*, 110 (6), 645–650. https,//.DOI: 10.1016/j.envres.2010.07.002

Westaby, D., Jiménez-Vacas, J. M., Figueiredo, I., Rekowski, J., Pettinger, C., Gurel, B., Lundberg, A., Bogdan, D., Buroni, L., Neeb, A., Padilha, A., Taylor, J., Zeng, W., Das, S., Hobern, E., Riisnaes, R., Crespo, M., Miranda, S., Ferreira, A., & Sharp, A. (2024). BCL2 expression is enriched in advanced prostate cancer with features of lineage plasticity. *The Journal of Clinical Investigation, 134*(18), e179998. Advance online publication. DOI: 10.1172/JCI179998 PMID: 39286979

White, M. P., Elliott, L. R., Gascon, M., Roberts, B., & Fleming, L. E. (2020). Blue space, health and well-being: A narrative overview and synthesis of potential benefits. *Environmental Research, 191*, 110169. DOI: 10.1016/j.envres.2020.110169 PMID: 32971082

Wild, C. P. (2005). Complementing the genome with an 'exposome': The outstanding challenge of environmental exposure measurement in molecular epidemiology. *Cancer Epidemiology, Biomarkers & Prevention, 14*(8), 1847–1850. DOI: 10.1158/1055-9965.EPI-05-0456 PMID: 16103423

Wild, C. P. (2012). The exposome: From concept to utility. *International Journal of Epidemiology, 41*(1), 24–32. DOI: 10.1093/ije/dyr236 PMID: 22296988

Wild, C. P., Scalbert, A., & Herceg, Z. (2013). Measuring the exposome: A powerful basis for evaluating environmental exposures and cancer risk. *Environmental and Molecular Mutagenesis, 54*(7), 480–499. DOI: 10.1002/em.21777 PMID: 23681765

Wild, J., Greenberg, N., Moulds, M. L., Sharp, M. L., Fear, N., Harvey, S., Wessely, S., & Bryant, R. A. (2020). Pre-incident Training to Build Resilience in First Responders: Recommendations on What to and What Not to Do. *Psychiatry, 83*(2), 128–142. DOI: 10.1080/00332747.2020.1750215 PMID: 32338579

Wirth, J. J., & Mijal, R. S. (2010). Adverse effects of low-level heavy metal exposure on male reproductive function. *Systems Biology in Reproductive Medicine, 56*(2), 147–167. DOI: 10.3109/19396360903582216 PMID: 20377313

Withrow, D. R., Freedman, N. D., Gibson, J. T., Yu, M., Nápoles, A. M., Berrington de Gonzalez, A., & Shiels, M. S. (2021). Leading cancers contributing to educational disparities in cancer mortality in the US, 2017. *Cancer Causes & Control, 32*(11), 1193–1196. DOI: 10.1007/s10552-021-01471-9 PMID: 34244895

Woodruff, T. J., Zota, A. R., & Schwartz, J. M. (2011). Environmental chemicals in pregnant women in the United States: Nhanes 2003-2004. *Environmental Health Perspectives, 119*(6), 878–885. DOI: 10.1289/ehp.1002727 PMID: 21233055

World Health Organization / International Programme on Chemical Safety (IPCS). (2002). *Global assessment of the state-of-the-science of endocrine disruptors*. Geneva, Switzerland: WHO/IPCS. https://www.who.int/ipcs/publications/new_issues/endocrine_disruptors/en/

World Health Organization/Food & Agriculture Organization. (2001). Safety Evaluation of Certain Food Additives & Contaminants, Dioxins. WHO Technical Report Series No. 909. *Geneva, WHO*. https,//www.who.int/publications/i/item/9241209094

Wright, R. O., & Hanson, H. A. (2022). A tipping point in cancer epidemiology: Embracing a life course exposomic framework. *Trends in Cancer, 8*(4), 280–282. DOI: 10.1016/j.trecan.2022.01.016 PMID: 35181274

Wu, C. T., Chiu, L. T., & Raturi, V. P. (2023). Investigation of the Correlation Between Mental Disorder and Cervical Cancer in Taiwan: A Nationwide Population-Based Cohort Study. *Indian Journal of Gynecologic Oncology, 21*(1), 29. DOI: 10.1007/s40944-022-00670-9

Wu, X., & Xiong, H. (2024). The role of pharmacogenetic-based pharmacokinetic analysis in precise breast cancer treatment. *Pharmaceutics, 16*(11), 1407. DOI: 10.3390/pharmaceutics16111407 PMID: 39598531

Wu, Y., Zhu, R. Y., Mitchell, L. A., Ma, L., Liu, R., Zhao, M., Jia, B., Xu, H., Li, Y. X., Yang, Z. M., Ma, Y., Li, X., Liu, H., Liu, D., Xiao, W. H., Zhou, X., Li, B. Z., Yuan, Y. J., & Boeke, J. D. (2018). In vitro DNA Scramble. *Nature Communications, 1*(1), 1935. Advance online publication. DOI: 10.1038/s41467-018-03743-6 PMID: 29789594

Xiao, W., & Goswami, P. C. (2015). Down-regulation of peroxisome proliferator activated receptor γ coactivator 1α induces oxidative stress and toxicity of 1-(4-Chlorophenyl)-benzo-2,5-quinone in HaCaT human keratinocytes. *Toxicology In Vitro, 29*(7), 1332–1338. DOI: 10.1016/j.tiv.2015.05.009 PMID: 26004620

Xia, W., Yuan, Z., Wang, S., Zheng, Q., Wu, Z., Zhong, M., Xu, F., Wang, Y. X. S., Zhang, Y., Zhang, L., Shi, Y., Huang, H., Xu, X., & Li, H. (2024). Neoadjuvant pegylated liposomal doxorubicin-containing chemotherapy in combination with trastuzumab and pertuzumab in patients with HER2-positive early breast cancer: A randomized phase II study (METIS). *Journal of Clinical Oncology, 42*(16_suppl), 596. Advance online publication. DOI: 10.1200/JCO.2024.42.16_suppl.596

Xu, K., Shimelis, H., Linn, D. E., Jiang, R., Yang, X., Sun, F., Guo, Z., Chen, H., Li, W., Chen, H., Kong, X., Melamed, J., Fang, S., Xiao, Z., Veenstra, T. D., & Qiu, Y. (2009). Regulation of androgen receptor transcriptional activity and specificity by RNF6-induced ubiquitination. *Cancer Cell, 15*(4), 270–282. DOI: 10.1016/j.ccr.2009.02.021 PMID: 19345326

Xu, K., Wu, Z. J., Groner, A. C., He, H. H., Cai, C., Lis, R. T., Wu, X., Stack, E. C., Loda, M., Liu, T., Xu, H., Cato, L., Thornton, J. E., Gregory, R. I., Morrissey, C., Vessella, R. L., Montironi, R., Magi-Galluzzi, C., Kantoff, P. W., & Brown, M. (2012). EZH2 Oncogenic Activity in Castration Resistant Prostate Cancer Cells is Polycomb-Independent. *Science, 338*(6113), 1465–1469. DOI: 10.1126/science.1227604 PMID: 23239736

Yadav, R., Petrunak, E. M., Estrada, D. F., & Scott, E. E. (2016). Structural Insights into the Function of Steroidogenic Cytochrome P450 17A1. *Molecular and Cellular Endocrinology, 441*, 68–75. DOI: 10.1016/j.mce.2016.08.035 PMID: 27566228

Yan, C., Brunson, D. C., Tang, Q., Do, D., Iftimia, N. A., Moore, J. C., Hayes, M. N., Welker, A. M., Garcia, E. G., Dubash, T. D., Hong, X., Drapkin, B. J., Myers, D. T., Phat, S., Volorio, A., Marvin, D. L., Ligorio, M., Dershowitz, L., McCarthy, K. M., & Langenau, D. M. (2019). Visualizing Engrafted Human Cancer and Therapy Responses in Immunodeficient Zebrafish. *Cell, 177*(7), 1903–1914.e14. DOI: 10.1016/j.cell.2019.04.004 PMID: 31031007

Yao, T. P., Ku, G., Zhou, N., Scully, R., & Livingston, D. M. (1996). The nuclear hormone receptor coactivator SRC-1 is a specific target of p300. *Proceedings of the National Academy of Sciences of the United States of America, 93*(20), 10626–10631. DOI: 10.1073/pnas.93.20.10626 PMID: 8855229

Yaqinuddin, A., Qureshi, S. A., Pervez, S., Bashir, M. U., Nazir, R., & Abbas, F. (2013). Frequent DNA Hypermethylation at the RASSF1A and APC Gene Loci in Prostate Cancer Patients of Pakistani Origin. *ISRN Urology, 627249*, 1–4. Advance online publication. DOI: 10.1155/2013/627249 PMID: 23431474

Yarima, A., Ali, R. S., Abdullahi, A. A., & Idris, Z. I. (2020). Nanotechnology: Review on emerging techniques in remediating water and soil pollutions. *Journal of Applied Science & Environmental Management, 24*(5), 933–941. DOI: 10.4314/jasem.v24i5.31

Yegnasubramanian, S., Haffner, M. C., Zhang, Y., Gurel, B., Cornish, T. C., Wu, Z., Irizarry, R. A., Morgan, J., Hicks, J., DeWeese, T. L., Isaacs, W. B., Bova, G. S., De Marzo, A. M., & Nelson, W. G. (2008). DNA hypomethylation arises later in prostate cancer progression than CpG island hypermethylation and contributes to metastatic tumor heterogeneity. *Cancer Research, 68*(21), 8954–8967. DOI: 10.1158/0008-5472.CAN-07-6088 PMID: 18974140

Ylitalo, E. B., Thysell, E., Landfors, M., Brattsand, M., Jernberg, E., Crnalic, S., Widmark, A., Hultdin, M., Bergh, A., Degerman, S., & Wikström, P. (2021). A novel DNA methylation signature is associated with androgen receptor activity and patient prognosis in bone metastatic prostate cancer. *Clinical Epigenetics, 13*(1), 1–15. DOI: 10.1186/s13148-021-01119-0 PMID: 34193246

Yoshimura, M., Kimura, T., Ishii, M., Ishii, K., Matsuura, T., Geshi, E., Hosokawa, M., & Muramatsu, M. (2008). Functional polymorphisms in carboxylesterase1A2 (CES1A2) gene involves specific protein 1 (Sp1) binding sites. *Biochemical and Biophysical Research Communications, 369*(3), 939–942. DOI: 10.1016/j.bbrc.2008.02.120 PMID: 18328811

Young, A. S., Mullins, C. E., Sehgal, N., Vermeulen, R., Kolijn, P. M., Vlaanderen, J., Rahman, M. L., Birmann, B. M., Barupal, D. K., Lan, Q., Rothman, N., & Walker, D. I. (2024). The Need for a Cancer Exposome Atlas: A Scoping Review. *JNCI Cancer Spectrum, 9*(1), pkae122. Advance online publication. DOI: 10.1093/jncics/pkae122 PMID: 39700422

Ystrom, E., Gustavson, K., Brandlistuen, R. E., Knudsen, G. P., Magnus, P., Susser, E., Davey Smith, G., Stoltenberg, C., Surén, P., Håberg, S. E., Hornig, M., Lipkin, W. I., Nordeng, H., & Reichborn-Kjennerud, T. (2017). Prenatal Exposure to Acetaminophen and Risk of ADHD. *Pediatrics*, *140*(5), e20163840. DOI: 10.1542/peds.2016-3840 PMID: 29084830

Yüksel, M. K., Öztürk, D., Öztaş, E., Özhan, G., Türker, A. A., Korkmaz, T., Okyar, A., & Kara, Z. P. (2019). Evaluation of the association of SNP in carboxylesterase enzyme (*CES1*) with pharmacokinetic and adverse effects of capecitabine in breast and colorectal cancer patients. *Istanbul Journal of Pharmacy*, *49*(2), 64–69. DOI: 10.26650/IstanbulJPharm.2019.19018

Yu, S. Y., Koh, E. J., Kim, S. H., Lee, S. Y., Lee, J. S., Son, S. W., & Hwang, S. Y. (2021). Integrated analysis of multi-omics data on epigenetic changes caused by combined exposure to environmental hazards. *Environmental Toxicology*, *36*(6), 1001–1010. DOI: 10.1002/tox.23099 PMID: 33438815

Yusufi, A. (n.d.). *Studies on Hexachlorobenzene (HCB) Induced Toxicity and Oxidative Damage in the Kidney and Other Rat Tissues*. Retrieved 3 April 2025, from https://www.academia.edu/127701788/Studies_on_Hexachlorobenzene_HCB_Induced_Toxicity_and_Oxidative_Damage_in_the_Kidney_and_Other_Rat_Tissues

Zaman, N., Giannopoulos, P. N., Chowdhury, S., Bonneil, E., Thibault, P., Wang, E., Trifiro, M., & Paliouras, M. (2014). Proteomic-Coupled-Network Analysis of T877A-Androgen Receptor Interactomes Can Predict Clinical Prostate Cancer Outcomes between White (Non-Hispanic) and African-American Groups. *PLoS One*, *9*(11), e113190. DOI: 10.1371/journal.pone.0113190 PMID: 25409505

Zarezadeh, M., Saedisomeolia, A., Shekarabi, M., Khorshidi, M., Emami, M., & Müller, D. (2020). The effect of obesity, macronutrients, fasting and nutritional status on drug-metabolizing cytochrome P450s: A systematic review of current evidence on human studies. *European Journal of Nutrition*, *60*(6), 2905–2921. DOI: 10.1007/s00394-020-02421-y PMID: 33141242

Zhan, F. B., Brender, J. D., Han, Y., Suarez, L., & Langlois, P. H. (2006). GIS-EpiLink: A Spatial Search Tool for Linking Environmental and Health Data. *Journal of Medical Systems*, *30*(5), 405–412. DOI: 10.1007/s10916-006-9027-y PMID: 17069004

Zhang, X., S. Wang, X. Zhou, Y. Tian, & T. Zhang. (2021). Endocrine Disruptor Global Policy, Review of Scientific Advances & Regulatory Practices. *Environmental Science & Policy*, 116, 1–7. https,//.DOI: 10.1016/j.envsci.2020.10.010

Zhang, A., Luo, X., Li, Y., Yan, L., Lai, X., Yang, Q., Zhao, Z., Huang, G., Li, Z., Wu, Q., & Wang, J. (2024). Epigenetic changes driven by environmental pollutants in lung carcinogenesis: A comprehensive review. *Frontiers in Public Health*, *12*, 1420933. Advance online publication. DOI: 10.3389/fpubh.2024.1420933 PMID: 39440184

Zhang, F., Ma, Y., Li, D., Wei, J., Chen, K., Zhang, E., Liu, G., Chu, X., Liu, X., Liu, W., Tian, X., & Yang, Y. (2024a). Cancer associated fibroblasts and metabolic reprogramming: Unraveling the intricate crosstalk in tumor evolution. *Journal of Hematology & Oncology*, *17*(1), 80. DOI: 10.1186/s13045-024-01600-2 PMID: 39223656

Zhang, H., De, T., Zhong, Y., & Perera, M. A. (2019). The Advantages and Challenges of Diversity in Pharmacogenomics: Can Minority Populations Bring Us Closer to Implementation? *Clinical Pharmacology &amp. Therapeutics*, *2*(2), 338–349. DOI: 10.1002/cpt.1491 PMID: 31038731

Zhang, H., Gao, H., Gu, Y., John, A., Wei, L., Huang, M., Yu, J., Adeosun, A. A., Weinshilboum, R. M., & Wang, L. (2022). 3D CRISPR screen in prostate cancer cells reveals PARP inhibitor sensitization through TBL1XR1-SMC3 interaction. *Frontiers in Oncology*, *12*, 999302. DOI: 10.3389/fonc.2022.999302 PMID: 36523978

Zhang, H., Gao, Y., Qian, P., Dong, Z., Hao, W., Liu, D., & Duan, X. (2019). Expression analysis of Rab11 during zebrafish embryonic development. *BMC Developmental Biology*, *19*(1), 25. DOI: 10.1186/s12861-019-0207-7 PMID: 31884948

Zhang, J., Wang, X., Vikash, V., Ye, Q., Wu, D., Liu, Y., & Dong, W. (2016). ROS and ROS-Mediated Cellular Signaling. *Oxidative Medicine and Cellular Longevity*, *4350965*(1), 4350965. Advance online publication. DOI: 10.1155/2016/4350965 PMID: 26998193

Zhang, L., & Shiverick, K. T. (1997). Benzo(a)pyrene, but not 2,3,7,8-tetrachlorodibenzo-p-dioxin, alters cell proliferation and c-myc and growth factor expression in human placental choriocarcinoma JEG-3 cells. *Biochemical and Biophysical Research Communications*, *231*(1), 117–120. DOI: 10.1006/bbrc.1997.6053 PMID: 9070231

Zhang, T., Ambrodji, A., Huang, H., Bouchonville, K., Etheridge, A., Schmidt, R., Nunez, J., Temesgen, Z., Innocenti, F., Diasio, R., Largiadèr, C., & Offer, S. (2022). Abstract 5420: DPYD enhancer variant confers increased risk of severe toxicity in 5-FU chemotherapy. *Cancer Research*, *82*(12_Supplement), 5420. Advance online publication. DOI: 10.1158/1538-7445.AM2022-5420

Zhang, Y., Han, L., He, Q., Chen, W., Sun, C., Wang, X., Chen, X., Wang, R., Hsiao, C. D., & Liu, K. (2017). A rapid assessment for predicting drug-induced hepatotoxicity using zebrafish. *Journal of Pharmacological and Toxicological Methods*, *84*, 102–110. DOI: 10.1016/j.vascn.2016.12.002 PMID: 27940076

Zhang, Y., Huang, Z., Li, K., Xie, G., Feng, Y., Wang, Z., Li, N., Liu, R., Ding, Y., Wang, J., Yang, J., & Jia, Z. (2024). TrkA promotes MDM2-mediated AGPS ubiquitination and degradation to trigger prostate cancer progression. *Journal of Experimental & Clinical Cancer Research : CR*, *43*(1), 16. Advance online publication. DOI: 10.1186/s13046-023-02920-w PMID: 38200609

Zhang, Y., Yin, X., & Zheng, X. (2023). The relationship between pm2.5 and the onset and exacerbation of childhood asthma: A short communication. *Frontiers in Pediatrics*, *11*, 1191852. Advance online publication. DOI: 10.3389/fped.2023.1191852 PMID: 37593445

Zhang, Z., Cheng, L., Li, J., Farah, E., Atallah, N. M., Pascuzzi, P. E., Gupta, S., & Liu, X. (2018). Inhibition of the Wnt/b-catenin pathway overcomes resistance to enzalutamide in castration-resistant prostate cancer. *Cancer Research*, *78*(12), 3147–3162. DOI: 10.1158/0008-5472.CAN-17-3006 PMID: 29700003

Zhao, F., Zhang, T., Wei, J., Chen, L., Liu, Z., Jin, Y., Liu, M., Zhou, H., Hu, Y., & Sheng, X. (2024). Integrated single-cell transcriptomic analyses identify a novel lineage plasticity-related cancer cell type involved in prostate cancer progression. *EBioMedicine*, *109*, 105398. DOI: 10.1016/j.ebiom.2024.105398 PMID: 39418984

Zhao, J., Shi, Y., & Cao, G. (2023). The Application of Single-Cell RNA Sequencing in the Inflammatory Tumor Microenvironment. *Biomolecules*, *13*(2), 344. DOI: 10.3390/biom13020344 PMID: 36830713

Zheng, H., Zhu, Y., Shao, X., Cai, A., Dong, B., Xue, W., & Gao, H. (2020). Distinct Metabolic Signatures of Hormone-Sensitive and Castration-Resistant Prostate Cancer Revealed by a 1H NMR-Based Metabolomics of Biopsy Tissue. *Journal of Proteome Research*, *19*(9), 3741–3749. DOI: 10.1021/acs.jproteome.0c00282 PMID: 32702989

Zheng, L., Zhang, X., Gao, Z., Zhong, C., Qiu, D., & Yan, Q. (2024). The association between polychlorinated dibenzo-p-dioxin exposure and cancer mortality in the general population: A cohort study. *Frontiers in Public Health*, *12*, 1354149. Advance online publication. DOI: 10.3389/fpubh.2024.1354149 PMID: 38410662

Zhong, W., Fan, B., & Zhang, L. (2015). Bisphenol A Impairs DNA Repair Capacity by Downregulating XRCC1 Expression via Epigenetic Mechanisms. *Journal of Applied Toxicology*, *35*(9), 1100–1108.

Zhou, J., L. Cai, & L. Zhu. (2010). Are Endocrine Disruptors among the Causes of the Deterioration of Aquatic Biodiversity?. *Integrated Environmental Assessment & Management,* 6 (1), 12–21. https,//.DOI: 10.1002/ieam.47

Zhou, L., Zhang, C., Zhang, Y., & Shi, C. (2021a). Application of Organoid Models in Prostate Cancer Research. *Frontiers in Oncology, 11*, 736431. DOI: 10.3389/fonc.2021.736431 PMID: 34646778

Zhou, W., Liotta, L. A., & Petricoin, E. F. (2012). Cancer Metabolism: What we Can Learn from Proteomic Analysis by Mass Spectrometry. *Cancer Genomics & Proteomics, 9*(6), 373. https://pmc.ncbi.nlm.nih.gov/articles/PMC5547437/ PMID: 23162076

Zhu, M., Huang, C., Ma, X., Wu, R., Zhu, W., Li, X., Liang, Z., Deng, F., Wu, J., Geng, S., Xie, C., & Zhong, C. (2018). Phthalates promote prostate cancer cell proliferation through activation of ERK5 and p38. *Environmental Toxicology and Pharmacology, 63*, 29–33. DOI: 10.1016/j.etap.2018.08.007 PMID: 30125794

Zhu, W., Liu, H., Wang, X., Lu, J., Zhang, H., Wang, S., & Yang, W. (2019). Associations of CYP1 polymorphisms with risk of prostate cancer: An updated meta-analysis. *Bioscience Reports, 39*(3), BSR20181876. Advance online publication. DOI: 10.1042/BSR20181876 PMID: 30765615

Zoeller, R. T., A. L. S. Dowling, C. T. A. Herzig, E. A. Iannacone, K. J. Gauger, & R. Bansal. (2002). Thyroid Hormone, Brain Development, & the Environment. *Environmental Health Perspectives*, 110 (3), 355–361. https,//.DOI: 10.1289/ehp.02110s3355

Zota, A. R., & B. Shamasunder. (2017). The Environmental Injustice of Beauty, Framing Chemical Exposures from Beauty Products as a Health Disparities Concern. *American Journal of Obstetrics & Gynaecology*, 217 (4), 418.e1–418.e6. https,//.DOI: 10.1016/j.ajog.2017.07.020

Zou, Z., Yoshimura, Y., Yamanishi, Y., & Oki, S. (2023). Elucidating disease-associated mechanisms triggered by pollutants via the epigenetic landscape using large-scale ChIP-Seq data. *Epigenetics & Chromatin, 16*(1), 1–15. DOI: 10.1186/s13072-023-00510-w PMID: 37743474

Zur Hausen, H. (2009). Papillomaviruses in the causation of human cancers—A brief historical account. *Virology, 384*(2), 260–265. DOI: 10.1016/j.virol.2008.11.046 PMID: 19135222

About the Contributors

Ramya Raghavan is an Assistant Professor at Sri Sathya Sai University for Human Excellence, Karnataka, India. Her recent editorial work focuses on advancing cancer treatment through spatial omics approaches, highlighting her commitment to innovation. She uniquely bridges complex scientific concepts with broader societal implications as an editor. Dr. Raghavan research caters to the need for a more integrated approach to understanding environmental health risks. Her expertise extends to the intersection of the exposome and Social Determinants of Health (SDOH). Currently working on various early developmental programming projects, aligning with the Developmental Origins of Health and Disease (DOHaD) paradigm and addressing health disparities and equitable approach to disease prevention. Dr. Raghavan's work has the potential to significantly inform and expedite progress toward the Sustainable Development Goals (SDGs) by identifying and mitigating environmental risk factors associated with cancer. Dr. Ramya Raghavan specializes in community health research that aligns seamlessly with the SDGs, aiming to promote health and well-being for all.

***

A. Sanjay Gandhi is currently serving as an Assistant Professor in Electronics at Sri Ramakrishna Mission Vidyalaya College of Arts and Science, Coimbatore. He earned his Ph.D. in Electronics from Karpagam Academy of Higher Education in August 2018 for his research on secure multicast routing and data integrity in wireless sensor networks. His academic journey includes an M.Phil. in Electronics and Instrumentation from Bharathiar University (2012), an M.Sc. in Applied Electronics from PSG College of Arts and Science (2010), and a B.Sc. in Electronics from Periyar University (2007). With over 10 years of teaching experience across reputed institutions, his research interests span wireless sensor networks, embedded systems, and medical electronics. Dr. Sanjay Gandhi has published multiple research papers in national and international journals and has actively participated in organizing seminars and workshops. He has also completed MOOCs and Faculty Development Programs focusing on ICT tools, Arduino, and digital education, demonstrating his commitment to academic and professional growth.

A. T. Rajamanickam is currently serving as an Associate Professor in Electronics at Sri Ramakrishna Mission Vidyalaya College of Arts and Science, Coimbatore. He earned his Ph.D. in Electronics from Bharathiar University in April 2017 for his research on the structural, optical, and photocatalytic properties of doped TiO_2 nanostructured thin films. With over 19 years of teaching experience across various reputed institutions, he has held multiple academic positions, ranging from Lecturer to Associate Professor. His academic credentials include an M.E. in Applied Electronics from Anna University, and an M.Phil., M.Sc., and B.Sc. in Electronics. He has published more than 20 Articles in various journals, reviewer of 5 journals. Dr. Rajamanickam's research interests lie in thin films, nanomaterials, gas sensors, and photocatalysis, and he has published extensively in high-impact journals like Optik, Journal of Materials Science: Materials in Electronics, and Inorganic Chemistry Communications. He has also guided research scholars, served as a Board of Studies member at several institutions, and contributed to numerous national and international seminars and workshops. He is a lifetime member of various professional bodies and has received a Best Teacher Award from the Deccan Environmental Research Organization, Karnataka.

S. Athinarayanan holds a strong academic background in the field of Electronics. He completed his B.Sc. in Electronics in 2003 from Manonmaniam Sundaranar University, followed by a M.Sc. in Electronics in 2005 from Bharathidasan University, where he also earned his M.Phil. in Electronics in 2022. Demonstrating a continuous passion for academic and research excellence, he is currently pursuing his Ph.D. in Electronics at Sri Ramakrishna Mission Vidyalaya College of Arts and Science, Coimbatore. His academic journey reflects a deep commitment to lifelong learning, with a focus on both foundational principles and emerging trends in electronics. He remains actively engaged in research and innovation, aiming to contribute meaningfully to the advancement of the field.

Duygu Aygunes-Jafari is currently affiliated with Ege University Faculty of Medicine, Izmir, Turkey where she works in the fields of cancer and psychiatric genetics, with a focus on molecular biology. Her research centers on the genetic and molecular mechanisms underlying complex diseases, including breast cancer, ADHD, and autism spectrum disorders. She has a particular interest in cell death pathways, especially apoptosis, and investigates how these mechanisms intersect with genetic variation and disease progression. Her work integrates experimental molecular biology with computational approaches, including bioinformatic analysis, artificial intelligence, and machine learning, to explore multi-level data and model disease processes.

Ankur Bhardwaj (Ph.D.) is working as Assistant professor in the Department of Biotechnology, Shri Vaishnav Institute of Sciences, Shri Vaishnav Vidyapeeth Vishwavidyalaya, Indore. He obtained Ph.D. (2021) in Molecular Biology and Microbiology from Mangalayatan University, Aligarh, Uttar Pradesh, India. He started his career as a Lecturer in Department of Biotechnology and Life Sciences, Mangalayatan University, Aligarh in 2014 and served there for more than 06 years. He has more than 10 years of teaching and research experience. He prominently has worked in the field of Plant Biotechnology, Molecular Biology, Immuno-informatics and Microbiology. He has published more than 11 research papers in peer reviewed journals and 14 book chapters. From 2017 to 2025, he received 03 young scientist award and best thesis award in 2021. Dr. Bhardwaj is a lifetime member of the Scholars Academic and Scientific Society and American Chemical Society and have published more than 05 conference abstracts. Recently Dr. Bhardwaj served as an editor for the book entitled "Exploring the Mycology and Parasitology of Plant Life: Roots and Rivals", that is going to be published by Cambridge Scholars Publisher, UK and received Prof. M.L. Khorana IJPS Best Paper Award in the area of Pharmaceutical & Medicinal Synthetic Chemistry and was a keynote speaker in National webinar series entitled "Current Trends in Infectious disease, Diagnosis and Therapeutics".

Sümeyya Çapuk is a dedicated PhD candidate in Immunology and currently serves as a research assistant at the Faculty of Medicine. With a strong academic foundation in the health sciences, she earned her Master's degree in Medical Microbiology, following a Bachelor's degree in Molecular Biology and Genetics. Her academic and professional journey reflects a deep commitment to understanding the complexities of the human immune system and its interactions with microbial pathogens and infectious agent-induced cancer. Throughout her graduate studies, Sümeyya has focused on exploring the immunological mechanisms involved in infectious diseases, autoimmune disorders, and host-pathogen interactions. As a research assistant, she actively contributes to various laboratory projects, assisting in experimental design, data analysis, and scientific publication. Her interdisciplinary background allows her to approach research questions from both a molecular and clinical perspective, bridging the gap between bench science and medical application.

Surendra Prakash Gupta is working as Associate Professor in the Department of Biotechnology, SVIS, Shri Vaishnav Vidyapeeth Vishwavidyalaya, Indore. He has 16 years of academic experience under various capacities in university. He has worked in Drug-DNA interactions, Bioenergy, and Computational Biology. He qualified for GATE in 2006 in Life Science. He has published 05 research papers in peer reviewed Journals, 14 book chapters, 05 conference papers and more than 35 conference abstracts. He has supervised B. Tech and M.Sc. Biotechnology students successfully. He is also a member of several reputed professional bodies like, IAENG, Education and Development Research and ASR etc. and Lifetime Member of IARA, and ISTD, Indore Chapter.

M. Robinson Joel received the Doctorate Ph.D degree in Computer and Information Technology from the Manonmaniam Sundaranar University, Tirunelveli in March 2019. He completed his M.Tech and MCA from the same university year 2008 and 2002 respectively. He is currently working as an Associate Professor in the Department of Computer Science and Engineering at KCG College of Technology, Chennai. He has 16 years of teaching experience.

K. Dhanakodi is currently serving as an Assistant Professor in Electronics at Sri Ramakrishna Mission Vidyalaya College of Arts and Science, Coimbatore. He holds a Ph.D. in Electronics from Bharathiar University, awarded in May 2017, for his research on Nebulizer Sprayed Doped and Undoped ZnO Thin Films for Gas Sensing Applications. With over 15 years of teaching experience, including service at K.S.G. College of Arts and Science and SRMV College, Dr. Dhanakodi has been actively engaged in academic research and supervision, currently guiding four Ph.D. scholars. His research interests include thin films, nanotechnology, and gas sensors, and he has published several papers in reputed journals such as Optik (Elsevier) and Journal of Materials Science: Materials in Electronics. Additionally, he has participated in various orientation and refresher programs and has contributed significantly to academic bodies such as Boards of Studies and university-level committees.

Sevgi Kalkanli Taş is the Head of the Department of Immunology, where she leads both academic and research initiatives with a focus on advancing the understanding of immune system function in health and disease. She holds a PhD in Immunology and completed her undergraduate education in Veterinary Medicine, providing her with a comprehensive background in health sciences. Prof. Kalkanlı Taş has developed extensive expertise in tumor immunology, with a particular interest in the complex interactions between cancer cells and the immune system. Over the years, she has contributed to numerous projects investigating how immunological pathways can be manipulated to enhance anti-tumor responses, including studies on checkpoint inhibitors, cancer vaccines, and the tumor microenvironment. As a department head, she oversees a multidisciplinary team engaged in both basic and translational immunology research. She is deeply committed to mentoring graduate students and early-career scientists, fostering an environment of scientific curiosity, collaboration, and innovation. Her long-standing dedication to cancer research and immune system science positions her as a leading figure in the field, with ongoing contributions aimed at improving therapeutic outcomes and understanding disease mechanisms at the molecular and cellular levels.

Buket Kosova is a faculty member at Ege University Faculty of Medicine, where she serves as a Professor of Medical Biology. She received her PhD in Germany and has since focused her research on the genetic and molecular mechanisms of cancer. Her areas of special interest include bioinformatics, cancer genomics, and the integration of computational approaches into medical biology.

Akhilesh Prajapati is a dedicated cancer biologist and academician with a Ph.D. in Biochemistry and extensive experience in teaching and research in Biotechnology. Currently serving at GSFC University, Dr. Prajapati leads projects focused on endocrine-related cancers, with a special emphasis on prostate and breast cancer. His research delves into cancer stem cells, metabolic vulnerabilities, ferroptosis, and therapeutic resistance, utilizing advanced tools such as CRISPR/Cas9, exosome-based delivery, and multi-omics integration. Dr. Prajapati has received prestigious funding, including grants from GSBTM, Government of Gujarat, for targeting mitochondrial OXPHOS in castration-resistant prostate cancer. In addition to academic responsibilities, He actively mentors students, organize International/ National-level symposia/ conferences, and engages in science communication. Dr. Prajapati is also a recognized reviewer for reputed journals such as Scientific Reports, Cell Signalling, and JOVE. He also served as guest editor and editorial member for many journals and regularly participates in interdisciplinary collaborations aimed at translational cancer research.

R. Kavitha is an accomplished academician and researcher in the field of Computer Science and Engineering, with over 12 years of teaching experience across reputed institutions including Vel Tech High Tech Engineering College, Annamacharya Institute of Technology, and PSN College of Engineering and Technology. She holds a Ph.D. in Computer Science and Information Technology (2024) from Manonmaniam Sundaranar University, with research focused on cervical cancer diagnosis using texture-based ensemble classification methods. Her academic background includes an M.E. in CSE from Anna University, an

M.Phil. in Computer Science from Madurai Kamaraj University, and a dual degree in M.Sc. and B.Sc. Computer Science from Mother Teresa Women's University. Dr. Kavitha has published over 12 international journal papers (including SCI and Scopus-indexed journals) and presented at several national and international conferences. She is a life member of IAENG, ISRD, and GERN, and has played key roles in academic committees such as Board of Studies, technical committees, and admission coordination. Her research interests lie in medical image processing, machine learning, and cancer diagnosis, and she brings strong technical expertise in tools like IDL, MATLAB, C++, Python, and Linux environments.

S. Athinarayanan is a seasoned academic and researcher in Computer and Information Technology, with over 16 years of teaching experience, including 7 years post-Ph.D. He currently serves as an Associate Professor in the Department of Computer Science and Engineering at Vel Tech Rangarajan Dr. Sagunthala R&D Institute of Science and Technology, Chennai. He holds a Ph.D. in Computer and Information Technology (2017) from Manonmaniam Sundaranar University, with a specialization in medical image processing, particularly focusing on cervical cancer detection using Pap smear images. His academic background includes M.Tech in Computer & IT, M.Sc. Electronics, and B.Sc. Electronics, with multiple university recognitions. Dr. Athinarayanan has published over 30 research papers in Scopus, Web of Science, and UGC CARE-listed journals, authored books and book chapters, filed patents, and has been a resource person in numerous FDPs and conferences. His core areas of research include machine learning, image processing, edge computing, and blockchain networks. A recognized reviewer for several reputed journals, he also actively guides research scholars and contributes to academic governance through roles such as BoS member, IQAC coordinator, and technical committee member. He is a lifetime member of professional bodies like ISTE, IAENG, ISRD, and GERN, and has received accolades including a Best Paper Award at an international conference.

S. Muthukumar holds a Ph.D. in Information and Communication Engineering from Anna University and has over 10 years of teaching experience as an Assistant Professor at PSN College of Engineering and Technology. He is proficient in several programming languages such as C, C++, Java, and Python, and has expertise in web development and database management. His research contributions include publications in national and international journals, focusing on topics like wireless sensor networks and image processing. He has actively participated in academic development by organizing and attending various seminars, workshops, and faculty development programs. Additionally, he has held key departmental roles such as NAAC, NBA, and ISO coordinator, as well as serving as HOD in-charge.

Canfeza Sezgin graduated from Ege University Faculty of Medicine in 1993. He completed his specialization in Internal Medicine in 1999 and in Medical Oncology in 2001 at the same institution. He was appointed Associate Professor of Medical Oncology in 2006 and became a Full Professor in 2013. In March 2016, he played a leading role in establishing the Department of Medical Oncology at Biruni University Faculty of Medicine Hospital. His work focuses not only on the medical treatment of cancer but also on integrative oncology, combining conventional therapies with evidence-based complementary approaches.

Mamta Singh MSc, PhD (Biochemistry) is a Professor of Biochemistry in the Department of Basic Sciences at Sri Ramachandra Faculty of Allied Health Sciences (SRMC & RI), Chennai, India. With over 14 years of pedagogical and scientific expertise, she has made substantial contributions to clinical biochemistry and molecular diagnostics. Dr. Singh obtained her Ph.D. in Medical Biochemistry from PGIMS, Pt. B.D. Sharma Health & Science University, Rohtak. Her scientific interests encompass oxidative stress, metabolic disorders, endocrinology, and hepatic illnesses. She has authored over 15 publications in esteemed national and international journals. Significant contributions encompass research on oxidative and nitrosative stress in chronic obstructive lung disease, biochemical analyses of polycystic ovarian syndrome, and metabolic dysregulation in coronary syndrome and diabetes. Dr. Singh has had academic roles in prestigious colleges around India, such as K.R. College of Health Sciences (Bangalore), PDM Dental College (Haryana), and Maitri College of Dentistry (Chhattisgarh). Her technical expertise includes molecular biology, RT-PCR, HPLC, spectrophotometry, and enzymatic tests. Dr. Singh, a fervent educator and mentor, perpetuates innovation in biomedical science and education via her commitment to research and student-focused learning.

Aylin Seher Uzunoglu is an experienced scientist with a solid academic foundation in the health sciences. She holds a PhD in Immunology, preceded by a Master's degree in Molecular Medicine and a Bachelor's degree in Biology. Over the years, she has cultivated a specialized focus on the immune system's response to infectious diseases and cancer. Her research is dedicated to uncovering the complex interactions between pathogens and the host immune system, with the goal of informing the development of innovative therapeutic and preventive approaches. With her interdisciplinary expertise, Dr. Uzunoglu integrates principles from molecular medicine and immunology to address pressing challenges in infectious disease research, demonstrating a strong commitment to advancing human health through science.

Merve Saide Uzunoglu is an accomplished researcher with a strong academic background in the health sciences. She earned her PhD in Immunology, building on a Master's degree in Molecular Medicine and a Bachelor's degree in Biology. Throughout her academic and professional journey, she has developed a deep expertise in the immunological mechanisms underlying infectious diseases and cancer. Her work focuses on understanding how the immune system responds to various pathogens and cancer, with the aim of contributing to the development of more effective diagnostics, treatments, and preventive strategies. Driven by a passion for biomedical research, Dr. Uzunoglu combines her multidisciplinary training to explore complex questions at the intersection of immunology, molecular biology, and infectious disease.

Index

A

B

C

D

E

G

H

I

M

N

O

P

R

S

T

www.ingramcontent.com/pod-product-compliance
Lightning Source LLC
LaVergne TN
LVHW062329300926
849161LV00007B/1629
9798337357966